**8e**

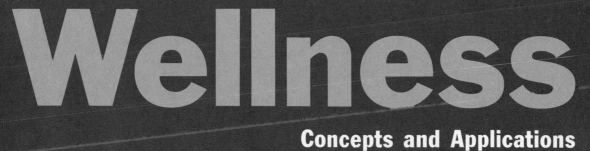

# Wellness

## Concepts and Applications

**David J. Anspaugh, PED, EdD, CHES, FAAHE**
PROFESSOR EMERITUS AT THE UNIVERSITY OF MEMPHIS
TRI-STATE UNIVERSITY

**Michael H. Hamrick, EdD, CHES, FAAHE**
THE UNIVERSITY OF MEMPHIS

**Frank D. Rosato, EdD**
THE UNIVERSITY OF MEMPHIS

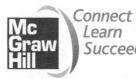

Connect
Learn
Succeed™

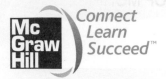

Published by McGraw-Hill, a business unit of The McGraw-Hill Companies, Inc., 1221 Avenue of the Americas, New York, NY 10020.

♻ This book is printed on recycled, acid-free paper containing 10% postconsumer waste.

1 2 3 4 5 6 7 8 9 0 QDB/QDB 1 0

ISBN: 978-0-07-802250-0
MHID: 0-07-802250-9

Vice President, Editorial: *Michael Ryan*
Director, Editorial: *Beth Mejia*
Executive Editor: *Christopher Johnson*
Director of Development: *Kate Engelberg*
Development Editor: *Lynda Huenefeld*
Editorial Coordinator: *Lydia Kim*
Marketing Director: *Allison Jones*
Marketing Manager: *Caroline McGillen*
Media Project Manager: *Rethuel Jabez*
Production Editor: *Ruth Sakata Corley*
Interior Designer: *Lisa Buckley*
Cover Designer: *Allister Fein*
Photo Researcher: *Poyee Oster*
Senior Buyer: *Laura Fuller*
Production Service: *Lachina Publishing Services*
Composition: *10/12 Sabon by Lachina Publishing Services*
Printing: *45# New Era Matte by Quad/Graphics*

Cover image: *Jupiterimages*

Credits: **Page 6:** © Corbis; **13, 17:** © Stockbyte/PunchStock; **52, 53:** © Photodisc; **92:** Michael Newman/PhotoEdit; **177, 181, 195:** © Photodisc; **251 (all):** Courtesy of Life Measurement Instruments. Concord, CA.; **281:** © The McGraw-Hill Companies, Inc./Christopher Kerrigan; **348, 372** © Photodisc; **377:** Missouri Chapter of MADD and the parents of Jason Bitter; **379:** © Felicia Montirez/PhotoEdit; **402:** © Corbis; **410:** © Dr. Ken Greer/Visuals Unlimited; **411:** © Steven J. Nussenblatt/Custom Medical Stock Photo; **412:** © Corbis; **429 left:** © J. E. Wilson/Photo Researchers, Inc.; **429 right:** © Biophoto Associates/Photo Researchers, Inc.; **431:** © Keith Brofsky/Getty Images; **442:** © David K. Crow/PhotoEdit; **476:** © The McGraw-Hill Companies, Inc./Christopher Kerrigan. All other photos author provided.

Library of Congress Cataloging-in-Publication Data

Anspaugh, David J.
   Wellness : concepts and applications / David Anspaugh, Michael Hamrick, Frank Rosato. — 8th ed.
      p. cm.
   ISBN 978-0-07-802250-0 (pbk.)
   1. Health. 2. Self-care, Health. 3. Medicine, Preventive. I. Hamrick, Michael H. II. Rosato, Frank D. III. Title.
   RA776.A57 2011
   613—dc22
                                    2010039610

www.mhhe.com

# Brief Contents

# Contents

# Preface

*Wellness is not a destination—it's a **journey**...*

*...one that begins with knowledge, self-awareness, and self-evaluation*

*...that requires health-related skills, attitudes, beliefs, and habits*

*...that includes behavior change*

*....and that serves you well throughout your life!*

Wellness is more than fitness and more than health—it involves a balance of the physical, emotional, intellectual, social, spiritual, occupational, and environmental aspects of life.

*Wellness: Concepts and Applications* focuses on the **lifestyle decision-making information** that builds knowledge and awareness:

- Learning Objectives identify the knowledge and comprehension goals for each chapter
- Student-centered topics and issues include the latest on overweight and obesity, techno stress, energy drinks, salt intake, commercial-break workouts, texting while driving, the HPV vaccine, steroid use, risk factors for cardiovascular disease among children and adolescents, and a host of others.
- Just the Facts boxes offer new information on intimacy, exercise intensity, exotic forms of smoking, vitamin B, the glycemic index, the obesity gene, and more.

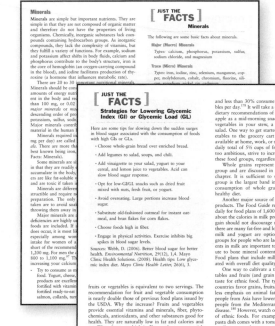

## [ JUST THE FACTS ]

### Estimating Calorie Source

Carbohydrates, fats, and protein yield 4, 9, and 4 calories per gram, respectively. These values can be used to estimate the percent of calories by energy source of a food. For example, a turkey sandwich on white bread yields 24 grams of protein, 14 grams of fat, and 29 grams of carbohydrate. Column 2 times column 3 produces the number of calories for each energy source. Total calories in a turkey sandwich equal 338. Percent protein is determined by dividing protein calories by total calories. Repeat the procedure for carbohydrates and fat. Conclusion: 28% of the calories in a turkey sandwich come from protein, 34% from carbohydrates, and 38% from fat.

*Wellness: Concepts and Applications* focuses on *lifestyle decision-making skills.*

- Goals for Behavior Change identify the behavioral applications of the material in each chapter.
- Coverage of such topics as substance abuse, STDs, personal safety, cancer, diabetes, and cardiovascular disease encourages personal responsibility for all areas of wellness.
- Real World Wellness boxes give practical advice for initiating behavior change, staying motivated, and overcoming lapses.
- Assessment Activities help you find out where you stand in relation to each wellness area and how you can move in positive directions.

---

Name _____    Date _____    Section _____

## Assessment Activity 8-3

### Walking Assessment

One way to monitor physical activity is to count the number of steps you take daily. This includes steps taken at home, work, play, or when performing chores, household tasks, yardwork, and so on. Experts recommend 10,000 steps a day to achieve health benefits associated with walking, 15,000 steps a day to lose weight, and 20,000 steps a day to maintain weight after a weight-loss goal has been reached. The purposes of this activity are to determine your "walking baseline," that is, the number of steps you take in your daily routine, excluding structured time set aside for exercise and sport activities, and start a walking program to achieve 10,000 steps per day. To complete this assessment, you will need to use or purchase a pedometer. Ask your instructor for his or her recommendation of a pedometer, or Google "pedometer" on the Internet, or shop for one at a

sports retail store. Inexpensive, accurate, and reliable digital pedometers can be purchased for less than $20. Follow the instructions for attaching the pedometer and put it on when you start the day. At the end of the day, record the number of steps in Part 1 of the log. Reset the pedometer the next morning. Repeat this for 5 days. Calculate a 5-day average to determine your walking baseline. Enter this number in the "baseline" column of Part 2. If you average 10,000 steps or more and you're not trying to lose weight, continue with your present routine. If you're short of the recommended 10,000 steps, add 300 steps a day during the first week and continue in 300-step increments each subsequent week until you build up to 10,000 steps per day. Chart your walking program in Part 2. Print or make extra copies of the log to cover at least a 6-week period.

#### Part 1. Walking Baseline Log

| Day | Number of Steps |
|---|---|
| 1 | |
| 2 | |
| 3 | |
| 4 | |
| 5 | |
| Total | |
| 5-Day Average (Walking Baseline) | |

#### Part 2. Walking Log (10,000 Steps a Day)*

| Week/Day | Baseline (from Part 1) | Add 300 | Daily Goal (Baseline + 300) | Actual** Steps |
|---|---|---|---|---|
| | | +300 | | |
| | | +300 | | |
| | | +300 | | |
| | | +300 | | |
| | | +300 | | |
| | | +300 | | |
| | | +300 | | |

*___ to monitor steps for 6 weeks (or more).
**___ se taken in structured workouts, sport activities, etc.

---

Name _____    Date _____    Section _____

## Assessment Activity 6-4

### Do You Have Fatty Habits?

Fat has earned a bad reputation because of the health problems it contributes to in high-fat diets. The following questionnaire will help you think about the amounts and types of fat that you generally eat. For each general type of food or food habit, circle the category that is most typical for your diet. If you never or almost never eat any items of a particular food type, skip it.

| Food Type/Habit | High-Fat | Medium-Fat | Low-Fat |
|---|---|---|---|
| Chicken | Fried with the skin | Baked, broiled, or barbecued with the skin | Baked, broiled, or barbecued without the skin |
| Fat present on meats | Usually | Sometimes | Never |
| Fat used in cooking | Butter, lard, bacon grease, chicken fat | Margarine, oil | Nonstick cooking spray or no fat used |
| Additions to rice, bread, potatoes, vegetables, etc. | Butter, lard, bacon grease, chicken fat, coconut oil | Margarine, oil, peanut butter | Butter-flavored granules or no fat used |
| Pizza toppings | Sausage, pepperoni, extra cheese, combination | Canadian bacon | Vegetables (e.g., peppers, onions, mushrooms) |
| Sandwich spreads | Mayonnaise or mayonnaise-type dressing | Light mayonnaise, oil and vinegar | Mustard, fat-free mayonnaise |
| Milk and milk products (e.g., yogurt) | Whole milk and whole-milk products | Low-fat dairy products | Skim milk and milk products |
| Sandwich side orders | Chips, potato salad, macaroni salad with creamy dressing | Coleslaw, pasta salad with clear dressing | Vegetable sticks, pretzels, pickle |
| Salad dressings | Blue cheese, Ranch, Thousand Island, other creamy type | Oil and vinegar, clear-base dressing | Oil-free dressing, lemon juice, flavored vinegar |
| Typical meat portion | 6–8 oz. or more | 4–5 oz. | 2–3 oz. |
| Sandwich fillings | Beef or pork hot dogs, salami, bologna, pepperoni, cheese, tuna or chicken salad | Turkey hot dogs, 85% fat-free lunch meats, corned beef, peanut butter, hummus (chick-pea paste) | 95% fat-free lunch meats, roast turkey, roast beef, lean ham |
| Ground meats | Regular ground beef, sausage meat, ground meat, ground pork (about 30% fat) | Lean ground beef, ground chuck, turkey sausage meat (20–25% fat) | Ground turkey, extra-lean ground beef, ground round (about 15% fat) |
| Deep-fried foods (e.g., french fries, onion rings, fish or chicken patties, egg rolls, tempura) | Eat every day. | Eat once a week. | Eat once a month or never. |
| Bread for sandwiches | Croissant | Biscuit | Whole-wheat, French, tortilla, pita or pocket bread, bagel, sourdough, English muffin |
| Cheeses | Hard cheeses (e.g., cheddar, Swiss, provolone, Jack, American, processed) | Part-skim mozzarella, part-skim ricotta, low-fat cheeses | Nonfat cheese, nonfat cottage cheese, no cheese |
| Frozen desserts | Premium or regular ice cream | Ice milk or low-fat frozen yogurt | Sherbet, Italian water ice, nonfat frozen yogurt, frozen fruit whip |

---

Date _____    Section _____

## ...essment Activity 12-2

### Sexually

...following sexual behav-
...y of the listed activities,
...racting a sexually trans-
...ctivity by checking the

There is no risk for activity 1. The risk is low for activity 2. The risk is high for activities 3, 4, 5, and 6. After reviewing the different categories of activities, are there areas of concern for you?

| Risk | Precautions |
|---|---|
| No risk: There is virtually no chance of getting an STD. | No precautions are necessary. |
| Low risk: If both partners have no other sex partners and no disease, there is almost no risk of getting an STD. | Remain monogamous. |
| High risk: Each time there is another partner, the risk increases. | Choose partners carefully, use condoms and spermicides, wash after sex, do not douche, and urinate after sex. |
| High risk: The more partners, the greater the risk an STD will be transmitted. | Be aware of symptoms. |
| High risk: If needles are shared, the risk is great, particularly of getting AIDS and hepatitis B. | Know the social and sexual history of your partner. |
| High risk. | Know your partner; do not engage in oral sex if you do not know the history of your partner. |

# Changes to the Eighth Edition:

## Chapter 1:

Information on the *2008 Physical Activity Guidelines for Americans* added; application of SMART approach to developing goals for a lifestyle change programs added; new Just the Facts box on intimacy added; new Just the Facts box on exercise intensity added; statistics updated.

## Chapter 2:

Information added on atrial fibrillation as a risk factor for stroke; new guidelines on salt intake from the CDC and *2010 Dietary Guidelines Advisory Committee Report* added; information added on Herbert Benson's relaxation techniques; new Just the Facts box on exotic forms of smoking added; information on risk factors for cardiovascular disease among children and teenagers added; new section on peripheral artery disease added; statistics updated.

## Chapter 3:

Information on the *2008 Physical Activity Guidelines for Americans* added; information on the FITT principle added; information on heat cramps added; statistics updated.

## Chapter 4:

Information on conjugated linoleic acid (CLA) added; information on steroid usage added; statistics updated.

## Chapter 5:

Information added on lifestyle behaviors that may reduce neck pain; information added on repetitive strain injuries; statistics updated.

## Chapter 6:

New Just the Facts box on hidden trans fats added; information added on fat intake for babies and children; new section on Vitamin D added; new Just the Facts box on Vitamin B added; new Just the Facts box on glycemic index and glycemic load added; new weight gain guidelines during pregnancy from the National Institutes of Medicine added; statistics updated.

## Chapter 7:

The ACSM recommendations body fat percentages for adult women and men added; information on intra-abdominal fat added; statistics updated.

## Chapter 8:

New Just the Facts box on healthy weight, ideal weight, and desirable weight added; new Just the Facts box on obesity percentages today versus 50 years ago added; New Just the Facts box on being overweight and healthy added; New Just the Facts box on the obesity gene added; information on volume eating added; a new overeating quiz added; new Just the Facts box on commercial-break workouts added; information on overcompensatory eating added; information on the *2008 Physical Activity Guidelines for Americans* added; New Just the Facts box on losing weight and keeping it off added; statistics updated.

## Chapter 9:

New Real World Wellness box on stress-free test preparation added; new Real World Wellness box on dealing with techno stress added; statistics updated.

## Chapter 10:

Information added on texting while driving; New Just the Facts box added on cell phone use while driving; statistics updated.

## Chapter 11:

Information on the use of energy drinks added; information on LSD added; statistics updated.

## Chapter 12:

Information on the HPV vaccine added; statistics updated.

## Chapter 13:

Information on the two main types of lung cancer added; information on gene therapy added; statistics updated.

## Chapter 14:

Information on hospitalists added; information on preparation for hospital discharge added; information on personal health records (PHR) added; information on the most common complementary and alternative therapies added; statistics updated.

## Teaching and Learning Tools

The *Wellness: Concepts and Applications* **Online Learning Center** (**www.mhhe.com/anspaugh8e**) provides many resources for instructors:

- **Course Integrator Guide**
- **Test bank**
- **PowerPoint slides**
- **Image bank**
- **Web links**

**Classroom Performance System (CPS)** brings interactivity into the classroom or lecture hall with "clickers." Instructors can get immediate feedback on polling or quiz questions from the entire class using this system. Questions for each chapter are included on the *Wellness: Concepts and Applications* Online Learning Center.

**Tegrity Campus** is a service that captures audio and computer screen shots from your lectures, allowing students to review class material when studying or completing assignments. Lectures are captured in a searchable format so that students can replay any part of any class across an entire semester of class recordings. With classroom resources available all the time, students can study more efficiently and learn more successfully.

**CourseSmart**, the largest provider of eTextbooks, offers students the option of receiving *Wellness: Concepts and Applications* as an eBook. At CourseSmart your students can take advantage of significant savings off the cost of a print textbook, reduce their impact on the environment, and gain access to powerful web tools for learning. CourseSmart eTextbooks can be viewed online or downloaded to a computer. The eTextbooks allow students to do full text searches, add highlighting and notes, and share notes with classmates. Visit **www.CourseSmart.com** to learn more and to try a sample chapter.

 **McGraw-Hill Create** allows you to create a customized print book or eBook tailored to your course and syllabus. You can search through thousands of McGraw-Hill texts, rearrange chapters, combine material from other content sources, and include your own content or teaching notes. Create even allows you to personalize your book's appearance by selecting the cover and adding your name, school, and course information. To register and to get more information, go to **http://create.mcgraw-hill.com**.

**Student Resources** available with *Wellness: Concepts and Applications* include the following:

- The *Daily Fitness and Nutrition Journal* (ISBN 0077349709) is a handy booklet that guides students in planning and tracking their fitness programs.
- NutritionCalc Plus (ISBN 0077312430) is a dietary analysis program that allows users to track their nutrient and food group intakes, energy expenditures, and weight control goals. NutritionCalc Plus is available on CD-ROM (Windows only) or in an Internet version.

## Acknowledgments

Many thanks to the reviewers of the Eighth Edition for their expertise and assistance:

Carol Allen
*Linn-Benton Community College*

Becca Battaglini
*University of North Carolina, Chapel Hill*

Stephen Burks
*Harding University*

Justin Byers
*Bethel University*

Mary Nelle Cook
*Southwest Tennessee Community College*

Deborah B. Dowdy
*North Georgia College & State University*

Jim Roberts, Jr.
*Edinboro University of Pennsylvania*

Tracy Yengo
*University of Wisconsin-Eau Claire*

Bonnie J. Young
*Georgia Perimeter College*

*David J. Anspaugh*
*Michael H. Hamrick*
*Frank D. Rosato*

# Wellness and Fitness for Life

## ONLINE LEARNING CENTER

Log on to our Online Learning Center (OLC) for access to these additional resources:

- Chapter key term flashcards
- Learning objectives
- Additional goals for behavior change
- Concentration game
- Self-scoring chapter quizzes
- Additional lab activities

The OLC also offers Web links for study and exploration of wellness topics. Access these links through **www.mhhe.com/anspaugh8e.**

## GOALS FOR BEHAVIOR CHANGE

- Implement four new health promoting behaviors.
- Increase physical activity to improve overall wellness.
- Choose and implement three countering strategies.
- Formulate a self-help plan for lifestyle change.
- Identify and discuss the main wellness challenges for Americans.
- Describe the 2008 Physical Activity Guidelines for Americans.
- Identify obvious and subtle factors that help shape behavior.
- Discuss some of the underlying assumptions of lifestyle change.
- Identify and describe the six stages of change.
- Describe strategies that can be useful in designing and implementing an action plan for change.
- Apply the S.M.A.R.T. approach to developing goals for a lifestyle change program.

## Objectives

After completing this chapter, you will be able to do the following:

- ✔ Discuss the wellness approach to healthy living.
- ✔ Identify benefits of living a wellness lifestyle.
- ✔ Describe the dimensions of wellness.
- ✔ Cite evidence of the relationship between physical health problems and social, emotional, and spiritual stressors.
- ✔ Identify health disparities that exist in the United States.
- ✔ Compare and contrast the major influences on the health of Americans today with those of Americans of the past.
- ✔ Differentiate between moderately intense and vigorously intense physical activities.
- ✔ Outline a plan for lifestyle change.
- ✔ Define and explain the S.M.A.R.T. approach to setting goals for a lifestyle change program.

## [ Key Terms ]

| | | |
|---|---|---|
| contracting | locus of control | S.M.A.R.T. |
| countering | moderate-intensity physical activity | social connectedness |
| health-behavior gap | | transtheoretical model of behavior change |
| health disparities | psychosomatic diseases | |
| intimacy | risk factors | vigorous-intensity physical activity |
| Leading Health Indicators (LHIs) | self-efficacy | wellness |
| | self-help | |
| lifestyle diseases | shaping up | |

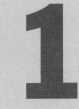

Good health is one of our most cherished possessions, one that is often taken for granted until it is lost. Some people convincingly argue that everything else in life is secondary to good health. For many, it is not difficult to recall instances when life's goals seemed unimportant because of sudden illness or a long-term debilitating health crisis.

Fortunately, the prospects of good health for Americans have never been better. The extent to which good health is realized is contingent on many factors. Chief among these factors are our actions and the choices we make. We can make choices that will promote health and well-being, prevent or delay the premature onset of many chronic illnesses, and improve our quality of life (see Real-World Wellness: Benefits of Living a Wellness Lifestyle). Staying healthy is not just a matter of common sense. Rather, it is a lifelong process that requires self-awareness, introspection, reflection, inquiry, accurate information, and action. This process relies on the concept of wellness and implies that each of us has the opportunity and the obligation to assume responsibility for factors that are under our control and to shape our health destiny. The wellness approach represents a formidable challenge because the processes leading to today's serious health threats are insidious, often originate in childhood or adolescence, flourish throughout adulthood, and finally culminate in full-blown disease in middle age or later. Lifestyle interventions initiated late in life produce limited success, but begun early in life they have maximum effect.

## Components of Wellness

**Wellness** is defined as an active process through which people become aware of, and make choices toward, a more successful existence.[1] Wellness is a process rather than a goal. It implies a choice, a way of life. It is positive and embraces people's strengths. It promotes feelings of self-worth. It is holistic and encompasses the body, mind, and spirit. It symbolizes acceptance of yourself. It suggests that what you believe, feel, and do have an influence on your health. It directs people to achieve their full potential. However, it does not imply that we make the best choice in every situation.

Consider the brief profiles of David, Susan, Carlos, and Maria. How would you rate each of them in terms of health and wellness?

David is physically active, places a high priority on his social life, barely makes passing grades in school, and engages in binge drinking almost every weekend. Susan is a perfectionist and her grades reflect it. To her, a *B* means failure. She spends an inordinate amount of time studying, regularly skips meals, has no physical activity outlet, and rarely socializes. Her family tells her to "get

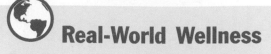

## Real-World Wellness

### Benefits of Living a Wellness Lifestyle

I am a full-time student, work 20 plus hours a week, and help with family responsibilities. At the same time, I'm trying to maintain my academic scholarship. There just isn't enough time in the day to be concerned about health and wellness. What am I to gain from a wellness lifestyle?

*A wellness lifestyle offers the following benefits:*

· Increases energy level and productivity at work and school

· Decreases absenteeism from school and work

· Decreases recovery time after illness or injury

· Supplies the body with proper nutrients

· Improves awareness of personal needs and the ways to meet them

· Expands and develops intellectual abilities

· Increases the ability to communicate emotions to others and to act assertively rather than aggressively or passively

· Promotes the attitude that life's difficulties are challenges and opportunities rather than overwhelming threats

· Acts from an internal locus of control

· Increases ability to cope with stress and resist depression

· Improves the cardiorespiratory system

· Increases muscle tone, strength, flexibility, and endurance

· Improves physical appearance

· Helps prevent or delay the premature onset of some forms of chronic disease

· Regulates and improves overall body function

· Promotes self-confidence

· Delays the aging process

· Promotes social awareness and the ability to reach out to, understand, and care about others

· Protects against cognitive decline in older persons[2]

· Reduces symptoms of depression and improves mood[3]

a life." She needs the entire weekend to recover from the stress of academics. Carlos runs 3 miles every day, works out with weights three times a week, eats a balanced diet almost every day, has a close circle of friends, refuses to use his seat belt when driving, and smokes an average of two packs of cigarettes daily.

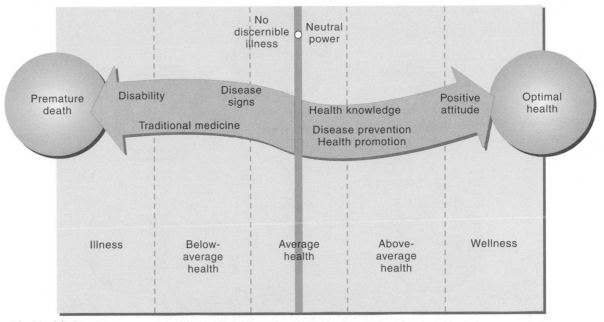

**FIGURE 1-1** The Health Continuum

Maria is a worrier. She makes good grades but is rarely satisfied. Her eating practices are exemplary, but she is constantly counting carb grams and calories and rarely looks forward to mealtime. She is self-conscious about her weight and occasionally engages in bulimic practices.

Figure 1-1 depicts how health moves along a continuum from optimal health to premature death. Your position on this continuum is always subject to change and is affected by many factors, including physical health, activity level, nutritional patterns, personal demands, career goals, time of year, and effectiveness in managing stress. Good health does not imply perfection. The human condition is highly imperfect. It has more to do with attitude, acceptance, adaptation, and lifestyles than it does with medicines or surgery. Good health is not automatic; it is partly a gift and partly a choice. The direction you move on the continuum and your place on the continuum at any time are largely determined by the activities you pursue and your attitudes toward these activities. These activities and attitudes can prevent illness and promote health or can destroy peace of mind and physical well-being. Because your behaviors are intrinsic to your health, you must learn to assume responsibility for your health by developing the skills and acquiring the knowledge to improve it.

In the past, medicine approached wellness from a different perspective. It emphasized the treatment of diseases rather than their prevention. It demanded no more than passive participation by the patient in the decision-making process. Now people are encouraged to become active participants in their health care, to exercise control over wellness **risk factors** (factors or

conditions that threaten wellness and increase the chances of developing or contracting disease), to shape their lifestyles to promote health, and to serve as partners with health care providers in making medical decisions. This approach places the responsibility for wellness on the individual.

Achieving a high level of wellness requires constant balance and maintenance of certain components (Figure 1-2 on page 4): spiritual, social, physical, emotional, intellectual, occupational, and environmental.

## Spiritual

Spirituality is a belief in a source of value that transcends the boundaries of the self but also nurtures the self. Everyone has a personal perception of spirituality. The spiritual component provides meaning and direction in life and enables you to grow, learn, and meet new challenges. Spiritual wellness includes developing a strong sense of values, ethics, and morals. It overlaps with the emotional component of wellness (described later). While spirituality may relate to religious precepts, it does not necessarily adhere to any particular religious structure. Spiritual support, in one form or another, is gaining favor among health care providers as a treatment strategy for patients and among researchers as a topic worthy of investigation.[4] For example, a recent study[5] randomly assigned college students to one of three groups regardless of their spiritual beliefs. Following weeks of meditation exercises, students in the spiritual meditation group had less anxiety and higher tolerance for pain than their peers in a secular meditation group and those in a relaxation group. While a study

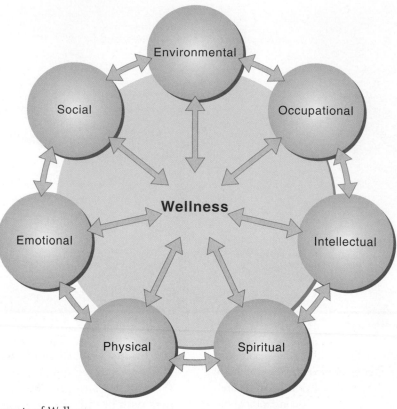

**FIGURE 1-2**   The Seven Components of Wellness

of this nature falls short of proving cause and effect, the growing interest among health researchers in the relationship between spirituality and a range of health conditions, including cancer, rheumatoid arthritis, cardiac surgery, drug abuse, sleep disorders, obesity, and psychological disorders, is unmistakable. Related to spiritual health is the act of forgiveness. Research indicates that harboring grudges and negative feelings about hurtful events and people may influence your psychological and physical health. Learning to forgive and move on is a better choice for overall health.[6] (See Nurturing Your Spirituality: Can Forgiveness Improve Your Health?)

## Social

Being social means having the ability to interact successfully with people and one's personal environment. Social health is the ability to develop and maintain **intimacy** with others and to have respect and tolerance for those with different opinions and beliefs. **Social connectedness** is the ability to establish and maintain relationships with other people. It is fundamental to health and well-being (see Just the Facts: Indicators of Social Connectedness). People are defined by their social roles, whether as roommates, fraternity or sorority members, teammates, children, friends, siblings, parents, employees, or countless other roles. Social relationships give people support, happiness, content-

ment, and a sense they belong and have a role to play in society. They also mean that people have support networks in place they can call on for help during difficult times. Studies have consistently found that social relationships contribute to a person's wellness regardless of age.[7,8] Conversely, loneliness and feelings of isolation have the opposite effect and can be detrimental to physical and emotional health.

## Physical

The physical component of wellness involves the ability to carry out daily tasks, develop cardiorespiratory and muscular fitness, maintain adequate nutrition and a healthy body fat level, and avoid abusing alcohol and other drugs or using tobacco products. In general, physical health is an investment in positive lifestyle habits. Separate chapters in this text are devoted to many of these physical dimensions of wellness.

## Emotional

Emotional wellness is the ability to control stress and to express emotions appropriately and comfortably. It is the ability to recognize and accept feelings and not be defeated by setbacks and failures. Achieving emotional wellness allows you to cope with life's ups and downs effectively.

# [ JUST THE FACTS ]

## Indicators of Social Connectedness

*The Social Report 2006*, published by the Ministry of Social Development in New Zealand, identifies five indicators of social connectedness:

1. **Telephone and Internet Access:** Both the phone and the Internet enable people to maintain contact with others without actually seeing each other. This means social connectedness can be maintained when people are in different cities or even different countries. Access to the Internet improves people's ability to obtain information and provides more opportunity to engage in society.
2. **Regular Contact with Family and Friends.** For most people, social networks center on family and friends.
3. **Trust in Others.** Trust enhances people's ability to develop positive relationships with others. People with high levels of trust expect others to act fairly and honestly toward them.
4. **Loneliness.** Feelings of isolation and loneliness undermine overall well-being.
5. **Contact Between Young People and Their Parents.** This indicator focuses on the needs of young people to get time each week with their parents and to receive nurturing and care.

Source: Ministry of Social Development. (*2008*). *The Social Report 2008*. Retrieved January 10, 2010, from http://www.socialreport.msd.govt.nz/2008/social-connectedness/index.html.

## Nurturing Your Spirituality

### Can Forgiveness Improve Your Health?

Forgiveness is a new topic of interest to health researchers. There is evidence that the ability to forgive contributes to psychological and physical well-being. In a study of college students, participants who focused on personal grudges had elevated blood pressures, pulse rates, muscle tension, and feelings of being less in control. Conversely, when participants learned to forgive, blood pressure, heart rates, and muscle tension returned to normal. Improvements in health and well-being have been observed in studies that included women who were abused as children, elderly people who were neglected, and people whose spouses were unfaithful.[9]

What is forgiveness? Forgiveness starts by acknowledging the hurtful event and how you feel. It does not mean condoning hurtful actions, forgetting what happened, looking the other way, excusing someone, or seeking revenge. However, at some point in time forgiveness means being able to let go of the pain even if there is no justice. In doing so, it is important to recognize that to let go, or forgive, does not forgive the act; it forgives the person, even if the act was cruel and extreme. "Forgiving the person is a way to take that person's power away. By forgiving the person, you choose to no longer define yourself as a victim in relation to the person." When this can be done, the process of healing begins.

The International Forgiveness Institute maintains that research on forgiveness may be as important to the treatment of emotional and mental disorders as the discovery of sulfa drugs and penicillin were to the treatment of infectious diseases. The Institute has developed a 20-step process model for forgiveness.[10,11] These steps are organized into four phases:

1. **Uncovering Phase.** In this phase the anger and emotional pain are confronted and acknowledged.
2. **Decision Phase:** In this phase the idea of forgiveness is considered. A prerequisite to forgiveness is to dismiss intentions of revenge toward the person who hurt you.
3. **Work Phase:** This phase is the essence of forgiveness and starts with the acceptance of the pain that was unjustly given and through active work moves toward forgiveness of the person who caused you pain. This may include finding new ways to think about that person, possibly even developing some compassion for his or her circumstances.
4. **Outcome/Deepening Phase:** In this phase the injured person begins to experience relief from the process of forgiving the injurer. The forgiving person may find meaning in the suffering he or she experienced.

Sources: The International Forgiveness Institute. (2010). Retrieved August 20, 2010, from http://www.forgiveness-institute.org/html/process model.htm; The International Forgiveness Institute. (2010). Retrieved August 20, 2010, from http://www.forgiveness-institute.org/html/about forgiveness.htm; Mayo Clinic. (2005). Forgiveness and health. *Mayo Clinic Health Letter*, 23(12), 6.

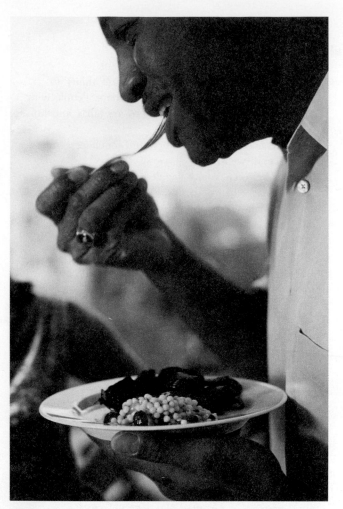

Behavior change, such as following a healthier diet, should be viewed as a lifetime goal, not a temporary fix.

Many studies report on the connection between wellness and emotional health. Anger, for example, is a powerful emotion that has been linked to heart attacks.

In a recent study, researchers followed medical students for 36 years following medical school. They found that students who became angry quickly under stress were three times more likely to develop premature heart disease and five times more likely to have an early heart attack.[12] Examples of anger tendencies include being quick-tempered, flying off the handle, saying nasty things when upset, and reacting aggressively and furiously when annoyed.

How does anger translate into heart attack risks? Anger induces a stress response that releases a myriad of chemicals that speed the development of fatty deposits in the heart and arteries. When you're angry, the body acts as if it is under attack and it prepares itself chemically and hormonally to defend itself. In our culture, we're warned against acting out on our anger. The result is an elevated level of stress hormones that may induce disease if anger pervades our daily lives.

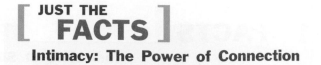

## [ JUST THE FACTS ]
### Intimacy: The Power of Connection

Often, when people think of intimacy they think of physical closeness. Physical closeness, and more specifically sexual closeness, is just one of the ways people connect on an intimate level. The editor of the highly respected *Mayo Clinic Health Letter* puts intimacy in perspective: "intimacy is a thread of connection that runs through your lifetime not only in a physical way but also in an emotional and spiritual way. It allows you to maintain meaningful relationships and connect with others. Physical, emotional and spiritual intimacy are interrelated with your feelings of wholeness, happiness and integration into the world."[16]

Source: Mayo Clinic Health Solutions. (2007). The power of connection: Physical, emotional and spiritual intimacy. *Mayo Clinic Health Letter*, 25(10), 1–8 (Supplement).

Anger may be as much of a risk factor for heart disease as smoking, obesity, and lack of exercise. People with a penchant for high levels of anger should consider anger management therapy.[13]

Another emotion vital to wellness is intimacy.[14] **Intimacy** refers to a special degree of closeness and trust between two or more people. It may include physical, emotional, social, and spiritual intimacy and is usually achievable only in certain relationships. Intimacy is an important part of wellness. Studies have shown that people who lack intimacy and feel lonely and isolated lead shorter and unhappier lives and experience significant health risks[15] (see Just the Facts: Intimacy: The Power of Connection).

Many other health problems are rooted in emotional stressors. Health conditions ranging from hives to cancer may have as their origin a breakdown in the body's immune system caused by the body's response to emotional stressors. These stressors, by disrupting the body's delicate balance of powerful hormones, may serve as the triggering mechanism for myriad health problems. The growing acceptance of stress-coping techniques, like those presented in Chapter 9 of this text, is evidence of the trend toward nonphysical strategies for preventing and treating many health problems.

## Intellectual

The intellectual component of wellness involves the ability to learn and use information effectively for personal, family, and career development. Intellectual wellness means striving for continued growth and learning to deal with new challenges effectively. It means acting on accepted principles of wellness and assuming responsibility for eliminating the discrepancy between knowl-

## [ JUST THE **FACTS** ]

### Laughter as Medicine

If it is true that powerful negative emotions, such as anger, have a deleterious effect on health, might it also be true that powerful positive emotions, such as humor and laughter, are good for health? Research has long associated anger and hostility with increased heart disease risk. Studies now suggest that laughter may be heart-protective. Researchers at the University of Maryland found that people with heart disease were 40% less likely to laugh in uncomfortable situations and were less likely to recognize humor, compared with people of the same age without heart disease.

A more recent 7-year study in Norway surveyed the role of humor in the lives of 54,000 Norwegians. Researchers found that people with a high sense-of-humor score were 35% less likely to die in the successive years than their peers with low humor scores. Of the more than 2,000 people with cancer, those with a sense of humor were 70% more likely to survive than those who were less lighthearted.[22]

The health-protective mechanism of laughter is not clearly understood. Several possible explanations include

1. Laughter decreases the secretion of serum cortisol, a stress hormone related to several diseases, including heart disease.
2. Laughing releases chemicals, such as nitric oxide (similar to laughing gas), that relax blood vessels.
3. Laughter increases blood levels of immunoglobulin A, an antibody that fights bacterial and viral infections.
4. Laughter may boost disease-fighting T-cells and natural killer cells, which are depressed during and after stressful experiences.
5. Laughter boosts good cholesterol (HDL) and lowers bad cholesterol (LDL).[23]
6. A hearty laugh involves the contraction and relaxation of muscles in the face, shoulders, abdomen, and diaphragm and may have a palliative effect on pain associated with arthritis.
7. Laughing changes the normal breathing pattern, ventilation, and circulation. Oxygen levels improve and help people with compromised breathing.
8. Laughter promotes fun and a sense of enjoyment with friends and family.
9. Laughter can improve your mood and help take your mind off your troubles. It is difficult to laugh and worry at the same time.

Sources: Consumers Union. (2001). Taking humor seriously. *Consumer Reports on Health*, 13(10), 7; The Week Publications. (2007). Laughing yourself healthy. *The Week*, 7(303), 26; Consumers Union. (2009). Laughter boosts "good" HDL cholesterol. *Consumer Reports on Health*, 21(7), 2.

---

edge and behavior, often referred to as the **health-behavior gap**. For example, people know that they should wear their seat belts and that they should not smoke, yet many people do not buckle up and continue to use tobacco products. For wellness to occur, people must internalize information and act on it.

An intellectually well person understands and applies the concepts of locus of control and self-efficacy. **Locus of control** refers to a person's view or attitude about his or her role in wellness and illness. A person's locus of control may be either internal or external. When people view problems concerning their health or other parts of their lives as generally out of their control (when they view themselves as being at the mercy of other people, places, and events), they have an external locus of control. They are reactive, rather than proactive, and are driven by factors out of their control. On the other hand, people who have an internal locus of control view their own behaviors as having significant effects, feel that they are at least partially the masters of their fate, and recognize that they can change the course of their health. People with an internal locus of control tend to be proactive and driven by factors within their control. They are more likely to succeed in wellness activities because they assume responsibility for their actions.

Locus of control serves as a simple but powerful yardstick of the relationship among attitudes, health perceptions, and wellness. People who appear optimistic about their health and believe they can have a direct influence on their well-being recover faster from surgery, have less heart disease, have better mental health, enjoy a higher quality of life, report more vitality and less pain, and live longer than people who have a pessimistic outlook.[17,18,19,20,21] Assessment Activity 1-2 at the end of this chapter will help you determine whether you have an internal or external locus of control.

Another influence on intellectual wellness is self-efficacy. **Self-efficacy** refers to a person's belief in his or her ability to accomplish a specific task or behavior. It means being confident of success. Perhaps the most important influence on the achievement of a wellness goal is the perception that it can be accomplished. Although the support of others is a source of encouragement, success is likely to require generating a personal sense of competence. Self-efficacy is not earned, inherited, or acquired; it is something you bestow on yourself.

For high-level wellness to be achieved, people must see themselves as successful and believe that they can accomplish a task. A recent weight-loss study illustrates the point. Obese men and women participated in an 8-week, very-low-calorie diet program. Those who had a high level of self-efficacy and thought they could control their eating behavior and didn't blame their weight on things outside of their control (e.g., low metabolism, heredity, etc.) lost more weight than their peers who experienced low self-efficacy. Researchers concluded that a strong self-efficacy was the best predictor of weight-loss success.[24] Other researchers maintain that self-efficacy is a potent predictor of treatment success for dozens of health behaviors and adds credibility to the old saying that "if you think you can succeed, you will, and if you don't, you won't."[25] Although locus of control establishes an attitude toward one's role in achieving wellness, self-efficacy establishes behavior. Self-efficacy links knowing what to do and accomplishing the task. Together, an internal locus of control and a strong sense of self-efficacy are powerful tools in promoting wellness and coping with illness.

## Occupational

Occupational wellness is the ability to achieve a balance between work, school, and leisure time. Attitudes about work, school, career, and career goals greatly affect work or school performance and interactions with others. Striving for occupational wellness adds focus to your life and allows you to find personal satisfaction in your life through work.

Occupational wellness does not come without its challenges. Changes in careers and jobs are common and are associated with psychosocial stress. Such stress may affect health, either through neuroendocrine pathways or through increases in high-risk behaviors. For example, an unstable employment history and shorter duration of current job are linked with a greater prevalence of smoking and greater alcohol consumption.[26] Careers of today demand increased levels of flexibility and mobility. A person's level of wellness is a key factor in carving out and maintaining a successful career path. Finding work is easier for healthy persons; also, people who need to find work repeatedly are likely to drop out of the workforce if their health deteriorates.[27]

## Environmental

Environmental wellness is the ability to promote health measures that improve the standard of living and quality of life in the community, including laws and agencies that safeguard the physical environment.

To illustrate the impact of environment on wellness, consider the differences in mortality (incidence of deaths) and morbidity (incidence of sickness) between earlier times and today. At the beginning of the 20th century, the average life span of Americans was 47 years. Today it is 77.9 years,[28] an all-time high. In 1900, communicable, or infectious, diseases (diseases that can be transmitted from one person to another) were the major causes of death. Influenza, pneumonia, tuberculosis, smallpox, polio, diphtheria, and dysentery were often fatal and were greatly feared. Only 50% of children were expected to reach their fifth birthday. Environmental conditions were appalling; water was dirty and food was often unsafe for consumption. People generally had little control over their health, and prospects for a long life were greatly influenced by fate and circumstance. By comparison, children born today have a 99% rate of survival to their fifth birthday. Governmental agencies at the federal, state, and local levels now assume responsibility for protecting health and preventing infectious diseases. Vaccinations have eradicated many dreaded diseases. The world food supply has improved. Adult literacy has increased. Mind-boggling advancements in medical technology have given rise to diagnostic and surgical procedures far beyond the wildest imaginations of early-20th-century physicians. Still, even with all of the discoveries of modern medicine, the greatest improvement in the health of Americans is due to a much more basic element of the environment: safe water. No other factor, not even vaccinations or antibiotics, has had as significant an impact on mortality reduction and population growth as safe water.[29]

Today, environmental influences include more than safe water, food, and air. Subtle influences, such as the socioeconomic factors of income, housing, poverty, and education, play a crucial role in the health status of various population groups. As a rule, the less education you have and the less money you earn, the shorter your life expectancy and the greater your chances of getting many diseases.[30] People with lower socioeconomic status are less likely to work and, when they do, they are more likely to be exposed to unhealthy conditions. They do not have health care coverage, are underweight or overweight, are smokers, have high blood pressure and diabetes, or do not participate in leisure activities, compared with their peers who enjoy a higher socioeconomic status. Regardless of socioeconomic status and education level, people can safeguard their health by making healthy lifestyle choices. But even more can be done through policies and environments that support healthy behaviors and promote quality of life for entire communities.[31] (See Just the Facts: Environmental Changes That Promote Wellness.)

The influence of environment on health is viewed more broadly today than in the past. The obesity epidemic is a case in point. Obesity has traditionally been viewed as a lifestyle problem caused by individual behaviors and choices. Experts now recognize that changes in environment are a major driving force and that the current environment encourages overconsumption of calories and discourages expenditure of energy.[32,33] Diet and lifestyle recommendations issued by the American Heart Association reinforce this point and call for substantial changes in the environment that target health care practitioners, restaurants, the food industry, schools, and local government, with specific recommendations about future policies that could be initiated by these groups. Examples include displaying caloric content prominently on menus, reducing portion size, limiting trans fatty acids, using low-saturated fatty-acid oils in food preparation, restricting nutrition-poor food choices in school vending machines, creating walking trails, building bicycle-friendly streets, integrating physical activity in the school curriculum, improving school playgrounds, creating user-friendly and safe neighborhood parks, and improving pedestrian infra-

structure (sidewalks, lighting, aesthetics). Most health problems are like obesity in that they are multifaceted in causes, interventions, treatments, and preventive measures.[34] Also, like obesity, they require substantial changes in the environment.

An important assumption of the wellness approach to living is that good health is best achieved by balancing each of the seven components. The body, mind, and spirit are inseparably linked. When they work together in a fully unified, integrated biological system, the body can ward off or overcome many diseases. When any of these components breaks down, wellness is threatened. Although the association between disease and physical causes (such as pathogens) is obvious, some people are reluctant to accept the association between illness and its mental, social, and spiritual aspects.

Nonphysical causes of illness are intangible and difficult to assess. Many people experience poor health because of guilt, anger, hostility, poor interpersonal skills, loneliness, anxiety, and depression. Any of these factors can interfere with the body's immune system and lay the foundation for the disease process. Medical records are replete with examples of **psychosomatic diseases,** in which physical (soma) symptoms are caused by mental and emotional (psycho) stressors. Such symptoms are just as real as if caused by disease-producing germs. Every disease involves interplay among the components of wellness. Fortunately, after a long-standing obsession with medical technology, many health care providers are beginning to focus on treating the whole person, and more people are demanding more than lab-test medical care.

Assessment Activity 1-1 at the end of this chapter provides an assessment of various aspects of wellness.

## Health Disparities

**Health disparities** are differences in the overall rate of disease incidence, prevalence, morbidity, mortality, or survival rates that exist among specific population groups in the United States.[35] Many different populations are affected by disparities including racial and ethnic minorities, residents of rural areas, women, children, the elderly, and persons with disabilities.[36] Racial and ethnic minorities include African Americans, Hispanics/Latinos, American Indians and Alaska Natives, Asian Americans, and Native Hawaiians and Pacific Islanders. These disparities may stem from many factors, including accessibility of health care, increased risk of disease from environmental and/or occupational exposure, increased risk of disease from underlying genetic, ethnic, or familial factors, substandard living conditions, inequities in education and income, discrimination, quality of health care, and shortage of racial and ethnic minority health professionals.[37,38] While progress in closing the disparity

# [ JUST THE FACTS ]

## Selected Health Disparities by Race, Ethnicity, Level of Education, and Gender

The gap in life expectancy according to race, ethnicity, and gender has narrowed during the past 15 years. Still, disparities persist. Some racial and gender disparities in mortality are not as large as reported in 2005, while others remain unchanged. Consider the following disparities by race and ethnicity, level of education, and gender:

*Race/Ethnicity*

1. The infant mortality rate is highest for infants of non-Hispanic black mothers and lowest for infants of mothers of Chinese origin.

2. Life expectancy at birth is 6 and 4 years longer for white men and women, respectively, than for black men and women.

3. African Americans, Hispanic Americans, Native Hawaiians, and American Indian and Alaska Natives are more likely to have diabetes than non-Hispanic whites. African Americans are also more likely to suffer complications from diabetes than non-Hispanic whites.

4. Prevalence of asthma in African American and Native American populations is 30% higher than that of non-Hispanic whites.

5. African Americans account for approximately 13% of the U.S. population, but represent almost half of new AIDS diagnoses. Hispanics/Latinos comprise 15% of the U.S. population, but represent 17% of new HIV infections.

6. The rate of chlamydia among African Americans is approximately 8 times higher than the rate among whites. Rates among Native Americans and His-

panic Americans are about 5 times and 3 times higher than whites, respectively.

7. More than 80% of new tuberculosis cases occur in racial minorities. Hispanic Americans account for 30% of these cases, followed in descending order by African Americans (27%), Asian Americans (24%), and non-Hispanic whites (17%).

8. Non-Hispanic white people are more likely to see a dental professional annually for a cleaning than are non-Hispanic black or Mexican-origin people.

9. Non-Hispanic black adults and non-Hispanic white adults experience more work-loss days due to injury and illness than Hispanic adults.

10. Diabetes is more prevalent among American Indian and Alaska Native adults and black adults compared with white adults.

11. Arthritis or chronic joint symptoms are less common among Asian adults than white adults, black adults, and American Indian or Alaska Native adults.

12. Fifty-seven percent of Asian adults are at a healthy weight and body mass index compared with 37% of white adults, 33% of American Indian or Alaska Native adults, and 28% of black adults. White adults are three times as likely as Asian adults to be obese; black adults and American Indian or Alaska Native adults are 3 to 4 times as likely to be obese as Asian adults.

13. Nine percent of Asian adults are cigarette smokers compared with 19% of black adults, 20% of white adults, and 28% of American Indian or Alaksa Native adults.

gap has been made during the past 15 years, many population groups remain disproportionally affected by health risks and diseases[39,40,41] (see Just the Facts: Selected Health Disparities by Race, Ethnicity, Level of Education, and Gender).

## The Wellness and Lifestyle Challenge

The most serious health problems of today are largely caused by the way people live and are referred to as **lifestyle diseases.** Lifestyle accounts for an increasing proportion of life expectancy, and this trend is likely to continue.[42] The leading causes of death in the United States among all age groups are heart disease, cancer, and stroke; they account for 56% of all deaths (Table 1-1 on page 12).[43] These are chronic diseases that are

often caused by behaviors established early in life. *Chronic diseases* are health conditions that often begin gradually, have multiple causes, and usually persist for an indefinite time. Heart disease, diabetes, arthritis, and hypertension are examples of chronic illnesses. By contrast, *acute illnesses* come on suddenly, often have identifiable causes, are usually treatable, and often disappear in a short time. Appendicitis, pneumonia, and influenza are examples of acute illnesses.

Diseases are not the only causes of death. Accidents, homicide, and suicide account for nearly three-fourths of deaths of Americans between the ages of 15 and 24. Most accidental deaths among this age group involve motor vehicle accidents, many of which are alcohol-related. For young adults 25 to 34 years old, accidents, cancer, heart disease, suicide, homicide, and human immunodeficiency virus (HIV) infection are the leading causes of death.

*Level of Education*

1. Education is inversely associated with heart disease, hypertension, and stroke: As the educational level increases, the percentages of adults with these conditions decrease.

2. Absence of all natural teeth is inversely associated with education. Fifteen percent of adults with less than a high school diploma have lost all of their natural teeth compared with 3% of adults with a bachelor's degree or higher.

3. Adults with at least a bachelor's degree are less likely than other adults to be current cigarette smokers and more likely never to have smoked.

4. Educational attainment and family income are positively associated with current regular alcohol consumption and inversely associated with being a lifetime abstainer.

5. Adults with higher educational attainment are more likely to have a personal doctor or health maintenance organization as their usual place of health care than those with lower educational attainment.

*Gender*

1. Seventy-four percent of women have visited or contacted a health professional within the past 6 months, compared to 60% of men. Men are more likely never to have contacted a doctor than are women. Men are more likely than women to consider a hospital emergency room or outpatient department to be their usual place of health care.

2. Overall, 37% of adults 18 years of age and over have been tested for HIV. Women are more likely to be tested than are men.

3. Women participate in leisure-time physical activity less often and less consistently than do men. Regarding participation in vigorous physical activities, 27% of men engage in such activities each week, compared to 22% of women.

4. Forty-four percent of women are at a healthy weight as measured by body mass index, compared with 30% of men. Forty-two percent of men are overweight (but not obese), compared with 28% of women. Women are nearly three times as likely to be underweight as are men. Obesity percentages are similar between men and women.

Sources: U.S. Department of Health and Human Services, The Office of Minority Health and Health Disparities. (2005). *What are health disparities?* Retrieved January 6, 2010, from http://minorityhealth.hhs.gov/templates/content.aspx?ID=3559; National Institute of Allergy and Infectious Diseases. (2009). *Minority health: What are health disparities?* Retrieved January 6, 2010, from http://www3.niaid.nih.gov/topics/minorityHealth/disparities.htm; National Institutes of Health. (2006). *Health disparities fact sheet.* Retrieved January 6, 2010, from http://www.nih.gov/about/researchresultsforthepublic/HealthDisparities.pdf; U.S. Department of Health and Human Services, National Partnership for Action to End Health Disparities. (2009). *Health disparities.* Retrieved January 6, 2010, from http://minorityhealth.hhs.gov/npa/templates/browse.aspx?lvl=1&lvlid=13; Pleis, J. R. (2009). Summary health statistics for U.S. adults: National health interview survey, 2007. National Center for Health Statistics. *Vital Health Statistics,* 10(240); National Center for Health Statistics. (2009). *Health, United States, 2008 with special feature on health of young adults.* Hyattsville, MD: U.S. Department of Health and Human Services.

For too many Americans these conditions reflect the dangers of negative lifestyle choices. Despite this, much of Americans' health-related anxiety involves exotic diseases. The current fear that some sort of strangely mutated disease will soon pose the greatest threat to life on Earth ironically coincides with a reduction in attention to chronic diseases that do kill in large numbers.

Although the appearance of terrorism is a genuine concern and the spread of new viruses, such as the 2009–2010 H1N1 virus (aka swine flu), in a global community is scary, the real threats to Americans are less sensational and less likely to be featured in the news media. The chances of getting them are remote, especially compared with the chance of getting lifestyle-related diseases that in many cases can be delayed, attenuated, or even prevented.

Healthy lifestyles that involve diet, physical activity, and personal health habits offer the most potential for preventing health problems or delaying them until much later in life. More specifically, the following 10 health issues have been identified in the landmark document *Healthy People 2010*[44] as priority areas. These priority areas are referred to as **Leading Health Indicators (LHIs)** and are discussed in detail in this text. The LHIs are

1. Physical activity
   - Vigorous physical activity in adolescents
   - Moderate physical activity in adults
2. Overweight and obesity
   - Overweight and obesity in children and adolescents
   - Obesity in adults

**TABLE 1-1    Ten Leading Causes of Death in 1900 and Today***

| | All Ages, 1900** | | All Ages, Today*** | | 15–24 Years, Today*** | | 25–34 Years, Today*** | |
| --- | --- | --- | --- | --- | --- | --- | --- | --- |
| Rank | Cause | % | Cause | %[+] | Cause | %[++] | Cause | %[+++] |
| 1 | Pneumonia & influenza | 12 | Heart disease | 27 | Accidents | 46 | Accidents | 33 |
| 2 | Tuberculosis | 11 | Cancer | 23 | Assault (homicide) | 16 | Cancer | 9 |
| 3 | Diarrhea & enteritis | 8 | Stroke | 6 | Intentional self-harm (suicide) | 12 | Heart disease | 8 |
| 4 | Heart disease | 8 | Chronic lower respiratory disease | 5 | Cancer | 5 | Intentional self-harm (suicide) | 12 |
| 5 | Stroke | 6 | Accidents | 5 | Heart disease | 3 | Assault (homicide) | 11 |
| 6 | Nephritis | 5 | Diabetes mellitus | 3 | Congenital problems | 2 | HIV disease | 3 |
| 7 | Accidents | 4 | Alzheimer's disease | 3 | Diabetes mellitus | 1 | Diabetes mellitus | 2 |
| 8 | Cancer | 4 | Influenza & pneumonia | 3 | Cerebrovascular disease | 1 | Cerebrovascular disease | 1 |
| 9 | Diphtheria | 2 | Nephritis | 2 | Pregnancy and childbirth | 0.4 | Congenital problems | 1 |
| 10 | Meningitis | 2 | Septicemia | 1 | HIV disease disease | 0.4 | Influenza & pneumonia | 1 |
| | All other causes | 38 | All other causes | 22 | All other causes | 13.2 | All other causes | 19 |

*Percentage mortality (i.e., percentage of all deaths by age group, rounded to nearest whole percent)

**Novartis Nutrition and McGraw-Hill. (2000). Obesity: A modern epidemic. *Innovations: Nutrition updates and applications*. New York: McGraw-Hill.

***Heron, M. P., and B. Tejada-Vera. (2009). Deaths: Leading causes for 2005. *National Vital Statistics Reports,* 58(8). Hyattsville, MD: National Center for Health Statistics.

+Total deaths, all ages: 2,488,017.

++Total deaths, 15–24 years: 34,234.

+++Total deaths, 25–44 years: 41,925.

3. Tobacco use
  - Cigarette smoking by adolescents
  - Cigarette smoking by adults
4. Substance abuse
  - Alcohol and illicit drug use by adolescents
  - Illicit drug use by adults
  - Binge drinking by adults
5. Responsible sexual behavior
  - Responsible adolescent sexual behavior
  - Condom use by adults
6. Mental health
  - Treatment for adults with recognized depression
7. Injury and violence
  - Deaths from motor vehicle crashes
  - Homicides
8. Environmental quality
  - Ozone pollution exposure
  - Exposure to environmental tobacco smoke
9. Immunization
  - Fully immunized children aged 19 to 35 months
  - Flu and pneumococcal vaccination in high-risk adults
10. Access to health care
  - Persons with health insurance
  - Source of ongoing care

  - Early prenatal care

In addition to the foregoing LHI, respected health and consumer organizations and newsletters offer similar but somewhat different health priorities. Most emphasize consuming a healthy diet, maintaining a healthy body weight, adopting a physically active lifestyle, and avoiding the use of tobacco products (see Just the Facts: Lifestyle Recommendations).

The risk factor most strongly associated with preventable death and chronic disease is cigarette smoking.[45] In a landmark study in the early 1990s that tried to pinpoint causes of death, tobacco use accounted for 400,000 deaths or nearly 1 in 5 deaths in the United States, with a 50% risk of premature mortality in cigarette smokers who do not successfully quit.[46,47,48,49,50] Following tobacco use as leading causes of death in descending order were poor diet and physical inactivity, obesity, excessive alcohol consumption, exposure to pathogens, toxic agents, motor vehicle crashes, firearms, risky sexual behavior, and illicit use of drugs. These risk factors persist today. In a 24-year study of the cause of death of 8,882 nurses, Harvard researchers calculated the contribution of five lifestyle factors to those deaths. Smoking cigarettes accounted for the highest percentage of deaths, fol-

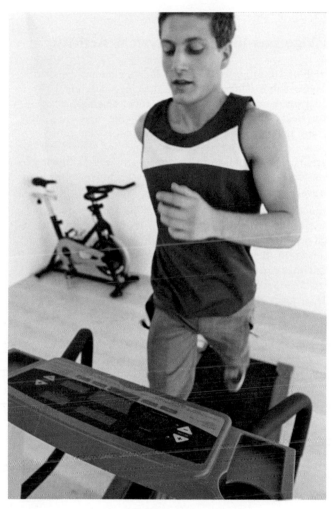

Running is a challenging activity that builds cardiorespiratory endurance.

lowed by physical inactivity, being overweight, having a bad diet, and not drinking moderate amounts of alcohol[51] (see Figure 1-3).

For the smoker, his or her primary wellness challenge is to stop smoking; if that proves impossible, significant reduction in the frequency and duration of smoking will attenuate some of the risk factors that threaten health. Second in importance to the smoker and first in importance to the nonsmoker as a wellness challenge are an increase in physical activity, maintenance of a healthy weight, and improvements in the diet. This is the most formidable challenge for Americans of all ages because obesity is the epidemic of the 21st century. Physical inactivity, overweight, and poor diet are inseparably linked and together account for 44% of deaths.

Americans' propensity for obesity and sedentary lifestyles comes at a time when evidence of the benefits of an active lifestyle is compelling. Adopting physically active lifestyles should be a priority for the nearly two-thirds of Americans who do not engage in regular leisure-time physical activity.[52] Physically active people outlive those who are inactive, and physical activity enhances the quality of life for people of all ages. Regular physical activity lessens the risk for heart disease, diabetes, colon cancer, high blood pressure, osteoporosis, arthritis, and obesity. It also improves symptoms associated with mental health, such as depression and anxiety.[53] Moderate amounts of physical activity improve health and reduce the incidence of premature death. Recognizing that being physically active is one of the most important steps we can take to improve our health, the Department of Health and Human Services established new physical activity guidelines in 2008.[54] Guidelines for adults, which are explained in more detail in Chapters 2–5 of this text, are as follows:

- All adults should avoid inactivity. Some physical activity is better than none, and adults who participate in any amount of physical activity gain some health benefits.

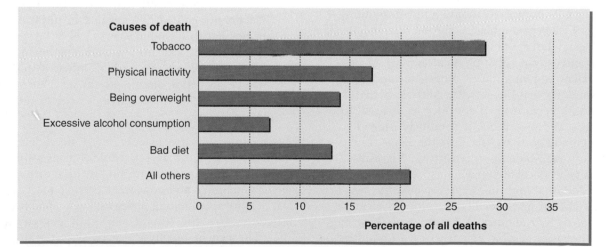

**FIGURE 1-3**   Contribution of Five Risk Factors as Causes of Death in the United States[51]

Source: Harvard Medical School. (2009). Lifestyle factors for longer life. Harvard Health Letter, 34(3), 7.

[ **JUST THE**
**FACTS** ]

## Light-Intensity vs. Moderate-Intensity vs. Vigorous-Intensity Physical Activity

Exercise intensity is one of the fundamental principles of exercise and is discussed in detail in Chapters 3 and 4 of this text. Exercise scientists express the intensity of exercise in METs, or metabolic equivalents. A MET is the ratio of the rate of energy expended during an activity to the rate of energy expended at rest. For example, 1 MET is the rate of energy expenditure while at rest. A 4-MET activity expends 4 times the energy used by the body at rest.[56] METs range between 0.9 and 18. Sleeping yields a MET of 0.9, sitting quietly has a MET of 1, and running 11 miles/hr has a MET of 18.[57,58] Because few people understand METs, *2008 Physical Activity Guidelines for Americans* expresses intensity in terms of minutes of exercise and types of exercise.[59,60,61]

**Light-Intensity Activities** have a MET of 1.1 to 2.9 and include light activities such as sitting, standing, shopping, cooking, or laundry. Light-intensity activities don't meet the guidelines because they don't sufficiently increase your heart rate.

**Moderate-Intensity Activities** have a MET of 3.0 to 5.9. Brisk walking at 3.0 miles per hour, for example, requires 3.3 METs. Other examples include water aerobics, riding a bike under 10 miles per hour on level ground, playing doubles tennis, general gardening, ballroom dancing, and engaging in any physical exertion that raises your heart rate and makes you break a sweat. In moderately intense activities you should be able to talk, but not sing the words to your favorite song.

**Vigorous-Intensity Activities** have a MET of 6.0 or more. For example, running a 10-minute mile has a

MET of 10. Other examples include swimming laps, playing tennis (singles), aerobic dancing, bicycling 10 miles per hour or faster, jumping rope, playing basketball, heavy gardening (continuous digging or hoeing), and hiking uphill or with a heavy backpack. In vigorously intense activities you're breathing hard and your heart rate increases significantly. If you're working at this level, you won't be able to say more than a few words without pausing for a breath.

Sources: Ainsworth, B. E. et al. (1993). Compendium of physical activities: Classification of energy costs of human physical activities. *Med Sci Sports Exerc*, 25(1), 71–80; Ainsworth, B. E. et al. (2000). Compendium of physical activities: An update of activity codes and MET intensities. *Med Sci Sports Exerc*, 32(9 Suppl), S498–504; Department of Health and Human Services. (2008). *2008 Physical activity guidelines for Americans*. Hyattsville, MD: U.S. Department of Health and Human Services; National Center for Health Statistics. (2009). *Health, United States, 2008 with special feature on the health of young adults*. Hyattsville, MD: U.S. Department of Health and Human Services; Centers for Disease Control and Prevention. (2009). How much physical activity do adults need? Retrieved January 6, 2010, from http://www.cdc.gov/physicalactivity/everyone/guidelines/index.html; Center for Disease Control and Prevention. (2009, December 28). Be physically active in the new year. *Healthy Lifestyle Newsletter*. Atlanta, GA: Division of Nutrition, Physical Activity and Obesity.

- For substantial health benefits, adults should do at least 150 minutes (2 hours and 30 minutes) a week of moderate-intensity aerobic activity, or 75 minutes (1 hour and 15 minutes) a week of vigorous-intensity aerobic physical activity or an equivalent combination of **moderate-** and **vigorous-intensity** aerobic activity. Aerobic activity should be performed in episodes of at least 10 minutes, and preferably, it should be spread throughout the week (see Just the Facts: Light-Intensity vs. Moderate-Intensity vs. Vigorous-Intensity Physical Activity).
- For additional and more extensive health benefits, adults should increase their aerobic physical activity to 300 minutes (5 hours) a week of moderate-intensity aerobic activity, or 150 minutes a week of vigorous-intensity aerobic physical activity or an equivalent combination of moderate-

and vigorous-intensity activity. Additional health benefits are gained by engaging in physical activity beyond this amount.
- Adults should also do muscle-strengthening activities that are moderate or high intensity and involve all major muscle groups on 2 or more days a week, as these activities provide additional health benefits.

For people who are inactive, even small increases in physical activity are associated with measurable health benefits. Since it is recent activity that offers health benefits, regular and consistent participation in physical activity is a lifelong endeavor[55] (see Wellness for a Lifetime: Tips for Staying Physically Active on page 17). The benefit of physical activity is the underlying theme of this text and, ideally, will serve as an impetus for you to establish an active lifestyle.

[ JUST THE **FACTS** ]

## Lifestyle Recommendations

Listed below are lifestyle recommendations from *Consumer Reports on Health*, the American Heart Association, and *Tufts University Health and Nutrition Letter*.

A healthy diet, physically active lifestyle, and avoidance of tobacco are common threads that run through these sets of recommendations.

| Consumer Reports on Health[+] | American Heart Association[++] | Tufts University Health and Nutrition Letter[+++] |
|---|---|---|
| 1. Engage in moderate physical activity for 30 minutes, five days a week. | 1. Minimize intake of beverages and foods with added sugars. | 1. Start the morning with whole-grain cereal. |
| 2. Get 7–8 hours sleep daily. | 2. Consume a diet rich in vegetables and fruits. | 2. Add 30 minutes of exercise per week. |
| 3. Maintain a healthy waist size. (Inches in waist size should be less than half those for your height.) | 3. Aim for a desirable lipid profile. Consume oily fish at least twice a week. Limit intake of saturated and trans fat and cholesterol. | 3. Choose a diet low in dairy, meat, and saturated fats. Opt for vegetable oils in preparing foods. |
| 4. Maintain a healthy lipid profile. | 4. Aim for a normal blood pressure. | 4. Eat more fruits and vegetables. |
| 5. Eat whole-grain foods. | 5. Be physically active. | 5. Have fish for dinner. |
| 6. Eat your colors: red, orange, yellow, green, purple, and white fruits and vegetables. | 6. Aim for a normal blood glucose level. | 6. Eat a colorful variety of produce, especially dark loafy greens. |
| 7. Eat fish high in omega-3 fatty acids twice weekly. | 7. Avoid tobacco products. | 7. Add vitamin D to your diet. |
| 8. Consume food in healthful portions; limit meat to 3-ounce servings and pasta to 1-cup servings. | 8. Aim for a healthy body weight. Balance caloric intake with caloric expenditure. | 8. Consume cold-water seafoods that are high in omega-3 fatty acids. |
| 9. Limit watching television to less than two hours a day. | 9. Choose whole-grain, high-fiber foods. | |
| 10. Challenge yourself each week. Do something meaningful. | 10. Choose and prepare foods with little or no salt. | |
| 11. Schedule time for pleasurable activities. Have some fun. | 11. If you consume alcohol, do so in moderation. | |

+Consumers Union. (2006). Power up your lifestyle. *Consumer Reports on Health*, 18(8), 1–3.

++American Heart Association Nutrition Committee: Lichtenstein, A. H. et al. (2006). Diet and lifestyle recommendations revision 2006: A scientific statement from the American Heart Association Nutrition Committee. *Circulation*, 114, 82–96.

+++Tufts University. (2006). Special report: From the lab to your lifestyle: 8 ways to be healthier in 2006. *Tufts University Health and Nutrition Letter*, 23(11), 4–5.

## Achieving Lifestyle Change: A Self-Help Approach

A fundamental assumption underlying lifestyle-change programs is that behavior is a learned response. For example, we are not born with a taste for some foods and a dislike for others. And using seat belts is not a function of heredity. Like most other behaviors, health behaviors are learned responses to both obvious and subtle influences. This learning begins at birth and continues throughout life. This is as true for behaviors that promote wellness as for behaviors that diminish it.

Examples of obvious influences that help shape behavior include parents and family, role models, advertising, and social norms. In many instances, these influences are combined to form a single powerful influence on behavior, such as exemplified by an advertisement for cigarettes using "ideal" masculine or feminine models, depending on the brand of cigarettes and the target population. Advertisers are successful not only at marketing products but also at influencing people to think they need those products.

Much of our behavior is also motivated by psychological needs. An infant whose main source of attention and stimulation comes during feeding time may learn to associate food with the deeper psychological

| | Stage | | | | | |
|---|---|---|---|---|---|---|
| | **1**<br>Precontemplation | **2**<br>Contemplation | **3**<br>Preparation | **4**<br>Action | **5**<br>Maintenance | **6**<br>Termination |
| **Characteristic** | Lack of awareness<br><br>Denial | Awareness of the need to change<br><br>Thinking about changing | Planning to change within a month<br><br>Thinking about the future | Engaging in strategies<br><br>Commitment to change | Greater difficulty than action stage<br><br>Duration from 6 months to a lifetime | Problem behavior no longer an issue |
| **Goal** | Feedback on need to change<br><br>Consciousness raising | More consciousness raising<br><br>Emotional arousal | Public affirmation of change<br><br>Development of a plan | Application of strategies<br><br>Changes in environment<br><br>Forming of or joining of support groups<br><br>Establishment of rewards<br><br>Countering | Application of same strategies as in action stage | Exit from cycle of change |

**FIGURE 1-4**   Stages, Characteristics, and Goals of Lifestyle Change

needs of love and affection. A parent who consistently uses food to appease an unhappy child may be inadvertently establishing a preoccupation with food that will endure far beyond childhood.

Sometimes, behavior is motivated in response to force or coercion. *Reactance motivation,* a theory of behavior that has been associated with drinking among college students, suggests that telling people to abstain completely from doing something often produces the opposite reaction. For many people, it isn't difficult to recall instances in their lives in which they behaved a certain way primarily because they were told that they could not or should not behave that way. Coercion, in particular, leads to the arousal of reactance, which in turn tends to reduce compliance.

These examples help explain the myriad complex forces that contribute to behavior and illustrate why successful lifestyle change is so difficult to achieve. The hope and promise of any lifestyle-change program is that, while easier said than done, bad habits can be unlearned and new habits can be learned.

## A Self-Help Plan

A **self-help** approach assumes that individuals can manage their lifestyle changes and can learn to control those features in the environment that are detrimental to health. In other words, expensive, long-term, professional help is not a prerequisite for everyone trying to

make a lifestyle change. The self-help approach puts you in control of your health, requires your involvement, and permits you to determine what to do and how and when to do it. However, to be successful, this approach requires considerable time and thought devoted to planning. Successful lifestyle change is almost impossible to achieve without a plan.

The self-help approach that follows is based on the **transtheoretical model of behavior change.**[62] This model of lifestyle change is presented in six stages (Figure 1-4), as described next, along with recommended strategies. In applying this model of change, it is helpful to remember several important assumptions:

1.  Each of the six stages is well defined and entails a series of tasks that need to be completed before moving to the next stage.

2.  Unquestionably, changing a habit that has been a part of your everyday lifestyle for years is a difficult challenge and may feel impossible to achieve. It is helpful to know that a linear progression through the stages of change, although possible, is rare. Most people lapse at some point, and it is possible to get stuck at one stage. However, the important thing is to formulate a plan and act on it. Trying to discard an unhealthy habit or adopt a healthy one may not succeed the first time. It often takes anywhere from three to 30 tries to succeed.[63] Even if a relapse takes you back temporarily to an earlier

## Wellness for a Lifetime
### Tips for Staying Physically Active

Here are some tips for starting and sticking with physical activity as a part of your daily routine.

1. Divide exercise and activity into 10- or 15-minute segments. Remember, exercise, to be good for health, does not have to be in one shot.
2. If you have stairs in your home or your dormitory (and don't have knee problems), go up and down a few extra times.
3. Use a pedometer to measure the steps you take. Work up to 10,000 a day (about 5 miles).
4. Consider housework and yard work as a workout.
5. Schedule your workout and keep a record of it. A daily or weekly log of time spent in exercise or steps or miles provides feedback of accomplishments and may reveal opportunities to add more activity to your daily routine.
6. Park farther away from your destination when you are shopping, going to class, meeting friends for lunch, and so forth.
7. Work out during television time. Do floor exercises while watching television or exercise on a treadmill or stationary bike, if one is available.
8. Establish realistic goals for your workout. Track your progress. Success is a great motivator. Make adjustments in your workout that ensure success.
9. Seek variety. Vary your activities so that you look forward to working out.
10. Make it convenient. Choose an activity that is doable on a regular basis and a venue that is near your home, school, or job.

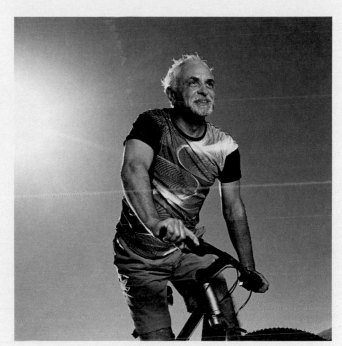

11. Have fun. If it's fun you're more likely to stay with it. If you stay with it for 6 months, you are more likely to make physical activity a habit for life.
12. Look at exercise as a positive addiction, one that becomes so integrated in your lifestyle that you miss it if you skip a session.

Source: Tufts University. (2006). 9 easy ways to add exercise to every day. *Tufts University Health and Nutrition Letter*, 24(6), 4–5.

stage, you are more likely to succeed than a person who never tried at all.[64]

3. A key to successful change is knowing what stage you are in for the health issue or behavior at hand. Behavioral research reveals that people who try to accomplish changes they are not ready for set themselves up for failure. Similarly, too much time spent on a task already mastered—such as understanding your problem—may result in an indefinite delay in taking action.
4. Although nearly all change begins with precontemplation, only the most successful ends in termination. But you cannot skip stages. Most people who succeed follow the same road for every problem. However, you may be at different stages of change for different problems.
5. Successful behavior change does not typically happen all at once; it takes time.

### Precontemplation Stage

In the precontemplation stage, individuals have no intention of changing in the near future. Precontemplators may be unaware of the health risks associated with their behaviors. Or they may feel a situation is hopeless; maybe they've tried to change before without success. They often use denial and defensiveness to keep from going forward. They feel safe in precontemplation because they can't fail there. A recent study on alcohol abuse among college freshmen and sophomores illustrates the tendency toward denial. Researchers found that 70% of freshmen and sophomores participating in the study were in the precontemplation stage. Less than 10% were aware of their problem-drinking behavior and in the preparation stage for stopping alcohol abuse.[65]

**Strategies.** Consciousness raising is a key strategy. If you do not perceive a problem or are too overwhelmed by other circumstances, you are not likely to be receptive to making a change.[66] The lack of awareness of a problem explains why many health improvement or behavioral intervention programs fail. Sometimes awareness comes from a visit to the doctor, a health-threatening diagnosis, a headline news story, or feedback from others. One way to encourage consciousness raising is to take an inventory of personal health habits and practices. A good way to start is to make a list of your health-promoting behaviors, practices you engage in to maintain or improve your level of wellness (see Just the Facts: Examples of Health-Promoting Behaviors). Make another list of health-inhibiting behaviors, practices that may be detrimental to your health (see Assessment Activity 1-3). If your lists are specific and identify behaviors that relate to wellness in its broadest sense (that is, the physical, social, emotional, and psychological aspects of health), comparing the two should give you insight into and information about your lifestyle.

Detailed, comprehensive lifestyle questionnaires, such as in Assessment Activity 1-1, can provide even more information about specific health practices and behavioral tendencies that can be targeted for change. These questionnaires also provide an opportunity to assess and/or reflect on your motivation for lifestyle change. This is important because experts believe "motivation is at the heart of any lifestyle change. It's what gets you going and keeps you at it. It serves as a barometer of your commitment to take action. Absent sufficient motivation, making a lifestyle change is almost always unsuccessful."[67]

## Contemplation Stage

Contemplators have a sense of awareness of a problem behavior and begin thinking seriously about changing it. However, it is easy to get stuck in the contemplation stage for years. Perhaps making a change requires more effort than someone is willing to expend, or the rewards or pleasures of the current behavior seem to outweigh the benefits of change.[68]

**Strategies.** Contemplators need more consciousness raising. Reading, studying, and enrolling in courses are good ways to promote an awareness of the potential problems associated with certain behaviors. (One goal of this text, for example, is to increase your consciousness of habits and practices that promote wellness and of risk factors that may threaten your health.) Getting involved in activities that expose you to information about various aspects of health and wellness allows you to focus on the negatives of your current health practices and to imagine the consequences down the line if your behavior doesn't change.

*Cognitive dissonance,* the internal conflict that occurs when people feel that their behavior is inconsistent with their intentions or values (such as exhibited by a smoking parent who doesn't want his or her child to smoke), helps in this stage. Also, *emotional arousal,* sometimes accomplished by watching a movie or news story on the subject in question (such as about the sudden death of a child caused by drunken driving), spurs someone to action. Social strategies also help. For example, a problem drinker might attend an Alcoholics Anonymous meeting as a way of experiencing social support for behaving differently.

## Preparation Stage

Most people in the preparation stage are planning to take action within a month. They think more about the future than about the past, more about the pros of a new behavior than about the cons of the old one. Many people motivate themselves by making their intended change public rather than keeping it to themselves. This stage involves developing a plan customized to a person's unique circumstances and personality.

Most people make three serious mistakes when starting a lifestyle change. First, they expect miracles and set unrealistic goals. Setting goals that are too ambitious often guarantees failure. For many people, the fear of failure easily discourages future efforts at a lifestyle change.

Second, people oversimplify the complexities associated with lifestyle change and view it as a willpower issue. The strategy of choice for these people is "cold turkey," which involves picking a day for the change and, through determination and willpower, refraining from the target behavior. Experts disagree on the effectiveness of this strategy for changing many health behaviors, arguing that, while it may work for some because it forces them to adopt new habits, it inflates the "hold" over people by assigning it more power than it deserves.[69] A dieter, for example, who decides to cold-turkey his consumption of high-fat, gourmet-style ice cream may actually encourage an obsession with this forbidden food. In this approach, little learning takes place, with the possible exception that willpower by itself is usually insufficient to cause a permanent change in behavior.

Third, people often view lifestyle change as a temporary goal rather than as a lifetime change. Perhaps more than anything else, this attitude accounts for the high *recidivism* (the tendency to revert to the original behavior) rate of many programs. One of the best examples is weight-loss programs. In weight-loss programs, for example, people typically set a goal, diet until they reach their goal, revert to their original eating habits, and invariably regain the lost weight. The proper way is to change eating habits, so that they will endure for a lifetime. When people try to change some aspect of behavior, they have to deny themselves something that feels comfortable or that provides enjoyment or pleasure. Denial often triggers a preoccupation that worsens the health behavior being changed. This is the reason dieters often become more interested in food during a diet (see Real-World Wellness: Are You Ready for a Lifestyle Change?).

No single strategy for lifestyle change is right for everyone. The key is to get involved in planning your personal program and to use your imagination to create the most suitable plan.

## Real-World Wellness

### Are You Ready for a Lifestyle Change?

*I've started an exercise program four times during the past 2 years. Each effort resulted in failure. I don't want to start again until I know I'm ready. How will I know that I'm ready to begin a lifestyle-change program?*

If you can answer yes to the following questions, you are ready to begin a lifestyle-change program:

- Do you view lifestyle change as a lifetime goal rather than as a temporary, short-term goal?
- Are you willing to get personally involved in planning a lifestyle-change program?
- Are you prepared for some disappointments?
- Are you willing to experiment with different ideas?
- Do you have the patience to accept success in small increments stretched over a long period?
- Are you willing to set modest, realistic goals?
- Are you willing to establish some time benchmarks for success?
- Are you willing to make some changes in the way you live?
- Are you willing to tell others about your goals?
- Can you accept a relapse as a temporary setback rather than as a full-blown failure?
- Are you willing to formulate a plan that makes provisions for countering, avoidance, contracting, shaping up, reminders, and support?

**Strategies.** In this stage, a firm, detailed plan is developed that involves (1) assessing behavior and (2) setting specific, realistic goals.

*Assess behavior.* Behavior assessment, the collection of data on target behaviors, is the lifeline of any lifestyle-change plan. It involves the process of counting, recording, measuring, observing, and describing. Any behavior that can be qualified is assessed.

Assessment tools provide objective data regarding behavioral patterns, health changes, and/or results. They may be daily logs, journals, and diaries or medical diagnostic tools (e.g., blood pressure machine). Data should be collected long enough to note trends, usually for a minimum of 1 to 2 weeks. Often, people are surprised at what they learn about themselves. One example is the amount of time people spend sitting still in front of a TV and/or computer. A 2008 study revealed that adults averaged watching TV more than

5 hours a day and in doing so substantially increased their chances for morbidity and mortality.[70] In a recent highly publicized study of 8,800 adults over a period of 6 years, researchers reported that people who watched TV 2 to 4 hours a day were 13% more likely to die of any cause and 19% more likely to die of cardiovascular disease than people who reported spending less than 2 hours a day in front of the TV. The percentages jumped exponentially for people who watched TV more than 4 hours a day with 46% and 80% higher mortality for "any cause" and cardiovascular disease, respectively.[71] For many adults, the simple act of assessing the amount of time in prolonged periods of inactivity such as TV viewing, playing video games, or browsing the Internet would quickly reveal the magnitude of their sedentary lifestyle and provide a basis for establishing specific goals.

Sometimes a behavior assessment will prompt a change in behavior without any other action. In most lifestyle-change programs, a plan of action is not started until it is clear that assessment alone will not be enough to alter the behavior completely. For example, some people attach an electronic pedometer to their waistband to count the number of steps taken each day. For some people the first step is the only step required. Counting serves as a sufficient intervention to behavior improvement.

The assessment phase also provides clues to a person's commitment to making a change in lifestyle. A thorough, detailed log is a good sign that a person has the motivation to carry out the plan.

When the assessment phase is finished, there should be sufficient information to form a behavioral profile, state specific goals, and customize an intervention program that matches goals and strategies to a person's unique circumstances and personality.

*Set specific, realistic, measurable goals.* Apply the **S.M.A.R.T.**[72] acronym in setting goals. "S.M.A.R.T." refers to 5 characteristics of effective goals: specific, measurable, accurate, realistic, and trackable.

*Specific.* Setting specific goals means stating goals that focus on concrete behaviors. If goals are specific, you know precisely what you are trying to accomplish and where, when, and how often. Specific goals also provide instant feedback on your progress. A behavioral goal to overcome shyness may be important, but it is general and lacks specificity. A specific goal might be to initiate a conversation with a different person each day for the next week. Another way to increase specificity is to establish a timetable for achieving goals. A timetable adds structure to the plan and provides a way to evaluate progress. In setting specific goals, avoid the temptation of setting too many goals. Focus on one or two goals that will command your attention. For complex lifestyle changes, break down long-range goals into a set of intermediate goals, beginning with the easier ones and then moving gradually to more difficult ones.[73]

*Measurable.* Objective, observable, and measurable goals are at the heart of a good lifestyle-change plan and go hand in hand with setting specific goals. Without measurable goals, it isn't possible to determine the extent to which goals are achieved. The assessment phase, done correctly, provides the foundation for establishing measurable goals.

*Attainable.* Achievable, attainable goals are reasonable and relate to personal circumstances. Setting attainable goals also means forming them in the context of correct information. For example, an informed dieter knows that setting a goal to lose 10 pounds in a week is not reasonable. A more attainable goal is 1 to 2 pounds. In identifying attainable goals, lean toward the side of conservative, easy goals. Setting a modest goal initially facilitates some degree of success, which increases confidence. Nothing breeds success like success. Conversely, setting overly ambitious goals that are difficult to attain breeds failure, which can be very demoralizing.

*Realistic.* Realistic behavioral goals are within your capabilities and relate to personal circumstances. If your goal is to walk 3 miles a day, does your school schedule and work schedule allow sufficient time, say an hour, to achieve this goal? If not in one time setting, do you have sufficient control of your schedule to walk in 10-to-15 minute increments throughout the day? Do you have access to walking facilities? Do you feel safe walking at night on your campus or in your neighborhood? Addressing these questions on the front end will help you formulate a realistic as well as attainable plan. Avoid setting extreme goals because they promote the erroneous attitude that lifestyle change is temporary. A 500-calorie-per-day diet is extreme and an example of a goal that cannot be sustained. Long-term failure is almost guaranteed. Other examples of extreme goals are cold-turkey or willpower approaches, which create a strong sense of denial, encourage preoccupation with target behaviors, and often lead to failure. Exceptions include cigarette smoking, alcoholism, and other drug dependence, for which abstinence continues to be a preferred treatment strategy.

*Trackable.* Keeping track of your goals provides instant feedback on your progress and requires some form of written record. A journal or log works for most people. Another option is a progress chart that is displayed on a wall to serve as a daily reminder of where you are in reaching your goal. Sometimes just the act of keeping a record promotes success. For example, a Duke University weight-loss study found that participants who kept daily food records lost twice as much weight as those who kept no records. The records were not restricted to food diaries. Some of the records were in the form of sticky notes, text messages, and e-mails.[4]

## Action Stage

In the action stage, a person overtly makes changes in behavior, experiences, or environment. This is the busiest stage of change. It's also the stage most visible to others. New behaviors, such as exercising, not smoking, or actively changing a dietary pattern, can be observed.

**Strategies.** People in the action stage implement their plan for change. In doing so, they apply their sense of commitment to the change. Rewards and incentives are important elements of this stage. **Countering,** or behavior substitution, in which a new behavior is substituted for the undesirable one, is the most common and one of the most powerful strategies available to people trying to make a change. When this technique is applied, the goal is to think of a behavior incompatible with the one being altered. Examples include chewing gum to suppress the urge to smoke, substituting diet colas for sweetened colas, and going for a walk instead of watching television. Some effective countering techniques are summarized in Just the Facts: Countering Strategies on page 20.

Making changes in the environment is another key element of the action stage. Avoidance, or the elimination of the circumstances associated with an undesirable behavior, is a fundamental technique of the control process. A smoker cannot smoke if there are no cigarettes, an ice cream binge is not possible if there is no ice cream parlor, and loud music cannot interfere with studying if the radio is put away.

Avoidance is not limited to objects. It may also include jobs, school, and even people. If taking 18 hours of coursework while working 20 hours per week is compromising your academics, you may feel justified in dropping several courses or withdrawing from school if a reduction in your workload isn't possible. By the same token, it may be necessary to associate less often with people who contribute to a problem behavior.

The use of reminders is also a key element of an action plan. These may be in the form of a daily planner, a calendar, clocks, sticky notes, signs on a door, or a to-do list. During times when behavior change is not an issue, the list might read "call home, library, 2:00–4:00 p.m.; racquetball, 4:30–5:30; dinner date, 6:00–8:30; study time, 9:00–11:00." If you are working on an action plan for lifestyle change, adding action goals is a natural extension. If, for example, you are working on social skills, you might add "initiate a conversation with a classmate" or "eat lunch with someone different." A positive benefit of reminders, in addition to their reinforcement of positive behaviors, is the satisfaction that results from checking something off a list.

**Contracting** is another common action strategy. Written contracts tend to be more powerful than spoken ones. They usually include a statement of long-range and intermediate health goals; target dates for completion of each goal; intervention strategies; and rewards and incentives, such as "I will deposit $5 in my new car savings account for every day that I attend all of my classes between now and the end of the semester." These contracts are not legal documents, so simplicity and creativity are in order.

**Shaping up** is another essential part of lifestyle change. It requires a person to allow him- or herself opportunities to practice desired behaviors, usually in small increments. The saying "Behavior begets behavior" is the essence of shaping up. This is also true for harmful behaviors. For example, cigarette smokers rarely enjoy their first cigarette; they learn to enjoy smoking by smoking. The same is true for most beer drinkers. Typically, shaping up occurs gradually until it becomes fully integrated into one's behavioral repertoire.

The acquisition of positive health behaviors occurs the same way. A step-by-step approach, with reinforcement following each successive movement, promotes success. In overcoming a fear of flying, a person might first visit the airport; the next step might be to tour an airplane; next the person may take a seat, fasten up, and visualize flying. Each step brings the person closer to flying, each step is reinforced, and any feelings of anxiety are countered with relaxation. People forget that problem behaviors are formed cumulatively and reflect many years of conditioning. It is only reasonable to expect that acquiring a preference for a new behavior will also require considerable time, thought, and reinforcement.

Another good strategy in an action plan is the formation of a support group, which may include a roommate, family, friends, classmates, or someone who can identify with the lifestyle goal. Dieting may be easier and more tolerable when done with a friend. Two people may accomplish their goals more effectively than either can alone. For example, two roommates may be more successful at maintaining their exercise regimen together than separately. Involving someone else in the process of change makes it easier to stick to your action plan, provides a source of encouragement, and holds you accountable for your goals. Social factors, such as the involvement of a support group, companion, or buddy system, are keys to success for health behavior improvement, particularly in the area of exercise and physical activity.[75]

## Maintenance Stage

The goal in the maintenance stage is to retain the gains made during the action and other stages and to try hard to prevent a relapse. Change never ends with action. Although people tend to view maintenance as a static stage, it is actually a continuation of the action stage and can last 6 months to a lifetime. Programs that promise easy change usually fail to acknowledge that maintenance is a long, ongoing process. This is why trendy, extreme programs, such as many diet programs, have a high recidivism rate. People may achieve their weight-loss goal, but they cannot maintain their strategy for losing weight for life. When this happens, a person may erroneously view the action plan as a temporary strategy. This is the opposite of maintenance and lifestyle change.

Most people experience a relapse and return to the precontemplation or contemplation stage of change, maybe several times, before eventually succeeding in maintaining the change. People move through the change process at different paces, and relapse is a part of behavior change. Learn from any relapse instead of reacting to it by giving up. It is important to remember that the real test of a program's success is not how many people reach their goals but how many people successfully maintain that goal for at least 2 years.

**Strategies.** Strategies used in the action plan should be continued in maintenance. Provisions for avoidance, reminders, contracting, countering, shaping up, and support groups apply during maintenance, just as they do during the action stage.

## Termination Stage

The termination stage is the ultimate goal for people trying to make a lifestyle change. In this stage, the problem behavior is no longer tempting. A person becomes confident that his or her problem behavior will never return; it becomes a nonissue. The cycle of change is exited.

**Strategies.** Some experts believe that termination is impossible, that the most anyone can hope for is a lifetime of maintenance. The key strategy is to be aware of early warning signs of relapse, such as overconfidence, that can recycle the problem behavior.

Regardless of the results, maintaining the proper perspective about success and failure is important. Many people have the attitude that they either completely succeed or completely fail. This way of thinking can be devastating to a person's motivation. When goals are not fully realized, the proper attitude is to view the shortcoming as justification for making adjustments in the program. The goals may have been too general or unrealistic. The intervention strategies may have lacked relevance. Look at relapse as a learning tool. Reshaping goals, setting a more realistic schedule, changing the rewards and penalties, or formulating different intervention strategies may be necessary.

Above all, you should maintain a healthy perspective about yourself and not burden yourself with guilt if you fall short of your goals. What seems important now becomes insignificant when viewed within a broader context. You may consider how significant this event is likely to be to you 2 years from now. Doing this helps establish the right perspective on your progress. More important than total success are the answers to the following questions: What did you learn from this experience? What did you learn about yourself? What can you do differently? Lifestyle change is a lifelong project that requires insight, skillful planning, and plenty of practice.

# Summary

- Wellness is an active process through which people become aware of, and make choices toward, a more successful existence. Wellness is a process rather than a goal. It is holistic and encompasses the body, mind, and spirit.
- Health is a constantly changing state of being that moves along a continuum from optimal health to premature death and is affected by an individual's attitudes and activities.
- Lifestyle diseases represent the major threat to the health and quality of life of Americans.
- Wellness requires the consistent balancing of spiritual, social, physical, emotional, intellectual, occupational, and environmental dimensions.
- Social connectedness is fundamental to health and well-being. Social relationships give people support, happiness, contentment, and a sense they belong and have a role to play in society.
- The ability to forgive someone for a hurtful event contributes to psychological and physical well-being. The International Forgiveness Institute maintains that research on forgiveness may be as important to the treatment of emotional and mental disorders as the discovery of sulfa drugs and penicillin were to the treatment of infectious diseases.
- An internal locus of control is the attitude that a person is in control of his or her life. An internal locus of control is consistent with the principles of wellness. An external locus of control is the belief that factors affecting health are outside one's control.
- *Self-efficacy* refers to the beliefs people have in their ability to accom-

plish specific tasks or behaviors. A strong sense of self-efficacy is consistent with the principles of wellness.
- The mind, body, and spirit are inseparably linked. A breakdown in any one of these can threaten health and wellness.
- Physical, emotional, and spiritual intimacy is an important part of wellness and is associated with happiness, longevity, and reduced risk of health problems.
- Psychosomatic diseases occur when physical symptoms are caused by psychological, social, spiritual, or emotional stressors.
- Most health problems are multifaceted in causes, treatments, and preventive measures. Successful interventions often require substantial changes in the environment.
- *Healthy People 2010* has as one of its goals the elimination of health disparities that exist among population groups.
- Lifestyle diseases are those caused by the way people live. The major lifestyle diseases are heart disease, cancer, and stroke. Together these account for 56% of all deaths among Americans.
- Chronic diseases are those that persist for an indefinite time.
- Accidents are the leading cause of death among Americans between 15 and 24 years of age.
- Healthy lifestyles that involve diet, physical activity, and personal health habits offer the most potential for preventing health problems or delaying them until much later in life.
- The risk factor most strongly associated with premature death and chronic disease in the United States is cigarette smoking.

- An increase in physical activity is the most formidable challenge for Americans of all ages.
- Adopting physically active lifestyles should be a priority for the nearly two-thirds of Americans who do not engage in any leisure-time periods of vigorous physical activity.
- Adults should participate in a minimum of 2 hours and 30 minutes a week of moderate-intensity, or 75 minutes a week of vigorous-intensity physical activities in episodes of at least 10 minutes each, preferably spread throughout the week.
- Adults should engage in muscle-strengthening activities that are moderate or high intensity and involve all major muscle groups on 2 or more days a week.
- Lifestyle change is one of the most pervasive human endeavors.
- A fundamental belief in lifestyle-change programs is that health behavior is a learned response and therefore can be changed.
- Health behavior is influenced by many complex forces, including family, role models, social pressure, advertising, and psychological needs.
- The six stages of change are precontemplation, contemplation, preparation, action, maintenance, and termination.
- In setting specific goals for improving wellness, the S.M.A.R.T. approach requires specific, measurable, attainable, realistic, and trackable goals.
- Action strategies include countering, avoidance, reminders, contracting, shaping up, and support groups.

# Review Questions

1. How are the health problems of today different from those of 50 years ago? Of 100 years ago?
2. This book suggests that wellness is a process rather than a goal. What does this mean? What are the implications of this statement?
3. What are the components of wellness? How are they similar? Dissimilar?
4. Define *psychosomatic diseases*. Cite four examples of psychosomatic conditions.
5. Cite some data that confirm the relationship between physical

health problems and the spiritual, social, and emotional dimensions of wellness.
6. Define *intimacy*. Explain the relationship between intimacy and wellness.
7. What are the differences between an internal locus of control and an

external locus of control? Which of the two is more consistent with the principles of wellness?

8. Define the concept of self-efficacy. What is the relationship between the concepts of locus of control and self-efficacy?
9. How does the impact of environmental improvements compare with advancements in medical technology in increasing health and longevity among Americans?
10. To what does the term *health disparities* refer? Give three examples.
11. How do the leading causes of mortality today compare with those of 100 years ago? How do the leading causes of mortality among all Americans compare with those of young adults between the ages of 25 and 44?
12. What is the relationship between "social connectedness" and well-being? Identify four indicators of social connectedness.
13. How is the ability to forgive someone for a hurtful event related to health and well-being? What are

the four phases in the International Forgiveness Institute's model for forgiveness?

14. To what does the term *Leading Health Indicator* refer? Identify 10 Leading Health Indicators.
15. What do medical experts consider the risk factor most strongly associated with premature death and chronic disease?
16. This book suggests that the most formidable wellness challenge for Americans of all ages is overcoming a sedentary lifestyle. Do you agree or disagree? Why?
17. Differentiate between light-intensity, moderate-intensity, and vigorous-intensity physical activities. Identify two examples of each.
18. List eight lifestyle recommendations for improving health and wellness. What lifestyle behaviors appear in each set of recommendations established by the American Heart Association, Consumers Union, and Tufts University, respectively?
19. Identify and briefly describe the six stages of change as presented in

the transtheoretical model of behavior change.

20. To what does the acronym S.M.A.R.T. refer? Explain the meaning of each letter.
21. What are some common mistakes people make in setting goals for health behavior change?
22. What is a major reason for the high recidivism rate in many lifestyle-change programs?
23. If a college student wants to use countering strategies as a way to cope with compulsive eating, what can he or she do or use?
24. Your roommate wants to improve his or her study habits. Identify for your roommate four strategies that apply the techniques recommended in the action stage of lifestyle change.
25. Give an example of a specific and realistic lifestyle goal.
26. Identify three strategies experts recommend for staying physically active.

## References

1. National Wellness Institute. (2010). Defining Wellness. Retrieved January 15, 2010, from http://www.nationalwellness.org/index.php?id–tier=2&id–c=26.
2. *New England Journal of Medicine.* (2006). Healthy brain in a healthy, social body. *HealthNews,* 12(5), 5.
3. Blumenthal, J. (2006). Exercise has physical and mental health benefits. *HealthNews,* 12(12), 1.
4. Hawks, S. (2004). Spiritual wellness, holistic health, and the practice of health education. *American Journal of Health Education,* 35(1), 14.
5. Hooper, R. (September 3, 2005). If meditation is good, God makes it better. *New Scientist,* 187(2515), 9.
6. Mayo Clinic Health Solutions. (2005). Forgiveness and health. *Mayo Clinic Health Letter,* 23(12), 6.
7. Ministry of Social Development. (2007). The Social Report 2008. Retrieved January 10, 2010, from http://www.socialreport.msd.govt.nz/2008/social-connectedness/index.html.

8. Tufts University. (2009). Social butterflies appear to age more gracefully. *Tufts University Health and Nutrition Letter,* 27(7), 1–2.
9. Mayo Clinic (2005).
10. The International Forgiveness Institute. (2010). Retrieved January 3, 2010, from http://www.forgiveness-institute.org/html/process model.htm.
11. The International Forgiveness Institute. (2010). Retrieved January 2, 2010, from http://www.forgiveness-institute.org/html/about forgiveness.htm.
12. The Cleveland Clinic Foundation. (2010). Angry young men become angry old men—with heart attacks. *Cleveland Clinic Magazine.* Retrieved January 4, 2010 from http://www.clevelandclinic.org/heartcenter/pub/guide/prevention/stress/anger.htm.
13. Ibid.
14. Mayo Clinic Health Solutions. (2007). The power of connection: Physical, emotional and spiritual intimacy. *Mayo Clinic Health Letter,* 25(10), 1–8 (Supplement).
15. Ibid.

16. Ibid.
17. Tufts University. (2003). Optimistic people live longer. *Tufts University Health & Nutrition Letter,* 20(11), 4.
18. Consumers Union. (2004). Happier and healthier? *Consumer Reports on Health,* 16(3), 1, 4.
19. *New England Journal of Medicine.* (2005). Attitude influences how you age. *HealthNews,* 11(2), 6.
20. Mayo Clinic Health Solutions. (2009). Optimism and health: Shift from the dark side *Mayo Clinic Health Letter,* 27(7), 4–5.
21. The Week Publications. (2007). Laughing yourself healthy. *The Week,* 7(303), 26.
22. Ibid.
23. Consumers Union. (2009). Laughter boosts "good" HDL cholesterol. *Consumer Reports on Health,* 21(7), 2.
24. Wamsteker, E. W., R. Geenen, J. Lestra, J. K. Larsen, P. M. J. Zelissen, & W. A. Van Staveren. (2005). Obesity-related beliefs predict weight loss after an 8-week low-calorie diet.

*Journal of the American Dietetic Association,* 105(3), 441–444.

25. Squires, S. (2005, March 22). To lose well, think positive. *The Washington Post,* p. HE01.

26. Metcalf, C., G. D. Smith, J. A. C. Sterne, P. Heslop, J. Macleod, & C. Hart. (2001). Individual employment histories and subsequent cause specific hospital admissions and mortality: A prospective study of a cohort of male and female workers with 21 years follow-up. *Journal of Epidemiology & Community Health,* 55(7), 503.

27. Ibid.

28. Xu, J., K. D. Kochanek, & B. Tejada-Vera. (2009). Deaths: Preliminary data for 2007. *National Vital Statistics Reports,* 58(1). Hyattsville, MD: National Center for Health Statistics.

29. Knox R. (1998). Longevity reshaping the globe. *The Commercial Appeal,* 159(132), 2.

30. Harvard Medical School. (2003). The Latino paradox. *Harvard Health Letter,* 28(8), 3.

31. Marks, J. S. (2003). We're living longer, but what about our quality of life? *Chronic Disease: Notes & Reports,* 16(1), 2–16.

32. American Heart Association Nutrition Committee of the Council on Nutrition, Physical Activity and Metabolism, Council on Cardiovascular Disease in the Young, Council on Arteriosclerosis, Thrombosis and Vascular Biology, Council on Cardiovascular Nursing, Council on Epidemiology and Prevention, and Council for High Blood Pressure Research: Gidding, S. S., et al. (2009). AHA Scientific Statement: Implementing American Heart Association Pediatric and Adult Nutrition Guidelines. *Circulation,* 119:, 1161–1175. Retrieved December 16, 2009, from http://circ.ahajournals.org/cgi/content/full/119/8/1161.

33. American Heart Association Nutrition Committee: Lichtenstein, A. H., et al. (2006). Diet and lifestyle recommendations revision 2006: A scientific statement from the American Heart Association Nutrition Committee. *Circulation,* 114, 82–96.

34. Ibid.

35. U.S. Department of Health and Human Services, The Office of

Minority Health and Health Disparities. (2005). *What are health disparities?* Retrieved January 6, 2010, from http://minorityhealth.hhs.gov/templates/content.aspx?ID=3559.

36. Ibid.

37. National Institute of Allergy and Infectious Diseases. (2009). *Minority health: What are health disparities?* Retrieved January 6, 2010, from http://www3.niaid.nih.gov/topics/minorityHealth/disparities.htm.

38. U.S. Department of Health and Human Services, National Partnership for Action to End Health Disparities. (2009). *Health Disparities.* Retrieved January 6, 2010, from http://minorityhealth.hhs.gov/npa/templates/browse.aspx?lvl=1&lvlid=13.

39. National Institutes of Health. (2006). *Health disparities fact sheet.* Retrieved January 6, 2010, from http://www.nih.gov/about/researchresultsforthepublic/HealthDisparities.pdf.

40. Pleis, J. R. (2009). Summary health statistics for U.S. adults: National health interview survey, 2007. *National Center for Health Statistics. Vital Health Statistics,* 10(240).

41. National Center for Health Statistics. (2009). *Health, United States, 2008 with special feature on the health of young adults.* Hyattsville, MD: U.S. Department of Health and Human Services.

42. Cappelen, A. W., & O. F. Norheim. (2005). Responsibility in health care: A liberal egalitarian approach. *Journal of Medical Ethics,* 31, 476–480.

43. Heron, M.P., & B. Tejada-Vera. (2009). Deaths: Leading causes for 2005. *National Vital Statistics Reports,* 58(8). Hyattsville, MD: National Center for Health Statistics.

44. U.S. Department of Health and Human Services. (2000). *Healthy people 2010. Understanding and improving health* (2nd ed.). Washington, DC: U.S. Government Printing Office.

45. Fryar, C. D., R. Hirsch, K. S. Porter, B. Kottiri, D. J. Brody, & T. Louis. (2006). Smoking and alcohol behaviors reported by adults, United States, 1999 2002. *Advanced Data From Vital and Health Statistics,* 378(November 29, 2006).

46. Mokdad, A. H., J. S. Marks, D. F. Stroup, & J. L. Gerberding. (2004).

Actual causes of death in the United States, 2000. *Journal of the American Medical Association,* 291(10), 1238–1245.

47. Duke Medicine. (2009). 4 healthy lifestyle factors help ward off chronic disease. *HealthNews,* 15(11), 4–5.

48. Koop, C. E. (2006). Health and health care for the 21st century: For all the people. *American Journal of Public Health,* 96(12).

49. Flegal, K. M., B. I. Graubard, D. F. Williamson, & M. H. Gail. (2005). Excess deaths associated with underweight, overweight, and obesity. *Journal of the American Medical Association,* 293(15), 1861–1867.

50. Tufts University. (2005). Fat chance? Making sense of the new research on weight and mortality. *Tufts University Health and Nutrition Letter,* 23(5), 1–2.

51. Harvard Medical School. (2009). Lifestyle factors for longer life. *Harvard Health Letter,* 34(3), 7.

52. National Center for Health Statistics (2009).

53. Ibid.

54. Department of Health and Human Services. (2008). *2008 Physical activity guidelines for Americans.* Hyattsville, MD: U.S. Department of Health and Human Services.

55. Tufts University. (2009). Even being a little more fit improves longevity. *Tufts University Health and Nutrition Letter,* 27(10), 2.

56. Department of Health and Human Services (2008).

57. Ainsworth, B. E. et al. (1993). Compendium of physical activities: Classification of energy costs of human physical activities. *Medicine and Science in Sports and Exercise,* 25(1), 71–80.

58. Ainsworth B. E. et al. (2000). Compendium of physical activities: An update of activity codes and MET intensities. *Medicine and Science in Sports and Exercise,* 32(9 Suppl), S498–504.

59. Department of Health and Human Services (2008).

60. Centers for Disease Control and Prevention. (2009). How much physical activity do adults need? Retrieved January 11, 2010, from http://www.cdc.gov/physicalactivity/everyone/guidelines/index.html.

61. Centers for Disease Control and Prevention. (2009, December 28). Be

physically active in the new year. *Healthy Lifestyle Newsletter.* Atlanta, GA: Division of Nutrition, Physical Activity and Obesity.

62. Prochaska J., J. C. Norcross, & C. C. DiClemente. (1994). *Changing for good.* New York: William Morrow.

63. Mayo Clinic Health Solutions. (2007). Changing unhealthy habits. *Mayo Clinic Health Letter,* 25(2 Special Report), 1–8.

64. Tufts University. (2003). New Year's resolution can start any day you want. *Tufts University Health and Nutrition Letter,* 21(1), 8.

65. Prochaska, J. M., J. O. Prochaska, F. C. Cohen, S. O. Gomes, R. G. Laforge, & A. L. Eastwood. (2004). The transtheoretical model of change for multi-level interventions for alcohol abuse on campus. *Journal of*

*Alcohol and Drug Education,* 48(13), 34–51.

66. American Heart Association Nutrition Committee of the Council on Nutrition, Physical Activity and Metabolism (2009).

67. Mayo Clinic Health Solutions (2007), p. 4.

68. Prochaska, J. (1996). "Just do it" isn't enough: Change comes in stages. *Tufts University Diet And Nutrition Letter,* 14(7), 4–6.

69. Tufts University. (2002). Is sugar really addictive? *Tufts University Health and Nutrition Letter,* 20(8), 5.

70. Winslow, R. (2010). Watching TV linked to higher risk of death. *The Wall Street Journal* January 12, 2010:D1,D4.

71. Dunstan, D. W., E. L. M. Barr, G. N. Healy, et al. (2010). Television view-

ing time and mortality: The Australian diabetes, obesity and lifestyle study. *Circulation,* 121(2), 384–391.

72. Mayo Clinic Health Solutions (2007), p. 6.

73. Harvard Health Publications. (2006). How to keep those New Year's resolutions. *Harvard Health Letter,* 31(3), 1–2.

74. De Bourdeaudhuij, I., & J. Sallis. (2002). Getting adults to exercise by modifying psychosocial variables. *Physical Activity Today,* 8(3), 3.

75. Hollis, J. F., C. M. Gullion, V. J. Stevens, et al. (2008). Weight loss during the intensive intervention phase of the weight-loss maintenance trial. *American Journal of Preventive Medicine,* 35(2), 118–126.

## Suggested Readings

Brownlee, Shannon. (2007). *Overtreated: Why too much medicine is making us sicker and poorer.* London, England: Bloomsbury Publishing Plc.

The thesis of this book is that much of the health care in the United States goes toward unnecessary care that patients don't need and would likely avoid if they were better informed. The case studies and patient profiles offered by the author challenge traditional beliefs about wellness, health, lifestyle diseases, morbidity, and mortality in the United States.

Federal Interagency Forum on Child and Family Statistics. (2009). *America's children: Key national indicators of well-being, 2009.* Federal Interagency Forum on Child and Family Statistics, Washington, DC: U.S. Government Printing Office.

Seven federal agencies joined forces to document leading indicators on the health challenges facing America's youth. Forty key indicators are presented under the headings of economic security, health, behavior and social environment, and education. Specific health indicators range from such topics as childhood immunization to childhood obesity. This book also includes statistics on population and family characteristics and special features on asthma, lead poisoning, emotional difficulties, and the influence of

family structure on children, infant, and adolescent well-being.

Gawande, A. (2009). *The checklist manifesto: How to get things right.* New York: Henry Holt and Company, LLC.

The author uses his experiences as a surgeon to simplify ways for people to deal with the increasing complexity of their lives, whether it relates to their professional careers, personal lifestyle issues, or consumer decisions. Examples on how the problems and challenges of modern medicine are similar to architecture, construction, aviation, performing arts, and nearly every aspect of the modern world are illustrated. Gawande offers a new and fresh perspective for accomplishing goals and preventing failures.

Goldberg, S. (2009). *Lessons for the living: Stories of forgiveness, gratitude, and courage at the end of life.* Boston: Shambhala Publications, Inc.

When Stan Goldberg was diagnosed with terminal cancer, he chose to face his fear of dying by serving as a hospice volunteer. He writes about his experiences with people he met in hospice and in doing so provides a poignant, insightful perspective on the human spirit and the power of forgiveness, gratitude, and letting go of anger.

National Center for Health Statistics. (2009). *Health, United States, 2008*

*with special feature on the health of young adults.* Hyattsville, MD: U.S. Department of Health and Human Services.

This book serves as a major reference on health trends and statistics. Charts, tables, and figures present current data on health risk factors, mortality, health care resources, chronic diseases, life expectancy, and much more. This edition includes a special feature on the health status, behaviors, and risk factors of young adults, ages 18 29 years. Data are compiled by the National Center for Health Statistics and Centers for Disease Control and Prevention.

Singer, M. (2009). *Introduction to syndemics: A critical systems approach to public and community health.* Hoboken, NJ: Jossey-Bass.

As a cultural and medical anthropologist, the author makes a compelling case for the interactions among disease that address underlying social and environmental issues. This interaction refers to the syndemic theory, a framework for the analysis and prevention of disease interactions. The thesis of the book is that health problems should not be viewed in isolation, but rather in the context of other diseases and the social, political, environmental, and economic factors that have an influence on them.

**Name** _____   **Date** _____   **Section** _____

# Assessment Activity 1-1

## Lifestyle Assessment Inventory

**Directions:**  Wellness involves a variety of components that work together to build the total concept. Following are some questions concerning the different aspects of wellness. Using the scale, respond to each question by circling the number that best represents you at this time. At the end of each section, add up your response numbers and transfer the total to the appropriate section in the Wellness Assessment Summary. Save your results. Your instructor may ask you to complete this assessment again toward the end of the semester.

10 Yes/almost always (at least 90% of the time)
 7 Very often (more than 50% but less than 90% of the time)
 5 Sometimes (about 50% of the time)
 3 Occasionally (less than 50% of the time but more than 10% of the time)
 1 No/almost never (less than 10% of the time)

### Physical Assessment

| | Yes/Almost Always | Very Often | Sometimes | No/ Occasionally | Almost Never |
|---|---|---|---|---|---|
| 1. I get at least 150 minutes of moderately intense physical activity each week. | 10 | 7 | 5 | 3 | 1 |
| 2. When participating in physical activities, I include stretching and flexibility exercises. | 10 | 7 | 5 | 3 | 1 |
| 3. When driving or riding (in a vehicle), I wear a seat belt. | 10 | 7 | 5 | 3 | 1 |
| 4. I engage in muscle-strengthening exercises at least two times per week. | 10 | 7 | 5 | 3 | 1 |
| 5. My physical fitness level is excellent for my age. | 10 | 7 | 5 | 3 | 1 |
| 6. My body composition is appropriate for my gender (men, 10 to 18% body fat; women, 17 to 25%). | 10 | 7 | 5 | 3 | 1 |
| 7. I have appropriate medical checkups regularly and am able to talk to my doctor and ask questions that concern me. | 10 | 7 | 5 | 3 | 1 |
| 8. I keep my immunizations up to date. | 10 | 7 | 5 | 3 | 1 |
| 9. When operating a vehicle, I avoid talking or texting on a cell phone. | 10 | 7 | 5 | 3 | 1 |
| 10. I get 7–9 hours of sleep each night. | 10 | 7 | 5 | 3 | 1 |

**Physical assessment score** _____

## Alcohol and Other Drugs Assessment

| | Yes/Almost Always | Very Often | Sometimes | No/ Occasionally | Almost Never |
|---|---|---|---|---|---|
| 1. I avoid smoking. | 10 | 7 | 5 | 3 | 1 |
| 2. I avoid using smokeless tobacco products. | 10 | 7 | 5 | 3 | 1 |
| 3. I avoid drinking alcohol or restrict my consumption to two drinks or fewer per day. | 10 | 7 | 5 | 3 | 1 |
| 4. I avoid drinking alcohol to the point of intoxication. | 10 | 7 | 5 | 3 | 1 |
| 5. I do not drive when drinking alcoholic beverages or taking medicines that make me sleepy. | 10 | 7 | 5 | 3 | 1 |
| 6. I avoid using mood-altering substances. | 10 | 7 | 5 | 3 | 1 |
| 7. I follow directions when taking medications. | 10 | 7 | 5 | 3 | 1 |
| 8. I thoroughly read labels before taking a nonprescription drug. | 10 | 7 | 5 | 3 | 1 |
| 9. I ask about warnings and side effects of prescription drugs before taking them. | 10 | 7 | 5 | 3 | 1 |
| 10. I keep in my wallet or purse a record of drugs to which I am allergic. | 10 | 7 | 5 | 3 | 1 |

**Alcohol and other drugs assessment score** _____

## Nutritional Assessment

| | Yes/Almost Always | Very Often | Sometimes | No/ Occasionally | Almost Never |
|---|---|---|---|---|---|
| 1. I eat at least 2½ cups of vegetables and 2 cups of fruits each day. | 10 | 7 | 5 | 3 | 1 |
| 2. My daily diet includes at least 3 ounces of whole-grain products each day. | 10 | 7 | 5 | 3 | 1 |
| 3. My daily intake of dairy products is 3 cups of fat-free or low-fat milk or milk equivalents. | 10 | 7 | 5 | 3 | 1 |
| 4. My daily intake of meats is limited to low-fat or lean selections that are baked, boiled, or grilled. | 10 | 7 | 5 | 3 | 1 |
| 5. I make a conscious effort to choose or prepare foods low in saturated fat. | 10 | 7 | 5 | 3 | 1 |
| 6. When purchasing a food item, I read the labels to identify foods high in salt, hidden sugars, tropical oils, and saturated fat. | 10 | 7 | 5 | 3 | 1 |
| 7. I avoid adding salt to my food without first tasting my food. | 10 | 7 | 5 | 3 | 1 |
| 8. I avoid eating unless I'm hungry. | 10 | 7 | 5 | 3 | 1 |
| 9. I stop eating before feeling completely full. | 10 | 7 | 5 | 3 | 1 |
| 10. I avoid binge eating. | 10 | 7 | 5 | 3 | 1 |

**Nutritional assessment score** _____

## Social Wellness Assessment

| | Yes/Almost Always | Very Often | Sometimes | No/ Occasionally | Almost Never |
|---|---|---|---|---|---|
| 1. I have at least one person in whom I can confide. | 10 | 7 | 5 | 3 | 1 |
| 2. I have a good relationship with my family. | 10 | 7 | 5 | 3 | 1 |
| 3. I have friends at work or school from whom I gain support and with whom I talk regularly. | 10 | 7 | 5 | 3 | 1 |
| 4. I am involved in school activities. | 10 | 7 | 5 | 3 | 1 |
| 5. I am involved in my community. | 10 | 7 | 5 | 3 | 1 |
| 6. I do something for fun and just for myself at least once a week. | 10 | 7 | 5 | 3 | 1 |
| 7. I am able to develop close, intimate relationships. | 10 | 7 | 5 | 3 | 1 |
| 8. I engage in activities that contribute to the environment. | 10 | 7 | 5 | 3 | 1 |
| 9. I am interested in the views, opinions, activities, and accomplishments of others. | 10 | 7 | 5 | 3 | 1 |
| 10. I provide social support to others. | 10 | 7 | 5 | 3 | 1 |

**Social wellness assessment score** _____

## Spiritual Wellness Assessment

| | Yes/Almost Always | Very Often | Sometimes | No/ Occasionally | Almost Never |
|---|---|---|---|---|---|
| 1. I know my values and beliefs. | 10 | 7 | 5 | 3 | 1 |
| 2. I live by my convictions. | 10 | 7 | 5 | 3 | 1 |
| 3. My life has meaning and direction. | 10 | 7 | 5 | 3 | 1 |
| 4. I derive strength from my spiritual life daily. | 10 | 7 | 5 | 3 | 1 |
| 5. I have life goals that I strive to achieve every day. | 10 | 7 | 5 | 3 | 1 |
| 6. I view life as a learning experience and look forward to the future. | 10 | 7 | 5 | 3 | 1 |
| 7. I have a sense of peace about my life. | 10 | 7 | 5 | 3 | 1 |
| 8. I am tolerant of the values and beliefs of others. | 10 | 7 | 5 | 3 | 1 |
| 9. I am satisfied with the degree to which my activities are consistent with my values. | 10 | 7 | 5 | 3 | 1 |
| 10. Personal reflection is an important part of my life. | 10 | 7 | 5 | 3 | 1 |

**Spiritual wellness assessment score** _____

## Emotional Wellness Assessment

| | Yes/Almost Always | Very Often | Sometimes | No/ Occasionally | Almost Never |
|---|---|---|---|---|---|
| 1. I feel positive about myself and my life. | 10 | 7 | 5 | 3 | 1 |
| 2. I am able to be the person I choose to be. | 10 | 7 | 5 | 3 | 1 |

| | | | | | |
|---|---|---|---|---|---|
| 3. I am satisfied that I am performing to the best of my ability. | 10 | 7 | 5 | 3 | 1 |
| 4. I can cope with life's ups and downs effectively and in a healthy manner. | 10 | 7 | 5 | 3 | 1 |
| 5. I am nonjudgmental in my approach to others. | 10 | 7 | 5 | 3 | 1 |
| 6. I feel there is an appropriate amount of excitement in my life. | 10 | 7 | 5 | 3 | 1 |
| 7. When I make mistakes, I learn from them. | 10 | 7 | 5 | 3 | 1 |
| 8. I can say no without feeling guilty. | 10 | 7 | 5 | 3 | 1 |
| 9. I find it easy to laugh. | 10 | 7 | 5 | 3 | 1 |
| 10. I avoid blaming others for my failures or problems. | 10 | 7 | 5 | 3 | 1 |

**Emotional wellness assessment score** _____

## Stress Control Assessment

| | Yes/Almost Always | Very Often | Sometimes | No/ Occasionally | Almost Never |
|---|---|---|---|---|---|
| 1. I am easily distracted. | 1 | 3 | 5 | 7 | 10 |
| 2. I tend to be nervous and impatient. | 1 | 3 | 5 | 7 | 10 |
| 3. I prepare ahead of time for events or situations that cause stress. | 10 | 7 | 5 | 3 | 1 |
| 4. I schedule enough time to accomplish what I need to do. | 10 | 7 | 5 | 3 | 1 |
| 5. I set realistic goals for myself. | 10 | 7 | 5 | 3 | 1 |
| 6. I can express my feelings of anger. | 10 | 7 | 5 | 3 | 1 |
| 7. I avoid putting off important tasks to the last minute. | 10 | 7 | 5 | 3 | 1 |
| 8. I participate in activities that provide relief from stress. | 10 | 7 | 5 | 3 | 1 |
| 9. When working under pressure, I stay calm and patient. | 10 | 7 | 5 | 3 | 1 |
| 10. I can make decisions with a minimum of stress and worry. | 10 | 7 | 5 | 3 | 1 |

**Stress control assessment score** _____

## Intellectual Wellness Assessment

| | Yes/Almost Always | Very Often | Sometimes | No/ Occasionally | Almost Never |
|---|---|---|---|---|---|
| 1. I believe my education is preparing me for what I would like to accomplish in life. | 10 | 7 | 5 | 3 | 1 |
| 2. I am interested in learning just for the sake of learning. | 10 | 7 | 5 | 3 | 1 |
| 3. I like to be aware of current social and political issues. | 10 | 7 | 5 | 3 | 1 |
| 4. I have interests other than those directly related to my vocation. | 10 | 7 | 5 | 3 | 1 |
| 5. I am able to apply what I know to real-life situations. | 10 | 7 | 5 | 3 | 1 |
| 6. I am interested in the viewpoint of others, even if it is very different from my own. | 10 | 7 | 5 | 3 | 1 |

| | Yes/Almost Always | Very Often | Sometimes | No/ Occasionally | Almost Never |
|---|---|---|---|---|---|
| 7. I seek advice when I am uncertain or uncomfortable with a recommended health or medical treatment. | 10 | 7 | 5 | 3 | 1 |
| 8. I ask about the risks and benefits of a medical test before its use. | 10 | 7 | 5 | 3 | 1 |
| 9. When seeking medical care, I plan ahead how to describe my problem and what questions I should ask. | 10 | 7 | 5 | 3 | 1 |
| 10. I keep abreast of the latest trends and information regarding health matters. | 10 | 7 | 5 | 3 | 1 |

Intellectual wellness assessment score _____

## Occupational Wellness Assessment

| | Yes/Almost Always | Very Often | Sometimes | No/ Occasionally | Almost Never |
|---|---|---|---|---|---|
| 1. I am aware of my skills, strengths, and weaknesses as they relate to possible occupational choices. | 10 | 7 | 5 | 3 | 1 |
| 2. I have a good work ethic at school, home, and work. | 10 | 7 | 5 | 3 | 1 |
| 3. I look for opportunities to learn about careers that may be of interest to me. | 10 | 7 | 5 | 3 | 1 |
| 4. I am aware of the demands that future occupational choices may make on my personal life. | 10 | 7 | 5 | 3 | 1 |
| 5. I am aware of the demands that future occupational choices may make on my family life. | 10 | 7 | 5 | 3 | 1 |
| 6. I try hard to connect academics to the needs and demands of occupational choices. | 10 | 7 | 5 | 3 | 1 |
| 7. I view occupational choices as a source of personal growth and fulfillment. | 10 | 7 | 5 | 3 | 1 |
| 8. I consider money the only criterion for choosing a career. | 1 | 3 | 5 | 7 | 10 |
| 9. I am aware of the need for continuing education in various careers of interest to me. | 10 | 7 | 5 | 3 | 1 |
| 10. I am willing to spend extra personal time acquiring skills and knowledge required for occupational success. | 10 | 7 | 5 | 3 | 1 |

Occupational wellness assessment score _____

## Environmental Wellness Assessment

| | Yes/Almost Always | Very Often | Sometimes | No/ Occasionally | Almost Never |
|---|---|---|---|---|---|
| 1. I try to conserve energy by turning off lights and electrical appliances when they are not being used. | 10 | 7 | 5 | 3 | 1 |

| | | | | | |
|---|---|---|---|---|---|
| 2. I repair or report leaking faucets. | 10 | 7 | 5 | 3 | 1 |
| 3. I avoid littering. | 10 | 7 | 5 | 3 | 1 |
| 4. I avoid disposing of toxic chemicals or petroleum products illegally. | 10 | 7 | 5 | 3 | 1 |
| 5. I look for recycled materials when purchasing products. | 10 | 7 | 5 | 3 | 1 |
| 6. I store toxic chemicals in their original containers and out of the reach of small children. | 10 | 7 | 5 | 3 | 1 |
| 7. I make sure that smoke detectors are in use and working properly. | 10 | 7 | 5 | 3 | 1 |
| 8. I make sure that carbon monoxide detectors are in use and working properly. | 10 | 7 | 5 | 3 | 1 |
| 9. I check for or inquire about radon concentrations when moving into a new house or apartment. | 10 | 7 | 5 | 3 | 1 |
| 10. I wash my hands with soap for at least 10 seconds after using the bathroom. | 10 | 7 | 5 | 3 | 1 |

**Environmental wellness assessment score** _____

**Wellness Assessment Summary** Transfer the total score for each section to the following spaces. Add the scores and divide by 10 to determine your average wellness score.

Physical assessment _____
Alcohol and other drugs assessment _____
Nutritional assessment _____
Social wellness assessment _____
Spiritual wellness assessment _____
Emotional wellness assessment _____
Stress control assessment _____
Intellectual wellness assessment _____
Occupational wellness assessment _____
Environmental wellness assessment _____
   Total _____
   Average wellness score
   (Divide total score by 10) _____

**90–100—Excellent.** You are engaging in behaviors and attitudes that can significantly contribute to a healthy lifestyle and a higher quality of life. If you scored in this range, you are an example to many.

**75–89—Good.** You engage in many health-promoting attitudes and behaviors that should contribute to good health and a more satisfying quality of life. However, there are some areas that could use some upgrading to provide optimal benefits. If you are at this level, you are showing how much you care about yourself and your life.

**65–74—Average.** You are typical of the average American who tends to act without considering the consequences of behaviors. Now is the time to consider your lifestyle and the ramifications it is having on you now and will have in the future. Maybe there are some positive actions that you could consider taking to improve your quality of life.

**45–64—Below average.** Perhaps you lack current information about behaviors and attitudes that can enhance your health and quality of life. Now is the time to begin to learn about positive changes that can improve your life.

**0–44—Needs improvement.** It's good that you are concerned enough about your health to take this test, but indications are that your behaviors and attitudes may be having detrimental effects on your health. You can easily begin to take action now to improve your prospects for the future.

**Follow-Up** Complete the following statements: In completing this wellness assessment,

1. I was surprised to learn that I _____

_____

2. I was disappointed that _____

_____

3. I have learned that the concept of wellness _____

_____

# Assessment Activity 1-2

## Health Locus of Control

Locus of control is an important component of individual wellness. This activity will assist you in identifying your locus of control and its ability to affect your health. This rating scale is an adaptation of the Multidimensional Health Locus of Control Scales. The test is composed of three subscales:

1. The *Internal Health Locus of Control Scale (I)* measures whether you feel that you have control over your health.

2. The *Powerful Others Health Locus of Control Scale (P)* measures whether you feel that powerful individuals, such as physicians or other health professionals, control your health.

3. The *Chance Health Locus of Control Scale (C)* measures whether you feel your health is due to luck, fate, or chance.

**Directions:** For each answer, choose a number from 1 to 5 that best describes your feelings.

5 = Strongly agree
4 = Agree
3 = Neither agree nor disagree
2 = Disagree
1 = Strongly disagree

### Subscale 1: Internal Health Locus of Control (I)

_____ If I get sick, my behavior determines how soon I get well.
_____ I am in control of my health.
_____ When I get sick, I am to blame.
_____ If I take care of myself, I can avoid illness.
_____ If I take the right actions, I can stay healthy.
_____ Total

### Subscale 2: Powerful Others Health Locus of Control (P)

_____ Having regular contact with my physician is the best way for me to avoid illness.
_____ Whenever I don't feel well, I should consult a medically trained professional.
_____ My family has a lot to do with my becoming sick or staying healthy.
_____ Health professionals control my health.
_____ When I recover from an illness, it's usually because other people, such as doctors, nurses, family, and friends, have been taking good care of me.
_____ Regarding my health, I can do only what my doctor tells me to do.
_____ Total

### Subscale 3: Chance Health Locus of Control (C)

_____ No matter what I do, if I am going to get sick, I will get sick.
_____ Most things that affect my health happen to me accidentally.
_____ Luck plays a big part in determining how soon I will recover from an illness.
_____ My good health is largely a matter of good fortune.
_____ No matter what I do, I am likely to get sick.
_____ If it is meant to be, I will stay healthy.
_____ Total

To obtain your score for each subscale, add the numbers you chose.

1. A score of 23 to 30 on any subscale means you have a strong inclination toward that subscale. For example, a high C score indicates you hold strong beliefs that your health is a matter of chance.

2. A score of 15 to 22 means you are moderate on that subscale. For example, a moderate P score indicates you have moderate belief that your health is due to powerful others.

3. A score of 6 to 14 means you are low on that subscale. For example, a low I score means you generally do not believe that you control your health.

**Name** _____   **Date** _____   **Section** _____

# Assessment Activity 1-3

## Assessing Your Health Behaviors

Before planning a lifestyle-change program, you should take an inventory of your health behaviors. This reveals important information about your lifestyle and should also help identify areas in need of improvement.

**Directions:**   In this assessment, you are asked to make two lists. In the left column, list the things you do to maintain or improve your level of health. These are

your health-promoting behaviors. In the right column, list the things you do that may be detrimental to your health. These are your health-inhibiting behaviors. Try to be specific. Include the things that affect your mental, emotional, social, spiritual, and physical health. If you have a difficult time thinking of specific activities, you can refer to Assessment Activity 1-1.

Health-Promoting Behaviors

1. _____
2. _____
3. _____
4. _____
5. _____
6. _____
7. _____
8. _____
9. _____
10. _____
11. _____
12. _____
13. _____
14. _____
15. _____

Health-Inhibiting Behaviors

1. _____
2. _____
3. _____
4. _____
5. _____
6. _____
7. _____
8. _____
9. _____
10. _____
11. _____
12. _____
13. _____
14. _____
15. _____

Which health-inhibiting behavior would you be willing to change right now? _____

# Preventing Cardiovascular Disease

##  ONLINE LEARNING CENTER

Log on to our Online Learning Center (OLC) for access to these additional resources:

- Chapter key term flashcards
- Learning objectives
- Additional goals for behavior change
- Concentration game
- Self-scoring chapter quizzes
- Additional lab activities

The OLC also offers Web links for study and exploration of wellness topics. Access these links through **www.mhhe.com/anspaugh8e.**

## GOALS FOR BEHAVIOR CHANGE

- Choose three high-fat foods that you regularly eat and replace them with low-fat, healthier foods.
- Find out your total cholesterol, LDL cholesterol, and HDL cholesterol. Select three or four lifestyle behaviors to change to improve your cholesterol profile.
- Find out your blood pressure. Select two or three behaviors to change (excluding taking medication) to lower it.
- If you use tobacco products, devise a plan for quitting the tobacco habit.
- If you are not currently active, make a list of physical activities to improve your health status and level of fitness. Determine how many calories you would attempt to expend per week.
- Plan and implement three strategies to help you deal with chronic stress.

## Objectives

After completing this chapter, you will be able to do the following:

- ✔ Describe the gross anatomy and function of the heart.
- ✔ Trace the development of cardiovascular disease during the 20th century in the United States.
- ✔ Identify and differentiate among several types of cardiovascular disease.
- ✔ Identify the risk factors for coronary heart disease and discuss ways to reduce them.
- ✔ Explain the lifestyle behaviors that contribute to health and longevity.

## [ Key Terms ]

| | |
|---|---|
| aneurysm | ischemia |
| angina pectoris | lipoprotein (a) |
| atherosclerosis | metabolic syndrome |
| cerebral hemorrhage | myocardial infarction |
| cholesterol | peripheral artery disease |
| C-reactive protein (CRP) | sedentary |
| embolus | sedentary death syndrome |
| fibrinogen | sleep apnea |
| homocysteine | thrombus |
| hypertension | |

Cardiovascular disease encompasses a group of diseases that affect the heart and blood vessels. Cardiovascular disease—the leading cause of death in the United States—accounts for 35.3% of deaths.[1] About 25% of Americans (approximately 80,000,000 people) have one or more forms of heart or blood vessel disease. While cardiovascular disease has been on the decline for many years, it still causes approximately as many deaths as cancer, chronic lower-respiratory diseases, accidents, and diabetes combined.

The most prevalent form of heart disease, coronary heart disease (CHD), also referred to as ischemic heart disease or coronary artery disease, kills more Americans than all other forms of heart disease combined. Approximately 445,687 people die annually of CHD, either in a hospital emergency room or before reaching the hospital. These deaths are usually the result of cardiac arrest (the heart stops beating due to interference of its electrical impulse).[2]

Coronary heart disease is but one of many types of heart disease, but it produces about half of all heart disease deaths in people under the age of 75. It is the leading cause of death for both men and women, although the development of CHD in women lags behind men about 10 years. With advancing age, however, the mortality rate between the sexes begins to equalize.[3]

The death rate from heart disease in the United States has been steadily declining for the last 50 years. The decline in death rate from heart disease has been largely responsible for the improvement in life expectancy. According to the U.S. Department of Health and Human Services, the average life expectancy (the number of years that a newborn can expect to live) has risen to 77.9 years.[4] If all major forms of cardiovascular disease were eliminated, life expectancy would increase by about 7 years.[5] One of the greatest public health successes of the 20th century has been the decline in the death rate from cardiovascular disease.[6] From 1970 to 2002, the death rate from heart disease declined by 52% while the death rate from strokes declined by 63%.[7]

Research has convincingly shown that following a heart-healthy lifestyle can significantly lower the risk for heart disease, and it has been a major contributor to the decline in heart disease mortality.[8] The medical profession, through the development and use of sophisticated diagnostic procedures and vastly improved after-the-fact treatments, has equally contributed to the downward trend in the death rate from cardiovascular disease.

## Circulation

Circulation is better understood if you are familiar with the basic anatomy and function of the heart. The heart consists of cardiac muscle and weighs between 8 and

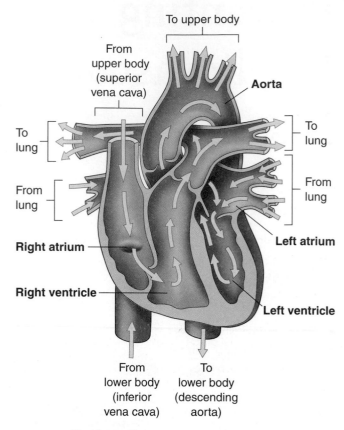

**FIGURE 2-1** Circulatory System

10 ounces. It is about the size of a fist and lies in the center of the chest. The heart is divided into two halves, or pumps, by a wall (the septum), and each half is subdivided into an upper chamber (the atrium) and a lower chamber (the ventricle). The right heart, or pulmonary pump, receives deoxygenated blood from all bodily tissues and pumps it to the lungs, so that carbon dioxide can be exchanged for a fresh supply of oxygen. From the lungs, the oxygen-rich blood is sent to the left heart, or systemic pump, so that the oxygenated blood can be pumped to all the tissues of the body. Both pumps work simultaneously. The systemic pump carries the heavier workload of the two and thus has a more muscular ventricular wall. Figure 2-1 illustrates the circulatory system.

The arteries carry oxygenated blood away from the heart, while the veins carry deoxygenated blood to the heart. There are two exceptions, one in the arterial system and one in the venous system. First, the pulmonary artery carries *deoxygenated* blood from the right heart to the lungs to exchange carbon dioxide for a fresh supply of oxygen. Second, the pulmonary vein carries *fully oxygenated* blood from the lungs to the left heart for distribution throughout the body.

The primary function of circulation is to provide a constant supply of blood and nutrients to the cells while removing their waste products. Under ordinary circumstances, the interruption of blood flow for as little as 4 to 6 minutes can result in irreversible brain damage due to oxygen deprivation.

The average heart beats 70 to 80 times per minute at rest. Endurance athletes often have resting heart rates in the 30- and 40-beat range, whereas some overweight and sedentary smokers have resting heart rates in the 90s.[9] The lowest documented resting heart rate ever recorded belongs to a Spanish cyclist named Miguel Indurain.[10] His resting heart rate is an incredible 28 beats per minute. The low heart rates of endurance athletes reflect physiological adaptations to training that represent normal values for this group. The Framingham Heart Disease Study showed that a rapid resting heart rate increased the risk for death from heart attack. Mortality increased progressively with higher resting heart rates, especially among men.[11] Men with resting heart rates greater than 75 beats per minute were 3.5 times more likely to die suddenly, compared with men whose heart rate was below 60. There are three plausible factors supporting the relationship between high resting heart rate and sudden death. First, medical researchers discovered that at least half of all heart attacks occur when atherosclerotic plaque is unstable. Unstable plaque has a thin, fibrous cap and is more likely to rupture than stable plaque. Blood rushing over unstable plaque threatens to rip off the fibrous cap. This situation is made more threatening by a high resting heart rate because more waves of blood rush over the cap in a given amount of time.[12] Second, a high resting heart rate is indicative of an inefficient heart that has less time between beats (the diastolic phase of the heart cycle) to deliver blood, oxygen, and nutrients to the myocardium (heart muscle). Third, a high resting heart rate could be an indicator of poor health habits, such as lack of exercise or diabetes, or could be the result of undiagnosed weakened heart muscle.

The heart is self-regulating; it contains its own conduction system fully capable of establishing and maintaining the heartbeat without outside neural stimulation. The heart's beating rate and rhythm are established by the sinoatrial node (SA node, or pacemaker), located in the right atrium, as shown in Figure 2-2. The atria contract, forcing blood into the ventricles as the electrical impulse travels from the SA node to the atrioventricular node (AV node), located between the right atrium and right ventricle. The electrical impulse pauses for one-tenth of a second at the AV node to allow the ventricles to fill with blood and then resumes down the system and spreads throughout the ventricular walls. The ventricles contract during this time, ejecting blood from these chambers.

Blood that enters the chambers of the heart does not directly nourish the heart muscle, because there are

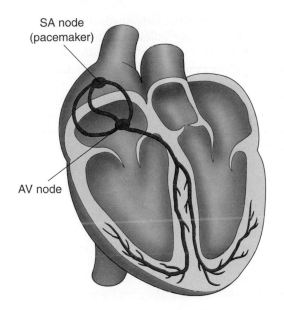

**FIGURE 2-2**  Electrical Conduction System of the Heart

no direct circulatory routes from the heart's chambers into its muscular walls. Instead, blood must first be ejected from the heart to the aorta (the largest artery in the body) and then to the coronary arteries that supply the myocardium (heart muscle) with blood and oxygen. The majority of blood is received by the myocardium during diastole (between beats) because the blood vessels dilate during this time, increasing their capacity to accept and deliver blood.

Coronary circulation is illustrated in Figure 2-3. The left coronary artery supplies a major portion of the myocardium with blood, whereas the right coronary

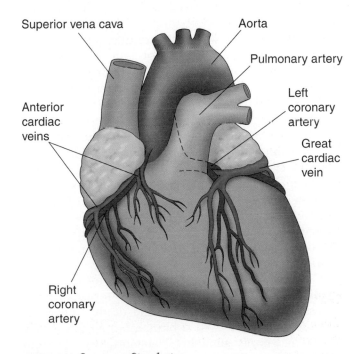

**FIGURE 2-3**  Coronary Circulation

artery serves less of it. Both vessels divide and subdivide downstream and eventually culminate in a dense network of capillaries (the smallest blood vessels in the body). Blood supply to the myocardium is so important that every muscle fiber is supplied by at least one capillary. The coronary veins return deoxygenated blood to the right atrium, so that it can enter pulmonary circulation. The veins bring deoxygenated blood from all tissues back to the right atrium.

Blood plasma is a clear, yellowish fluid that carries approximately 100 chemicals. Plasma represents 55% of the blood content. The remaining 45% consists of blood solids—the erythrocytes (red blood cells), the leukocytes (white blood cells), and the blood platelets. The red blood cells are the most abundant of the blood solids, composing about 99% of the total. These cells carry oxygen and carbon dioxide attached to hemoglobin, an iron-rich protein pigment and a main component of red blood cells. The white blood cells are an important part of the body's defense system against invading microorganisms and other foreign substances. The blood platelets are involved in the complex processes that lead to the formation of clots for repairing damaged blood vessels.

# Cardiovascular Disease: A 20th-Century Phenomenon

Cardiovascular disease, a relatively rare event 100 years ago, reached epidemic proportions during the middle of the 20th century. The term **angina pectoris** (chest pain) was introduced into the medical literature by William Heberden, a British physician, in the latter part of the 18th century, but he was unable to offer any treatment for this strange malady. It was not until 1910 that physicians made the connection between recurrent episodes of angina pectoris and heart disease. Chest pain and other manifestations of a heart attack were not identified with obstructions of the coronary arteries until the early 1900s. An American physician gave the first accurate description of the events associated with a heart attack in 1912. The illness he described, which afflicted a 55-year-old man with no previous evidence of disease, is now a common occurrence in American life. The man died three days after the onset of symptoms. A postmortem examination of the heart revealed that a clot had occluded, or blocked, one of the major coronary arteries. In 1912, this was a medical rarity.

Coronary heart disease is responsible for the majority of heart attack deaths, but other forms of heart disease contribute to disability and death. Congenital heart defects, which exist at birth, affect approximately 36,000 newborns annually. The mortality rate from congenital heart defects in 2005—the latest year for this

statistic—was 3,637. Heart defects account for more than 30% of all mortality from birth defects.[13] The most common type of birth defect is abnormalities in the development of the heart. Heart defects affect nearly 1% of all newborns, and 10 times as many occur in spontaneously aborted pregnancies.[14] Rheumatic heart disease, caused by a streptococcal infection of the throat or ear, is virtually 100% preventable. Antibiotic treatment during the infection stage arrests the processes that could lead to rheumatic heart disease. Congestive heart failure occurs when the heart muscle is so damaged that it can no longer contract with sufficient force to pump blood throughout the body. The leading causes of congestive heart failure are poorly controlled or uncontrolled long-standing hypertension, a history of heart attacks, or both. Approximately 5.7 million Americans have congestive heart failure, and it is an underlying or contributing cause of 292,000 deaths!

## Coronary Heart Disease

Coronary heart disease, also known as coronary artery disease or ischemic heart disease, is a disease of the arteries that supply the heart with blood and nutrients. A diagnosis of coronary artery disease is made if any artery is narrowed by 60%. A heart attack, or **myocardial infarction** (death of heart muscle tissue), occurs when an obstruction or a spasm disrupts or blocks blood flow to a portion of the heart muscle. The amount of heart muscle damage is determined by the location of the obstruction or spasm and the speed with which medical intervention is begun. A spasm occurs when an artery temporarily contracts and either substantially reduces or interrupts blood flow to a portion of the heart muscle. Heart attacks of any magnitude produce irreversible injury and myocardial tissue death. It usually takes 5 to 6 weeks to form a fibrous scar around dead cardiac tissue. This area of dead tissue can no longer contribute to the pumping of blood, resulting in a less efficient heart. Massive heart attacks that cause extensive muscle damage result in death.

Although most heart attacks occur after the age of 65, the dysfunctions leading to them often begin before adolescence. These processes occur most often without symptoms and often go undetected until, without warning, a heart attack occurs. The attack is sudden, but the circumstances leading to it develop over many years. There is considerable evidence that the silent phase of coronary heart disease begins as early as childhood.[15,16]

Risk factors are genetic predispositions, lifestyle behaviors, and environmental influences that increase one's susceptibility to disease. Elevated blood pressure and blood fats (cholesterol and triglycerides) that occur during adulthood can often be traced back to childhood. See Wellness for a Lifetime: Childhood Origins of Heart Disease for more information about this connection.

# Wellness for a Lifetime

## Childhood Origins of Heart Disease

Behavior patterns established during childhood that increase the likelihood of coronary heart disease often persist into adulthood. A physically inactive child is likely to become a physically inactive adult, and conversely, active children usually become active adults.[19] Only 35% of high school students (grades 9–12) meet the currently recommended physical activity guideline developed by the American Heart Association, which states that children and adolescents should participate in at least 60 minutes of moderate to vigorous daily physical activity.[20,21] Physical inactivity is a primary contributor to the unprecedented explosion of overweight and obesity among children in the United States. The percentage of overweight adolescents today has tripled since 1980, and this trend shows no signs of abating or reversing in the near future.[22] Various organizations have deleted the term *obesity* when describing the body composition of children and adolescents, and instead use the term *overweight* for all. Children ages 6–11 and adolescents ages 12–19 whose body mass index (BMI) is equal to or greater than the 95th percentile on the Centers for Disease Control growth charts are considered overweight.[22] Using these charts as criterion, overweight is at an all-time high for both groups: 17% for children and 17.6% for adolescents. Overweight adolescents have an 80% chance of becoming overweight adults if one or both parents are overweight or obese.[23] One of the serious consequences of early obesity has been the emergence of Type 2 diabetes—a disease with life-threatening complications that in the recent past occurred almost exclusively in middle-aged adults—which is currently occurring among American adolescents.[24] The two major reasons for this trend are (1) overweight/obesity and (2) physical inactivity.[25] The American Diabetic Association and the American Academy of Pediatrics recommend that at-risk children be screened with a blood test every 2 years starting at the age of 10.[26] A second, and related, concern is the emergence of **metabolic syndrome** among overweight and obese adolescents. This cluster of events—visceral fat deposition, insulin resistance, high blood pressure, elevated triglycerides, and low HDL cholesterol—together are a potent risk for coronary artery disease.[27]

Smoking is a major risk for many diseases that tend to track into adulthood. In 2007, 21.3% of male high school students and 18.7% of female high school students were smoking cigarettes on a regular basis.[28]

Leading health authorities presented a list of 10 high-priority public health concerns in *Healthy People 2010*. Topping the list was the need for Americans, young and old, to become more physically active. The second concern was the unprecedented number of overweight and obese people in the United States.[29]

In a recent study using sophisticated measuring techniques, children 9 to 11 years old whose cholesterol was higher than normal had blood vessels stiffer than expected for their young age. Arterial dilation was less than normal in these children, while resistance to blood flow was greater than normal in response to the heart's contractions.[30]

Obese children show blood vessel abnormalities that can lead to premature heart disease later in life.[31]

Attempts to prevent heart disease need to begin in childhood. Knowledgeable parents can serve as role models who practice, rather than just talk about, healthy behaviors. Active parents should be the strongest influence, but they are not the only influence. Schools need to offer quality physical education programs throughout the 12 years of precollege education, and communities should offer opportunities and provide facilities for active participation in games and recreational play.

---

The ongoing Framingham Study, which began in 1949, identified the risk factors connected with heart disease.[17] Cigarette smoking, high blood pressure, elevated cholesterol levels, diabetes, obesity, stress, physical inactivity, age, gender, and family history were found to be highly related to heart attack and stroke. As the risks were discovered, the realization evolved that heart disease is not the inevitable consequence of aging or bad luck but a preventable, acquired disease. After a few years, researchers realized that preventive efforts should begin in childhood.

Autopsy studies of 18-year-olds who died in accidents have shown a positive relationship between blood cholesterol levels and the prevalence of fatty streaks on the walls of the coronary arteries and aorta. The evidence indicates that the average cholesterol level in children in overfed, underexercised societies, such as the United States, is too high.[18]

Autopsy studies of American combat battle casualties, whose average age was 22 years, in the Korean and Vietnam wars showed obstructions in the coronary arteries. These obstructions are caused by **atherosclerosis**, a slow, progressive inflammatory disease of the arteries that can originate in childhood.[32] It is characterized by the deposition of plaque beneath the lining of the artery (Figure 2-4). Plaque consists of fatty substances, cholesterol, blood platelets, fibrin, calcium, and cellular debris. The atherosclerotic process is responsible for 80% of the coronary heart disease deaths in the United States. The current theory of the development of atherosclerosis is explained in the section dealing with cholesterol as a risk factor.

Between 3 and 4 million people have silent **ischemia**, or silent heart attacks.[33] These people typically do not experience chest pain or chest discomfort, nor

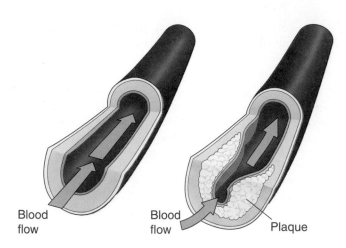

Blood
flow

Blood
flow

Plaque

**FIGURE 2-4**  Progressive Narrowing of a Normal Coronary Artery (Atherosclerosis)

do they have arm, neck, or jaw pain.[34] Those most likely to experience a silent heart attack are older people, diabetics, females, those who have had a prior stroke or heart failure, nonwhites, and those who are under chronic stress or who are lonely, angry, and

## [ JUST THE FACTS ]
### Heart Attack: The Warning Signs

#### The Warning Signs

- Uncomfortable pressure, fullness, a squeezing sensation as if a band were being tightened around the chest, pain in the center of the chest lasting longer than 10 minutes
- Pain that spreads to the shoulders, arms, or neck
- The preceding warning signs accompanied by dizziness, fainting, sweating, nausea, and shortness of breath

#### What to Do If These Signs Appear

If you have chest discomfort lasting more than 10 minutes,

- Do not deny what may be occurring.
- Call emergency services first; if they cannot respond, then have a friend or family member drive you to the nearest hospital that has 24-hour emergency cardiac care.
- Know in advance which hospitals have emergency cardiac care.
- Prominently display in your home the telephone number of the emergency rescue service, and carry a copy with you.

negative most of the time.[35] The absence of chest pain, a hallmark of heart attacks, can more than double the risk of dying, probably because these people wait longer before seeking medical treatment. Three to four million Americans experience cardiac ischemia without knowing it. Ischemia (reduced blood flow) occurs as the result of arterial disease or arterial spasms that restrict blood flow to any part of the body, including the heart.[36] Silent ischemia can initiate heart attacks without warning. However, the typical heart attack is obvious, and the symptoms are pronounced. See Just the Facts: Heart Attack: The Warning Signs.

## Stroke (Brain Attack)

Strokes or brain attacks are the third leading cause of death in the United States.[37] About 795,000 people suffer a stoke each year, resulting in approximately 185,000 deaths. The majority of strokes (cerebrovascular accidents, or brain attacks) follow the same sequence of events that results in coronary heart disease. A stroke is essentially the result of diseased blood vessels that supply the brain. It shares the same risk factors as coronary heart disease, and it takes years to develop.[38]

Strokes are caused by a **thrombus** (a clot that forms and occludes an artery supplying the brain) or an **embolus** (a clot that forms elsewhere in the body and fragments, dislodges, and is transported to one of the cerebral blood vessels that is too small for its passage). **Cerebral hemorrhage** (the bursting of a blood vessel in the brain caused by trauma, arterial brittleness, or aneurysm) is also a cause of stroke. An **aneurysm** is a weak spot in an artery that forms a balloonlike pouch, which can rupture. It may be a congenital defect or the result of uncontrolled or poorly controlled hypertension.

Eighty-seven percent of all strokes are due to a thrombus or an embolus.[39] Brain cells once supplied by these blood vessels die and do not regenerate. As a result, the functional losses that occur (e.g., paralysis on one side of the body, difficulty speaking) cannot be fully recovered. That brain cells die also means that treatment will not be very effective. Many stroke victims are unable to return to a normal lifestyle unless the stroke was mild, in which case a full recovery is possible.

Strokes caused by hemorrhages result in a 50% mortality rate. Victims die from the pressure imposed by blood leaking into or around the brain. Those who survive this type of stroke are likely to recover more of their normal functions than are those whose strokes were caused by a blood clot. The blood that spills in and on the brain during a hemorrhagic stroke produces pressure, which gradually abates as the blood is absorbed by the body. Function is regained as the pressure relents.

On many occasions a stroke is preceded by warning signs and signals days, weeks, or months before a

## [ JUST THE ] FACTS
### Stroke: The Warning Signs

The American Heart Association suggests that people be familiar with the following warning signs:

- Temporary loss of speech or difficulty in speaking or understanding speech
- Unexplained dizziness, unsteadiness, or sudden falls
- Temporary dimness or loss of vision, particularly in one eye
- Sudden, temporary weakness or numbness of the face, arm, and leg on one side of the body
- Occurrence of a series of minor strokes, or transient ischemic attacks (TIAs)

The symptoms or warning signs of a stroke are difficult for a layperson to identify. But a quick screening test that bystanders can use to recognize a stroke in progress was presented at the 2003 International Stroke Conference.[40] The test is called the "Smile Test" and consists of asking three questions of the potential stroke victim: (1) ask the individual to smile, (2) ask the person to raise both arms, and (3) ask the person to speak a simple sentence. If the person has difficulty performing any of these simple acts, call 9-1-1 immediately. While this sounds logical and plausible, the American Stroke Association has not endorsed this test.

major stroke. These must be recognized and then acted on, so that prompt medical and lifestyle interventions can be instituted to prevent or delay a stroke. A full-blown stroke is often preceded by a transient ischemic attack or TIA.[41] These are "mini strokes" that produce strokelike symptoms, are temporary, and usually do no lasting damage. People who have one or more TIAs are much more likely to have a stroke than are those who have never experienced a TIA.

It is extremely important to learn the warning signs of a stroke or TIA and to receive medical attention as quickly as possible. The sooner medical intervention is started (within 3 hours after the onset of symptoms), the less brain damage and the better the outlook for the patient.

Preventing a stroke is similar to preventing coronary heart disease. Both involve blood pressure and cholesterol control, smoking cessation, weight management, exercise, and proper nutrition. A risk factor commonly associated with a stroke rather than a heart attack is atrial fibrillation. This rhythm disorder raises the risk for a stroke by approximately five times above normal.[42] Atrial fibrillation is characterized by an exceptionally rapid heart rate of the upper chambers

of the heart.[43] The high heart rate causes the atria to quiver (fibrillate) instead of beating rhythmically and effectively. As a result, blood that remains or pools in the atria has a tendency to clot. If a clot forms and/or fractures and dislodges with fragments entering the bloodstream, there is a good chance that an artery supplying the brain will be blocked resulting in an ischemic stroke. See Just the Facts: Stroke: The Warning Signs, which identifies the major warning signs.

## Risk Factors for Heart Disease

The major risk factors for heart disease are increasing age, male gender, heredity, and race.[44] While these risk factors cannot be changed, their impact on heart disease can be reduced by a heart-healthy lifestyle. Tobacco smoke, high blood cholesterol, high blood pressure, physical inactivity, obesity and overweight, and diabetes mellitus are major risk factors that can be modified by a heart-healthy lifestyle and medication if needed. Other contributing risk factors include an individual's response to stress, hormonal factors, birth control pills, and excessive alcohol consumption. See Figure 2-5 (page 44) for the major risk factors.

These risk factors account for the majority of cardiovascular disease in the United States. However, there are many other factors that can be involved, some backed by a sound and growing body of evidence. These include high serum homocysteine, lipoprotein (a), high blood fibrinogen, and high blood insulin levels. Other possible risk factors, supported by inconclusive evidence, include short stature, baldness, ear lobe creases, and high serum uric acid level. A few of the more important of these risk factors are covered later in this chapter.

## Major Risk Factors That Cannot Be Changed

### Age

Cardiovascular disease is the leading cause of death and disability among the elderly because atherosclerotic disease is usually more advanced late in life. Approximately 55% of heart attacks occur in people 65 years of age or older. This age group accounts for more than 80% of fatal heart attacks.[45]

### Male Gender

Until recently, the incidence of coronary heart disease among women was largely unexplored. Men have been the primary subjects in coronary heart disease and risk factor studies because of the high incidence of both among men. Males are more likely to have a heart attack than females and to suffer such an attack at an earlier time in life.[46] A man in his forties is four times more likely to die from heart disease than a woman of

**Risk factors that cannot be changed**

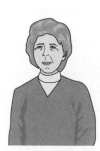

Increasing age

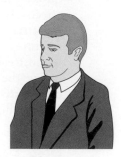

Male gender

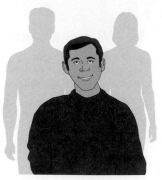

Heredity

**Risk factors that can be changed**

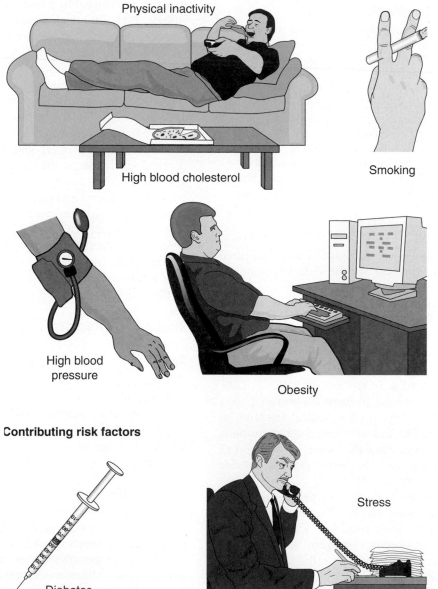

Physical inactivity

High blood cholesterol

Smoking

High blood pressure

Obesity

**Contributing risk factors**

Diabetes

Stress

**FIGURE 2-5** Cardiovascular Disease Risk Factors

## Wellness for a Lifetime

### Women and Coronary Heart Disease: Pre- and Postmenopause

Heart attacks are relatively rare among premenopausal women because of the production and presence of estrogen (the female sex hormone responsible for the development of secondary sexual characteristics and the various phases of the menstrual cycle and essential for bone formation). Estrogen is also protective in that it lowers LDL cholesterol (the harmful form), raises HDL cholesterol (the protective form), and may increase blood flow to the heart.

During and after menopause, the production of estrogen decreases and eventually stops, and the protection from heart disease diminishes. Women tend to develop coronary heart disease about 10 years later than men. At age 65, the risk for men and women equalizes.[48]

A survey of women conducted by the American Heart Association indicated that most respondents perceived breast cancer as their greatest threat to health, even though heart disease kills and disables more women. Breast cancer deaths were estimated to reach 40,170 in 2009,[49] while 454,600 women are estimated to die from cardiovascular disease in the same year.[50] Heart attack

symptoms—such as nausea; shortness of breath; fatigue; and jaw, shoulder, and back pain—tend to be far less dramatic in women. Women also present with symptoms such as extreme tiredness, flulike symptoms, and abdominal pain, with one or a constellation of symptoms that last for hours or days.[51] Such nonspecific symptoms may induce women to delay seeking medical treatment long enough to render angioplasty or blood-thinning drugs ineffective.

Because women are typically older than men when they develop heart disease, they usually have comorbid conditions, such as diabetes or high blood pressure. These complications interfere with post-heart-attack healing processes.

Women should not take hormone replacement treatment for heart protection. This was standard treatment just a few years ago. But the results of two large placebo-controlled, randomized studies showed that hormone replacement therapy did not prevent heart disease; in fact, those subjects who were in the hormone replacement group had a higher incidence of heart attacks and strokes than the subjects who were taking a placebo.[52]

the same age. However, coronary heart disease is also the leading cause of death and disability among women, accounting for almost 214,000 deaths annually.[47] Women have less heart disease than men, particularly before menopause. See Wellness for a Lifetime: Women and Coronary Disease: Pre- and Postmenopause.

An alarming trend is the increased incidence of heart attacks in premenopausal women who have been smoking cigarettes long enough for it to affect their health, especially when combined with oral contraceptive use.

### Heredity

According to the American Heart Association, "a tendency toward heart disease or atherosclerosis appears to be hereditary, so children of parents with cardiovascular disease are more likely to develop it themselves."[53] A history of first-degree male relatives (father, grandfather, and brothers) who have coronary heart disease or who died of coronary heart disease before the age of 55, or first-degree female relatives (mother, grandmother, and sisters) who have coronary heart disease or who died of coronary heart disease before the age of 65, indicates a strong familial tendency.[54] If the family history is positive, the modifiable risk factors must be controlled.

### Race

Some minority groups have a higher rate of heart disease than would be expected. For example, African Americans have a high incidence of hypertension. One

in three African American adults is hypertensive, compared with one in four adults in the general public. They also experience higher rates of morbidity (illness) and mortality (death) from consequences of hypertension, such as strokes and kidney failure.[55] Other minority groups—Mexican Americans, Native Americans, Native Hawaiians, and some Asian Americans—have high rates of heart disease primarily due to rampant obesity and one of its major consequences, diabetes.[56]

Although age, male gender, heredity, and race are major risks not under our direct control, we can modify their effects by living a wellness lifestyle. Abstaining from tobacco products; exercising regularly; controlling blood pressure, cholesterol, and body weight; managing stress; and maintaining a social support system can lessen the impact of these unchangeable risk factors.

## Major Risk Factors That Can Be Changed

A well-designed study, whose results were reported in 2003, showed that approximately 90% of all coronary heart disease victims had one or more of the following risk factors: cholesterol abnormalities, high blood pressure, cigarette smoking/tobacco use, physical inactivity, obesity, and diabetes.[57] The data examined in this investigation came from three major heart disease studies that featured thousands of subjects. The authors of the current study stated that the evidence gathered in the three previous studies convincingly challenges the frequently made claim that only 50% of heart attacks occur to those with known risk factors. The facts indicate quite the opposite. The data showed that 90% of all heart attack victims had one or more of the five risk factors. Heart attacks don't occur unless there are reasons for their occurrence.

This conclusion was reinforced by a study that sampled more than 27,000 subjects from 52 countries.[58] They found that the causes of heart disease were similar from country to country, and, secondly, nine risk factors accounted for more than 95% of the risk for future cardiovascular disease.

## Cholesterol

**Cholesterol** is a steroid that is an essential structural component of neural tissue; it is used in the construction of cell walls and for the manufacture of hormones and bile (for the digestion and absorption of fats). A certain amount of cholesterol is required for good health, but high levels in the blood are associated with heart attacks and strokes.

The National Heart, Lung, and Blood Institute suggests that Americans reduce cholesterol consumption to less than 200 milligrams per day (200 mg/day) for those at high risk for cardiovascular disease and less than 300 mg/day for all other Americans[59] Fat intake may be increased to a maximum of 35% of the total calories consumed, but saturated fat plus trans fats should be reduced to no more than 10% of the total calories. (See Just the Facts: Guidelines for Fat and Cholesterol.) Many authorities are convinced that limiting total fat and saturated fat is more important than being overly restrictive of cholesterol.

Americans should consume no more than 7 to 8% of their total calories in the form of saturated fat and trans fatty acids.[60] Monounsaturated and polyunsaturated fats should make up the remainder—up to 25% of the total fat intake—in approximately equal proportions.[61] Monounsaturates and polyunsaturates are heart-healthy fats, while saturates and trans fats are very harmful.

The average American male consumes about 337 mg/day of cholesterol, while average female consumption is 217 mg/day.[62] Dietary cholesterol comes from animal flesh and animal products (eggs, milk, cheese). Plant foods contain no cholesterol. The average consumption of total fat is approximately 33% of total calories; 13% is saturated fat, 3% is trans fats, and the remainder consists of monounsaturated and polyunsaturated fats.[63]

Cholesterol is consumed in the diet (exogenous, or dietary cholesterol), but it is also manufactured by the body from saturated fats (endogenous). Cholesterol synthesis in the body would occur even if a cholesterol-free diet were consumed. The liver manufactures about 80% of endogenous cholesterol, with the remainder being synthesized in the intestinal and arterial walls.

The liver alone produces enough cholesterol to meet the body's needs. Therefore, consuming cholesterol is not necessary to maintain health. Table 2-1 lists some common foods that contain cholesterol and saturated fat.

A number of population studies during the last 35 years have indicated a positive relationship between

## [ JUST THE ] FACTS

### Guidelines for Fat and Cholesterol

The National Cholesterol Education Program through the auspices of the National Heart, Lung, and Blood Institute released its newest recommendations for detecting and lowering high cholesterol in adults in May 2001. This revision represents the first major change since 1993. The following are some selected highlights recommended by a panel of 27 experts:

1. Physicians are strongly encouraged to pay more attention to the "metabolic syndrome," representative of a significant risk for heart disease. This syndrome is a combination of excessive abdominal fat, high blood pressure, high blood glucose, elevated triglycerides, and low HDL cholesterol.

2. HDL cholesterol is considered a major risk if it is below 40 mg/dL for men and below 50 mg/dL for women.

3. Dietary intake of cholesterol should be less than 200 mg/day for those at high risk and less than 300 mg/day for all others.

4. There should be more aggressive treatment of triglycerides.

5. Less than 10% of calories should come from saturated fat and trans fats together.

6. Dietary fat may be increased to 35% of the total daily calories instead of the previous 30%, provided that the majority of these come from monounsaturated and polyunsaturated sources.

7. The new recommendations strongly urge the necessity of attaining and maintaining normal body weight, as well as consistent participation in physical activity.

Table 2-1   Sources of Dietary Cholesterol and Saturated Fat

| | Cholesterol (mg)* | Saturated Fat (g)** | | Cholesterol (mg)* | Saturated Fat (g)** |
|---|---|---|---|---|---|
| **Meats (3 oz.)** | | | **Seafood (3 oz.)** | | |
| Beef liver | 372 | 2.5 | Squid | 153 | .4 |
| Veal | 86 | 4.0 | Oily fish | 59 | 1.2 |
| Pork | 80 | 3.2 | Lean fish | 59 | .3 |
| Lean beef | 56 | 2.4 | Shrimp (6 large) | 48 | .2 |
| Chicken (dark meat) | 82 | 2.7 | Clams (6 large) | 36 | .3 |
| Chicken (white meat) | 76 | 1.3 | Lobster | 46.4 | .08 |
| Egg | 215 | 1.7 | | | |
| **Dairy Products (1 Cup; Cheese, 1 oz.)** | | | **Other Items of Interest** | | |
| Ice cream | 59 | 8.9 | Pork brains (3 oz.) | 2,169 | 1.8 |
| Whole milk | 33 | 5.1 | Beef kidney (3 oz.) | 683 | 3.8 |
| Butter (1 tsp.) | 31 | 7.1 | Beef hot dog (1) | 75 | 9.9 |
| Yogurt (low-fat) | 11 | 1.8 | Prime ribs of beef (3 oz.) | 66.5 | 5.3 |
| Cheddar | 30 | 6.0 | Doughnut | 36 | 4.0 |
| American | 27 | 5.6 | Milk chocolate | 0 | 16.3 |
| Camembert | 20 | 4.3 | Green or yellow vegetable or fruit | 0 | Trace |
| Parmesan | 8 | 2.0 | Peanut butter (1 tbsp.) | 0 | 1.5 |
| | | | Angel food cake | 0 | 1.96 |
| **Oils (1 tbsp.)** | | | Skim milk (1 cup) | 4 | .3 |
| Coconut | 0 | 11.8 | Cheese pizza (3 oz.) | 6 | .8 |
| Palm | 0 | 6.7 | Buttermilk (1 cup) | 9 | 1.3 |
| Olive | 0 | 1.8 | Ice milk, soft (1 cup) | 13 | 2.9 |
| Corn | 0 | 1.7 | Turkey, white meat (3 oz.) | 59 | .9 |
| Safflower | 0 | 1.2 | | | |

*There are 1,000 mg in a gram.

**There are 28 g in an ounce and 454 g in a pound

serum cholesterol (the level of cholesterol circulating in the blood) and the development of coronary heart disease. The National Heart, Lung, and Blood Institute reviewed this evidence and concluded that high circulating levels of serum cholesterol cause heart disease.

Values of serum cholesterol above 200 milligrams per deciliter (mg/dL) of blood are higher than the average risk. Table 2-2 shows the values of risk associated with total cholesterol (TC), LDL and HDL cholesterol (to be discussed shortly), and another serum lipid (blood fat), the triglycerides.

An important collaborative study involving 12 research centers throughout the United States provided clinical evidence implicating cholesterol as a culprit in coronary heart disease[64] The researchers concluded that each 1% reduction in cholesterol level results in a 2% reduction in the risk for coronary heart disease.

A later follow-up of this study indicated that the reduction in coronary heart disease is probably closer to 3% for every 1% that cholesterol is lowered[65] The strategies for lowering cholesterol in the blood are presented in Real-World Wellness: Strategies for Lowering Cholesterol.

**The Cholesterol Carriers.** The amount of cholesterol circulating in the blood accounts for only part of the total cholesterol in the body. Unlike sugar and salt, cholesterol does not dissolve in the blood, so it is transported by protein packages, which facilitate its solubility. These transporters are the lipoproteins manufactured by the body. They include the chylomicrons, very low-density lipoprotein (VLDL), intermediate-density lipoprotein (IDL), low-density lipoprotein (LDL), and high-density lipoprotein (HDL). Dietary cholesterol enters the body from the digestive system attached to the chylomicrons. The chylomicrons shrink as they give up their cholesterol to the cells of the body. The fragments that remain are removed by the liver and used to manufacture and secrete VLDLs, triglyceride-rich lipoproteins. The triglycerides represent 95% of the stored fats in the body. The VLDLs are degraded as their cargo of triglycerides is either used by the cells for energy or stored in adipose cells (fat cells). The

**TABLE 2-2**   Risk Profile–Lipid and Lipoprotein Concentrations

| Total Cholesterol | Category of Risk |
| --- | --- |
| < 200 mg/dL* | Desirable |
| 200–239 mg/dL | Borderline |
| ≥ 240 mg/dL** | High |

| LDL Cholesterol | Category of Risk |
| --- | --- |
| < 100 mg/dL | Optimal |
| 100–129 mg/dL | Near optimal/above optimal |
| 130–159 mg/dL | Borderline high |
| 160–189 mg/dL | High |
| ≥ 190 mg/dL | Very high |

| HDL Cholesterol | Category of Risk |
| --- | --- |
| ≤ 40 mg/dL*** | Increased risk |
| ≥ 60 mg/dL | Heart-protective |

| Triglycerides | Category of Risk |
| --- | --- |
| < 150 mg/dL | Normal |
| 150–199 mg/dL | Borderline high |
| 200–499 mg/dL | High |
| ≥ 500 mg/dL | Very high |

Source: Adapted from American Heart Association. (2009). *Heart and stroke facts*. Dallas, TX: American Heart Association.

\* < less than

\*\* ≥ equal to or greater than

\*\*\* ≤ equal to or less than

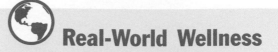

## Real-World Wellness

### Strategies for Lowering Cholesterol

*My doctor told me that my cholesterol level is too high. How can I lower it to reduce my risk of having a heart attack or stroke?*

First, establish a realistic goal, such as about how much you think you can lower your cholesterol. Second, identify the lifestyle changes that can lower cholesterol. Third, attempt to do all of the following that apply to you:

- Reduce your fat consumption to less than 30% of total calories (25% would be better).
- Reduce your saturated fat and trans fats consumption to less than 10% of total calories (8% would be better).
- Reduce your dietary cholesterol to less than 300 mg/day (less than 200 mg/day would be better).
- Lose weight if you are overweight.
- Stop smoking cigarettes and/or stop using other tobacco products.
- Increase your consumption of soluble fiber, found in fruits, vegetables, and grains.
- Do aerobic exercise at least three times per week for at least 30 minutes each time.
- If these strategies fail to normalize your cholesterol level in 6 months, you may have to consider taking cholesterol-lowering drugs.

VLDL remnants may be removed by the liver or converted to LDLs (Figure 2-6).

LDLs are the primary transporters of cholesterol—they carry 60 to 80% of the body's cholesterol—and the most capable of producing atherosclerosis. Michael S. Brown and Joseph L. Goldstein won a 1985 Nobel Prize in medicine and physiology for discovering that the liver and the cells of the body have receptor sites that bind LDLs, removing them from circulation. The liver contains 50 to 75% of these sites; the remainder are in other cells of the body. When LDL concentrations are excessive, the liver sites become saturated, and further removal of them from the blood is significantly impeded. As a result, plasma levels of cholesterol rise, leading to the conditions that are conducive to the development of atherosclerosis.

The development of atherosclerosis in the coronary arteries is complex. Since the early 1990s, the medical community has been seriously investigating the connection between disease and inflammation. Inflammation represents the body's major mechanism of defense against infection. Atherosclerosis—responsible for 80% of coronary disease—is a chronic inflammatory disease.

The initial event in the atherosclerotic process is an injury (lesion) that occurs to the inner lining (endothelium) of the arteries. Such injuries occur because of prolonged exposure to tobacco smoke, high blood pressure, elevated LDL cholesterol, diabetes mellitus, high amounts of serum homocysteine, and viral and bacterial infections.[66] These injuries, which occur at multiple sites, resulting in endothelial dysfunction and a vulnerable artery, allow LDL cholesterol to infiltrate under the artery lining, where they become oxidized (come in contact with oxygen). Oxidized LDLs become toxic. Oxidized LDLs resemble an infection, which triggers the immune system to initiate defensive actions. This is the connection between atherosclerosis and inflammation.[67] Monocytes from the immune system enter the artery wall and act as macrophages (long-lived cells that ingest foreign substances) to engulf and destroy oxidized LDLs.[68] The fat-filled macrophages become bloated with oxidized LDLs; in this state, they actually contribute to the formation of plaque. Plaque grows steadily over many years. The process initiates and maintains a low-grade inflammatory response by

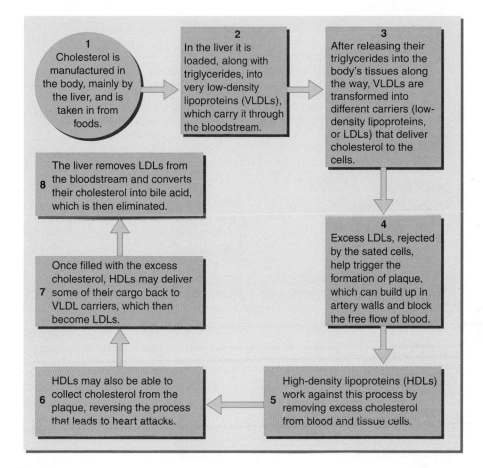

**FIGURE 2-6**   Cholesterol Carriers

the body. Chronic inflammation damages the cells lining the arteries and can cause an acute heart attack by destabilizing plaque. Destabilized plaque has a thin, fibrous cap that is likely to rupture, causing a blood clot that can block blood flow in an artery and result in a heart attack. Inflammation also contributes to the growth of the fibrous cap that seals over the plaque.[69]

Cigarette smoke, lack of regular exercise, high blood pressure, cholesterol abnormalities, excessive body weight, an unhealthy diet, and a rapid heart rate result in continued inflammation and the growth of plaque. Many plaques are unstable, meaning that they have a thin, fibrous cap. These plaques are under constant threat of rupturing at any time. When a break in the cap occurs, plaque spews out through the opening, triggering further inflammatory responses by the body, which result in the formation of a blood clot. Often the clot is large enough to block the entire opening of the artery, the culmination of which is the stoppage of blood flow and oxygen to a portion of the heart muscle. This is a heart attack. See Figure 2-7 for an illustration of this process.

Physicians can test for chronic low-grade inflammation of the type that might be indicative of coronary heart disease. This is a simple blood test called high-sensitivity C-reactive protein (hs-CRP) test. This test

has become a useful biomarker for assessing cardiovascular disease, and in several studies it predicted future heart attacks more accurately than LDL cholesterol.[70] C-reactive protein is produced by the liver in response to an increase in the blood of interleukin 6 (IL-6), which is the principal initiator of the inflammatory response. People who are overweight or obese or who have metabolic syndrome may spontaneously secrete sufficient IL-6 to mimic low-grade systemic inflammation, complete with an elevation of inflammatory proteins such as C-reactive protein.[71] Interleukin 6 increases with age. CRP levels of 3.0 milligrams per liter of blood (3 mg/L) or higher can triple the risk of having heart disease. The risk is higher for females than males. People whose CRP is less than 0.5 mg/L rarely have heart attacks.[72]

Heart attacks are less likely to occur when LDL values are below 100 mg/dL. The average LDL level in the United States, according to the latest figures available at this writing, is 123 mg/dL. A cursory examination of Table 2-2 indicates that this level is too high.[73] However, LDL cholesterol consists of a varied mixture of particle types that range in their impact on atherosclerosis from neutral to very harmful.[74] LDL particles also vary in size from small to medium or large. It is

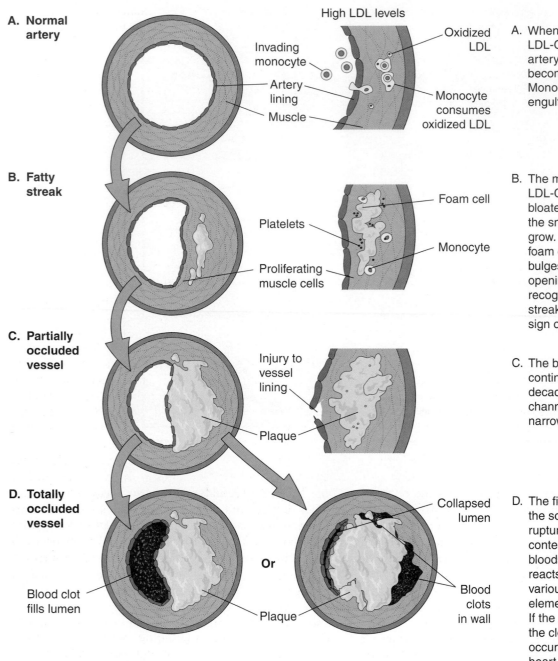

**A. Normal artery**

High LDL levels

Invading monocyte

Oxidized LDL

Artery lining

Monocyte consumes oxidized LDL

Muscle

A. When a lesion occurs, LDL-Cs infiltrate below the artery lining, where they become oxidized and toxic. Monocytes follow and engulf the toxic LDLs.

**B. Fatty streak**

Platelets

Foam cell

Monocyte

Proliferating muscle cells

B. The monocytes swell with LDL-C and become bloated. Platelets stimulate the smooth muscle cells to grow. Monocytes become foam cells. The growth bulges into the artery opening (lumen) and is recognized as a fatty streak (the first noticeable sign of atherosclerosis).

**C. Partially occluded vessel**

Injury to vessel lining

Plaque

C. The bulge (now plaque) continues to grow over decades and the artery channels continue to narrow.

**D. Totally occluded vessel**

Collapsed lumen

Blood clot fills lumen

Or

Blood clots in wall

Plaque

D. The fibrous cap covering the soft arterial plaque ruptures, spewing its contents into the bloodstream. The body reacts by stimulating various immune system elements to seal the break. If the artery is occluded by the clot, a heart attack occurs and a portion of the heart muscle dies.

**FIGURE 2-7** Progression of Atherosclerosis and Coronary Artery Disease

the small, dense particles that are the most athero-genic—that is, the most capable of penetrating the wall of an injured artery and therefore the greatest contributor to the development of atherosclerosis. A national panel of experts has developed guidelines for safe and unsafe levels of LDL, and these appear in Table 2-2. A high circulating level of LDL cholesterol is positively related to cardiovascular disease. Weight loss, a diet low in saturated fat and total fat and high in soluble fiber, exercise, and medication (if needed) will lower LDL levels in the blood.

HDLs are involved in reverse transport; they accept cholesterol from the blood and tissues and transfer it to the liver, where it can be degraded and disposed of in the feces. This is a major route for removal of cholesterol. HDLs protect the arteries from atherosclerosis by clearing cholesterol from the blood.[75] Cardiovascular health depends greatly on low levels of total cholesterol and LDLs and a high level of HDLs. Cigarette smoking, diabetes, elevated triglyceride levels, and anabolic steroids lower HDL, whereas physical exercise, weight loss, the B vitamin niacin, and moderate alcohol consumption raise it.[76]

Moderate alcohol consumption (no more than two drinks per day for males and no more than one drink per day for females) increases HDL cholesterol.[77] However, recent evidence has shown that three to four alcoholic drinks per week is sufficient to modestly raise HDL cholesterol. Caution should be exercised regarding alcohol intake because the health hazards associated with it far outweigh its few advantages. Alcohol consumption, even in moderate amounts, is not an acceptable way to raise HDL unless prescribed by a physician who is well aware of the patient's health and family history. An alcoholic drink is defined as a 5-ounce glass of wine, a 12-ounce beer, or 1½ ounces of 80-proof spirits. However, alcohol is a depressant that impairs judgment and removes inhibitions, so that people under its influence behave in ways they ordinarily would not while sober. Excessive alcohol intake is three drinks or more per day. Health is compromised at consumption levels above two drinks per day. The risks increase for heart disease, high blood pressure, cirrhosis of the liver, breast cancer, and osteoporosis; also, the immune system weakens, red blood cell production slows down, and the brain is adversely affected. (See Chapter 10 for a more complete discussion of the effects of alcohol.)

Table 2-2 presents the current guidelines for HDL cholesterol levels in the blood. The higher the HDL, the greater the protection from cardiovascular disease. The average value for men is 46 mg/dL, and for women it is 56 mg/dL.[78] This biological difference in HDL levels between genders partly explains the lower incidence of heart disease in premenopausal women as compared with men. After menopause, HDL levels in women begin to decrease, as does their protection provided by this subfraction of cholesterol. The ratio between total cholesterol (TC) and HDL (TC/HDL) should also be considered when the risk is interpreted. This ratio is determined by dividing TC by HDL (Table 2-3).[79]

Another blood fat, the serum triglycerides, is involved in the development and progression of atherosclerosis. Normal serum triglycerides range from 50 mg/dL to 150 mg/dL. Table 2-2 identifies the risk associated with various serum triglyceride levels.

High serum triglycerides usually coexist with low HDL cholesterol, a proven risk factor for cardiovascular disease. Teasing out the independent effect of serum triglyceride levels has been difficult. But recent evidence has shown that high levels are a modest independent risk factor for heart disease and a reliable predictor when coupled with low HDL cholesterol.[80] Serum triglycerides greater than 190 mg/dL increase blood viscosity (blood thickness), resulting in sluggish blood flow and increasing the risk for blood clots. Viscous blood is more difficult to circulate, so oxygen and nutrients are not delivered as efficiently to the body's tissues, and these include the heart muscle.[81]

Table 2-2 shows the relative risk posed by high serum triglycerides. Levels below 150 mg/dL are in the normal category, but evidence suggests that an optimal level is below 100 mg/dL.[82]

A number of studies have shown that sedentary people with high triglycerides can reduce serum triglycerides substantially when they participate in moderately intense aerobic exercise for 45 minutes 4 days per week.[83] Physically fit people metabolize serum triglycerides more effectively than do sedentary people and are able to clear these triglycerides from the blood more rapidly after a high-fat meal.[84] Fatty acids, stored in the body as triglycerides, are the primary type of fat used by muscle cells for energy.[85] This is the reason that exercise significantly lowers the triglyceride level in the body.

Other strategies for lowering serum triglycerides include weight loss; reductions in dietary sugar, fat, and alcohol; and the substitution of fish for meat a couple of times during the week. Increasing fish consumption, as long as it is not fried, lowers the dietary intake of calories and saturated fat and increases the intake of omega-3 fatty acids, which tend to lower serum triglycerides.

## Blood Pressure

*Blood pressure*, recorded in millimeters of mercury (mmHg), is the force exerted against the walls of the arteries as blood travels through the circulatory system. Pressure is created when the heart contracts and pumps blood into the arteries. The arterioles (smallest arteries) offer resistance to blood flow, and if the resistance is persistently high, the pressure rises and remains high. The medical term for high blood pressure is **hypertension.**

Hypertension is a silent disease that has no characteristic signs or symptoms, so blood pressure should be checked periodically. Blood pressure can be measured quickly with a sphygmomanometer. A cuff is wrapped around the upper arm and inflated with enough air to compress the artery, temporarily stopping blood flow. A stethoscope is placed on the artery below the cuff, so that the sound of blood coursing through the artery

| **TABLE 2-3** Ratio of Total Cholesterol to HDL Cholesterol | | |
|---|---|---|
| **Risk** | **Men** | **Women** |
| Very low (one-half average) | < 3.4 | < 3.3 |
| Low risk | 4.0 | 3.8 |
| Average risk | 5.0 | 4.5 |
| Moderate risk (two times average) | 9.5 | 7.0 |
| High risk (three times average) | > 23.0 | > 11.0 |

can be heard when the air in the cuff is released. The first sound represents the systolic pressure (the maximum pressure of blood flow when the heart contracts), and the last sound heard is the diastolic pressure (the minimum pressure of blood flow between heartbeats).

The guidelines for prevention and treatment of high blood pressure were revised in 2003 for the first time since 1997. The new guidelines were developed by a panel of experts under the direction of the National Heart, Lung, and Blood Institute.[86] The panel established a new category of blood pressure called "prehypertension." This category includes blood pressures ranging from 120/80 to 139/89. Fifty-eight million American adults have hypertension and 59 million are prehypertensive.[87] The blood pressures in the new category were considered normal under the old guidelines. The upgrade was made because a growing body of evidence showed that a blood pressure of 135/85 doubles the risk of having a heart attack or stroke when compared with a reading of 115/75. The risk for death from heart disease or stroke begins to increase at 115/75 and doubles for each 20 mmHg systolic or every 10 mmHg diastolic. Further, prehypertensive pressures between 120/80 and 129/84 mmHg increase the risk of cardiovascular disease by 181%, while upper levels of prehypertension of 130/85 to 139/89 mmHg increase the risk by 233%.[88] Prehypertension presents the greatest risk among African Americans, diabetics, and the overweight/obese. See Table 2-4 for the new versus the old guidelines.

Table 2-4 represents the latest thinking among medical researchers about the stages of blood pressure values. The higher the blood pressure, the greater the risk. The lower the blood pressure, the better. However, blood pressure can be too low if it causes symptoms such as lightheadedness or fainting. A low systolic blood pressure (less than 140 mmHg) in the very old (aged 85 and older) increases the risk of dying, possibly

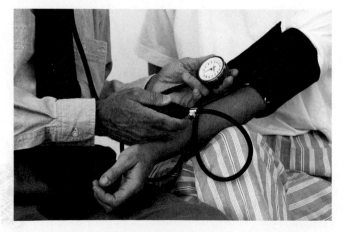

Keeping your blood pressure under control helps keep your heart healthy.

**TABLE 2-4   New vs. Old Blood Pressure Guidelines**

| Category | Now (2001) | Before (1997) |
|---|---|---|
| No hypertension | Less than $\frac{120}{80}$ | Less than $\frac{140}{90}$ |
| Prehypertension | $\frac{120}{80}$ to $\frac{139}{89}$ | —— |
| Hypertension | $\frac{140}{90}$ or higher | $\frac{140}{90}$ or higher |

The numerator (upper number) is the systolic blood pressure and the denominator (lower number) is the diastolic blood pressure.

Source: Editors. (2003, July). Why it pays to lower even "normal" blood pressure. Heart Advisor, 6(7), 2.

because it is a sign of decreased vitality, poor health, and diminished driving force needed to adequately supply the brain with blood and oxygen.[89] Recent evidence indicates that an increase in systolic blood pressure (SBP) accompanied by a decrease in the diastolic blood pressure (DBP) doubles the risk of dying from cardiovascular disease.[90] This combination seems to be more dangerous than when both pressures increase. The DBP decreases when the large arteries stiffen.

The difference between the SBP and DBP is called the "pulse pressure" (SBP minus DBP).[91] The SBP increases because age and poor lifestyle habits cause the arteries to lose their resilience. At the same time, the DBP decreases because the stiff arteries aren't as responsive to blood flow between heartbeats. A pulse pressure of 60 mmHg or more is associated with the development and progression of atherosclerosis. Some researchers are convinced that pulse pressure is the most effective predictor of cardiovascular mortality when compared to age, physical activity, total serum cholesterol, obesity, and smoking.[92] Other researchers do not agree with this assessment.

Approximately 73,600,000 American adults have high blood pressure, and another 56,600,000 are prehypertensive. Hypertension was listed as the primary or contributing cause of death in about 319,000 deaths in 2005 (the latest year in which these data were available).[93] The cause of high blood pressure is not known in 90 to 95% of the cases. This is referred to as *essential hypertension. Essential* is a medical term that means "of unknown origin or cause." Essential hypertension cannot be cured, but it can be treated and controlled. The other 5 to 10% of the cases of hypertension have a specific cause. If the cause can be determined and eliminated, blood pressure will return to normal.

The heart is adversely affected by uncontrolled or undiagnosed hypertension of long duration. Pumping blood for years against high resistance in the arteries increases the workload of the heart, and it becomes enlarged in response to the strain. The heart receives

## [ JUST THE FACTS ]
### Hypertension Is Color Blind

Prevalence rates of hypertension and severe hypertension in African Americans is among the highest in the world.[96] Also, the complications of hypertension are more severe in African Americans compared to white people as indicated by (1) an 80% higher mortality rate from strokes, (2) a 50% higher heart disease death rate, and (3) a 320% greater rate of kidney failure. While the causes are unknown, contributing factors include genetics, salt sensitivity, and higher rates of obesity and diabetes.[97]

inadequate rest because the resistance to blood flow is consistently high, and this produces overly stretched muscle fibers. They progressively lose the ability to rebound. The result is that they contract less forcefully. At this point the heart loses its efficiency and weakens. If intervention does not occur early, congestive heart failure is inevitable. Hypertension also damages the arteries and accelerates atherosclerosis.

Hypertension is the most important risk factor for brain attacks (strokes) as well as a major risk for heart disease. More than 795,000 brain attacks occur every year.[94] Certain segments of the population are at higher risk, such as African Americans, who are more likely to suffer a stroke or experience kidney damage than are whites, Latinos, or Asian Americans.[95] See Just the Facts: Hypertension Is Color Blind.

**Treatment for Hypertension.** Treatment for hypertension may include all or some of the following: weight loss; salt and alcohol restriction; adequate intake of calcium, potassium, and magnesium; voluntary relaxation techniques; exercise; and medication. Excess body weight increases the work of the heart because it must meet the nutrient demands of the extra tissue.

High salt intake increases the blood pressure in those who are salt sensitive. The Centers for Disease Control and Prevention estimates that approximately 70% of adult Americans should be consuming a low-salt diet. This is the first time that the total at-risk population has been quantified.[98] Salt is an acquired taste that can be modified. Curbing salt consumption while blood pressure is still normal cannot hurt and it may help.[99]

Salt consists of sodium and chloride. Sodium, which makes up 40% of salt, is the culprit involved in raising blood pressure. According to the Institute of Medicine, Americans on average consume too much sodium. The average American consumes 3,500 mg/day (3.5 g/day) of sodium, while the recommended amount is no more than 2,300 mg/d (2.3 g/d). Actually, the human body

needs only 200 mg/d (0.2 g/d) of sodium. The Institute of Medicine has issued recommendations for sodium intake based on age in the following manner: the upper limit is 1,500 mg/day; less than 1,300 mg/day for people 50–69 years of age; and less than 1,200 mg/day for people over 70 years of age.[99] Because these recommendations are very restrictive, many experts would rather apply them to individuals who already are hypertensive while loosening up to some extent the restrictions on those who aren't.

Dietary Approaches to Stop Hypertension (DASH) was specifically developed to lower blood pressure.[100] The diet emphasizes fruits, vegetables, low-fat dairy products, and low sodium intake. This diet has reduced systolic pressure by 10 to 12 mmHg. According to nutrition experts, the effectiveness of the diet is due to its rich content of calcium, potassium, and magnesium.

The daily potassium requirement has been increased to 4.7 g/day,[101] the calcium requirement is 1,200–1,500 mg/day,[102] and the magnesium requirement is 320 mg/day.[103]

Yoga, meditation, hypnotherapy, biofeedback, and other relaxation techniques can lower the pressure of hypertensive people. They can also reduce the pressure of normotensive people (those with normal blood pressure). Practicing relaxation techniques on a daily basis for a few minutes per session can lower the systolic blood pressure by as much as 10 mmHg.[104] There are many voluntary relaxation methods to choose from, but one developed by Harvard psychologist Herbert Benson is effective and easy to learn. Here is how to do it:

1. Select a neutral word such as *one* or a word that is meaningful such as *peace* (your mantra) to focus on.
2. Sit quietly in a comfortable position, feet flat on the floor, and close your eyes.

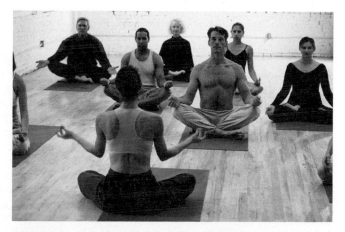

Stress-relieving activities, such as meditation, soothe the spirit and may even lower your risk for heart disease and other chronic illnesses. How do you manage stress?

3. Breathe slowly through your nose, silently repeating your focus word with each exhalation.

4. When other thoughts intrude, simply refocus on your mantra.

5. Do this for 10 to 20 minutes once or twice per day.

6. Sit quietly for a minute or so at the end of the session and then open your eyes.

Many people drink alcohol because it relaxes them, but the ingestion of more than 2 ounces of alcohol per day raises blood pressure in some people. The same precautions regarding the use of alcohol and HDL cholesterol apply for hypertension.[105]

The American College of Sports Medicine (ACSM) has developed a position paper on the relationship between exercise and hypertension.[106] Some of the more important conclusions follow:

1. Endurance exercises lower blood pressure by 5 to 7 mmHg. This is a significant reduction because small decrements in systolic blood pressure, as little as 2 mmHg, reduce the risk for stroke by 14% and coronary heart disease by 9%; a 2 mmHg decrease in diastolic blood pressure reduces the risk for stroke by 17% and coronary heart disease by 6%.

2. Blood pressure is reduced for up to 22 hours after a single bout of endurance exercise, with the greatest decreases occurring in those with the highest baseline blood pressures.

3. Moderate-intensity endurance exercise (40 to 60% of the heart rate reserve—explained in Chapter 3) will lower blood pressure.

4. The recommended exercise prescription for lowering blood pressure is as follows:

(a) Frequency: on most, preferably all days of the week

(b) Intensity: moderate

(c) Time: 30 minutes or more

(d) Type: endurance exercise supplemented with resistance training

Several mechanisms have been proposed to explain how endurance exercise can lower blood pressure. Endurance exercise

1. Lowers the blood levels of the catecholamines (epinephrine, norepinephrine, and dopamine), which are vasoconstrictors that increase resistance to blood flow

2. Lowers total peripheral resistance to blood flow by dilating blood vessels

3. Lowers body weight; evidence suggests that systolic blood pressure is lowered by 5 to 22 mmHg for every 22 excess pounds lost.[107]

4. Improves cellular sensitivity to insulin, which encourages the kidneys to excrete sodium

Medications that control blood pressure have been developed. However, they have side effects, including weakness, leg cramps, stuffy nose, occasional diarrhea, heartburn, drowsiness, anemia, depression, headaches, joint pain, dizziness, impotence, and skin rash. The side effects are unique to the drugs being used to control blood pressure. Despite these side effects, many people find it easier to take the medicine than to make the difficult lifestyle changes that lower blood pressure. However, the effort to control blood pressure with medication should not negate the importance of controlling the lifestyle factors that contribute to hypertension. Medicine and lifestyle efforts are not mutually exclusive—each contributes to blood pressure management. The effects of selected lifestyle behaviors on reducing systolic blood pressure appear in Table 2-5.

**TABLE 2-5** Lifestyle Behaviors That Work

| Behavior | Recommended Amount | Drop in Systolic B.P. |
| --- | --- | --- |
| DASH diet | Eat a diet high in fruits and vegetables, low-fat dairy products, low in fat and salt | 8 to 14 points |
| Lose excess weight | For every 20 lbs lost | 5 to 20 points |
| Exercise daily | Get at least 30 minutes a day of moderately intense aerobic exercise | 4 to 9 points |
| Limit alcohol intake | Upper limit is 2 drinks per day for males; 1 drink per day for females. 3 drinks per week should suffice | 2 to 4 points |

Source: Chobanian, A. V. et al. (2003, December). Seventh report of the Joint National Committee on Prevention, Detection, Evaluation, and Treatment of High Blood Pressure. *Hypertension*, 42(6), 1206–1252.

## Cigarette Smoking/Tobacco Use

Many medical authorities consider cigarette smoking the most harmful of the preventable risk factors associated with chronic illness and premature death.[108] More than 46 million adults in the United States currently smoke (approximately 21% of adults).[109] About half of those who continue to smoke will die from disease related to it. Tobacco usage (all forms) causes nearly one in five deaths, or about 443,600 Americans annually. The Centers for Disease Control and Prevention estimate that smoking shortens the lives of males by 13.2 years and females by 14.5 years. Compared to people who have never smoked, those who do smoke are more likely to die during middle age (between 35 and 69 years of age).[110]

Smoking accounts for 30% of all cancer deaths in America and is a causal factor in 87% of lung cancer deaths.[111] Lung damage begins early to smokers, and it continues to worsen as long as smoking continues. Smoking causes several types of lung disease, two of which—emphysema and chronic bronchitis—are nearly as bad as lung cancer. These two diseases make breathing difficult and diminish quality as well as quantity of life. Smoking also causes or is related to the development of many other forms of cancer.

**Harmful Products in Cigarettes.** Nicotine; carbon monoxide; and other poisonous gases, tars, and chemical additives for taste and flavor are the hazardous products in cigarettes. Carbon monoxide and nicotine have a devastating effect on the heart and blood vessels. Nicotine is an addictive stimulant that increases the resting heart rate, blood pressure, and metabolism. For this reason, it should be reclassified as a drug and placed under the jurisdiction of the Food and Drug Administration (FDA).

A brief summary of nicotine's effects on the cardiovascular system is found in Just the Facts: Nicotine. Carbon monoxide, a poisonous gas that is a by-product of the combustion of tobacco products, displaces oxygen in the blood because hemoglobin has a greater affinity for it than for oxygen. The diminished oxygen-carrying capacity of the blood is partly responsible for the shortness of breath that smokers experience with mild physical exertion.

Cigarettes and other tobacco products are not regulated by the FDA because tobacco is not classified as a food or drug. The tobacco industry is under no mandate to disclose the nature and type of chemicals added to tobacco products. Some of these additives are harmful. The public has a right to know, but the tobacco industry has successfully resisted attempts by governmental agencies and consumer groups to force disclosure.

The harmful effects of cigarette smoking are insidious and take time to appear. The medical profession

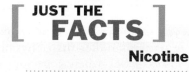

## [ JUST THE FACTS ]

### Nicotine

Nicotine is a powerful stimulant that

• Increases LDL and lowers HDL levels.

• Causes the platelets to aggregate, increasing the probability of arterial spasms.

• Increases the oxygen requirement of cardiac muscle.

• Constricts blood vessels.

• Produces cardiac dysrhythmias (irregular heartbeat).

• Is a causative agent in the 30% of coronary heart disease deaths related to smoking.

• Increases the viscosity of the blood.

measures the damage from smoking in pack years. Smoking one pack of cigarettes per day for 15 years is equal to 15 pack years (15 years × 1 pack per day = 15 pack years). Two packs per day for 15 years is equal to 30 pack years (15 × 2 = 30). Medical problems become evident after 25 to 30 pack years.

**The Challenge of Quitting.** To quit the tobacco habit, you have to simultaneously break the addiction to nicotine and the psychological dependence on smoking.[112] This involves changing behavior and effectively dealing with the social and situational stimuli that promote the desire to smoke. One-third of current cigarette smokers attempt to stop smoking every year but less than 10% of them succeed. In fact, most of them fail within 48 hours of their last cigarette.[113] Most quitters make 4 to 10 unsuccessful attempts and try several stop-smoking methods before finally succeeding. Quitting the smoking habit is a formidable challenge. However, 50% of active smokers have managed to stop smoking in the last 50 years. While exceedingly difficult, it can be done if one finds the right motivation. Since 1964, more men than women have quit, more whites than African Americans, and more non-Hispanics than Hispanics. More elderly people and more educated people also have higher quit rates.[114]

Complicating the effort to quit, particularly among young women, is the fear of gaining weight. Women who quit tend to gain slightly more weight than do men.[115] Approximately 65% of those who quit do gain weight, but the physiological adaptations that occur may account for only a 10-pound weight gain. The physiological mechanisms responsible are probably associated with a slowing of metabolism, a slight increase in appetite, and slower transit time of food in the digestive system, so that more is absorbed by the body. Weight gain beyond 10 pounds is probably caused by altered eating patterns rather than physiology. Food smells and tastes better when a person is not smoking. Food may substitute for a cigarette, especially during social activities. It may provide some of the oral gratification previously obtained from smoking, and it may relieve tension. Weight gain can be avoided by eating sensibly and exercising moderately and frequently; however, for best results, these new lifestyle habits need to be established before one attempts to quit smoking. It is very difficult to establish major lifestyle habits while attempting to quit another major habit.

Cigarette smoking increases the risk for many chronic diseases because of the direct effects of nicotine, carbon monoxide (CO), tars, and more than 4,000 chemicals that are inhaled with every puff.[116] Several studies have shown that smokers have higher blood levels of CRP, fibrinogen, and homocysteine than nonsmokers.[117] Fibrinogen and CRP are both involved with inflammation. Fibrinogen and homocysteine are risk factors that are covered later in this chapter. Both of these are components in the formation of blood clots.[118] Elevations of these three factors appear to be important mechanisms by which smoking promotes atherosclerotic disease. The totality of the harmful effects of cigarette smoking has been calculated, and biostatisticians have determined that male smokers lose an average of 13.2 years of life while females lose 14.5 years of life.[119] This loss of life from smoking represents a reduction in the life expectancy of approximately 18%. Smoking exacts a heavy price.

Smoking encourages the accumulation of visceral fat (abdominal fat), which, from a health perspective, is the most harmful way to store fat. Visceral fat can be determined by a circumferential measurement of the waist. Evidence indicates that a waist circumference of 35 inches or more for females and 40 inches or more for males predisposes one to coronary heart disease, stroke, diabetes, and some forms of cancer. Visceral fat also leads to a constellation of risk factors, collectively referred to as metabolic syndrome (insulin-resistance syndrome). Metabolic syndrome begins with abdominal fat, which leads to insulin resistance, high blood pressure, low HDLs, high triglycerides, and elevated inflammatory proteins that substantially increase the risk for diabetes and cardiovascular disease.[120] An estimated 75 million of American adults have metabolic syndrome.

**Passive Smoking and Smokeless Tobacco.** Involuntary, or passive, smoking (inhaling the smoke of others) is associated with premature disease and death. Estimates indicate that 46,000 nonsmoking adults die annually of heart disease due to breathing the smoke of others, and another 3,400 die of lung cancer for the same

reason.[121] There is a dose-response relationship between breathing secondhand smoke (passive smoke) and illness and death from smoke-related diseases.

Children of smoking parents are more likely to experience a higher incidence of influenza, colds, bronchitis, asthma, and pneumonia. The impact of passive smoking on them can last a lifetime and ranges from delayed physical and intellectual development to the hazards associated with prolonged exposure to carcinogenic substances.[122]

An alarming trend is the escalating sale of smokeless tobacco products. Chewing tobacco and dipping snuff have become popular among high school and college men. The World Health Organization (WHO) has described the growing use of smokeless tobacco as a new threat to society. Nicotine is an addictive drug regardless of the method of delivery. Its effects are similar whether it is inhaled, as in smoking, or absorbed through the tissues of the oral cavity, as in dipping and chewing. The incidence of oral cancer may be 50 times higher among long-term users of smokeless tobacco products than among nonusers.[123] Smokeless tobacco is addictive and deadly, and its use is rising among adolescent males.

Cigar sales in the country had been flat for 25 years until 1994, when sales began to increase as the result of a marketing campaign by the magazine *Cigar Aficionado*, cigar invitation-only dinners, and celebrity endorsements of cigar smoking, characterizing it as sophisticated and glamorous. Cigar smoking is no longer looked upon as the sole dominion of males; many women have taken up the habit. Cigar sales increased from 3.4 billion in 1993 to 5.1 billion in 1997. This period of time represented a rejuvenation for the cigar industry.

Cigars were not specifically included in the 1984 law that required tobacco companies to place labels on packages of cigarettes warning that they are hazardous to health. But in the year 2000, the Federal Trade Commission (FTC) announced a settlement with the largest U.S. cigar companies requiring that health warnings be displayed on cigar products.[124] Five warning statements were developed, and each warning must be displayed an equal number of times on a rotating basis. See Table 2-6 for the surgeon general's warning statements. See also Just the Facts: Cigar Smoking: A Hazard to Health for more facts on cigar smoking.

### Some Exotic Forms of Smoking [125]

1. Clove cigarettes. Also called Kreteks, these cigarettes are imported mainly from Indonesia. They consist of 30 to 40% ground cloves, clove oil, and other additives, plus 60 to 70% tobacco. These cigarettes are not a safe alternative to smoking tobacco; in fact, they deliver on average more nicotine, carbon monoxide, and tars than conventional cigarettes.

## [ JUST THE FACTS ]

### Cigar Smoking: A Hazard to Health

A common assumption is that cigar smoking is not as hazardous as cigarette smoking because people usually don't inhale cigar smoke. Here are the facts regarding the dangers of cigar smoking:

- Nicotine reaches the brain by being absorbed through the lining of the mouth rather than from the lungs, but the effect is the same.[126] See Just the Facts: Nicotine for a summary of nicotine's harmful effects on the heart and blood vessels.

- Cigars have larger quantities of nicotine, carbon monoxide, hydrogen cyanide, and other chemicals than cigarettes.

- Nicotine is more easily absorbed by the cells lining the mouth and nose because cigar smoke is more acidic than cigarette smoke.[127]

2. Bidis. Referred to as "beedies," these flavored cigarettes are imported primarily from India. These cigarettes have grown in popularity, particularly among young people, because they are cheaper than regular cigarettes and because they come in multiple candy-like flavors, such as strawberry, vanilla, grape, and licorice. Beedies may be more harmful than regular cigarettes because they deliver more toxic products (i.e., nicotine, tars, carbon monoxide, and ammonia).

3. Hookah (water pipes). Water-pipe smoking originated in the Middle East. Flavored tobacco is burned in a water pipe and inhaled through a long hose. It is gaining in popularity on college campuses. The claim that water-pipe smoking is safer than cigarettes is based on the false assertion that water filters out many of the toxins found in tobacco. It does not, as evidenced by the fact that water-pipe smoking produces more toxins in the form of nicotine, carbon monoxide, tars, and other harmful substances. The reality is, there is no safe way to smoke.

**Some benefits of quitting the cigarette smoking habit._** There are many benefits to quitting the tobacco habit. Some occur within 20 minutes; others may take years. Following are a few of the benefits that occur after smoking the last cigarette.[128]

1. Blood pressure and heart rate decrease, and the temperature of hands and feet returns to normal in 20 minutes.

**TABLE 2-6**   The Surgeon General's Warning Statements

1. Cigar smoking can cause cancers of the mouth and throat even if you do not inhale.
2. Cigar smoking can cause lung cancer and heart disease.
3. Tobacco use increases the risk of infertility, stillbirth, and low birth weight.
4. Cigars are not a safe alternative to cigarettes.
5. Tobacco smoke increases the risk of lung cancer and heart disease even in nonsmokers.

Source: CDC. (2004, August 2). Warning label fact sheet (http://www.cdc.gov/tobacco/sgr_2000/factsheets/factsheet_labels.htm).

2. The risk for a sudden heart attack decreases in the first 24 hours.
3. Circulation improves and lung function increases up to 30% within 2 weeks to 3 months of quitting.
4. The risk for coronary heart disease declines by 50% after 1 year.
5. Stroke risk reduces to that of a nonsmoker 5 to 15 years after quitting.
6. The lung cancer death rate reduces by 50% 10 years after quitting.
7. The risk for coronary heart disease drops to that of a nonsmoker 15 years after quitting.

### Physical Inactivity

Physical inactivity has been officially recognized as a major risk factor for cardiovascular disease by the American Heart Association.[129] The upgrading of physical inactivity, which appeared in the AHA's 1993 report, reflects the importance of participating in physical activities regularly. The AHA made the upgrade because the weight of the evidence that has been accumulating in the last few decades shows that exercise produces many important health benefits. This is good news for those who have been physically active, and it may motivate some **sedentary** people to become active. People who do not engage in 30 minutes of moderately intense physical activity on most days of the week are considered to be sedentary.

Physical inactivity (hypokinesis) is debilitating to the human body. A couple of weeks of bed rest or chair rest produce muscle atrophy, bone demineralization, and decreases in aerobic capacity and maximum breathing capacity. The human body was constructed for and thrives on physical exertion. The rapid deterioration of the human body from physical inactivity was exemplified in the 1966 Dallas Bed Rest study and follow-up 30 years later in 1996.[130] In 1966, five healthy 20-year-old males volunteered to remain in bed for 3 weeks for the cause of science. Those 3 weeks resulted in significant losses in muscle size and strength, a large decrease in maximal oxygen consumption, substantial losses in breathing capacity, and loss of bone mineral density. Bed rest was followed by 8 weeks of vigorous aerobic exercise training, which completely reversed the declines experienced during the bed-rest phase of the study.

The atrophy that bed rest produced in the young, healthy volunteers had an influence on the way cardiologists began to treat heart attack patients. The new philosophy emphasized rehabilitation and exercise instead of extended bed rest.

Thirty years later, the five subjects, then age 50, returned to the lab for follow-up testing. They had gained an average of 50 pounds, their body fat had doubled, and they exercised irregularly, if at all. In spite of these negative physical changes, as well as 30 years of aging, their cardiorespiratory endurance was higher at age 50 than it was at age 20 after 3 weeks of bed rest. The men then consented to participate in a 6-month training program featuring jogging, brisk walking, and stationary cycling. At the end of the training program, the men became almost as physically fit as they were after 8 weeks of training in 1966. In other words, the training program almost completely reversed a 30-year decline in fitness. Many experts have been proclaiming that the closest thing to a fountain of youth is exercise. According to the results of the Dallas Bed Rest study, exercising like a 20-year-old can make you almost as fit as one.

Two major reviews have shown that physical inactivity poses a significant risk of developing heart disease. In one review, the researchers critiqued 43 studies and concluded that physical inactivity increased the risk for coronary heart disease by 1.5 to 2.4 times.[131] The risk associated with physical inactivity is similar to that of the other major risk factors. According to the Centers for Disease Control and Prevention, the need for regular exercise by the general public should be promoted as vigorously as efforts to control blood pressure, lower cholesterol, and stop smoking. A later review by another team of researchers concluded that inactive people have a 90% greater risk of developing coronary heart disease than do active people.[132] With few exceptions, the results of later studies are consistent with the results of these two reviews. Some of the more recent studies have indicated a dose-response relationship between level of physical activity and cardiovascular disease.[133] This means that (1) men at high risk who regularly participate in light- to moderate-intensity physical activity expending about 1,500 calories per week will likely lower their risk for coronary heart disease by about 25 to 50%, and (2) men who engage regularly in more intense physical activity (above the moderate level) lower their risk for coronary heart disease by 60 to 70% and experience greater longevity.

Several studies examined the effect on coronary heart disease of level of physical fitness rather than of total numbers of calories expended per week in physical activity. These studies corroborated the results of the calorie expenditure studies that physically fit people are less inclined to develop coronary heart disease than are unfit people.[134] A later study indicated that people in the lowest 20th percentile of physical fitness had a significantly higher risk for coronary heart disease than those whose fitness level was in the top 20th percentile and their CRP and fibrinogen levels were also significantly higher[135] In another study, subjects who performed below the 20th percentile on a maximal graded treadmill test were three to six times more likely to develop diabetes, hypertension, and metabolic syndrome than subjects who performed at or above the 60th percentile on the same test[140] Physical fitness is protective because it increases the pliability of the blood vessels, it increases the efficiency of the heart, and it has an ameliorating effect on hypertension, diabetes, and dyslipidemias (cholesterol and triglycerides)[136]

People actively engaged in leisure-time or occupational physical activity as well as those who participate in physical activities for the purpose of developing fitness are at a lower risk for death from cardiovascular disease and all-cause mortality. Major studies have supported the view that people who regularly engage in physical activities of moderate intensity have significantly fewer heart attacks and experience fewer deaths from all causes than do people who exercise little or not at all. Moderate activity was described as the equivalent of walking 1 to 2 miles per day for a total of 5 to 10 miles per week at a speed of 3 to 4 mph. The greatest health benefits were gained by those who expended 2,000 or more calories per week (20 miles of walking) in physical activity. A total of 17,000 men were followed for more than 30 years.[137] Those who regularly walked, climbed stairs, or participated in sports activities decreased their risk from all causes of mortality. Those who expended a minimum of 500 calories per week (5 miles of walking or its equivalent) to a maximum of 3,500 calories per week (35 miles of walking or its equivalent) experienced a progressive increase in longevity.

Investigators at the Cooper Institute for Aerobics Research studied the relationship between physical fitness and mortality from all causes.[138] The uniqueness of this study was twofold: first, the researchers measured the physical fitness levels of all subjects by treadmill testing; second, more than 3,000 of the 13,344 subjects were women. Because of their lower risk for cardiovascular disease, women have essentially been neglected as subjects in heart disease studies. The results of this study indicated that a low physical fitness level increased the risk for both men and women for death from cardiovascular disease, cancer, and all other forms of disease. The difference in all-cause mortality was greatest between those in the moderately fit category and those in the low-fit category. The difference between the moderately fit and the highly fit was insignificant. Physical inactivity increases the risk for coronary heart disease at a rate that is comparable to that observed for high blood pressure, high blood cholesterol, and cigarette smoking.[139]

In 2004, two prominent researchers examined the literature regarding the effect of exercise on the prevention of heart disease in women.[140] Numerous studies were identified and discussed. The evidence overwhelmingly indicated that physically active women of all ages benefited from mild, moderate, and vigorous exercise and experienced risk reduction for heart disease.

Graded treadmill tests of males hooked to an electrocardiograph have been used effectively as a diagnostic test for coronary heart disease. The effectiveness of this test for women has been less than desirable because it produces too many false-positive tests (the test shows they have heart disease, when in reality they do not).[141] However, graded maximal treadmill tests for women are more effective in predicting future heart disease when physicians assess fitness level and recovery heart rate.[142] Women who had higher fitness levels and faster recovery heart rates posttest had the lowest risk of dying from coronary heart disease during several years of follow-up.

Evidence also suggests that physical fitness is an important factor in the cardiovascular health of males.[143] Lower exercise capacity is a reliable predictor of mortality among normal men and men with existing cardiovascular disease.

People who consistently exercise above the moderate level not only receive the health benefits but also develop a higher level of physical fitness. There is an inverse relationship between physical activity and coronary artery disease, meaning that higher levels of physical activity invoke an incremental reduction in the risk for developing heart disease.[144]

The health and longevity returns from exercise and a physically active lifestyle are significant. Estimates indicate that longevity is increased by 1 minute for every minute spent walking and by 2 minutes for every minute spent jogging.[145] The message is clear: daily physical activity is healthy, a sedentary lifestyle is not. Many health professionals are attempting to focus the nation's attention on the relationship between a sedentary lifestyle and the dramatic increase in the number of deaths observed from chronic diseases.[146] As a result, the term **sedentary death syndrome** (SeDS) has been created to illustrate the burgeoning list of health disorders that are exacerbated by a lack of physical activity. SeDS relates to 23 diseases and conditions including elevated blood fats, Type 2 diabetes, hypertension, heart disease, obesity, osteoporosis, weak skeletal muscles, low physical endurance, resting tachycardia, and many

more. An estimated 60% of Americans are at risk for SeDS, and an estimated minimum of 250,000 will die annually for the next 10 years. Its proponents consider SeDS to be the second-greatest threat to public health.

In summary, much information supports the need for exercising regularly in order to prevent or delay the onset of cardiovascular disease and other diseases. Add this to the list: increasing and maintaining cardiorespiratory fitness throughout life may preserve endothelial function as we age.[147] Atherosclerosis begins with injuries that cause endothelial dysfunction in the coronary and other arteries. Physical exercise, on the other hand, protects the arteries and thereby plays a role in the prevention of atherosclerosis.

## Obesity

Obesity strains the heart and coexists with many of the modifiable risk factors that promote cardiovascular disease. Obese people who have no other risk factors are still more likely to develop heart disease or stroke. Obesity continues to rise precipitously in the United States. A total of 66.7% of adults (people over 20 years of age) are overweight or obese.[148] *Overweight* is defined as carrying excess weight for one's height regardless of body composition. *Obesity* is defined as carrying an excess of body fat regardless of height.[149] The trend in the last couple of decades is that the number of overweight/obese, physically inactive Americans is continuing to rise.[150] More alarming is the increase in the number of people who are 100 pounds overweight (this is extreme, or morbid, obesity). There are four times as many people in this category today than 15 years ago and five times as many people who are 150 pounds overweight than 15 years ago.[151] The rate of illness and death from obesity increases in proportion to the amount of excess weight. Obesity is a chronic, severe condition that can also worsen other medical conditions and disabilities. Not only is obesity associated with an increased risk for heart disease, but the manner in which fat is distributed in the body might also accentuate the risk.[152] Fat that accumulates in the upper half of the body (referred to as *visceral* or *central abdominal obesity*) is likely to be accompanied by high triglycerides, low HDL cholesterol, insulin resistance, and hypertension. This cluster of factors is called metabolic syndrome, and it is associated with a significant increase in the likelihood of developing cardiovascular disease.[153]

Risk factors for cardiovascular disease among American children and teenagers have been increasing from the last few decades. High blood pressure, lipid abnormalities, overweight/obesity, physical inactivity, use of tobacco products, metabolic syndrome, and Type 2 diabetes are all on the rise.[154] Children and adolescents need treatment to reduce these risks to prevent them from tracking into adulthood.

Obese people can lower their risk with a modest weight loss of 5 to 10%.[155] This is a realistic, attainable goal. But the risk remains lower only if the loss of weight is maintained. Approximately 95% of people who lose weight regain it in a few years. Although calorie restriction is the primary method for losing weight, regular exercise is the most effective method for maintaining the loss. Diet and exercise are not mutually exclusive; instead, they complement each other, and both are important players in weight management.

## Diabetes Mellitus

*Diabetes mellitus* is a metabolic disorder in which the body cannot make use of sugar (glucose) as a fuel. The hormone insulin must be produced and secreted into the bloodstream, so that blood sugar can be transported into the cells. The cells have receptor sites, to which insulin attaches, making the cell amenable to the entrance of sugar.

Diabetes mellitus has numerous long-range complications. These primarily involve degenerative disorders of the blood vessels and nerves. Diabetics who die prematurely are usually the victims of cardiovascular lesions and accelerated atherosclerosis. The incidence of heart attacks and strokes is higher among diabetics than nondiabetics. Diabetes increases the risk for coronary artery disease by 10 times that of nondiabetics.

In fact, diabetes is such a potent risk factor for coronary heart disease that, by itself, it is the risk equivalent of having had a previous heart attack.[156] See Chapter 13 for more details about diabetes.

## Stress

The effects of stress are difficult to quantify because two people in the same stressful environment may react quite differently. It is one's response to a stressor (events or situations that cause stress) that empowers its effect. See Nurturing Your Spirituality: Can Stress Cause a Heart Attack? Chapter 9 covers stress in depth.

# Preventing and Reversing Heart Disease

Preventing heart disease is much preferred to treating it after the fact. Prevention includes regular exercise, maintenance of optimal body weight, sound nutritional practices, abstinence from tobacco products, nonuse of alcohol (or use in moderation), and abstinence from drugs. Dealing with stress in constructive ways, removing oneself as much as possible from destructive and disease-producing environmental conditions, and having periodic medical examinations are other aspects of prevention. It is much better physically, psychologi-

 **Nurturing Your Spirituality**

### Can Stress Cause a Heart Attack?

A convincing body of evidence suggests that chronic anger, anxiety, loneliness, or depression can be catastrophic for people with coronary artery disease.[157] At the same time, emerging evidence shows that the same mood states and feelings in healthy people may increase the likelihood of developing heart disease in the future.

Scientists are beginning to unravel the connection between mood states and heart disease. Consistently high levels of stress hormones circulating in the bloodstream suppress the immune system by interfering with the normal repair and maintenance functions of the body. This increases one's vulnerability to infections and disease.[158] Continuing high levels of cortisol and norepinephrine stimulate a prolonged fight-or-flight response, which can eventually lead to wear and tear on the heart and arteries. Frequent and prolonged periods of stress increase blood pressure, and that usually leads to injuries of the artery walls. These injuries are the first step in the development and ultimate progression of atherosclerosis.[159] Data indicate that exaggerated responses to stress may be a triggering mechanism for heart attack and stroke.

Regular exercise promotes relaxation, reduces the response to stress, enhances emotional well-being, and lowers cardiac reactivity (high heart rate, blood pressure, and resistance to blood flow). Cardiac reactivity occurs when modest stressors produce physiological responses by the heart and circulatory system that are out of proportion to the stressor. If these occur frequently, the development of atherosclerosis may well be the result.

Exercise acts as a safety valve that enables people to "let off steam" in a constructive way. Jogging, swimming, cycling, weight training, racquetball, and other physical activities focus our energies in worthwhile pursuits that rid the body of stress products that have accumulated. Exercise training, a physiological stressor, helps build tolerance to psychological and emotional stressors. In other words, the "physiological toughness" developed through exercise training enables us to cope more effectively with other types of stressors.[160]

Does stress cause heart attacks? The answer is a qualified yes. We should have a more definitive answer after a few more years of research.

cally, and economically to make the effort to enhance health now than to reject or ignore health-promotion principles and treat disease later. It is never too late to change behavior. Even patients with coronary artery disease can benefit from lifestyle changes.

Until recently, medical thinking indicated that established atherosclerotic plaques in the coronary arteries were there to stay. Progression of the disease seemed inevitable unless medical corrective procedures were employed. But evidence has surfaced indicating that reversal of the disease is possible with appropriate lifestyle behaviors and/or medication.

Dean Ornish showed that comprehensive behavior changes are required to reverse established coronary artery disease. Ornish devised a program that included a vegetarian diet in which only 6.8% of the calories came from fat; 4.4 hours of moderate aerobic exercise per week; stress management techniques consisting of stretching exercises, practicing of breathing techniques, meditation, progressive relaxation, and the use of imagery; smoking cessation; and attendance at regular group support meetings. The subjects in this study were evaluated against a control group who received "usual and customary" care.[161]

At the end of the first year, 82% of the subjects in the Ornish program showed regression of atherosclerosis, compared with only 10% of the usual care group. Over the following 4 years, the Ornish subjects showed further regression, whereas the usual care group experienced progression of atherosclerosis.[162]

Other investigators have examined the effect of less stringent interventions than those advocated by the Ornish program on the regression of atherosclerosis. These attempts have been less successful than the Ornish program but more successful than the usual care program.

The main criticism of the Ornish program was that lifelong compliance would be difficult. Twenty-nine percent of the study participants dropped out during the last 4 years of the program. It is not easy to permanently change bad habits, but the hard work associated with following a low-fat diet, exercising consistently at a moderately intense level, and giving up smoking can make people with coronary artery disease feel better and may allow them to avoid surgery.

Refer to Assessment Activity 2-1 at the end of this chapter. Respond to each of the risk questions about factors to determine your risk status.

## Other Risk Factors

### Homocysteine

**Homocysteine** is a sulphur-containing amino acid produced as a normal by-product of methionine metabolism. Methionine is an essential amino acid that must

**TABLE 2-7**  Homocysteine

| Blood Level Micromoles/Liter | Risk |
|---|---|
| 5–15 | Normal |
| 16–30 | Moderate |
| 31–100 | Intermediate |
| > 100 | Severe |

> greater than

be obtained through the diet.[163] Under normal conditions, homocysteine is either converted back to methionine or it splits into two harmless nonessential amino acids that are easily flushed from the body through the urine. These conversions are accomplished by adequate intakes of folic acid, vitamin B6, and vitamin B12. Inadequate consumption of these three vitamins, folic acid in particular, results in a buildup of homocysteine in the blood. Homocysteine contributes to atherosclerosis because (1) it has a direct toxic effect, resulting in lesions that damage the cells lining the inside walls of the arteries; (2) it interferes with clotting factors; and (3) it oxidizes low-density lipoprotein (LDL).[164]

Homocysteine is measured by drawing blood after a 12-hour fast. See Table 2-7 for a breakdown of the categories of risk.

Two major meta-analyses were reported in the *Journal of the American Medical Association,* indicating that elevated homocysteine may not be as dangerous a risk factor as earlier studies suggested. Meta-analysis is a procedure using statistics to interpret the results of many studies, often with conflicting conclusions, by treating the results of each investigation as a discrete bit of data. These two studies led to the conclusion that elevated homocysteine appears to be a modest risk factor at best for heart disease and stroke.[165] It is also unclear at this time whether lowering homocysteine actually reduces the incidence of heart attacks and strokes. Further research is needed in order to shed more light on this risk factor.

### Lipoprotein (a)

**Lipoprotein (a)** is a molecule of bad LDL cholesterol with an extra protein attached.[166] A high level of Lp(a) may be harmful because it appears to interfere with the body's clot-busting system. However, cardiologists are not sure that elevated Lp(a) translates into an increase in heart attacks and strokes. The research is still equivocal on this point.[167]

Lp(a) values above 30 milligrams per deciliter (mg/dL) of blood are considered to be high, and a very high value is above 50 mg/dL.[168] Lp(a) blood levels are determined primarily by one's genetic makeup, as opposed to lifestyle factors.[169] While lifestyle behaviors can lower the risk for cardiovascular disease by impacting blood pressure, blood lipid levels, obesity, and so on, they appear to have no effect on Lp(a). At this point, prescription strength niacin (one of the B vitamins) is the only treatment reputed to lower Lp(a).

Lp(a) is not routinely measured by physicians. It is likely to be measured when physicians need more information regarding the diagnosis of heart disease. For now, most physicians will continue to rely on the tried-and-true risk factors previously covered in this chapter.

## High-Sensitivity C-Reactive Protein (hs-CRP)

C-reactive protein (CRP), a biomarker for inflammation, was discovered 75 years ago. CRP is elevated in many diseases that have an inflammatory component, such as colorectal cancer, hypertension, rheumatoid arthritis, sepsis (blood poisoning), diabetes mellitus, and metabolic syndrome.[170] CRP is made by the liver in response to infection, inflammation, injury, or stress, and elevations can be detected by a blood test. This test has been available for many years but it was not sensitive enough to detect low levels of inflammation that are indicative of atherosclerosis.[171] The new and improved version, high-sensitivity C-reactive protein (hs-CRP), can identify inflammation earlier and at lower levels than its predecessor. Atherosclerosis, the underlying cause of 80% of coronary heart disease, is a low-level inflammatory process. The newer, more sensitive test shows promise as a diagnostic tool for detecting atherosclerosis early, so that an intervention program can be developed and put in place early in the process.

While many major prospective studies in the United States and other countries have found CRP to be a strong, robust, independent risk factor for cardiovascular disease, others are questioning their results. A large European meta-analysis has provided data indicating that CRP is a relatively moderate predictor of future coronary heart disease and that it adds only marginally to the predictive value of the major risk factors.[172] On the other hand, many other studies have found that CRP is more predictive of heart disease than are high LDLs. While LDL, HDL, and total cholesterol are established risk factors for heart disease, hs-CRP provides information regarding inflammation in the arteries. Lipid testing cannot produce this type of important information.[173] More research is needed to resolve this issue.

## Fibrinogen

An elevated **fibrinogen** level in the blood is positively correlated with heart disease and stroke. Fibrinogen adds to the viscosity (thickness or stickiness) of the blood and enhances the formation of blood clots.[174] High fibrinogen levels are more common in men than women, in smokers than nonsmokers, in those physically inactive than those who are active, and in those with high serum triglycerides than those with low levels.

## Peripheral Artery Disease (PAD)

**Peripheral artery disease**, also called peripheral vascular disease (PVD), affects between 8 and 12 million people.[175] Peripheral artery disease is defined as the narrowing or occlusion of arteries in the periphery (outside of the heart and brain) resulting from atherosclerotic plaque that leads to heart attacks and strokes. This disorder commonly occurs in the legs.[176] Clogged leg arteries limit or deprive muscles of blood and oxygen, which accounts for the leg pain (intermittent claudication) that occurs during walking, climbing stairs, or other weight-bearing activities. The pain ceases a few minutes after stopping the activity.[177] Peripheral artery disease is a symptom of heart disease and a warning that atherosclerosis in the legs is probably, and concurrently, occurring in the heart, brain, and other areas of the body.

Prevention and/or treatment of PAD follows the same prescription for preventing or treating atherosclerosis anywhere in the body. The regimen includes a coordinated approach featuring lifestyle behaviors and medical supervision. Regular exercise, control of blood pressure, glucose, cholesterol, stress, and body weight, and cessation of tobacco products are required.[178] Medical intervention such as medication and/or surgery may also be required.

Peripheral artery disease should be taken seriously as a predictor of heart attack or stroke by patient and physician alike.

## Metabolic Syndrome

The term *metabolic syndrome* represents an extremely high level of risk for cardiovascular disease and stroke because it is not one, but a collection of risk factors.[179] The cumulative effect of multiple risk factors depicts an increased vulnerability to atherosclerosis. A diagnosis of metabolic syndrome is made when three or more of the following are present:

1. Abnormal obesity: weight circumference greater than 40 inches for males and 35 inches for females.
2. Insulin resistance or diabetes: fasting blood glucose level of 100 mg/dL or higher.
3. Triglycerides: 150 mg/dL or higher.
4. HDL cholesterol: below 40 mg/dL for males or below 50 mg/dL for females.
5. Blood pressure: systolic pressure 130 mm Hg or higher, or diastolic pressure 85 mmHg or higher.

## Sleep Apnea

Obstructive **sleep apnea** (OSA) affects approximately 12 million Americans, most of whom are men between the ages of 40 and 70.[180] It is characterized by periodic interruption in breathing while asleep. Each episode lasts 20–30 seconds and may occur several hundred times per night. These episodes occur because the soft tissues of the throat collapse and partially or totally block the airway. As a result, the lungs receive an inadequate supply of oxygen, which causes a strain on the heart that may culminate in arrhythmias, high blood pressure, heart attack, and stroke.[181] The risk of death for those who suffer with sleep apnea is 40% higher compared to nonsufferers.

The major risk factor for sleep apnea is overweight. Contributing risk factors include cigarette smoking and regular use of alcohol and sedatives.[182] The symptoms include loud snoring, gasping for breath, interrupted sleep, daytime drowsiness, irritability, and heartburn.

The most effective and widely recommended treatment for sleep apnea is CPAP (continuous positive airway pressure). This device includes a mask that delivers pressurized air during sleep to prevent the airway from collapsing. Evidence indicates that CPAP is 95% effective.[183] The drawback is that it is uncomfortable and inconvenient to wear while trying to sleep. Severe cases may require surgery to remove tonsils and tissues from the roof of the mouth and back of the throat. Refer to Assessment Activity 2-1 to obtain an estimate of the probability of having a heart attack.

## Medical Contributions

### Diagnostic Techniques

Diagnosing cardiovascular disease is becoming more sophisticated. Diagnosis begins with a medical examination and patient history. This procedure may be supplemented with a variety of tests, which may confirm or refute the physician's suspicions of the presence of cardiovascular disease. Graded exercise tests (GXTs) using a motor-driven treadmill with the patient hooked to an electrocardiogram (ECG) have gained popularity in the medical community. Such noninvasive tests use surface electrodes on the chest that are sensitive to the electrical actions of the heart. Mechanical abnormalities of the heart produce abnormal electrical impulses displayed on the ECG strip. These are read and interpreted by the physician.

The treadmill "road tests" the heart as it works progressively harder to meet the increasing oxygen requirement as the exercise protocol becomes more physically demanding. This test is more accurate for men than women. The gender difference in response to the treadmill test is not completely understood, but it is believed that women's breasts and extra fat tissue interfere with the reception of electrical impulses by the chest electrodes. But the treadmill test is still a useful tool in diagnosing potential heart problems for women if attention

is shifted to a woman's physical fitness level; that is, how well she performs on the test, and how quickly her heart rate recovers immediately after the test ends.[184]

In some cases, a thallium treadmill test is required because it is more sensitive; however, it is also much more expensive. This involves the injection of radioactive thallium during the final minute of the treadmill test. Thallium is accepted, or taken up, by normal heart muscle but not by ischemic heart muscle.[185] The absorption or nonabsorption of thallium can be seen on a monitor. The thallium stress test increases diagnostic sensitivity to cardiovascular disease to approximately 81%.[186]

*Echocardiography* is a safe, noninvasive technique that uses sound waves to determine the size of the heart, the thickness of the walls, and the function of the heart's valves.[187] *Cardiac catheterization* is an invasive technique in which a slender tube is threaded from a blood vessel in an arm or a leg into the coronary arteries. A liquid contrast dye that can be seen on X-ray film is injected into the coronary arteries. X-ray films are taken throughout the procedure to locate where and how severely the coronary arteries are narrowed.[188]

### Medical Treatment

A variety of drugs are used in cardiovascular therapies. These drugs lower blood pressure and cholesterol level, minimize the likelihood of blood clotting, and dissolve clots during a heart attack.

Daily aspirin therapy lowers the risk for having a heart attack or stroke, but it may not be appropriate for everyone.[189] Aspirin use is contraindicated for bleeding disorders, asthma, stomach ulcers, and heart failure. It is indicated for those who have had a heart attack or stroke and for all others who have significant risk factors for either. However, the guidelines for aspirin usage differ somewhat for men and women.[190] (See Just the Facts Box for Current Guidelines for Daily Aspirin Use for Men and Women).

Aspirin is a drug and as such carries some degree of risk—discuss aspirin usage with your physician, who will determine the need for or the appropriate dose for your circumstance. Evidence indicates that a dosage as low as 71 milligrams may be as effective as larger doses. A baby aspirin is 81 milligrams while a full dose is 325 milligrams.

You should not stop aspirin therapy without consulting with your physician, because sudden stoppage can result in a rebound effect that can precipitate the formation of a blood clot.[191] Aspirin is effective because it is an anti-inflammatory agent and atherosclerosis is an inflammatory disease.[192] Aspirin also plays a role in the prevention of blood clots that might form in arteries. Additionally, there is growing evidence that aspirin may help reduce the risk for colorectal, esophageal, stomach,

## [ JUST THE FACTS ]

### Current Guidelines for Daily Aspirin Use for Men and Women

| Daily Aspirin Intake May: | Women under 65 years of age | Women over 65 years of age | Men all ages |
|---|---|---|---|
| Prevent first heart attack | No | Yes | Yes |
| Prevent second heart attack | Yes | Yes | Yes |
| Reduce heart disease risk | Yes | Yes | Yes |
| Prevent first stroke | Yes | Yes | No |

prostate, and ovarian cancer because it may inhibit the chemical pathways that fuel tumor growth.

Should people chew and swallow an aspirin if they think they are in the midst of having a heart attack? The answer is yes. The proper protocol is to call 9-1-1 within 5 minutes of the onset of symptoms and chew and swallow a 325-mg aspirin while you wait.[193]

Surgical techniques have also affected the treatment of cardiovascular disease. *Coronary artery bypass graft (CABG) surgery* is designed to shunt blood around an area of blockage by removing a leg vein and sewing one end of a leg vein into the aorta and the other end into a coronary artery below the blockage, thereby restoring blood flow to the heart muscle (Figure 2-8). The internal mammary arteries also are used for bypass grafts. Many authorities consider these to be the ideal grafts. There are two internal mammary arteries, but the one in the left side of the chest is preferable because it is nearer to the coronary arteries. Many surgeons would rather not use both arteries in the same patient because the diminished flow of blood to the chest impairs healing of the surgical wound. Also, fashioning bypass grafts out of these arteries is time-consuming precision surgery, there are only two of them, and they don't reach all parts of the heart. The advantage is that 95% of them remain open 20 to 30 years after surgery.[194]

In 2006, 448,000 CABG surgical procedures were performed, at an average cost of $99,700 each.[195] This procedure requires the surgical team to place the patient on a heart-lung machine, which pumps blood to the body's tissues while the heart is stopped for repairs. Postsurgical complications, primarily temporary short-term memory loss, may occur. Research indicates that this loss probably occurs because the heart-lung bypass machine produces microemboli (tiny blood clots), which flow to the brain and reduce its oxygen supply.

A new off-pump procedure has been developed that does not require stoppage of the heart while the surgeon sews the bypass grafts. This procedure is accomplished laparoscopically—that is, long, slender surgical instruments are inserted through several small incisions. There are fewer complications and a shorter rehabilitation with off-pump procedures. Also, studies indicate that off-pump bypass surgery is at least as effective as traditional bypass procedures.[196]

Balloon angioplasty, laser ablation, coronary atherectomy, and coronary stents are collectively referred to as percutaneous coronary interventions (PCIs). In 2006, an estimated 1,313,000 PCI procedures were performed in the United States at an average cost of $48,399 each.[197] More than 70% of PCI procedures involved the insertion of a drug-eluting stent as opposed to a bare metal stent.

*Balloon angioplasty* uses a catheter with a doughnut-shaped balloon at the tip. The catheter is positioned at the narrow point in the artery, and the balloon is inflated, which cracks and compresses the plaque, stretches the artery wall, and widens the blood vessel to allow greater blood flow (Figure 2-9). Laser ablation uses heat to burn away plaque if the catheter can be maneuvered into the correct position. This technology appears to be useful for patients with certain types of atherosclerotic narrowings or blockages. Coronary atherectomy, one of the newest techniques, uses a specially tipped catheter equipped with a high-speed rotary cutting blade to shave off plaque.

Catheterization techniques are also used to implant a coronary stent in a diseased artery. The stent is a flexible, metallic tube that functions as a scaffold to support the walls of diseased arteries, thus maintaining an open pas-

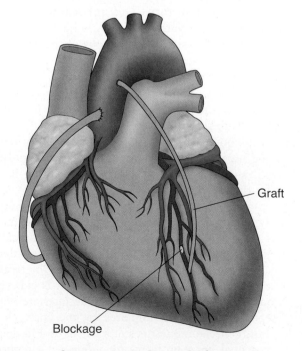

Figure 2-8   Coronary Artery Bypass Graft

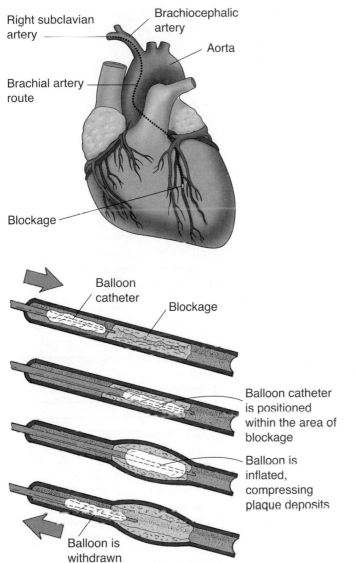

FIGURE 2-9  Balloon Angioplasty

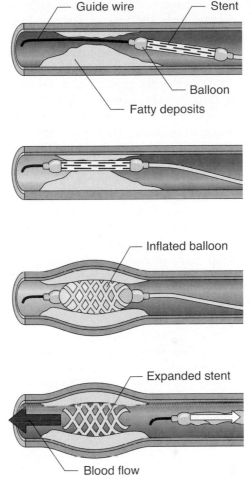

FIGURE 2-10  Coronary Stent

sage for blood flow (Figure 2-10). Stents are positioned in such arteries by a catheter. When correctly positioned, a balloon inside the stent is inflated, causing the stent to expand. This action stretches the artery. Then the balloon is withdrawn, leaving the expanded stent behind to keep the blood vessel open. The problem with this procedure is the damage that occurs to the fragile inner lining of the artery during the placement of the stent. The body's response to this injury is inflammation, accompanied by rampant cell growth, which is needed to heal the wound. Cell growth occurs around and into the stent, narrowing the artery and reducing blood flow. To circumvent this occurrence, stents coated with drugs that stop prolific muscle cell growth have been developed. These drug-eluting stents show great promise in averting restenosis (renarrowing of the artery), compared with stents without the drug. In fact, follow-up studies have shown that drug-eluting stents reduce the probability of restenosis by about 50% when compared to bare metal stents.[198] But, a problem unique to drug-eluting stents surfaced in 2006 when studies found that a small number of recipients suffered blood clots months and years after implantation. This prompted the American Heart Association to recommend that two anticlotting medications be prescribed: aspirin for an indefinite period of time, and Plavix for at least 1 year or longer. The next few years should determine the effectiveness of this approach.

Artificial valves have been developed to replace defective heart valves, and these work well. The cost of replacing a valve in 2006, the latest year for which we have data, was $141,210.[199] In the summer of 2001, the first successful self-contained mechanical heart was implanted in the chest of a male patient whose life expectancy was literally being measured in days. This device, the Abio-Cor artificial heart, is considered experimental and its long-term success rate has yet to be demonstrated.[200] However, it is a technological giant step forward, compared with its predecessors, and with modifications it seems to have great potential for extending the lives of people whose hearts are so severely damaged that conventional medical treatments are ineffective. Fourteen severely ill patients have received the AbioCor artificial heart, and all 14 have died. The longest survivor lived for 17 months after implantation. There are two major problems with the AbioCor: (1) its size—it weighs about 2 pounds and can be used only in relatively large people, and (2) there is a concern that the plastic and metal parts may wear out in 2 to 5 years necessitating additional surgery to replace them. The developers of the AbioCor are diligently working to overcome these problems.[201]

The current cost of the AbioCor is $250,000 plus hospital stay.

Mechanical devices (left ventricular assist devices) have been used to aid the failing hearts of patients awaiting donor hearts. These devices take over the burden of pumping blood throughout the body and may keep patients alive for several months or more.[202]

Heart transplants have prolonged many lives. The outlook for patients has improved considerably because of the development and use of medicines to suppress the immune system in such patients and because of refinements in the prevention and early detection of the body's attempts to reject donor hearts. As a result, about 87.5% for males and 85.5% for females live longer than 1 year, and more than half survive at least 12 years.[203] The longest living survivor has lived for 18 years with a transplanted heart. The longest survivor, who has recently died, survived 27 years with a transplanted heart.[204]

Candidates for transplants are those whose hearts are irreversibly damaged with disease that does not respond to conventional treatment. Without a new heart, these people will die. The main problems associated with heart transplantation are insufficient numbers of donors, the difficulty of procuring compatible donor hearts, and the constant threat of organ rejection by the recipient.

## Summary

- Approximately 1.5 million heart attacks occur each year, and 500,000 of these result in death.
- The heart is two pumps in one: the pulmonary pump, which sends deoxygenated blood to the lungs, and the systemic pump, which sends oxygenated blood to all tissues of the body.
- Blood plasma is a clear, yellowish fluid that makes up about 55% of the blood. The remaining 45% consists of blood solids—red blood cells, white blood cells, and blood platelets.
- Strokes are caused by a thrombus, an embolus, or a hemorrhage.
- Coronary heart disease is a disease of the coronary blood vessels that take nourishment and oxygen to the heart.
- Many of the risk factors for heart disease originate in childhood.
- The treatment of heart disease includes the development of appropriate lifestyle habits and medical intervention.
- The major risk factors that cannot be changed are age, male gender, and heredity.

- The major risk factors that can be changed are elevated cholesterol levels, hypertension, cigarette smoking, physical inactivity, obesity, diabetes mellitus, and stress.
- The other contributing risk factors are homocysteine, lipoprotein (a), high-sensitivity CRP, fibrinogen, peripheral artery disease, metabolic syndrome, and sleep apnea.
- Cholesterol is a steroid that is essential for many body functions, but too much circulating in the blood creates a risk for cardiovascular disease.
- Low-density lipoproteins are associated with the development of atherosclerotic plaque.
- High-density lipoproteins protect the arteries from the formation of plaque.
- Blood pressure is the force exerted against the walls of the arteries as blood is pumped from the heart and travels through the circulatory system.
- *Hypertension* is the medical term for high blood pressure.
- Cigarette smoking may be the most potent of the risk factors associated

with chronic illness and premature death.
- Involuntary, or passive, smoking is associated with premature disease and death.
- Obesity is a major risk factor that often coexists with many of the other risk factors for cardiovascular disease.
- Diabetes mellitus must be controlled to reduce the accompanying cardiovascular complications.
- Regular exercise significantly reduces the risk for Type 2 diabetes mellitus.
- Stress predisposes a person to illness and may hasten the disease process.
- Elevated levels of homocysteine and of Lp(a) in the blood are proving to be important risk factors for heart disease.
- Medical research has made a significant contribution to reducing the incidence of heart disease through the development of sophisticated technological advances in diagnosis and treatment.

## Review Questions

1. Define *pulmonary pump* and *systemic pump* and discuss the function of each.
2. Describe the advent of heart disease in the United States.
3. Identify and describe the causes of stroke.

4. What is coronary heart disease? Discuss the available treatment options.
5. What are the risk factors for heart disease and how are they categorized by the AHA?
6. What is cholesterol? LDL? HDL?

7. What is the relationship between total cholesterol and HDL?
8. What is essential hypertension?
9. What ingredients in cigarettes increase the risk for cardiovascular disease? Describe their effect on the heart and blood vessels.

# References

1. American Heart Association. (2009a). *Heart disease and stroke statistics—2009 update*. Dallas, Texas: American Heart Association.
2. Ibid.
3. Gerstenblith, G., & S. Margolis. (2008). *Coronary heart disease*. Baltimore, MD: Johns Hopkins Medicine.
4. Xu, Jiaquan, et al. (2009). Deaths: Preliminary data for 2007. *Vital Statistics Reports*, 58(1). Washington, DC: U.S. Department of Health and Human Services.
5. American Heart Association (2009a).
6. Editors. (2006, January). Longevity Report. *U.C. Berkeley Wellness Letter* 22(4), 8.
7. Ibid.
8. Gerstenblith, G. (2008).
9. Nieman, D. C. ( 2007). *Exercise testing and prescription* (6th ed.). Boston: McGraw-Hill.
10. Editors. (2006, July 6). Aerobics and cardio information. Retrieved from http://www.neverstoptrying.com/aerobics-cardio/35374.php.
11. Editors. (2009, December 15). Heart rate. Retrieved from Wikipedia, The Free Encyclopedia, at http://en.wikipedia.org/wiki/Heart_rate.
12. American Heart Association. (2009b). *Heart and stroke facts*. Dallas, Texas: American Heart Association.
13. American Heart Association (2009a).
14. Ibid.
15. Squires, R. W. (2006). Pathophysiology and clinical features of cardiovascular diseases. In *ACSMs Resource Manual* (5th ed.), edited by L. A. Kaminsky. Philadelphia: Lippincott Williams and Wilkins.
16. Blumenthal, R. S., & S. Margolis. (2008). *Heart attack prevention*. Baltimore, MD: Johns Hopkins Medicine.
17. Kannell, W. B., et al. (1968). Epidemiology of acute myocardial infarction: The Framingham Study. *Medicine Today*, 2, 50.
18. Staff. (2009, December 16). Heart disease risk factors for children and teenagers. Retrieved from Texas Heart Institute at http://www.texasheartinstitute.org/hic/topics/hsmart/children_risk_factors.cfm
19. Ibid.
20. American Heart Association. (2009, December 16). Exercise (physical activity) and children: AHA Scientific Position. Retrieved from http://www.americanheart.org/presenter.jhtml?identifier=4596.
21. American Heart Association (2009a).
22. American Heart Association. (2009, December 16). Overweight in children, AHA Recommendations. Retrieved from http://www.americanheart.org/presenter.jhtml?identifer=4670.
23. American Heart Association (2009a).
24. Zieve, D., & N. K. Kaneshiro. (2009, October 1). Weight problems in children. Retrieved from *Medline Plus* at http://www.n/m.nih.gov/medlineplus/ency/article/001999.htm.
25. Ogden, C. L., et al. (2006, April 5). Prevalence of overweight and obesity in the United States 1999–2004. *Journal of the American Medical Association*, 295, 1549.
26. Tufts University. (2000). More kids are getting diabetes and more should be screened for it. *Tufts University Health and Nutrition Letter*, 18(2), 2.
27. American Heart Association (2009a).
28. Ibid.
29. U.S. Department of Health and Human Services. (2000). *Healthy people 2010: Understanding and improving health* (2nd ed.). Washington, D.C.: U.S. Government Printing Office.
30. Editors. (2006, August 24). Cardiovascular disorders: High blood pressure in children and adolescents. Retrieved from Lucille Packard Children's Hospital at Stanford, at http://www.pch.org/diseaseHealthInfo/HealthLibrary/cardiac/hbpca.html.
31. Zieve & Kaneshiro (2009).
32. Squires (2006).
33. American Heart Association (2009a).
34. Gerstenblith & Margolis (2008).
35. Waldstein, S. R., et al. (2004). Stress induced blood pressure reactivity and silent cardiovascular disease. *Stroke*, 35, 1294.
36. American Heart Association (2009b).
37. American Heart Association (2009a).
38. American Heart Association (2009b).
39. American Heart Association (2009a).
40. American Stroke Association. (2006, July 21). A simple test for stroke. A Division of the American Heart Association. Retrieved from http://www.strokeassociation.org/presenter.jhtml?identifier=3032226.
41. American Heart Association (2009b).
42. American Heart Association (2009a).
43. American Heart Association (2009b).
44. Ibid.
45. Ibid.
46. Gerstenblith & Margolis (2008).
47. American Heart Association (2009a).
48. Editors. (2009, September). His and hers heart disease. *Harvard Health Letter*, 34(11), 1.
49. American Cancer Society. (2009). How many women get breast cancer? Retrieved from http://www.cancer.org/docroot/CRI/content/CRI_2_2_IX_How_many_people_get_breast_cancer_5.asp.
50. American Heart Association (2009a).
51. Editors (2009, September).
52. Bhatt, D. L. (2006). *Coronary heart disease*. Norwalk, CT: Belvoir Media Group
53. American Heart Association (2009b).
54. Ibid.
55. Ibid.
56. Ibid.
57. Ibid.
58. Greenland, P., et al. (2003). Major risk factors as antecedents of fatal and non-fatal coronary heart disease events. *Journal of the American Medical Association*, 290(7), 891.
59. Sharma, A. (2006). Further analysis of interheart: What do the data tell clinicians? *Medscape Cardiology*. Retrieved from http://www.medscape.com/viewarticle/520569_print.
60. American Heart Association (2009b).
61. Editors. (2009, July). The new skinny on fats. *Tufts Health and Nutrition Letter*, 27(5), 4.
62. Editors. (2007, September). Time to fatten up our diets. *Harvard Health Letter*, 32(11), 1.
63. Editors. (2008, July). Egg-cellent news for most, but not those with diabetes. *Harvard Health Letter*, 33(9), 6

64. Editors. (2006, July). To make an omelet you have to break some eggs. *Harvard Heart Letter,* 16(11), 3–4.

65. Editors. (1984). The lipid research clinics coronary primary prevention trial results. 1. Reduction in incidence of coronary heart disease. *Journal of the American Medical Association,* 251, 351.

66. LaRosa, J. C., et al. (1990). The cholesterol facts: A summary of the evidence relating dietary facts, serum cholesterol, and coronary heart disease: A joint statement by the American Heart Association, and the National Heart, Lung, and Blood Institute. *Circulation,* 81, 1721.

67. Editors. (2009, January). Changing picture of atherosclerosis. *Harvard Heart Letter,* 19(5), 4–5.

68. Cunningham, D. S. (2004, July). Quenching the flames of inflammation. *Life Extension,* 10(7), 27–34.

69. Editors (2009, January).

70. Bhatt (2006).

71. Editors. (2009, January). Changing the cardiovascular prevention game. *Harvard Health Letter,* 34(3), 6.

72. Cannon, C. P. (2006, June 22). The reasons and uses of C-reactive rrotein (CRP). *Medscape Cardiology.* Retrieved from http://www.medscape.com/viewarticle/531852_print.

73. Ibid.

74. Editors. (2005, December). Bad cholesterol: Very low is better—and safe. *Cleveland Clinic Heart Advisor,* 8(2), 2.

75. American Heart Association (2009b).

76. Boggs, W. (2006, June 23). Increasing HDL level independently reduces cardiovascular risk. *Medscape.* Retrieved from http://www.medscape.com/viewarticle/535816.

77. Nagelkirk, P. (2010). Pathophysiology and treatment of cardiovascular disease. In *ACSMs Resource Manual* (6th ed.), edited by J. K. Ehrman. Philadelphia: Walters Kluwer/Lippincott Williams and Wilkins.

78. Barcley, L. & D. Lie. (2005, January 28). HHS, USDA issue new dietary guidelines. *Medscape* Medical News. Retrieved from http://www.medscape.com/viewarticle/494517_print.

79. Nieman (2007).

80. Ibid.

81. Squires (2006).

82. Gerstenblith & Margolis (2008).

83. Editors. (2009, December 29). What is blood triglyceride? Retrieved from http://www.fatfreekitchen.com/cholesterol/triglycerides.html.

84. Thomas, T. R. & T. P. Lafontaine. (2001). Exercise nutritional strategies, and lipoproteins. In *ACSMs Resource Manual* (4th ed.), edited by J. L. Roitman. Philadelphia: Lippincott Williams and Wilkins.

85. Nieman (2007).

86. Ibid.

87. American Heart Association (2009a).

88. Ibid.

89. Kshirsager, A. V., et al. (2006, February). Blood pressure usually considered normal is associated with an elevated risk of cardiovascular diseases. *American Journal of Medicine,* 119(2), 133–141.

90. Vidt, D. (2009, June). Hypertension treatment in the elderly needs careful scrutiny. *Heart Advisor,* 12(6), 3.

91. Gerstenblith & Margolis (2008).

92. Radecki, T. E. (2009, December 30). Pulse pressure. Retrieved from http://www.modern-psychiatry.com/pulse_pressure.htm.

93. Ibid.

94. American Heart Association (2009a).

95. Ibid.

96. Ibid.

97. Ibid.

98. Ibid.

99. Editors. (2009, May). New reasons to be wary of hidden salt. *Tufts University Health and Nutrition Letter,* 27(3), 4–5.

100. Liebman, B. (2005, July/August). Pressure cooker—The scoops on salt. *Nutrition Action Health Letter,* 32(6), 1, 3.

101. Editors. (2008, August). DASH diet ignored, *Harvard Heart Letter,* 18(12), 6.

102. Liebman (2005, July/August).

103. Editors. (2004, April). New consumption guidelines issued for water, sodium, and potassium. *Tufts University Health and Nutrition Letter,* 22(2), 4.

104. Byrd-Bredbenner, C., et al. (2009). *Wardlaw's perspectives in nutrition.* New York: McGraw Hill Companies, Inc.

105. Editors. (2009, December). Blood pressure: How low should you go? *Harvard Heart Letter,* 20(4), 4.

106. Gerstenblith & Margolis (2008).

107. Editors. (2003, July). What was normal blood pressure is now considered too high. *Tufts University Health and Nutrition Letter,* 21, 4.

108. Pescatello, L. S., et al. (2004). Position stand—Exercise and hypertension. *Medicine and Science in Sports and Exercise,* 533–553.

109. American Heart Association (2009b).

110. American Cancer Society. (2010, January 4). Questions about smoking, tobacco, and health. Retrieved from http://www.cancer.org/docroot/PED/content/PED_10_2x_Questions_About_Smoking_Tobacco_and_Health.asp?sitearea=PED&viewmode=print&.

111. Ibid.

112. Ibid.

113. Ibid.

114. Glaxo Smith Kline Consumer Health Care. (2006, July 12). More than 5 million smokers successfully smoke-free since therapeutic nicotine made available over-the-counter a decade ago. Retrieved from http://www.committedquiters.com.

115. American Cancer Society. (2009). *Cancer prevention and early detection facts and figures.* Atlanta, GA: American Cancer Society.

116. American Cancer Society. (2009, November 23). Guide to quitting smoking. Retrieved from http://www.cancer.org/docroot/PED/content/PED_10_13x_Guide_for_Quitting_Smoking.asp?sistearea=PED&viewmode=print&.

117. Ibid.

118. American Heart Association (2009b).

119. Ibid.

120. American Heart Association (2009a)

121. Ibid.

122. Ibid.

123. American Cancer Society (2010, January 4).

124. American Cancer Society (2009).

125. Ibid.

126. American Cancer Society. (2009, October 1). Cigar smoking. Retrieved from http://www.cancer.org/docroot/PED/content/PED_10_2x_Cigar_Smoking.sap?siterea=PED&viewmode=print&.

127. American Cancer Society (2010, January 4).

128. American Cancer Society (2009, November 23).

129. American Heart Association (2009b).

130. Ibid.

131. Ibid.
132. Editors. (2002, January). Dallas bed rest study. *Harvard Heart Letter,* 12(5), 6.
133. Powell. K. E. (1987). Physical activity and the incidence of coronary heart disease. *Annual Review of Public Health,* 8, 253.
134. Berlin, J. A., & G. A. Colditz. (1990). A meta-analysis of physical activity in the prevention of coronary heart disease. *American Journal of Epidemiology,* 132, 612.
135. Katzmarzyk, P. T. (2006). Physical activity status and chronic diseases. In *ACSMs Resource Manual* (5th ed.), edited by L. A. Kaminsky. Philadelphia: Lippincott Williams and Wilkins.
136. Blair, S. N., et al. (1995). Changes in physical fitness and all-cause mortality: A prospective study of healthy and unhealthy men. *Journal of the American Medical Association,* 273, 1093.
137. Barclay, L., & D. Lie. (2004, January). Fitness important for cardiovascular health. *Medscape Medical News.* Retrieved from http://www.medscape.com/viewarticle/466028.
138. Ibid.
139. Editors. (2010, January). Exercise can improve arterial elasticity. *Heart Advisor,* 13(1), 2.
140. Paffenbarger, R. S., et al. (1993). The association of changes in physical activity level and other lifestyle characteristics with mortality among men. *New England Journal of Medicine,* 328, 538.
141. Blair, S. N., et al. (1989). Physical fitness and all-cause mortality—Prospective study of healthy men and women. *Journal of the American Medical Association,* 262, 2395.
142. American Heart Association (2009b).
143. Bussuck, S. S., & J. E. Manson. (2004). Preventing cardiovascular disease in women: How much physical activity is good enough? *PCPFS Research Digest,* 5(4), 1.
144. ACSM. (2010). *ACSM's guidelines for testing and prescription* (8th ed.). Philadelphia: Walters Kluwer/ Lippincott Williams and Wilkins.
145. Ibid.
146. Katzymarzyk (2006).
147. Kraus, W. E. (2010). Physical activity status and chronic diseases. In *ACSMs Resource Manual* (6th ed.), edited by J. K. Ehrman. Philadelphia: Walters Kluwer Lippincott Williams and Wilkins.
148. Lee, I. M., & R. S. Raffenbarger. (2000). Associations of light, moderate, and vigorous intensity physical activity with longevity: The Harvard Alumni Health Study. *American Journal of Epidemiology,* 151, 293.
149. Booth, F. (2002, March). Costs and consequences of sedentary living: New battleground for an old enemy. *PCPFS Research Digest,* 3(16), 1.
150. Bussuck & Manson (2004).
151. American Heart Association (2009a).
152. National Institute of Diabetes and Digestive and Kidney Diseases (NIDDK). (2009, October 21). Statistics related to overweight and obesity. Retrieved from http://win.niddk.nih.gov/statistics/.
153. American Heart Association (2009a).
154. Editors. (2003, December). Americans getting heavier still. *Tufts University Health and Nutrition Letter,* 21(10), 2.
155. American Heart Association (2009b).
156. Ibid.
157. Ibid.
158. Ibid.
159. Ryan, A., & L. Joseph. (2010). Pathophysiology and treatment of metabolic diseases in *ACSMs Resource Manual* (6th ed.), edited by J. K. Ehrman. Philadelphia: Walters Kluwer/ Lippincott Williams and Wilkins.
160. Heart disease and stress. (2010, January 12). *Web-MD.* Retrieved from http://www.webmd.com/heart-disease/stress_heart_attack_risk?print=true).
161. Miller, N. H. (2010). Psychosocial status and chronic disease. In *ACSMs Resource Manual* (6th ed.), edited by J. K. Ehrman. Philadelphia: Walters Kluwer/Lippincott Williams and Wilkins.
162. Gerstenblith & Margolis (2008).
163. Sime, W. W., & K. Helleoeg. (2001). Stress and coping. In *ACSMs Resource Manual* (4th ed.), edited by J. L. Roitman. Philadelphia: Lippincott Williams and Wilkins.
164. Ornish, D., et al. (1990). Can lifestyle changes reverse coronary heart disease? *The Lancet,* 333, 129.
165. Ornish, D., et al. (1993). Can lifestyle changes reverse atherosclerosis? Four-year results of the lifestyle heart trial. *Circulation,* 88(Suppl.), 2064.
166. Byrd-Bredbenner (2009).
167. Gerstenblith & Margolis (2008).
168. Collberg. S. R. (2010). Nutritional status and chronic diseases. In *ACSMs Resource Manual* (6th ed.), edited by J. K. Ehrman. Philadelphia: Walters Kluwer/ Lippincott Williams and Wilkins.
169. Lam, M. (2010, January 13). Lipoprotein(1)—How to reduce. Retrieved from http://www.drlam.com/opinion/Lp(a).asp.
170. Gerstenblith & Margolis (2008).
171. Lipoprotein (a). (2010, January 1). *Wikipedia.* Retrieved from http://www.enwikipedia.org/wiki/Lipoprotein(a).
172. Ibid.
173. Lee, R. T. (2005, October). Should my CRP level change from test to test? *Harvard Heart Letter,* 16(2), 8.
174. C-reactive protein. (2010, January 13). *Medline Plus.* Retrieved from http://www.nlm.nih.gov/medlineplus/ency/article/003356.htm.
175. Danesh. J., et al. (2004, April 1). C-reactive protein and other circulating markers of inflammation in the production of coronary heart disease. *New England Journal of Medicine,* 350, 1387.
176. Mayo Clinic Staff. (2010, January 13). Blood tests for heart disease. Retrieved from http://www.mayoclinic.com/health/heart-disease/HB00016/Methon=print.
177. Bruner, C., & M. Marmot. (2010, January 25). Fibrinogen Is a candidate measure of allostatic load. Retrieved from http://www.macses.ucsf.edu/research/allostatic/notebook/fibrinogen.html.
178. Editors. (2009, July). Protect yourself from peripheral arterial disease. *Heart Advisor,* 12(7), 4.
179. Editors. (2009, June). Exercise equals angioplasty for leg pain. *Harvard Heart Letter,* 19(10), 2.
180. Editors. (2009, March). Exercise benefits clogged leg arteries. *Harvard Health Letter,* 19(7), 7.
181. Editors. (2009, December). Healthy lifestyle choices can slow the progression of PAD. *Heart Advisor,* 12(12), 2.
182. American Heart Association (2009a).

183. Sleep apnea raises risk of death, especially for men: Report. *Medline Plus*. Retrieved from http://www.n/m.nih.gov/medlineplus/print/news/fullstory_88271.html.

184. Editors. (2009, November). Treat sleep-disordered breathing to protect your heart. *Heart Advisor,* 12(11), 4.

185. Ibid.

186. Ohio State Medical Center. (2009, November 4). Sleep apnea considered dangerous. Retrieved from http://www.internalmedicine.osu.edu/Pulmonary/3636.cfm.

187. Foster, C., & J. P. Porcari. (2010). Clinical exercise testing procedures. In *ACSMs Resource Manual* (6th ed.), edited by J. K. Ehrman. Philadelphia: Walters Kluwer/ Lippincott Williams and Wilkins.

188. Ibid.

189. Editors. (2010, January 18). Cardiac stress test. *Wikipedia, the Free Encyclopedia*. Retrieved from http://enwikipedia.org/wiki/Cardiac_stress_test.

190. American Heart Association (2009b).

191. Ibid.

192. Mayo Foundation for Education and Research. (2010, January 18). Daily aspirin therapy: Understand the benefits and risks. Retieved from http://www.mayoclinic.com/health/daily_aspirin_therapy/HB00073.

193. U.S. Department of Health and Human Services. (2009, March 16). Task force recommends using aspirin to prevent cardiovascular diseases when the benefits outweigh the harms. Retrieved from http://ww.ahrq.gov/news/press/pr2009/aspcvdpr.htm.

194. Mayo Foundation for Education and Research (2010, January 18).

195. Ibid.

196. Gerstenblith & Margolis (2008).

197. Ibid.

198. American Heart Association (2009a).

199. Gerstenblith & Margolis (2008).

200. American Heart Association (2009a).

201. Gerstenblith & Margolis (2008).

202. American Heart Association (2009a).

203. Kessel, A. (2010, January 19). The AbioCor artificial heart. Retrieved from http://signularityhub.com/2009/06/30/the_abiocor_artificial_heart_plastic_and_metal_mimics_real_life_function/.

204. Chan, B. W., et al. (2007, December 3). AbioCor Artificial Heart. Retrieved from http://courses.ece.illinois.edu/ECE317/presentations/Art_Heart_Pres.pdf.

205. Editors. (2009, May).Ventricular assist devices give failing hearts a boost. *Heart Advisor*, 12(5), 5.

206. American Heart Association (2009a).

207. Aleris-Banks, D. (2006, February 26). Defying the odds. *The Roanoke Times*. Retrieved from http://www.roanoke.com/news/roanoke/wb/wb/xp_54372.

## Suggested Readings

Editors. (2008, April). Small price to pay for an extra 14 years. *Harvard Heart Letter*, 18(8), 6.
Research indicates that people who exercise, eat plenty of fruits and vegetables, drink alcohol in moderation, and do not smoke may add 14 years to their lives. Much of the gain comes from a reduction in deaths from cardiovascular disease.

Editors. (2009, December). Another reason to get a flu shot: Your heart. *Harvard Heart Letter*, 20(4), 1.
Infections of any type can affect the heart and circulatory system. Influenza (the flu) is no different. It can make breathing more difficult, increases blood pressure, increases heart rate, and stirs up inflammation. Infection can cause unstable plaques to rupture. The clot that forms to seal the break can block the artery, causing a heart attack or sudden death. The message is: get a seasonal flu vaccine every year.

It is important to know your systolic blood pressure and your total and HDL cholesterol to obtain the most accurate estimate of cardiac risk. The estimate loses a substantial amount of predictive accuracy without these three values. Blood pressure can be measured in class, at the student health center, or by your health care provider. Total cholesterol and HDL testing requires a fasting blood draw and laboratory analysis that your health care provider can do and that the campus health center may be able to do.

Editors. (2009, August). Know the risks when blood pressure is too low. *Heart Advisor* ,12(8), 5.
Low blood pressure can be as dangerous as high blood pressure because the blood supply to such vital organs as the heart, brain, kidneys, liver, and so on, could be affected by hypotension. The symptoms associated with low blood pressure include dizziness, fainting, blackouts, tunnel vision, chest pain, fatigue, and a decrease in exercise tolerance.

Physicians agree that a pressure of 140/90 is the point where hypertension begins, but there is not a corresponding number that defines hypotension. If an individual experiences some of the symptoms listed above, then he or she may have low blood pressure.

Editors. (2009, March). A little weight loss or exercise makes a big difference in heart-failure risk. *Tufts University Health and Nutrition Letter*, 27(1), 1.
A new study found that body weight and physical activity level affected heart-failure risk independently but when they were combined, their effect increased dramatically. When compared to men who were both lean and physically active, the risk of heart failure increased by:
- 18% for the lean but inactive
- 49% in the overweight and active
- 8% in the overweight and inactive
- 168% in the obese and active
- 293% in the obese and inactive

Snowden, R.V. (2009, December 22). Obesity to outweigh public health gains of declining smoking rates. *ACS News Center*. Retrieved from http://www.DecliningSmokingRates.asp?sitenrea=MWS&viewmode=print&.
Over the past 15 years, smoking rates in the United States have declined by 20%, while obesity rates have risen by 48%. If these trends continue, obesity will soon cancel out the life expectancy and quality-of-life benefits gained by declining smoking rates. If all U.S. adults became normal weight nonsmokers by 2020, life expectancy would increase by 3.76 years.

**Name** _____   **Date** _____   **Section** _____

# Assessment Activity 2-1

## What's Your Heart Attack Risk?

**Directions:** By answering questions in the following 12 items, you can calculate your odds of having a heart attack within the next 10 years. The test is based on data from four of the most extensive American studies of coronary risk. (The test is not accurate for people who already have a history of coronary disease. For definitive advice, ask your doctor.) Advice on improving your odds follows this test.

It is important to know your systolic blood pressure and your total and HDL cholesterol to obtain the most accurate estimate of cardiac risk. The estimate loses a substantial amount of predictive accuracy without these three values. Blood pressure can be measured in class, at the student health center, or by your health care provider. Total cholesterol and HDL requires a fasting blood draw and laboratory analysis that your health care provider can do and that the campus health center may be able to do.

**The Test** For every yes answer to items 1 through 9, add or subtract points as shown.

| Question | Men | Women |
|---|---|---|
| 1. Do you get little or no regular exercise? | Plus 2 | Plus 6 |
| 2. Calculate your body mass index (BMI) as follows: Multiply your weight in pounds by 704. Divide the result by your height in inches. Divide that result by your height in inches again and round to the nearest whole number. | | |
| Is your BMI from 21 to 24? | Plus 0 | Plus 2 |
| Is your BMI from 25 to 28? | Plus 2 | Plus 3 |
| Is your BMI 29 or over? | Plus 4 | Plus 6 |

| | Men | Women |
|---|---|---|
| 3. Do you have Diabetes? | Plus 8 | Plus 11 |
| 4. If you're an ex-smoker, did you quit in the past 5 years? | Plus 1 | Plus 4 |
| If you smoke, do you smoke fewer than 15 cigarettes a day? | Plus 2 | Plus 8 |
| Do you smoke 15 to 24 cigarettes a day? | Plus 4 | Plus 15 |
| Do you smoke more than 24 cigarettes a day? | Plus 6 | Plus 18 |
| 5. Did either of your parents have a heart attack before age 60? | Plus 9 | Plus 9 |
| 6. Do you take medicine to control blood pressure? (This is a sign that your pressure was once elevated.) | Plus 1 | Plus 1 |
| 7. If you are a postmenopausal woman, are you currently taking estrogen alone? | | Minus 5 |
| Are you currently taking estrogen plus progestin? | | Minus 3 |
| If you don't currently take estrogen, did you previously take it (with or without progestin)? | | Minus 2 |
| 8. Do you take low doses of aspirin at least every other day? (A low dose is between one-quarter and one whole 325-mg tablet.) | Minus 4 | Minus 4 |
| 9. Do you drink alcohol in moderation? ("Moderate" drinking is 2 to 14 drinks per week. A "drink" is 12 ounces of beer, 5 ounces of wine, or 1½ ounces of liquor.) | Minus 4 | Minus 4 |

Add up your points so far.          SUBTOTAL _____  _____

Add up your
points so far.          SUBTOTAL _____ _____

Now calculate items
10 through 12, rounding
to the nearest whole
number.

10. Multiply your systolic          Plus ___   Plus ___
    pressure (the higher
    number) by 0.14 if you
    are a man, by 0.15 if
    you are a woman.

11. Multiply your age by            Plus ___   Plus ___
    0.51 if you are a man,
    by 0.8 if you are a
    woman.

12. Multiply your total             Plus ___   Plus ___
    cholesterol level by 0.07
    if you are a man, by 0.06
    if you are a woman. Multi-
    ply your HDL level by 0.25
    if you are a man, by 0.3 if
    you are a woman.
    If you don't know your          Minus ___  Minus ___
    cholesterol levels and
    want to assume they're
    about average, you could
    substitute 205 for total
    cholesterol and 51 for
    HDL. Adults 20 and over
    should have cholesterol
    testing at least every
    5 years.

Add up your points
for items 10
through 12.       SUBTOTAL _____         _____

Add the two
subtotals to
get your score    TOTAL _____         _____

## Probability* of Having a Heart Attack

**Men**

| Score | 1 Year | 5 Years | 10 Years |
|-------|--------|---------|----------|
| 0–35  | < 0.1% | < 0.4%  | < 1%     |
| 36–45 | 0.1–0.2 | 0.4–   | 1–3      |
| 46–55 | 0.2–0.6 | 1–3    | 3–7      |
| 56–65 | 0.6–2  | 3–8     | 7–17     |
| 66–70 | 2      | 8–13    | 17–27    |
| 71–75 | 2–4    | 13–20   | 27–40    |
| 76–80 | 4–6    | 20–30   | 40–56    |

**Women**

| Score | 1 Year | 5 Years | 10 Years |
|-------|--------|---------|----------|
| 0–60  | < 0.1% | < 0.4%  | < 1%     |
| 61–45 | 0.1–0.2 | 0.4–1  | 1.3      |
| 71–70 | 0.2–0.5 | 1–3    | 3–7      |
| 81–85 | 0.5–1  | 3–5     | 7–12     |
| 86–90 | 1      | 5–8     | 12–19    |
| 91–795 | 1–2   | 8–13    | 19–29    |
| 96–100 | 2–4   | 13–20   | 29–43    |

*"Probability" indicates the percentage of people like you who will have
a heart attack during the period cited. If your probability is 7% for the
10-year column, for example, it means that, out of a random sampling
of 100 people with the same score as yours, 7 will have a heart attack
within a decade of today.

**Name** _____ **Date** _____ **Section** _____

# Assessment Activity 2-2

## A Case Study of Bill M.

**Directions:** To determine your understanding of cardiovascular health and wellness, read the following case study and answer the accompanying questions. Bill, a 38-year-old man who is 5′8″ tall and weighs 205 lbs., has the following history:

- His father died of a heart attack at age 48 years; his grandfather died of a heart attack at age 52 years.

- His cholesterol level is 256 mg/dL, LDL is 172 mg/dL, and HDL is 40 mg/dL.

- His blood pressure is consistently in the 150/95 range.

- He smokes one pack of cigarettes per day.

- He drinks six to eight brewed cups of coffee daily.

- He eats two eggs with bacon or sausage and buttered toast daily.

- Meat is a major part of supper; he skips lunch.

- His favorite snacks are ice cream, buttered popcorn, and salted peanuts.

- He occasionally plays tennis on Sunday afternoons.

- He owns his own business and often works 55 to 60 hours per week.

**Answer the following:**

What are Bill's risk factors for coronary heart disease? _____

Which risk factors can he control? _____

What suggestions can you give him regarding his current diet? _____

_____

What effect may a change in diet have on his coronary risk profile? _____

What suggestions can you make regarding Bill's need for exercise, and how might a change in his activity level affect his coronary risk profile? _____

_____

What are the risks associated with obesity? _____

_____

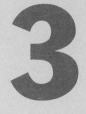
# Increasing Cardiorespiratory Endurance

## ONLINE LEARNING CENTER

Log on to our Online Learning Center (OLC) for access to these additional resources:

- Chapter key term flashcards
- Learning objectives
- Additional goals for behavior change
- Concentration game
- Self-scoring chapter quizzes
- Additional lab activities

The OLC also offers Web links for study and exploration of wellness topics. Access these links through **www.mhhe.com/anspaugh8e.**

## GOALS FOR BEHAVIOR CHANGE

- List three physical activities you normally do every week (exclusive of structured, planned exercise) and find and implement ways of making them more challenging.
- If you do not exercise regularly, list several factors that will motivate you to begin a cardiorespiratory endurance program. Begin a simple walking or other exercise program with these factors in mind.
- If you are physically active, list the main factors that will encourage you to improve the frequency, intensity, or duration of your activity. To help you stay motivated, post this list in a place where you will see it every day.
- Choose a piece of home exercise equipment that seems well suited to your exercise preferences and goals.

## Objectives

After completing this chapter, you will be able to do the following:

✔ Identify and define the health-related components of physical fitness.
✔ Discuss the principles of conditioning.
✔ Calculate your target heart rate for exercise by two methods.
✔ Identify and discuss the health benefits of consistent participation in exercise.
✔ Describe the problems associated with exercise in hot and cold weather.

## [ Key Terms ]

| | |
|---|---|
| aerobic | hyperthermia |
| aerobic capacity | hyponatremia |
| cardiorespiratory endurance | hypothermia |
| cross-training | performance-related fitness |
| exercise | physical activity |
| health-related fitness | physical fitness |

Technology has affected the lives of Americans by increasing productivity while reducing and in some cases eliminating the amount of physical work for the labor force. Therefore, physical fitness for most of the population can no longer be attained on the job, and leisure hours represent the only time for its development. Dozens of physical activities, exercise regimens, sports, games, and household and other physical chores that may contribute to health enhancement and fitness development are available. These activities are sufficiently different from each other, running the gamut from low- to high-skill requirement, so that almost anyone can find one or two enjoyable, fun, and challenging activities. This chapter focuses on the principles and concepts that have evolved for developing cardiorespiratory endurance for the purposes of health enhancement and physical fitness.

## Components of Physical Fitness

According to the American College of Sports Medicine (ACSM), **physical fitness** is defined "as a set of attributes that people have or achieve that relates to the ability to perform physical activity."[1] **Physical activity** is an umbrella term defined as "bodily movement that is produced by the contraction of skeletal muscle and that substantially increases energy expenditure."[2] **Exercise** is a subset of physical activity. It is defined as "planned, structured, and repetitive bodily movement done to improve or maintain one or more components of physical fitness."[3]

Physical activity includes exercise and all other types of human movements, such as mowing the lawn, raking leaves, vacuuming the floors, climbing stairs, washing the car by hand, chopping wood, and shoveling snow.[4] These activities, many of which are daily chores, may improve physical fitness for some unfit sedentary people, but when engaged in regularly, are health-enhancing for most people. Health improvement can be attained with regular participation in lower-intensity physical activities, whereas higher-intensity physical activities that sustain an exercise target heart rate are necessary for improving physical fitness. In addition to the development of a higher level of physical fitness, the extra effort involved in more vigorous exercise includes a significant bonus. Greater exercise intensity lowers the risk for heart disease, more so than lower-intensity levels.[5]

Most physical fitness experts have accepted the concept of performance-related and health-related fitness. **Performance-related fitness**, or sports fitness, consists of the following components: speed, power, balance, coordination, agility, and reaction time. These are essential for sports performance, but they may or may

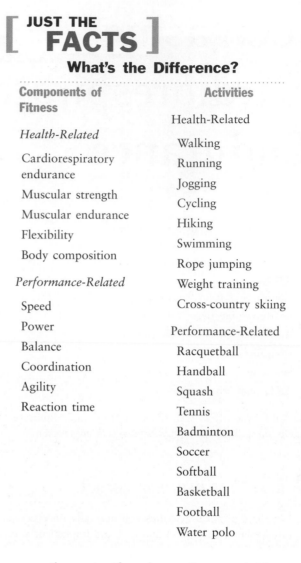

not contribute significantly to those activities performed for health enhancement (see Just the Facts: What's the Difference?).

*Speed* is velocity, or the ability to move rapidly. *Power* is the product of force and velocity and the rate at which work is performed. *Balance*, or equilibrium, is the ability to maintain a desired body position, either statically or dynamically. *Coordination* is the harmonious integration of the body parts to produce smooth, fluid motion. *Agility* is the ability to change direction rapidly. *Reaction time* is the time required (usually measured in hundredths of a second) to respond to a stimulus.

The components of **health-related fitness** are cardiorespiratory endurance, muscular strength, muscular endurance, flexibility, and body composition. In this text the exercise emphasis is on health-related fitness.

Performance-related and health-related fitness, although different, clearly are not mutually exclusive. For example, competitive athletes require an abundance of the performance-related components of fitness, but the natures of their sports may also require the simultaneous development of the health-related components. Athletes who play racquetball, tennis, basketball, soccer, and handball are some that fall within this category. Conversely, the same sports are appropriate for health and fitness enthusiasts who prefer to achieve their goals through friendly competition.

However, the development and maintenance of health-related fitness do not necessarily depend on athletic ability or activities high in the performance components. Fitness for health purposes can be achieved with minimal psychomotor ability through activities such as walking, jogging, cycling, hiking, backpacking, orienteering, swimming, rope jumping, and weight training. These are self-paced activities; that is, the exerciser selects a relatively comfortable pace that can be sustained for a minimum of 10 minutes. No competing opponent pushes the exerciser beyond his or her physiological limits.

Remember the adage "No pain, no gain"? Trying to comply with it has done more harm than good to sedentary adults attempting to become physically active. The health benefits of exercise begin to occur when exercise is somewhat uncomfortable but not painful. Only the most dedicated health enthusiasts and competitors can face exercise that periodically produces pain. Although exercise for health enhancement should stress cardiorespiratory development, the other components of fitness should not be neglected. Flexibility exercises can be a part of warm-up and cooldown procedures. Flexibility exercises may be performed three to five times per week, and the best results occur after the cooldown period following the cardiorespiratory workout.[6] Stretching is most effective at this time because muscle temperature is elevated. Warm muscles respond well to stretching, and the likelihood of muscle injury while stretching is decreased. Resistance/strength training plays an important role and should be an integral part of a well-rounded fitness program.

As with all components of wellness, developing and sustaining an exercise program are the responsibilities of each individual. This text provides convincing evidence of the need for regular exercise and provides guidelines for initiating a sound program or reinforcement for those currently exercising.

## Cardiorespiratory Endurance

**Cardiorespiratory endurance** is the ability to take in, deliver, and extract oxygen for physical work—that is, the ability to persevere at a physical task at a given intensity level.[7] Cardiorespiratory endurance improves with regular participation in aerobic activities, such as speed walking, jogging, cycling, swimming, cross-country skiing, and many others. The term **aerobic** means "with oxygen," but when applied to exercise, it refers

to activities in which oxygen demand can be met continuously during performance.[8] Aerobic performance depends on a continuous and sufficient supply of oxygen to burn the carbohydrates and fats needed to fuel such activities. In other words, someone performing aerobically has the capacity to sustain the intensity or the energy requirement for longer than a couple of minutes,[9] a phenomenon known as *steady state*. Steady state can be achieved only during aerobic exercise, and it represents a level of exertion that feels relatively comfortable to the exerciser. It is also referred to as a *pay as you go system*, in that the oxygen cost of an activity is paid in full by the body during the activity. Steady state oxygen consumption can be maintained for an average of 10 to 60 minutes during submaximal continuous exercise. This may not apply for exercise during hot and humid weather. The stress of exercising during these conditions causes a steady upward drift in oxygen consumption.[10]

Cardiorespiratory endurance is also referred to as **aerobic capacity**, or maximum oxygen consumption. Symbolized by "$VO_2$ max." It is the most important component of physical fitness and is the foundation of total fitness.

The physiological changes that result from cardiorespiratory training are referred to as the *long-term*, or *chronic, effects of exercise*. The effects of training are measurable and predictable.

## Heart Rate

A few months of aerobic training lowers the resting heart rate by 10 to 15 beats per minute (bpm).[11] It also lowers the heart rate for a given workload. For example, a slow jog may produce a heart rate of 165 beats per minute before training and 140 beats per minute after a few months of training. The trained heart is a stronger, more efficient pump capable of delivering the required blood and oxygen with fewer beats.

## Stroke Volume

*Stroke volume* is the amount of blood that the heart can eject in one beat. Aerobic training increases the stroke volume by (1) increasing the size of the cavity of the ventricles, which results in more blood filling the heart, and (2) increasing the contractile strength of the ventricular wall, so contraction is more forceful and a greater amount of blood is ejected from the ventricles.[12] The increase in stroke volume, both at rest and during exercise, is one of the primary effects of endurance training and one of the major mechanisms responsible for improvement in aerobic fitness (see Just the Facts: Stroke Volume).

# [ JUST THE **FACTS** ]
## Stroke Volume

For the average person, stroke volume rises with incremental aerobic exercise (exercise where the intensity is systematically increased); it plateaus or levels off at 40 to 50% of maximum oxygen uptake even though the intensity of exercise continues to increase. Leveling off is due to the reduced amount of time for filling the ventricles with blood at higher exercise heart rates; therefore, the amount of blood available for pumping is also reduced.[13] However, new evidence indicates that highly trained endurance athletes do not experience similar stroke volume plateaus during incremental exercise. The explanation for this phenomenon comes from echocardiographic studies that show superior ventricular filling among highly trained endurance athletes in spite of very high heart rates during maximum-effort exercise.[14]

## Cardiac Output

*Cardiac output* is the amount of blood ejected by the heart in 1 minute. Cardiac output ($Q$) is the product of heart rate ($HR$) and stroke volume ($SV$) ($Q = HR \times SV$). Cardiac output increases with aerobic training during maximal effort—it does not increase at rest or during submaximal exercise. Cardiac output does not change during rest or submaximal exercise because the lowered resting heart rate compensates for the increase in stroke volume. What does change is the manner in which cardiac output is achieved. This is illustrated by the following example: An untrained 25-year-old man has a resting heart rate of 72 bpm and a stroke volume of 70 mL of blood per beat. His cardiac output at rest is calculated as follows:

$$Q = HR \times SV$$
$$= 72 \times 70$$
$$= 5{,}060 \text{ mL (5.1L)}$$

The same person after 2 years of aerobic training has the same cardiac output at rest, but it is achieved differently: The resting heart rate is now decreased to 55 bpm and the stroke volume is increased to 92 mL of blood per beat.

$$Q = HR \times SV$$
$$\frac{5{,}060}{55} = \frac{55 \times SV}{55}$$
$$92 = SV$$

The average cardiac output at rest is 4 to 6 liters of blood per minute. During maximal exertion, cardiac output reaches values of 20 to 22 liters per minute for college-age untrained males and 18 liters per minute for college-age untrained females. The cardiac output of trained endurance athletes averages 34 liters per minute for males and 24 liters per minute for females.[15] The maximum cardiac output of a few large, well-conditioned endurance athletes is an exceptional 40 liters of blood per minute—what an incredible performance by an organ that weighs less than 1 pound. To put this in perspective, imagine 40 one-liter cola bottles filled with blood. Maximal cardiac output improves with training primarily because of the resulting increase in stroke volume.[16] Maximal heart rate is essentially unaffected by training; therefore, its influence on maximal cardiac output is relatively constant. However, maximal heart rate declines with age by about 1 bpm per year after age 20. Training cannot stop the decline; it can only slow the process.

## Blood Volume

Aerobic training increases total blood volume, plasma volume (the liquid portion of the blood), and blood solids (the red blood cells, white blood cells, and blood platelets). The increase is greatest in plasma volume, so the blood becomes more liquid. The increase in the ratio of plasma volume to red blood cell volume is an adaptation to exercise that lowers the viscosity, or thickness and stickiness, of the blood. This change decreases the resistance to blood flow, allowing it to circulate more easily through the blood vessels.[17]

Blood is automatically shunted by the body to areas of greatest need. At rest, a significant amount is sent to the digestive system and kidneys. During vigorous exercise, as much as 85% of the blood is sent to the working muscles, reducing the amount sent to the digestive and urinary systems.[18]

## Heart Volume

The muscles of the body respond to exercise by growing larger and stronger. As a muscular pump, the heart's volume and weight increase with endurance training.[19] Training that lowers the resting heart rate stimulates greater filling of the ventricles, whose muscle fibers respond to the increased pool of blood by stretching. This produces a recoil effect in the muscle fibers, which results in a stronger contraction with more blood ejected per beat. Continued training causes the ventricles to enlarge and grow stronger, so the weight and the size of the heart increase. The hypertrophied (enlarged) heart is a normal response to endurance training that has no long-term detrimental effects. Although maintaining this effect for life is beneficial, several months of inactivity will reduce heart weight and size to pretraining levels. The atrophy (wasting away) associated with physical inactivity is inevitable.

## Respiratory Responses

The chest muscles that support breathing improve in both strength and endurance with exercise.[20] Vital capacity, the amount of air that can be expired maximally following a maximal inspiration, increases slightly. A corresponding decrease occurs in "dead space" air, or residual volume, the amount of air remaining in the lungs after a maximal expiration.

Training substantially increases maximal pulmonary ventilation (the amount of air moved in and out of the lungs).[21] Before training, the lungs can ventilate approximately 110 liters of air per minute. Pulmonary ventilation increases to about 135 liters of air following a few months of training. Highly trained athletes commonly ventilate 180 to 200 liters of air per minute.

Blood flow to the lungs, particularly to the upper lobes, appears to increase after training. This results in a larger and more efficient surface for the exchange of oxygen and carbon dioxide.[22]

## Metabolic Responses

Aerobic endurance training improves aerobic capacity by 5 to 25% in previously untrained, healthy adults. The magnitude of improvement is primarily dependent on the initial level of physical fitness. The lower the fitness level, the greater the gain from aerobic training.[23] A gain of 15 to 20% in aerobic capacity is typical for an average person who trains at 75% of maximal oxygen intake ($VO_2$ max), 3 days per week, for 30 minutes per workout over a 6-month training period. Two to 3 years of highly intense training of greater frequency and longer duration has resulted in increases in $VO_2$ max in excess of 40% in some people.[24]

The improvement in aerobic capacity is the result of several physiological adaptations that increase the body's production of energy. First, adenosine triphosphate (ATP), the actual unit of energy for muscular contraction, is produced in greater quantities. The mitochondria, specialized organelles responsible for manufacturing ATP, respond to training by increasing in size and number to increase their output. Second, oxidative enzymes within the mitochondria that accelerate the production of ATP increase in quantity. Third, cardiac output and blood perfusion of the muscles performing the work increase. Fourth, training facilitates and increases the extraction of oxygen by the exercising muscles. These are some of the major adaptations that combine to enhance aerobic endurance.[25]

### Effects of Heredity on VO₂ Max

Aerobic capacity ($VO_2$ max) is limited by heredity and is finite. Studies of identical and fraternal twins and studies that examined family groups (parents and children) have produced estimates of the role of genetics in the development of maximal cardiorespiratory endurance. Separating the influence of genetics from the influence of training is very complex. As a result, the estimates of the genetic predisposition for maximal cardiorespiratory endurance ranges from a low of 25% to a high of 93%. At this point, the majority of the evidence indicates that the genetic component is probably closer to 40 to 50%.[26,27,28] Whatever the actual percentage turns out to be, the consensus among exercise scientists is that the role of genetics represents a substantial potential for the development of maximal cardiorespiratory endurance. The sensitivity of the $VO_2$ max response to aerobic training is to a significant degree dependent on heredity. If those who inherit the genetic potential for endurance events also train diligently, they become capable of exceptionally high levels of performance. But diligent training with an average genetic potential results in average or slightly above-average performance. Only a select few inherit the ability to produce world-class endurance performances. Most people are in the average category, but all can achieve their aerobic *potential* with training. However, the expectation that regularity of training will produce a fitness payback that is proportional to the effort is logical, albeit inaccurate. The relationship between genetics and sensitivity to training is complicated by the fact that some people are "responders" (capable of making significant improvement from consistent training), while others are "nonresponders" (their improvement is minimal, even though they are exposed to the same training program).[29] Therefore, two people who are the same age, height, weight, and gender who train together and are equally compliant may obtain results that are very different, based on their response to training. The sensitivity to training is genetic, and evidence indicates that it is dependent on mitochondrial mass and mitochondrial DNA.[30] Evidence also indicates that the mother's genes are responsible for mitochondrial mass.[31]

Then we have the dilemma of a very small group of people who have exceptionally high aerobic capacities without the benefit of training. See Just the Facts: The Conundrum for a possible explanation of this anomaly.

Genetic potential is extremely important for those who aspire to become serious competitors in endurance events. But it is essentially unimportant for those who are exercising for health and physical fitness purposes. The bottom line is that almost everyone can benefit physically, emotionally, and mentally from exercise regardless of their inheritance. So find an activity or activities that you enjoy, and participate regularly.

Three methods for assessing your cardiorespiratory endurance are presented in the Assessment Activities.

## [ JUST THE FACTS ]

### The Conundrum: No Training— High VO₂ max

The phenomenon of a high aerobic capacity with no training was investigated several years ago. More than 1,900 subjects were tested and only six demonstrated this anomaly. Their aerobic capacities were comparable to those of endurance-trained athletes. The researchers found that three subjects possessed a higher than normal volume of blood, which in turn resulted in a high stroke volume and cardiac output during maximal exercise. Collectively, these physiological factors seemed to account for their extraordinarily high aerobic capacity. The researchers hypothesized that the high volume of blood was genetically determined.[32]

These include the Rockport Fitness Walking Test, the 1.5-Mile Run/Walk Test, and the 3-Minute Bench Step Test. Each is accompanied by norms, so you can compare your performance against the standards.

### Effects of Training on VO₂ Max

Aerobic capacity reaches a peak after 6 months to 2 years of steady endurance training. At this point, it levels off and remains unchanged for a number of years, even if training is intensified. However, aerobic performance continues to improve with harder training, because a higher percentage of the aerobic capacity can be maintained for a longer period. For example, 6 months of appropriate training may allow you to jog 3 miles at 60% of your aerobic capacity. Another year of harder training may allow you to run 3 miles at 85% of your capacity. Capacity has changed little, if at all, during this time; but physiological adaptations have occurred that enable the body to function at progressively higher percentages of maximum capacity.

### Effects of Deconditioning on VO₂ Max

The effects of training persist as long as training continues. Training of moderate intensity may increase the $VO^2$ max by 10 to 20%. However, the $VO_2$ max returns to pretraining levels within a few months if training is discontinued.[33] Most of the decline occurs during the first month and slows down during the next 2 months.[34] Fitness developed through years of continuous training can be lost in months if training is interrupted or discontinued. Highly conditioned athletes respond to detraining in a similar manner. In a study, subjects who suspended training for 84 days after 10 years of active participation experienced a significant decline in aerobic capacity after 3 weeks of inactivity. They returned to pretraining levels

in most fitness parameters by the end of the study. The exceptions to complete reversal were muscle capillary density and mitochondrial enzymes, which remained 50% higher than levels measured in sedentary control subjects. This study indicated that the results of inactivity are variable and affect some systems more quickly than others. Physical decline with physical inactivity cannot be prevented.

### Effects of Age on VO₂ Max

Aerobic capacity decreases with age. During adulthood, peak aerobic energy steadily declines by an average of about 1% per year between the ages of 25 and 75.[35] A significant portion of the decline is related to the lack of physical activity that accompanies aging: Those who are physically active throughout their lifetimes experience declines in aerobic capacity but not at the same rate as those who are inactive. See Wellness for a Lifetime: Exercise Is for Everyone for more details about the impact of exercising on aging.

## Cardiorespiratory Endurance and Wellness

Most Americans believe that exercise is good for them, but the majority cannot explain how or why. This section provides some of the answers.

Consistent participation in exercise is necessary to improve health status. Sporadic exercise does not promote physical fitness or contribute to health enhancement. Infrequent participation increases the risk for sudden death during the time of exercise.[41] As discussed in Chapter 2, physical inactivity is a major risk factor for coronary heart disease. The risk is approximately equal to that imposed by cigarette smoking, high blood pressure, and elevated serum cholesterol. National surveys indicate that 37% of adults are not physically active. Only 30%, or 3 in 10 American adults, equal or exceed the amount of exercise recommended by the American College of Sports Medicine (ACSM) and the American Heart Association (AHA).[42] Therefore, 70% of the adult population is either inactive or not active enough for physical activity to improve their health.

The recently released physical activity guidelines for Americans by the U.S. Department of Health and Human Services recommended 60 minutes of moderate to vigorous physical activity daily for youngsters age 6 to 19.[43] More than 82% in this age group do not meet this recommendation, and 25% of adolescents, grades 9–12, did not participate in 60 minutes of physical activity on any given day. Only 25.6% of high school girls and 43.7% of high school boys meet the recommendation.[44] The number of physically inactive people exceeds the combined total of those who smoke, are hypertensive, and

## Wellness for a Lifetime

### Exercise Is for Everyone

The ability of the body to take in, transport, and extract oxygen for physical work and exercise declines with age. On the average, aerobic capacity declines by about 8 to 10% every decade after the age of 25 in both males and females. One of the major sources of this decline in the United States is the decreasing level of physical activity that tends to accompany aging. This trend toward inactivity also results in a loss of muscle weight, an increase in fat weight, and a decrease in metabolic rate, all of which contribute to the decline in aerobic capacity. Although physiological aging does lower aerobic capacity, at least 50% of the decline is due to "disuse atrophy" caused by inactivity.[36] But recent studies have indicated that aging may have less effect than the deconditioning that accompanies inactivity as people age.[37]

Biological aging cannot be stopped. We cannot live forever. However, exercise comes as close to an anti-aging pill as anything else available. Even older people who have been sedentary for decades can benefit from aerobic exercise and weight training.[38]

The beneficial outcomes of regular exercise for older people include an increase in energy, a favorable change in body composition (loss of fat, gain of muscle), an increase in muscular strength and endurance, an increase in metabolism, and significant improvements in cardiovascular and musculoskeletal health.[39] All of these changes translate into a higher quality of life and longevity.

Physically fit 60- and 70-year-olds have the aerobic capacity of unfit 25-year-olds.[40] This means that physically fit elderly people have the energy to live independently during their later years. The ability to perform the daily chores of living and to participate in an active lifestyle with energy to spare develops confidence that contributes to the enjoyment of life.

---

have high serum cholesterol.[45] Based on these numbers, promoting regular exercise for the general public should be an important priority of public health policy.

Coronary heart disease is rarely responsible for sudden cardiac death during or after exercise among people under the age of 30.[46] Congenital heart defects or other cardiac abnormalities, such as faulty valves, enlarged hearts, heart muscle disease, and fatal cardiac arrhythmias are the usual culprits for this age group.[47] Most exertional deaths occur among older Americans and are due to coronary heart disease and cardiomyopathy (wasting of cardiac muscle due to disease).[48] New evidence indicates that a substantial proportion of sudden exertional deaths among asymptomatic people are due to coronary plaque rupturing.[49] The increased rate of blood flow during physical exertion results in greater bending and flexing of the coronary arteries. This exaggerated arterial motion leads to the cracking of atherosclerotic plaque, the formation of a blood clot, and subsequent heart attack. A study by Harvard medical researchers found that heavy physical exertion, such as shoveling snow, gardening, walking fast, jogging, playing softball, and playing tennis, can trigger a heart attack.[50] For the physically unfit, the risk of incurring a heart attack during and in the first hour after strenuous exertion increased by 107 times. The risk for physically fit people increased only 2.7 times.

Adult males have been the subject of most investigations of cardiac death due to physical exertion because males are more susceptible to this phenomenon than females.[51] Even so, exertional deaths among males occur infrequently, yielding one death per 1.51 million hours of vigorous exertion. The Nurses Health Study with nearly 85,000 subjects found that the rate of exertional deaths among adult females is one per 36.5 million hours of moderate to vigorous physical activity.[52] A common finding between males and females was that regular exercisers were less likely to experience sudden exertional death than nonexercisers and were less likely to die prematurely of any cause.[53]

The benefits received from physical training far outweigh the minimal risk associated with one bout of strenuous exercise. A similar study conducted at the same time in Germany found amazingly similar results.[54]

One and one-half million heart attacks occur every year in the United States. The Harvard researchers concluded that 75,000 of these are exertional and they usually occur after strenuous exercise. Most of these heart attacks occur among those who are physically inactive and at high risk.[55] See Just the Facts: Exercise-Related Considerations (page 90) for some tips on reducing the hazards associated with regular exercise. Some selected health benefits of regular exercise are listed in Table 3-1. If these benefits could be distilled and sold in pill form, the American public would line up to pay any reasonable price to attain them, yet all of these benefits are readily available to anyone willing to commit the time and effort. While millions of people are exercising, 70% of the adult population is either inactive or marginally active.

## Table 3-1    Health-Related Benefits Associated with Regular Aerobic Exercise

**Reduces the Risk of Cardiovascular Disease**

- Increases HDL cholesterol
- Decreases LDL cholesterol
- Favorably changes the ratios between total cholesterol and HDL-C and between LDL-C and HDL-C
- Decreases triglyceride levels
- Promotes relaxation; relieves stress and tension
- Decreases body fat and favorably changes body composition
- Reduces age-related accumulations of central body fat
- Reduces blood pressure, especially if it is high
- Makes blood platelets less sticky
- Decreases the incidence of cardiac dysrhythmias
- Increases myocardial efficiency
   1. Lowers resting heart rate
   2. Increases stroke volume
- Increases oxygen-carrying capacity of the blood
- Reduces the risk for colon cancer and breast cancer

**Helps Control Diabetes**

- Makes cells less resistant to insulin
- Reduces body fat

**Develops Stronger Bones Less Susceptible to Injury**

**Promotes Joint Stability**

- Increases muscular strength
- Increases strength of the ligaments, tendons, cartilage, and connective tissue

**Contributes to Fewer Lower-Back Problems**

**Acts as a Stimulus for Other Lifestyle Changes**

**Improves Self-Concept**

**May Delay the Onset of Alzheimer's Disease**

Sources: American College of Sports Medicine. (2010). *ACSM's guidelines for exercise testing and prescription* (8th ed.). Philadelphia: Walters Kluwer/ Lippincott Williams and Wilkins.

Kraus, W. E. (2010). Physical activity status and chronic disease. In *ACSM's guidelines for exercise testing and prescription* (6th ed.), edited by J. K. Ehrman. Philadelphia: Walters Kluwer/Lippincott Williams and Wilkins.

Powers, S. K., & E. T. Howley. (2009). *Exercise physiology.* Boston: McGraw-Hill.

U.S. Department of Health and Human Services. (2008). *2008 physical activity guidelines for Americans.* www.health.gov/paguidelines.

American Institute for Cancer Research. (2008, Summer). Physical activity may curb abnormal cell growth. *Newsletter on Diet, Nutrition and Cancer Prevention,* 5.

## Exercise Recommendations

Exercise recommendations for the general public have evolved and changed over many years. Driven by research-based evidence, the guidelines changed as research advanced. What follows is a brief review of the ongoing process that highlights where we once were compared to where we are now.

The American College of Sports Medicine (ACSM) issued its first exercise recommendation in 1975. It recommended that healthy adults should exercise for 20–30 minutes per workout, at least 3 days per week, at an intensity level equal to 60 to 90% of their maximum heart rate. The objective was to improve the physical fitness of an unfit nation. Even though many people were turned off by or unable to sustain such a formidable challenge, many new converts were turned on. The incipient exercise movement was off and running.

This exercise guideline permeated and set the standard for the exercise community for 20 years, until ACSM produced its first revision that introduced mod-

erate-intensity physical activity for the purpose of improving the health of the nation. In 1995, the ACSM and the Centers for Disease Control and Prevention (CDC) developed and promoted the following recommendation for exercise: Every U.S. adult should accumulate 30 minutes or more of moderately intense physical activity on most and preferably all days of the week.[56] The recommendation refers to *physical activity* rather than *exercise*. This is an umbrella term that includes many types of physical exertion, including structured exercise. *Moderate intensity* refers to walking at a 3- to 4-mile-per-hour pace (15 to 20 minutes per mile) or engaging in any activity that burns a similar number of calories at a similar rate. The 30 minutes of activity can be split up into two or three bouts of 10 to 15 minutes each throughout the day.

The recommendation for health enhancement is a minimum guideline designed to motivate and recruit the 70% of the population not physically active. It is not intended to lower the standard for those who currently exercise at a higher level or whose primary goal is the development of physical fitness. Programs designed primarily to improve health may not improve or may minimally improve physical fitness. It takes higher-intensity exercise to significantly improve physical fitness. In fact, intensity is the most important principle for the development and maintenance of physical fitness.[57] The higher the intensity, up to a point, the greater the return. Those who exercise for physical fitness purposes also derive health benefits in a two-for-one deal. It takes a higher level of training to achieve both.

In September 2001, the Institute of Medicine (IOM), a private, nonprofit organization established by the U.S. Congress 150 years ago to advise the federal government on matters requiring technical and scientific expertise, issued an exercise recommendation of 60 minutes of brisk physical activity per day.[58] This recommendation was based on evidence indicating that successful weight loss occurs at this level of physical activity. *Brisk exercise* was defined as walking 4 miles per hour (a 15-minute-per-mile pace). The IOM also suggested that the cumulative effect of exercise is important for weight loss, so the 60 minutes does not have to be performed continuously—that is, it can be broken into segments scattered throughout the day. The caveat is that all segments need to be performed at a brisk intensity level. The issuance of this recommendation produced some confusion on the part of the general public. The ACSM recommended 30 minutes per day; the IOM recommended 60 minutes per day. Then in 2005, the Department of Agriculture issued "Dietary Guidelines for Americans." The department produces these guidelines every 5 years. One of the recommendations is that 60 minutes of moderate to vigorous intensity activity on most days of the week is needed to prevent gradual weight gain in adulthood, and 60 to 90 minutes of daily moderate-intensity activity is needed to sustain weight loss in adulthood.[59] The American Heart Association weighed in a year later in 2006 agreeing with the Institute of Medicine and recommending 60 minutes of physical activity for those who wish to lose weight.[60]

In 2007, ACSM and the American Heart Association collaborated on a set of exercise recommendations for healthy adults, healthy older adults (age 65 and beyond), and adults (age 50 to 64) with clinically significant chronic conditions and/or functional limitations. The objective for all groups is to improve and maintain health through consistent participation in moderate- to vigorous-intensity physical activity.[61] In 2008, the U.S. Department of Health and Human Services issued the latest guidelines that are being discussed in this chapter.[62]

Which recommendation is correct? The answer is that they are all correct because the programs are designed to meet different goals for different populations. The ACSM recommendation is a starter program for the purpose of health enhancement for sedentary adults. Thirty minutes of physical activity per day will make only a minimum contribution to weight loss, hence the IOM recommendation of 60 minutes of exercise per day buttressed by similar guidelines from the American Heart Association and the Dietary Guidelines for Americans.[63,64] The current guidelines define and differentiate between moderate and vigorous physical activity. Also, the recommendations are somewhat different from those who are under 65 years of age and those who are older than 65. Additionally, exercise recommendations for improving balance are provided for the first time.

## Principles of Conditioning

Becoming familiar with the principles of exercise is necessary to maximize the results of a physical fitness program. Your health and fitness objectives can be met through the appropriate manipulation of the FITT principle—frequency, intensity, time, (duration), and type (mode)—plus the principles of overload, progression, and specificity. See Table 3-2 for a summary of the current guidelines. Setting of objectives, warm-up, cooldown, and careful selection of activities are important elements that add to the enjoyment and effectiveness of exercise.

### Frequency

The *frequency* of exercise is the number of days of participation each week. The recommended number of days per week for aerobic training is dependent primarily on the intensity of each workout. Those pursuing a moderate-intensity program should exercise a minimum of 3 days per week to achieve health and fitness benefits.[65] Less than three workouts per week is not enough of a stimulus for improvement. An optimal moderate-intensity aerobic training program would have a frequency of 5 days per week. An optimal training program results in the greatest gain for the time and effort invested. A frequency greater than 5 days per week represents a point of diminishing returns, plus it increases the likelihood of increasing an exercise-related injury.

Vigorous-intensity exercise produces significant health and fitness benefits with less time (20–25 minutes per workout) and lower frequency (3 days per week) but at a higher level of energy expenditure (intensity).

An exercise program that combines moderate and vigorous physical activity is an excellent way to achieve health and fitness benefits. A brisk 30-minute walk 2 days per week plus a 20-minute jog on 2 other days for a total of 100 minutes of exercise, fits the bill very nicely. See Table 3-2 for a summary of the 2008 physical activity guidelines.

Table 3-2    Summary of 2008 Physical Activity Guidelines

| Frequency | Intensity | Time (Duration)[c] |
|---|---|---|
| 1. At least 5d/wk | Moderate (40 to 59% HRR)a weight-bearing plus flexibility exercises | a minimum of 30 min/d or 150 min/wk |
| 2. At least 3d/wk | Vigorous ( $\geq$ 60% HRR)b weight-bearing plus flexibility exercise | a minimum of 20–25 min/d or 75 min/wk |
| 3. 3–5 d/wk | Combination of moderate- and vigorous-intensity aerobic exercises plus weight-bearing and flexibility exercises | a minimum of 20–30 min/d or 75–150 min/wk |
| 4. 2–3 d/wk | Strength training: resistance exercises, calisthenics, plus balance and agility training | 2–4 sets, 8 12 repetitions 2–3 minutes rest between sets |

1. Numbers 1 through 3 refer to aerobic activities.
   a. HRR is the heart rate reserve.
   b. $\geq$ equal or greater than.
   c. The amount of time devoted to activity as suggested in Table 3-2 will enhance health and fitness but exercisers should be encouraged to do more to get greater benefits.

Source: Adapted from U.S. Department of Health and Human Services. (2008). 2008 Physical Activity Guidelines for Americans. http://www.health.gov/paguidelines.

## Intensity

*Intensity* refers to the degree of vigorousness of a single session of exercise.

$HR_{max}$ can be measured by a physical work capacity test on a treadmill or cycle ergometer. Because most people do not have access to such tests, $HR_{max}$ can be estimated by the following formula: $HR_{max} = 206.9 - (0.67 \times AGE)$.[66] For example, to estimate the maximum heart rate of a 20-year-old male, do the following:

$$HR_{max} = 206.9 - (0.67 \times 20)$$
$$= 206.9 - 13.4$$
$$= 193.5, \text{ or } 194 \text{ bpm}$$

ACSM considers this formula the most accurate way to estimate the maximum heart rate.

After the $HR_{max}$ has been determined, the target for exercise may be calculated. The easiest method for determining the target zone for exercise is to use the percentage of $HR_{max}$ recommended by ACSM (see the example that follows). The target zone for exercise provides the desirable heart rate for the development of physical fitness. For the 20-year-old person whose $HR_{max}$ is 194 beats per minute, the target zone for exercise is calculated as follows:

$$194 \text{ (estimated } HR_{max})$$
$$\underline{\times 0.70} \text{ (70\% of } HR_{max})$$
$$136 \pm 5 \text{ beats per minute}$$

Range 131–141 bpm (heart rate maintained during exercise)

This 20-year-old person should exercise at a heart rate range of 131–141 beats per minute, depending on objectives and level of fitness. A 20-year-old person who is sedentary, and possibly overweight, should exercise at a lower percentage of $HR_{max}$ (55%). A same-age subject who is at an average physical fitness level should exercise at 70 to 75% of the $HR_{max}$, and a 20-year-old person who is fit should exercise at 80 to 90% of the $HR_{max}$. The target for a person who has an average level of fitness is 140 to 150 beats per minute for exercise. The training effect occurs at heart rate levels below the maximum.

A slightly different emphasis was proposed by the ACSM concerning the prescription of exercise in the latest "position stand."[67] The suggestion was that exercise intensity should be monitored by the VO2 Reserve (VO2R) method. This approach is based on a given percentage of the VO2R (the difference between VO2 max and VO2 rest). This is an excellent way to generate an exercise prescription, but it requires that an individual perform a maximal aerobic test on a treadmill or cycle ergometer. Realistically, most people don't opt for such testing, so this method will be used on a limited basis. But the good news is that the heart rate reserve method (the Karvonen formula) simulates the VO2 Reserve without the measurements, and it is much more applicable for the general public.

The Karvonen formula considers fitness level and resting heart rate. The training heart rate is calculated with this formula by using a percentage of the heart rate reserve (cardiac reserve), which is the difference between the $HR_{max}$ and the resting heart rate. The way to determine the resting heart rate is to count your pulse rate for 15 seconds after sitting quietly for 5 to 10 minutes. Then multiply your 15-second heart rate by 4

Table 3-3 Guidelines for Selecting Exercise Intensity Level

| Fitness Level | Intensity Level (%) |
|---|---|
| Low | 60 |
| Fair | 65 |
| Average | 70 |
| Good | 75 |
| Excellent | 80–90 |

to obtain the heart rate for 1 minute. Next, you should estimate your level of fitness based on your exercise habits and select a category from Table 3-3 to determine the appropriate exercise intensity level. If you cannot decide which category is the most appropriate, take one of the fitness tests at the end of this chapter. Your performance on this test should place you in a category that reflects your physical fitness level.

The Karvonen formula is

$$THR = (MHR - RHR) \times TI\% + RHR$$

where *THR* is the training heart rate, or the heart rate that should be maintained during exercise; *MHR* is the maximum heart rate; *RHR* is the resting heart rate; and *TI%* is the training intensity (see Table 3-3). Therefore, the exercise heart rate for a 25-year-old with a resting heart rate of 75 beats per minute and an average fitness level is calculated as follows:

$$
\begin{aligned}
HR_{max} \quad &= 206.9 - (0.67 \times AGE) \\
&= 206.9 - (0.69 \times 25) \\
&= 206.9 - 16.8 \\
&= 190 \text{ bpm} \\
THR \quad &= (190 - 75) \times 0.70 + 75 \\
&= 115 \times 0.70 + 75 \\
&= 156 \pm 5 \text{ bpm}
\end{aligned}
$$

The training heart rate for this 25-year-old subject is 156 beats per minute. Assessment Activity 3-4 will enable you to determine your target heart rate for exercise.

Learning to take the pulse rate quickly and accurately is necessary to monitor exercise intensity by heart rate. Two of the most commonly used sites for taking the pulse rate are the radial artery on the thumb side of the wrist and the carotid artery at the side of the neck (Figure 3-1a and 3-1b). Use the first two fingers of your preferred hand to palpate (examine by touch or feel) the pulse. At the wrist, the pulse is located at the base of the thumb when the hand is held palm up. To find the carotid pulse, slide your fingers downward at the angle of the jaw below the earlobe to the side of the neck. You apply only enough pressure to feel the pulse, particularly at the carotid artery.

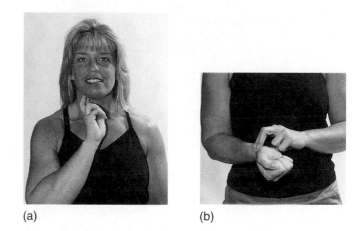

(a)                          (b)

**FIGURE 3-1** Sites for Taking a Pulse
The two sites for measuring pulse are (a) at the neck (carotid artery) and (b) at the wrist (radial artery).

Excessive pressure at this point stimulates specialized receptors that automatically slow the heart rate, leading to an underestimation of the rate achieved during exercise. The wrist is the preferred site for the palpation of the pulse rate. Palpate the carotid pulse if you cannot feel your pulse at the wrist.

Locate and count the pulse rate immediately after exercise stops. Count the beats for 10 seconds and multiply by 6 to get beats per minute. Regardless of which site you use, be consistent in its application. Some practice is required to locate the pulse quickly and count it accurately.

Another method for monitoring the intensity of exercise is to rate your subjective perception of the effort. On some days, exercise seems easier than normal, and on other days it may seem more difficult; therefore, it is important to adjust the intensity according to the perception of the effort. According to the ACSM, "the appropriate exercise intensity is one that is safe, is compatible with a long-term active lifestyle for that individual, and achieves the desired caloric output given the time constraints for the exercise session."[68]

The "Talk Test" is a simple subjective estimate that clearly demonstrates whether the individual is exercising too intensely. The intensity is excessive when the exerciser is unable to carry on a conversation without gasping for breath between each word or two. The remedy for such an occurrence is simple—*slow down the pace.*

## Time (Duration)

*Duration* refers to the length of each exercise session. Intensity and duration are inversely related—the more intense the exercise, the shorter its duration. Many fitness experts employ the acronym "FITT Principle" as a way for people to remember the major exercise principles of frequency, intensity, time, and type. Type refers to the physical activities that comprise the program. Intensity is the most important consideration for the development of physical fitness. But reducing the intensity somewhat while increasing the frequency and duration is the safest and most beneficial method for novice exercisers to attain physical fitness and health enhancement.

The number of minutes devoted to exercise is dependent upon intensity and one's objectives. Table 3-2 illustrates the time requirements for different exercise intensities. Calculating calories expended or steps counts are two alternative methods for monitoring duration. Expending 1,000 calories per week represents an initial goal for most healthy adults. This level of exercise translates to approximately 150 minutes per week. The recommended number of calories expended is 2,000 per week because this number returns greater health and fitness benefits, and it is sufficient to promote and sustain weight loss. Two thousand calories per week takes about 250 to 300 minutes per week or 50 to 60 minutes per day.[69]

Using a pedometer to count the number of steps per workout is gaining in popularity. Walking at a moderate-intensity pace for 30 minutes per day equals about 3,000 4,000 steps.[70] The recommended goal is to work your way up to 10,000 steps per day (approximately 5 miles).

## Type of Activity (Exercise Modality)

Select an aerobic activity or activities that you enjoy. You don't have to be an athlete or athletic to receive the benefits associated with a lifetime commitment to physical activity. Simple self-paced activities such as walking, jogging, cycling (overland or stationary), water activities, and so on will suffice. For those who are more skilled and enjoy the challenge of competing against others, lifetime sports such as racquetball, tennis, basketball, handball, and the like may be more appealing. Tables 3-4 and 3-5 present some physical activities and sports that may be included in an exercise program. See Real-World Wellness: Choosing Fitness Equipment for the Home for helpful advice for exercising in the privacy of your home.

Armed with knowledge of the principles of exercise, warm-up and cooldown procedures, along with advice on how to select your own exercise equipment, you should be able to design an exercise program for yourself using Assessment Activity 3-5 as a guide.

## Progression, Overload, and Specificity

As people attain a level of fitness that meets their needs and when further improvement is not desired, the program switches from developing fitness to maintaining it.

## Real-World Wellness
### Choosing Fitness Equipment for the Home

*I'm a working mother with two young children. My only chance to exercise is at home after the children have been put to bed. I'm most interested in purchasing a good piece of cardio equipment that will burn calories and increase my energy level. What advice can you give me for selecting such equipment?*

Here are some helpful hints:

1. Some of the most effective cardio equipment includes motor-driven treadmills, stationary exercise bikes, stationary rowers, stair climbers, elliptical trainers, cross-country skiing machines, videotape aerobic workouts (with or without stepping benches), and jump ropes.

2. Selecting the right piece of equipment is important. Many well-intentioned home exercisers become bored with the equipment they purchase or find that it is not meeting their needs, so they quit exercising.

3. Try out a piece of equipment before buying it. Make sure it feels comfortable, is easy to use, and is the right size for you.

4. Give equipment the 3-week test: Before making your purchase, borrow or rent the piece of equipment and use it three to five times per week for 3 weeks. At the end of 3 weeks, you should know whether you enjoy it well enough to use it regularly and whether it will meet your needs and goals. The best equipment in the world is useless unless you use it regularly.

5. Check the construction of equipment to make sure that it is sturdy. The machine should not rock or wobble, and it should perform smoothly.

6. Equipment made of lightweight sheet metal or with many plastic parts may not withstand regular use.

7. Do not buy the least expensive machine. Think of this purchase as a long-term investment. Usually a middle-of-the line product will do very well. These carry a 90-day warranty for parts, and the warranty may be extended to include service.

8. Shop at a reputable sports equipment store that has a knowledgeable sales staff who can answer your questions and help you make the appropriate choice.

9. Make sure that the store will deliver and set up the equipment.

10. If marketing and promotional claims made for the equipment sound too good to be true, they probably are.

At this point, the principles of overload and progression may be set aside, but both are necessary for the improvement phase of fitness. *Overload* involves subjecting the body to unaccustomed stress. Challenging the body to periodically accept a slightly increased level of work forces it to adapt by attaining a higher level of fitness. Deciding when to impose each new challenge involves the principle of *progression*. The workload is increased only when the exerciser is ready to accept a new challenge. For aerobic exercise, target heart rate or perceived exertion may be used to establish criteria for scheduling the progression. For example, if you jog, swim, or cycle a certain distance, the exercise heart rate will decrease over time as your body adapts to training. When the exercise heart rate drops to a predetermined level or the effort required becomes comfortable, you should adjust the pace or distance to return to the original target zone. However, the new physical challenge should not exceed the current amount of exercise by more than 10%. This should ensure that the new workload is not excessive.

The principle of *specificity* of training suggests that the body adapts according to the specific type of stress placed on it. The muscles involved in any activity are the ones that adapt, and they do so in the specific way in which they are used. For example, jogging prepares one for jogging but is poor preparation for cycling. Cycling does not prepare one for swimming. Although these activities stress the cardiorespiratory system, they are sufficiently different in that there is little fitness carryover among them.

The principle of specificity is particularly important for competitive athletes. Competitors attempt to maximize the returns from their training effort; therefore, runners must train by running, swimmers must swim, and cyclists must cycle. The focus is on maximal improvement in one activity, so that the body is trained in a specific manner. This locks athletes into regimented training programs, but noncompetitors who exercise for health and physical fitness reasons are not under such constraints. They can vary activities and prevent the boredom of participating in the same activity day after day, week after week. Cycling, jogging, swimming, racquetball, cross-country skiing, weight training, and other activities may be used in any combination or order for the development of physical fitness. This is the essence of **cross-training**. Not only does cross-training relieve boredom, but it may reduce the incidence of injury because it does not stress the same muscles in the same way during every workout.[71]

Cross-training has many advantages and is an excellent technique for attaining the health benefits of exercise. Variety, the major attraction of cross-training, can also be a disadvantage, however. By participating in many different activities, you seldom become proficient in any one. However, if the objective is physical fitness or health enhancement and not competition, proficiency is incidental.

Identifying goals provides some direction for the activities selected and the way the principles of exercise are to be manipulated to increase the probability of success. Only one or two major goals should be selected, and these should be as specific as possible, so that an effective exercise program can be devised. Activities, objectives, and exercise principles must match.

When you have identified the objectives and know what you wish to achieve from an exercise program, identify the means for sustaining the program. The resolve to exercise is shakiest during the early stages of the program, usually because people push untrained bodies beyond their limits. This results in sore muscles, stiffness, and possible injury. Consequently, the dropout rate is highest in the beginning of any exercise program. The irony is that the greatest return for the effort is attained during this phase.[72] Some tips for sustaining that effort are presented in Just the Facts: Motivational Tips.

## Other Exercise Considerations

### Warming Up for Exercise

Warming up prepares the body for physical action. The process involves physical activities that gradually heat the muscles and elevate the heart rate. It is a transitional stage that bridges the gap between rest and physical activity. For aerobic activities, the procedure involves physical movements that gradually raise muscle temperature, increase heart rate, and increase circulation. The intensity of the warm-up should be gradually increased over 5 to 10 minutes, ultimately reaching 50% of the planned exercise intensity.[73] Breaking out in a sweat is usually an indicator that the appropriate intensity has been achieved. The suggested warm-up for simple repetitive activities, such as jogging, cycling, and brisk walking, is to perform the specific activity at a lower intensity. For example, joggers should jog at a slower than exercise pace during the warm-up, gradually increasing the pace as the warm-up progresses. This procedure gradually warms up the muscles that are to be used during exercise in the specific way in which they are to be used. Additionally, it reduces the oxygen deficit that normally occurs at the beginning of exercise. The oxygen deficit is the result of the body's inability to meet the oxygen demand of the exercise. It takes 2 to 3 minutes for the aerobic system to catch up and thus supply the oxygen needed to support the exercise. At this point, the exercise will feel more comfortable and can be maintained for a period of time. The oxygen deficit can be attenuated and possibly eliminated with a well-structured warm-up.

Increasing the heart rate gradually during the warm-up is most important. This allows the circulatory system

Follow these tips to stay motivated to exercise:

- Exercise with a friend. Make sure both of you have compatible goals and are similar in fitness level. Friends can help each other sustain a program, particularly during busy times when the temptation is high to push exercise out of an already crowded schedule.

- Exercise with a group. Exchange ideas and literature about exercise with group members.

- Elicit the support of friends and family. Their support is a powerful source of reinforcement.

- Associate with other exercisers. They represent an enthusiastic, positive, and informative group—and their values are contagious.

- Join an exercise class or a fitness club. This gives you a place to go and meet people who want to exercise.

- Keep a progress chart. This will give you an objective account of your improvement.

- Exercise to music. Music makes the effort appear easier.

- Set a definite time and place to exercise. This is particularly important during the early days of the program. Schedule exercise as you would any other activity of importance and then commit to the schedule.

- Participate in a variety of activities. Cross-training is excellent for the person who exercises for health or recreation.

- Do not become obsessive about exercise. Skipping exercise is not a good practice normally, but skipping is appropriate at times. Do not exercise when you are sick or overtired. Do not feel guilty about missing exercise for a day or two. Resume exercise as soon as you can.

to adjust to the load. If the heart rate elevates suddenly, circulation cannot adjust rapidly enough to meet the oxygen and nutrient demands of the heart muscle. The effects of this lag time are abolished in about 2 minutes, but increasing the heart rate quickly can be hazardous even during those 2 minutes, particularly for those with compromised circulation. Even a healthy heart may be affected when the gradual phase of warm-up has been eliminated. Abnormal electrocardiographic (ECG) responses were reported in several studies when the exercise sessions were not preceded by an active warm-up. Sudden strenuous physical exertion produced temporary left ventricular dysfunction and possible ventricular arrhythmias that were evident on the ECG.[74,75,76] However, another study failed to confirm the cardiovascular abnormalities cited in the previous studies.[77] The reason for the disparity in the results may very well be the difference in the assessment techniques used. In light of the equivocal nature of these data, a proper warm-up should precede exercise. The logic of this position has not been refuted.

Passive warm-up techniques, such as massage, sauna baths, steam baths, hot showers, hot towels, and heating pads, should not be used as substitutes for an active warm-up. These techniques may precede an active warm-up if a person feels stiff and sore from the previous workout.

Stretching exercises may be performed after the warm-up is completed. At this point, muscle temperature is elevated, so that stretching is more effective and muscle, tendon, and joint injuries are less likely to occur. Stretching performed prior to exercise may not reduce the risk of musculoskeletal injury during exercise. The evidence in support of or against this supposition is equivocal at best.[78] Stretching is most effective during the cooldown following the workout because (1) muscles are heated and receptive to stretching, and (2) muscles that have contracted repeatedly during exercise need to be stretched. Figures 5-1 through 5-8 in Chapter 5 illustrate some typical stretching exercises that may be used before and after the workout period.

## Cooling Down from Exercise

The cooldown is as important as the warm-up. Cooldown should last 8 to 10 minutes and consist of two phases. The first phase involves approximately 5 minutes of walking or other light activities to prevent blood from pooling in the muscles that have been working. Light activity causes rhythmic contractions of the muscles, which in turn act as a stimulus to circulate blood from the muscles back to the heart for redistribution throughout the body. This boost to circulation following exercise, often referred to as the *muscle pump*, is essential for recovery and shares some of the burden of circulation with the heart. The muscle pump effect does not occur if a period of inactivity follows exercise. An inactive cooldown forces the heart to work at a high rate to compensate for the reduced volume of blood returning to it because of blood pooling in the muscles. Exercisers run the risk of a hypotensive response (a sharp drop in blood pressure), which may result in dizziness and fainting. Also, elevated blood levels of catecholamines (epinephrine and norepinephrine) during the first couple of minutes of recovery may produce fatal heart arrhythmias.[79]

Light physical activity after exercise also speeds the removal of lactic acid that has accumulated in the mus-

## Table 3-4   Rating 14 Sports and Exercises

| Excercise | Cardio-respiratory Endurance (Stamina) | Muscular Endurance | Muscular Strength | Flexibility | Balance | General Well-Being | | | | Total |
|---|---|---|---|---|---|---|---|---|---|---|
| | | | | | | Weight Control | Muscle Definition | Digestion | Sleep | |
| Jogging | 21* | 20 | 17 | 9 | 17 | 21 | 14 | 13 | 16 | 148 |
| Bicycling | 19 | 18 | 16 | 9 | 18 | 20 | 15 | 12 | 15 | 142 |
| Swimming | 21 | 20 | 14 | 15 | 12 | 15 | 14 | 13 | 16 | 140 |
| Skating (ice or roller) | 18 | 17 | 15 | 13 | 20 | 17 | 14 | 11 | 15 | 140 |
| Handball/ squash | 19 | 18 | 15 | 16 | 17 | 19 | 11 | 13 | 12 | 140 |
| Skiing— nordic | 19 | 19 | 15 | 14 | 16 | 17 | 12 | 12 | 15 | 139 |
| Skiing— alpine | 16 | 18 | 15 | 14 | 21 | 15 | 14 | 9 | 12 | 134 |
| Basketball | 19 | 17 | 15 | 13 | 16 | 19 | 13 | 10 | 12 | 134 |
| Tennis | 16 | 16 | 14 | 14 | 16 | 16 | 13 | 12 | 11 | 128 |
| Calisthenics | 10 | 13 | 16 | 19 | 15 | 12 | 18 | 11 | 12 | 126 |
| Walking | 13 | 14 | 11 | 7 | 8 | 13 | 11 | 11 | 14 | 102 |
| Golf** | 8 | 8 | 9 | 9 | 8 | 6 | 6 | 7 | 6 | 67 |
| Softball | 6 | 8 | 7 | 9 | 7 | 7 | 5 | 8 | 7 | 64 |
| Bowling | 5 | 5 | 5 | 7 | 6 | 5 | 5 | 7 | 6 | 51 |

*The ratings are on a scale of 0 to 3; thus, a rating of 21 is the maximum score that can be achieved (a score by 3 of all 7 panelists). Ratings were made on the following basis: frequency, four times per week minimal; duration, 30 to 60 minutes per session.

**The rating was made on the basis of using a golf cart or caddy. If you walk the course and carry your clubs, the values improve.

## Table 3-5  Rating Selected Sports

| Sport | Cardiorespiratory Endurance | Muscular Strength/Endurance | | Flexibility | Body Composition |
|---|---|---|---|---|---|
| | | Upper | Lower | | |
| Badminton | M-H* | L | M-H | L | M-H |
| Football (touch) | L-M | L-M | M | L | L-M |
| Ice hockey | H | M | H | L | H |
| Racquetball | H | M | H | M | H |
| Rugby | H | M-H | H | M | H |
| Soccer | H | L | H | M | H |
| Volleyball | M | M | M | L-M | M |
| Wrestling | H | H | H | M-H | H |

*H, high; M, medium; L, low. The values in this table are estimates that vary according to the skill and motivation of the participants.

cles. *Lactic acid* is a fatiguing metabolite resulting from the incomplete breakdown of sugar. It is produced by exercise of high intensity or of long duration.

The second phase of cooldown should focus on the stretching exercises performed during the warm-up. Most participants find that stretching after exercise is more comfortable and more effective because the muscles are heated and more elastic. Attention should also be given to the information that appears in Just the Facts: Exercise-Related Considerations.

## Environmental Conditions

People work and exercise in a variety of environmental conditions. Hot and cold weather produce unique problems for people who function outdoors. Their safety and comfort depend on their knowledge of the ways the body reacts to physical activity in different climatic conditions.

Heat is produced in the body as a by-product of metabolism. Physical activities significantly increase metabolism, generating more heat than normal. Heat must be dissipated efficiently, or it may build up, result-

# [ JUST THE FACTS ]

## Exercise-Related Considerations

Many health, fitness, and cosmetic benefits occur to those who exercise on a regular basis. Although they are outweighed by the benefits, risks are associated with such behavior. Despite precautions, injuries occasionally occur. Beginning exercisers are particularly susceptible to injury because of their lack of knowledge about training coupled with their misguided attempts to achieve their goals too quickly. The following suggestions should result in safer workouts:

1. Dress according to the weather: shorts, T-shirt, mesh baseball-type cap in warm weather; layers of light clothing, hat, gloves, ear protection, and windbreaker in cold weather.
2. Wear appropriate shoes for the activity in which you participate: jogging shoes, walking shoes, aerobic shoes, or cross-trainers. In general, exercise shoes should be ½ to ¾ of an inch longer than your longest toe. There should also be room enough for the toes to spread out. The soles of most exercise shoes consist of three layers. The outer sole that contacts the floor or ground should be made of hard rubber. The next layer is the midsole, which protects the midfoot and toes. The last layer is made of a thick, spongy substance that absorbs most of the shock when the foot strikes the surface.
3. Warm up and cool down properly before and after exercise.
4. Exercise within your capacity—it should feel a little uncomfortable but not painful. According to the American College of Sports Medicine (ACSM), the initial stage of an exercise program should last a minimum of 4 weeks at a low intensity (50 to 60% of the maximal heart rate, or HRmax). Each exercise session should last for 15 to 20 minutes during the first week and increase to 25 to 30 minutes during the fourth week. At this point, the exerciser is ready to increase the intensity, frequency, and duration of each session.

5. While following these simple guidelines reduces the possibility of incurring pain or injury, beginning exercisers may experience, as a result of overuse, shin splints, side stitch, blisters, chafing, muscle cramps, muscle soreness, Achilles tendon injuries, and lower-back pain.
   a. Muscle soreness following exercise usually occurs among beginners who have yet to adapt to physical exertion or to those at any level of fitness who exceed their physical capabilities. Following the ACSM guidelines reduces exposure to muscle pain.
   b. Side stitches occur primarily among walkers and joggers. They consist of severe pain in the upper right quadrant of the abdomen. Side stitches may be caused by reduced blood flow to the diaphragm (a large, dome-shaped muscle that separates the abdominal cavity from the chest cavity), or they may be due to the collection of gas in the intestines. In either case, deep breathing and direct pressure applied with both hands at the site of the pain may provide relief. Sometimes, stopping the activity for a few minutes is required for the pain to subside.
   c. A common injury occurring among beginners is shin splints. Shin splints produce a burning pain that radiates along the inner surface of the large bones of the lower leg. These are nagging, painful injuries better prevented than treated. The causes of shin splints include training demands that exceed a person's capacity to perform. High-impact activities, such as jogging or aerobics to music; poor-quality exercise shoes; hard exercise surfaces; and walking or jogging on hilly surfaces are other contributing causes. Treatment includes applying ice, resting, wrapping or taping the affected shin, and placing heel lifts in the shoes.

ing in **hyperthermia**, abnormally high body temperature that can cause illness or even death. Human beings are homeotherms, which means that we function within a narrow range of internal body temperatures. Normal temperature ranges from 97° to 100° Fahrenheit (F). The average temperature is 98.6 °F. Temperature control, or thermoregulation, represents a balance between heat produced by the body's metabolically active tissues plus heat gained from the environment compared to loss. The hypothalamus (a brain structure that maintains a constant internal environment) functions as a thermostat by decreasing heat production when the body tem-

perature rises and increasing heat production when it falls. When heat is gained more rapidly than it is lost—such as during vigorous exercise—the temperature may rise to the point where heat-stress illnesses may occur. Proteins that build body tissues and direct virtually all chemical processes can tolerate only small fluctuations in body temperature or they get too hot, change shape, and stop functioning.[80] At this juncture, heat-stress illness may occur and may run the gamut from a relatively minor problem, heat syncope (loss of consciousness), to a major life-threatening medical emergency, heat stroke. Heat cramps are painful muscle cramps that usually occur in the abdominal muscles or in fatigued leg muscles.[81] Treatment includes rest accompanied by drinking a cool, salted (0.5%) fluid. Heat syncope is characterized by feeling faint or fainting. Treatment involves moving subjects to a cool environment where they can lie down and drink cool, salted fluids. *Heat exhaustion* is a serious condition but not an imminent threat to life. It is characterized by dizziness, weakness, fainting, rapid pulse, profuse sweating, and cool skin. Treatment includes immediate cessation of activity. The victim should be moved to a cool, shady place; placed in a reclining position; and given cool fluids to drink.

Heat stroke is the most severe of the heat-induced illnesses. The symptoms include a high temperature (greater than 104 °F) and dry skin caused by the cessation of sweating. These symptoms are accompanied by delirium, convulsions, or loss of consciousness. The early warning signs include chills, nausea, headache, and general weakness. Victims of heat stroke should be rushed immediately to the nearest hospital for treatment.

## Mechanisms of Heat Loss

Heat is lost from the body by conduction, convection, radiation, and evaporation of sweat. Conduction, convection, and radiation are mechanisms responsible for heat loss *and* heat gain. These three depend on the difference between the temperature of the body and that of the environment. These mechanisms do not function alone to effect heat loss or gain.

*Conduction* occurs when direct physical contact is made between objects of which one is cooler than the other. The greater the difference in temperature between the objects, the greater the transfer of heat. An example is entering an air-conditioned room from outdoors on a summer day and sitting in a cool leather chair. Heat is lost through contact with the cooler chair, as well as the cooler air that is in contact with the skin. By the same token, sitting in a hot tub in which the temperature of the water is several degrees warmer than skin temperature results in the transfer of heat to the body rather than away from it.

Conductive heat loss occurs even more rapidly in water.[82] Water is not an insulator but a conductor. It absorbs 26 times more heat than does air at the same temperature. Air is an excellent insulator but a poor conductor. This is the reason that sitting at poolside is more comfortable than sitting in the pool, even if the temperatures of air and water are equal.

Heat loss or gain by *convection* occurs when a gas or water moves across the skin. Heat is transferred from the body to the environment more effectively if a breeze is blowing. Convective heat loss in water is increased when a person is swimming rather than floating because of the increased movement of the water

across the body. The same principle applies to running outdoors because of the air flow over the body.

Humans, animals, and inanimate objects constantly transmit heat by electromagnetic waves to cooler objects in the environment. This heat loss through *radiation* occurs without physical contact between objects. Heat is transferred on a temperature gradient from warmer objects to cooler ones.[83]

Heat loss by radiation is effective when the air temperature (ambient temperature) is well below skin temperature. This is one of the main reasons that outdoor exercise in cool weather is better tolerated than the same exercise in hot weather. Muscles fatigue more rapidly when exercise occurs in hot weather.[84] Exercise is more difficult to sustain in hot weather because higher amounts of lactic acid are produced and greater amounts accumulate in the muscles, promoting fatigue and making muscle contraction more difficult.[85] Temperatures in the upper 80s and 90s often result in heat gain by radiation.

*Evaporation* of sweat is the main method of heat loss during exercise, and this process is most effective when the humidity is low.[86] High humidity significantly impairs the evaporative process because the air is saturated and cannot accept much moisture. If both temperature and humidity are high, losing heat is difficult by any of these processes. Under these conditions, adjusting the intensity and duration of exercise or moving indoors, where the climate can be controlled, may be beneficial.

Heat loss by evaporation occurs only when the sweat on the surface of the skin is vaporized—that is, converted to a gas. The conversion of liquid to a gas at the skin level requires heat supplied by the body. As liquid sweat absorbs heat from the skin, it changes to a gaseous vapor carried away by the surrounding air, resulting in the removal of heat generated from exercise.[87] Small amounts of evaporative sweat remove large quantities of heat. For example, each pint of sweat that evaporates removes approximately 280 calories of heat. Beads of sweat that roll off the body do not contribute to the cooling process—only sweat that evaporates does.

Exercise in hot and humid conditions forces the body to divert more blood than usual from the working muscles to the skin in an effort to carry the heat accumulating in the deeper recesses to the outer shell. The result is that the exercising muscles are deprived of a full complement of blood and cannot work as long or as hard. Exercise is therefore more difficult in hot and humid weather.

Heat loss by evaporation is seriously impeded when a person wears nonporous garments, such as rubberized and plastic exercise suits. These garments encourage sweating, but their nonporous nature does not allow sweat to evaporate. This practice is dangerous because it may easily result in heat buildup and *dehydration* (excessive water loss), leading to heat-stress illnesses. You should dress for hot-weather exercise by wearing shorts and a porous top. A mesh, baseball-type cap is optional. It is effective in blocking the absorption of radiant heat if you exercise in the middle of the day, because the sun's rays are vertical. You do not need to wear a cap when exercising in the cooler times of the day or if the sun is not shining.

## Guidelines for Exercise in the Heat

Guidelines for exercising in heat and humidity have been developed for road races, but these guidelines can be applied to any strenuous physical activity performed outdoors during warm weather. Ambient conditions are considered safe when the temperature is below 70 °F and the humidity is below 60%.[88] Caution should be used and people sensitive to heat and humidity should reconsider exercising when the temperature is greater than 80 °F or the humidity is over 60%. People who are trained and heat acclimated can continue to exercise in these conditions, but they should be aware of the potential hazards and take precautions to prevent heat illness.

The keys to exercising without incident in hot weather are acclimating to the heat and maintaining the body's normal fluid level. Acclimation to heat is characterized by physiological adjustments that occur naturally from repeated exposure to exercise in the heat.[89] Acclimation includes the early onset of sweating, an increase in the rate of sweating, and the reduction of sodium in sweat. These adjustments result in less cardiovascular strain and a lower body temperature for a specific amount of exercise. Most healthy people become fully acclimated to heat in 10 to 14 days. The main consequence of dehydration (excessive fluid loss) is a reduction in blood volume. This results in sluggish circulation, which decreases the delivery of oxygen to the exercising muscles. Lowered blood volume results in less blood that can be sent to the skin to remove the heat generated by exercise. If too much of the blood volume is lost, sweating stops and the body temperature rises, leading to heat-stress illness. Heat stress illness is a serious problem that can be avoided by following these guidelines designed to preserve the body's fluid level:

*Estimating Water Loss*

- Weigh yourself nude before and after exercise.
- Towel off sweat completely after exercise and then weigh yourself.
- Each pound of weight loss represents about 1 pint of fluid loss. Be sure to drink that and more after exercise. See Just the Facts: Fluid Consumption Before, During, and After Exercise.[90]

*Other Considerations*

- Modify the exercise program by (1) working out during cooler times of day, (2) choosing shady

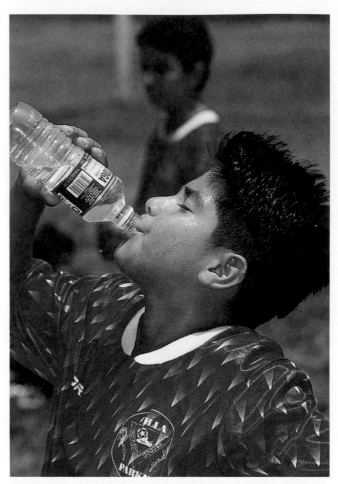

In hot, humid weather, drinking water and wearing loose clothing help prevent hyperthermia and heat-stress illnesses.

routes where water is available, (3) slowing the pace or shortening the duration of exercise on particularly oppressive days, and (4) wearing light, loose, porous clothing to facilitate the evaporation of sweat.
- Never take salt tablets. They are stomach irritants, they attract fluid to the gut, they sometimes pass through the digestive system undissolved, and they may perforate the stomach lining.
- Exercise must be prolonged, produce profuse sweating, and occur over a number of consecutive days to reduce potassium stores. For the average bout of exercise, you do not need to worry about depleting potassium or make a special effort to replace it. The daily consumption of fresh fruits and vegetables, as suggested by the food pyramid, is all that is needed (see Chapter 6).
- Remember to use a sunscreen lotion when the weather is sunny or hazy. Be sure that the sunscreen you select has a sun protection factor (SPF) of at least 15, and apply it liberally over exposed skin.

## [ JUST THE FACTS ]

### Fluid Consumption Before, During, and After Exercise

The American College of Sports Medicine has issued the following recommendations about fluid consumption:

1. Make a special effort to drink plenty of fluid every day, so that you will be fully hydrated prior to exercise.

2. The daily water needs of most moderately fit active people range between 3 and 5 liters (a little more than 3 to 5 quarts).

3. It is a common occurrence that fluid losses exceed fluid replacement during intense physical exercise for a variety of reasons.

4. Drink fluids during exercise that contain carbohydrates (sugars) and sodium because these will enhance performance and delay fatigue more effectively than an equal amount of plain water for exercises lasting 45 to 50 minutes or during high-intensity intermittent exercises.

5. It is imperative to consume carbohydrate/sodium fluids during prolonged physical activity. Replacing with plain water, combined with sweat loss, reduces blood levels of sodium. If the sodium deficit becomes excessive, it will lead to exertional **hyponatremia**. The symptoms of hyponatremia include progressively worsening headache, confusion, disorientation, nausea, vomiting, aphasia (impair-

ment of speech or understanding speech), muscle cramps, and muscle weakness. It sometimes results in death.

6. Women are at greater risk of incurring exertional hyponatremia because their fluid intake is more likely to exceed their sweat rate and because they have less body water than males and a smaller body mass that is more readily affected by overdrinking.

7. The general rule after exercise is to drink until thirst is satisfied and then drink a bit more in order to satisfy your tissue needs.

8. Rehydration after exercise requires fluid replacement of 125 to 150% of the loss of body mass (weight) during exercise. Each pound lost during exercise represents the loss of one pint of fluid. The loss of 3 pounds of body mass would require the consumption of 3.75 pints (125%) to 4.5 pints (150%) of fluid. The replacement fluid should be tasty and contain sugar, sodium, and possibly potassium and magnesium in amounts that can be found, for example, in sports drinks.

9. Caffeine, alcohol, and protein can modestly increase urine water loss and should not be consumed immediately after exercise. This is counterproductive because rapid and complete hydration is desirable at this point.

Sources: Casa, D. J., P. M. Clarkson, & W. O. Roberts. (2005). *American College of Sports Medicine Roundtable on Hydration and Physical Activity: Consensus statements.* Storrs, CT: Current Science Inc.

American College of Sports Medicine. (2007, February). Exercise and fluid replacement. *Medicine and Science in Sports and Exercise,* 39(2), 377.

Quinn, E. (2007, December 2). ACSM clarifies indicator for fluid replacement. *Sports Medicine.* http://sportsmedicine.about.com/cs/hydration/a/022504.htm.

## Guidelines for Exercise in the Cold

Problems related to exercise in cold weather include frostbite and **hypothermia** (abnormally low body temperature). *Frostbite* can lead to permanent damage or loss of a body part from gangrene. This can be prevented by adequately protecting exposed areas, such as fingers, nose, ears, facial skin, and toes. Gloves, preferably mittens or thick socks, should be worn to protect the fingers, hands, and wrists. Blood vessels in the scalp do not constrict effectively, so a significant amount of heat is lost if a head covering is not worn. A stocking-type hat is the best head covering because it can be pulled down to protect the ears. In very cold or windy weather, use surgical or ski masks and scarves to keep facial skin warm and to moisten and warm inhaled air. All exposed or poorly protected flesh is vulnerable to frostbite when the temperature is low and the windchill high. Air temperature plus wind speed equals the windchill index. This value will help you know how to dress appropriately for outdoor exercise.

People often experience a hacking cough for a minute or two after physical exertion in cold weather. This is a normal response and should not cause alarm. Very cold, dry air may not be fully moistened when it is inhaled rapidly and in large volumes during exercise, so the lining of the throat dries out. When exercise is discontinued, the respiratory rate slows and the volume of inhaled air decreases, allowing enough time for the body to fully moisturize it. Coughing stops within a couple of minutes as the linings are remoistened.

*Hypothermia* is the most severe of the problems associated with outdoor activity in cold weather. Hypothermia occurs when body heat is lost faster than it can be produced. This can be a life-threatening situation. The adjustments made by the body to avoid excessive heat loss include shivering, nonshivering thermogenesis, and peripheral vasoconstriction. Shivering is the involuntary contraction of muscles. These contractions increase the body's heat production by four to five times that produced under normal resting conditions.[91] Nonshivering thermogenesis raises body temperature through neural stimulation that increases metabolic rate. Peripheral vasoconstriction occurs from the neurally mediated contraction of smooth muscles located subcutaneously (beneath the skin). The contractions of these muscles constrict the small arteries beneath the skin, leading to decreased blood flow to the skin. This adjustment prevents unnecessary heat loss. However, hypothermia may still occur because these adjustments can be overcome by excessive exposure to cold.

Exercise in cold weather requires insulating layers of clothing to preserve normal body heat. Without this protection, body heat is quickly lost because of the large temperature gradient between the skin and environment. A layer or two of insulating clothing can be discarded if you get too hot.

Hypothermia can occur even if the air temperature is above freezing.[92] The rate of heat loss for any temperature is influenced by wind velocity. Wind velocity increases the amount of cold air molecules that come in contact with the skin. The more cold molecules, the more effective the heat loss. The speed of walking, jogging, or cycling into the wind must be added to the speed of the wind to properly evaluate the impact of windchill.

You should wear enough clothing to stay warm, but not so much as to induce profuse sweating. Knowing how much clothing to wear comes from experience exercising in various environmental conditions. Clothing that becomes wet with sweat loses its insulating qualities. It becomes a conductor of heat, moving heat from the body quickly and potentially endangering the exerciser.

If you exercise or work outdoors in cold weather, you may want to wear polypropylene undergarments. Polypropylene is designed to whisk perspiration away from the skin, so that evaporative cooling does not rob heat from the body. You should wear a warm outer garment, preferably made of wool, over this material. If it is windy, wear a breathable windbreaker as the third, outer layer.

If you follow the guidelines for activity in hot and cold weather, you can usually participate comfortably all year long. Other hazards associated with outdoor exercise are discussed in Real-World Wellness: Exercising Safely in an Urban Environment.

# Real-World Wellness

## Exercising Safely in an Urban Environment

*I live in a large city and like to jog outdoors in my neighborhood. How can I limit the risks associated with exercising in the heart of the city?*

You can start by becoming familiar with the risks to avoid or lessen their impact. Some of the major hazards follow:

1. Traffic volume is one of the primary risks associated with jogging in a large city. This risk can be reduced by wearing reflective clothing, jogging during daylight hours, and jogging on the sidewalks rather than the streets. The best way to handle the problem is to find a nearby park or outdoor running track.

2. A second risk comes from air pollution, primarily carbon monoxide and ozone. The Centers for Disease Control and Prevention has identified outdoor exercisers as one group at high risk for the effects of ozone, carbon monoxide, and other air pollutants. Rapid, deep breathing during exercise results in inhaling more pollutants more deeply into the lungs. Some studies have shown that 30 minutes of jogging during heavy traffic conditions increased carbon monoxide levels in the blood to the equivalent of smoking half a pack of cigarettes.

Carbon monoxide interferes with the delivery of oxygen to the body's tissues and, when inhaled in high quantities, can cause illness and death. Carbon monoxide emissions from cars, trucks, and buses are most prevalent during rush hours, so avoid jogging on busy streets during these times.

Ozone causes lung inflammation and injury. The long-term effects of exercising in high ozone conditions are not known. Ozone tends to accumulate in the atmosphere after 10:00 a.m. It is heaviest during bright, sunny days because it is produced by the photochemical reaction of sunlight with hydrocarbons and nitrogen dioxide from motor vehicle exhaust.

Jogging before the rush hour begins will (1) help control your exposure to motor vehicle emissions and (2) allow you to exercise prior to the buildup of ozone in the atmosphere.

3. Joggers and other outdoor exercisers can be targets for crime. Carry no visible money or valuables, such as watches or jewelry. Carry an I.D. tag with your name and the telephone number of a family member or friend in case you are involved in an accident. Do not carry addresses, yours or your family's, in case you are mugged.

# Summary

- *Physical fitness* is defined in terms of performance-related and health-related fitness.
- Cardiorespiratory endurance is the most important component of health-related fitness.
- The long-term effects of physical training include modifications in heart rate, stroke volume, cardiac output, blood volume, heart volume, respiration, and metabolism.
- Aerobic capacity is finite, improves by 5 to 25% with training, and decreases with aging; this decrease is slower in those who are physically fit.
- The training effect is lost in stages if exercise is interrupted or discontinued.
- Exercise affects cholesterol levels, blood pressure, and triglyceride levels; may reduce the risks for diabetes mellitus and stress; and is an alternative method for quitting use of tobacco products.
- The principles of exercise can be manipulated to meet any exercise objective.
- Exercising by varying the activities per exercise session or during exercise sessions is cross-training.
- The heat generated by exercise is lost from the body by conduction, convection, radiation, and evaporation.
- Evaporation of sweat is the major mechanism for ridding the body of heat that develops during exercise.
- Hypothermia is the most severe problem associated with exercise in cold weather.

# Review Questions

1. What are the physiological changes that occur from regular participation in aerobic exercise?
2. What are the health benefits that occur from regular participation in aerobic training?
3. Name and define the physiological changes that occur with exercise training.
4. Identify and define the principles of physical conditioning.
5. Define *cross-training* and give some examples.
6. Why should you warm up before exercise?
7. Identify and define the mechanisms of heat loss. Which of these is most important during exercise and why?
8. Describe fluid replacement before, during, and after exercise.

# References

1. American College of Sports Medicine. (2010). *ACSM's Guidelines for Exercise Testing and Prescription* (8th ed.) Philadelphia: Walters Kluwer/Lippincott Williams and Wilkins.
2. Ibid.
3. Ibid.
4. Bassett, D. (2010). Assessment of physical activity. In *ACSM's resource manual* (6th ed.), edited by J. K. Ehrman. Philadelphia: Walters Kluwer/Lippincott Williams and Wilkins.
5. Powers, S. K., & E. T. Howley. (2009). *Exercise physiology* (7th ed.). Boston: McGraw-Hill Higher Education.
6. Wilmore, J., H., D. L. Costill, & W. L. Kenney. (2009). *Physiology of sport and exercise* (4th ed.). Champaign, IL: Human Kinetics.
7. Ibid.
8. Powers & Howley (2009).
9. Ibid.
10. Ibid.
11. ACSM (2010).
12. Powers & Howley (2009).
13. Brawner, C. A., S. J. Keteyian, & M. Sawal. (2010). Adaptations to cardiovascular exercise training. In *ACSM's Resource Manual* (6th ed.), edited by J. K. Ehrman. Philadelphia: Walters Kluwer/Lippincott Williams and Wilkins.
14. Powers & Howley (2009).
15. Ibid.
16. Keteyian, S. J., & C. A. Brawner. (2006). Cardiopulmonary adaptations to exercise. In *ACSM's Resource Manual* (5th ed.), edited by L. A. Kaminsky. Philadelphia: Lippincott Williams and Wilkins.
17. Wilmore et al. (2008).
18. Ibid.
19. Ibid.
20. Powers & Howley (2009).
21. Ibid.
22. Ibid.
23. Baird, R. (2010, January 28). Tips to improve aerobic capacity. Retrieved from http://www.Selfgrowth.com/articles/Tips To Improve Aerobic Capacity.html.
24. Powers & Howley (2009).
25. Ibid.
26. Ibid.
27. Brooks, G. A., T. D. Fahey, T. White, & K. M. Baldwin. (2002). *Exercise physiology* (3rd ed.). Mountain View, CA: Mayfield.
28. Bouchard, C., et al. (1999). Familial aggregation of $VO_2$ max response to exercise training: Results from the Heritage Family Study. *Journal of Applied Physiology*, 87, 1003.
29. Wilmore et al. (2008).
30. Powers & Howley (2009).
31. Ibid.
32. Martino, M., N. Gledhill, & V. Jamnik. (2002). High $VO_2$ max with no history of training is due to high blood volume. *Medicine and Science in Sports and Exercise,* 34, 966.
33. Graves, B. S., M. Whitehurst, & B. W. Findlay. (2006). Physiologic effects of aging and deconditioning. In *ACSM's Resource Manual* (5th ed.), edited by L. A. Kaminsky. Philadelphia: Lippincott Williams and Wilkins.
34. Powers & Howley (2009).

35. Graves, B. S., M. Whitehurst, & B. W. Findlay. (2010). Lifespan effects of aging and deconditioning. In *ACSM's Resource Manual* (6th ed.), edited by J. K. Ehrman. Philadelphia: Walters Kluwer/Lippincott Williams and Wilkins.

36. Wilmore et al. (2008).

37. Ibid.

38. ACSM (2010).

39. Nieman, D. C. (2007). *Exercise testing and prescription* (6th ed.). Boston: McGraw-Hill.

40. Ibid.

41. ACSM (2010).

42. The President's Council on Physical Fitness and Sports. (2008, April 23). Physical Activity Facts. Retrieved from http://www.fitness.gov/resources/facts/index.html.

43. DHHS. (2008, March 20). 2008 Physical Activity Guidelines for Americans. Retrieved from http://www.health.gov/PAGuidelines/.

44. Centers for Disease Control. (2010, February 2). Physical activity school and community guidelines. Retrieved from http://www.cdc.gov/HealthyYouth/physicalactivity/guidelines/summary.htm.

45. Beckman, S. (2001). Emergency procedures and exercise safety. In *ACSM's Resource Manual* (4th ed.), edited by J. L. Roitman. Philadelphia: Lippincott Williams and Wilkins.

46. Beckman, S. (2010). Exercise program safety and emergency procedures. In *ACSM's Resource Manual* (6th ed.), edited by J. K. Ehrman. Philadelphia: Lippincott Williams and Wilkins.

47. Powers & Howley (2009).

48. Tucker, R., & J. Dugas. (2007, November). Sudden death during exercise—What does it mean for you? Retrieved from www.sportsscientists.com/2007/11/sudden death during ecercise what does.html.

49. ACSM (2010).

50. Mittleman, M. A., et al. (1993). Triggering of acute myocardial infarction by heavy physical exertion. *New England Journal of Medicine*, 329, 1677.

51. Whang, W., et al. (2006, March 22, 29). Physical exertion, exercise, and sudden cardiac death in women. *Journal of the American Medical Association*, 295, 1399.

52. Ibid.

53. ACSM (2010).

54. Willich, S. N., et al. (1993). Physical exertion as a trigger of acute myocardial infarction. *New England Journal of Medicine*, 329(23), 1684.

55. Mittleman et al. (1993).

56. Pate, R. R., et al. (1995). Physical activity and public health. A recommendation from the Centers for Disease Control and Prevention and the American College of Sports Medicine. *Journal of the American College of Sports Medicine*, 273, 402.

57. ACSM (2010).

58. Food and Nutrition Board, National Academy of Science. (2002). *Dietary reference intakes for energy, carbohydrates, fiber, fat, protein, and amino acids*. Washington, DC: National Academies Press.

59. U.S. Department of Health and Human Services and U.S. Department of Agriculture. (2005). (6th ed.). Washington, DC: U.S. Government Printing Office.

60. Barclay, L., & D. Lie. (2006, June 28). AHA dietary and lifestyle recommendations revised. *Medscape Medical News*. Retrieved from http://www.medscape.com/viewarticle/536831.

61. Nelson, M. E., W .J. Rejeski, S. N. Blair, et al. (2007). Physical activity and public health in older adults: Recommendation from the American College of Sports Medicine and the American Heart Association. *Medicine and Science in Sports and Exercise*, 39(8), 1435.

62. U.S. Department of Health and Human Services. (2008). *2008 physical activity guidelines for Americans*. Hyattsville, MD: Department of Health and Human Services.

63. U.S. Department of Health and Human Services (2005).

64. Barclay & Lie (2006).

65. ACSM (2010).

66. Ibid.

67. Ibid.

68. Ibid.

69. Ibid.

70. Wallace, J. (2006). Principles of cardiorespiratory endurance programming. In *ACSM's Resource Manual* (5th ed.), edited by L. A. Kaminsky. Philadelphia: Lippincott Williams and Wilkins.

71. King, A. C., & C. Castro. (2006). Factors associated with regular physical activity participation. In *ACSM's Resource Manual* (5th ed.), edited by L. A. Kaminsky. Philadelphia: Lippincott Williams and Wilkins.

72. Kravitz, L. (2006). Applied exercise programming. In *ACSM's Resource Manual* (5th ed.), edited by L .A. Kaminsky. Philadelphia: Lippincott Williams and Wilkins.

73. ACSM (2010).

74. Foster, C., J. D. Anholm, & C. K. Hellman. (1981). Left ventricular function during sudden strenuous exercise. *Circulation*, 63, 592.

75. Foster, C., et al. (1982). Effects of warm-up on left ventricular response to strenuous exercise. *Journal of Applied Physiology*, 53, 380.

76. Chelser, R. M., et al. (1997). Cardiovascular response to sudden strenuous exercise: An exercise echocardiographic study. *Medicine and Science in Sports and Exercise*, 29(10), 1299.

77. Kravitz (2006).

78. Howley, E. T., & B. D. Franks. (2007). *Health fitness instructor's handbook* (5th ed.). Champaign, IL: Human Kinetics.

79. Editors. (2003). Don't let the heat beat your heart." *Harvard Heart Letter*, 13(10), 2.

80. Harris, C., & K. J. Adams. (2010). Exercise physiology. In *ACSM's Resource Manual* (6th ed.), edited by J. K. Ehrman. Philadelphia: Walters Kluwer/Lippincott Williams and Wilkins.

81. Wilmore et al (2008).

82. Ibid.

83. Powers & Howley (2009).

84. Ibid.

85. Wilmore et al. (2008).

86. Ibid.

87. Nieman (2007).

88. ACSM (2010).

89. American College of Sports Medicine. (2007). ACSM position stand on exercise and fluid replacement. *Medicine and Science in Sports and Exercise*, 39, 377.

90. Wilmore et al (2008).

91. ACSM (2010).

92. Ibid.

# Suggested Readings

Editors. (2010, February). Know the warning signs of worsening PAD. *Heart Advisor,* 13(2), 4.

The authors of this article define and discuss peripheral artery disease (PAD. They identify the risk factors, explain who is at risk for PAD, and describe treatments. The role of exercise is also discussed.

Editors. (2009, February). Two-way street between depression and heart disease. *Harvard Heart Letter,* 19(6), 4.

People who are depressed are more likely to develop heart disease than those who aren't. People who have previously had a heart attack or some other cardiovascular problem are more susceptible to depression. Regular exercise appears to improve mood by nurturing the growth of new nerve cells in the brain while simultaneously improving existing connections.

Editors. (2009, April). Make every exercise minute count. *Consumer Reports on Health,* 21(4), 8.

This article provides many tips on how to start and maintain an exercise program. Included is advice on both aerobic and musculoskeletal exercise. Also included is how to equip a home gym for less than $100.

Editors. (2009, December). To live to a biblical old age, stay physically active. *Tufts University Health and Nutrition Letter,* 27(10), 1.

People over the age of 70 live longer and with higher quality if they are physically active at least 4 hours per week. In a recent study, physically active seniors were 31 to 58% less likely to die during the study compared to their inactive peers, and were 72 to 92% more likely to maintain their independence while performing the activities of daily living. Even seniors who did not engage in physical activity until 70 years of age and beyond improved their odds of survival.

Editors. (2008, September). Let's talk to an expert. *Harvard Health Letter,* 33(11), 8.

The expert referred to in the title is Dr. I-Min Lee, who is an authority on the epidemiology of physical activity and health. When asked to elaborate on the benefits of regular exercise, she replied that physical activity can prolong life as well as reduce risks of heart disease, stroke, Type 2 diabetes, colon cancer, and breast cancer; it improves blood pressure, glucose tolerance, and lipid profile; it reduces risks of fracture from falls; and it decreases depression. An impressive list—and all you have to do is to become, and stay, active.

**Name** _____ **Date** _____ **Section** _____

# Assessment Activity 3-1

## The Rockport Fitness Walking Test

**Directions:** This walking test estimates aerobic capacity based on the variables of age, gender, time required to walk 1 mile, and heart rate achieved at the end of the test. The guidelines for taking the test are as follows:

1. Count your heart rate for 15 seconds and multiply by 4 to get beats per minute.

2. The course should be flat and measured, preferably a 440-yard track.

3. Use a stopwatch or a watch with a second hand.

4. Warm up for 5 to 10 minutes before taking the test. Preparation for the test should include a 0.25-mile walk followed by the stretching exercises.

5. During the test, walk at a brisk pace, covering 1 mile as rapidly as possible.

6. Take your pulse rate immediately after the test. On the following pages, mark this rate on the chart that is appropriate for your age and gender.

7. Draw a vertical line through your time and a horizontal line through your heart rate. The point where the lines intersect determines your fitness level.

Rockport provides a series of 20-week walking-for-fitness programs based on the results of the walking test. These may be obtained for a nominal fee by sending a request to Rockport Fitness Walking Test, 72 Howe Street, Marlboro, MA 01752.

The charts on the following pages are designed to tell you how fit you are compared with other individuals of your age and gender. For example, if your coordinates place you in the "above average" section of the chart, you are in better shape than the average person in your category.

The charts are based on weights of 170 lbs. for men and 125 lbs. for women. If you weigh substantially more, your relative cardiovascular fitness level will be slightly overestimated. If you weigh substantially less, your relative cardiovascular fitness level will be slightly underestimated.

## 20- to 29-year-old men

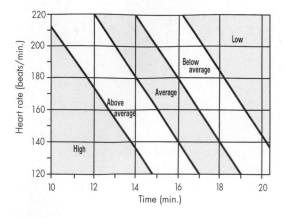

## 30- to 39-year-old men

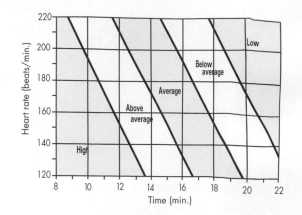

## 40- to 49-year-old men

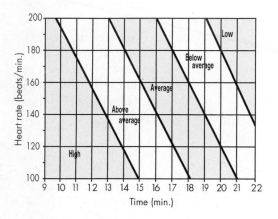

## 50- to 59-year-old men

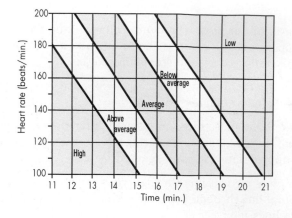

## 60-year-old and older men

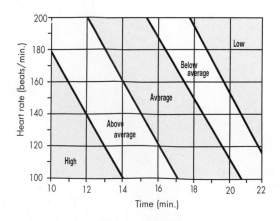

## 20- to 29-year-old women

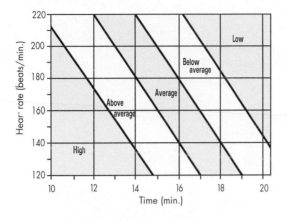

## 30- to 39-year-old women

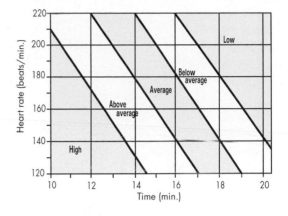

## 40- to 49-year-old women

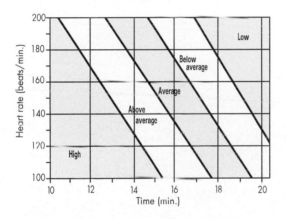

## 50- to 59-year-old women

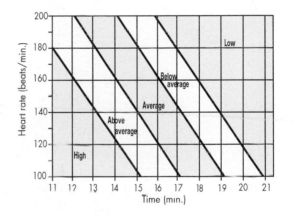

## 60-year-old and older women

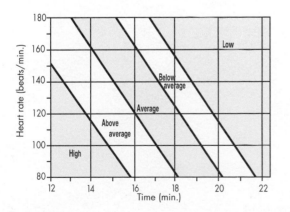

# Assessment Activity 3-2

## The 1.5-Mile Run/Walk Test

**Directions:** Select a measured course, preferably a running track, so that the starting and finishing points are at the same location for ease of timing and recording. Cover the distance as rapidly as possible to attain a realistic estimate of fitness level. You will perform better if you take the opportunity to practice running the course first, so that you can learn how to pace yourself.

If you cannot run the entire distance, walk until you recover enough to continue running again. Allow a 5- to 10-minute warm-up before the test and an equal amount of time for cooling down after the test. Use the following charts to compare your performance with the norm.

### Aerobic Physical Fitness Classification

**Men**

| Fitness Category | 13–19 Yrs. | 20–29 Yrs. | 30–39 Yrs. | 40–49 Yrs. |
|---|---|---|---|---|
| Very poor | > 15:31* | > 16:01 | > 16:31 | > 17:31 |
| Poor | 12:11–15:30 | 14:01–16:00 | 14:46–16:30 | 15:36–17:30 |
| Fair | 10:49–12:10 | 12:01–14:00 | 12:31–14:45 | 13:01–15:35 |
| Good | 9:41–10:48 | 10:46–12:00 | 11:01–12:30 | 11:31–13:00 |
| Excellent | 8:37–9:40 | 9:45–10:45 | 10:00–11:00 | 10:30–11:30 |
| Superior | < 8:37 | < 9:45 | < 10:00 | < 10:30 |

**Women**

| Fitness Category | 13–19 Yrs. | 20–29 Yrs. | 30–39 Yrs. | 40–49 Yrs. |
|---|---|---|---|---|
| Very poor | > 18:31* | > 19:01 | > 19:31 | > 20:31 |
| Poor | 16:55–18:30 | 18:31–19:00 | 19:01–19:30 | 19:31–20:30 |
| Fair | 14:31–16:54 | 15:55–18:30 | 16:31–19:00 | 17:31–19:30 |
| Good | 12:30–14:30 | 13:31–15:54 | 14:31–16:30 | 15:56–17:30 |
| Excellent | 11:50–12:29 | 12:30–13:30 | 13:00–14:30 | 13:45–15:55 |
| Superior | < 11:50 | < 12:30 | < 13:00 | < 13:45 |

\* > greater than; < less than

Name _____   Date _____   Section _____

# Assessment Activity 3-3

## The 3-Minute Bench Step Test

**Directions:**   The equipment needed includes a sturdy 12-inch-high bench; a metronome; a stopwatch; and, if possible, a stethoscope. The metronome should be set at 96 beats per minute for a total of 24 cycles. One cycle consists of four steps as follows: up left foot, up right foot, down left foot, down right foot.

Step up and down in time with each beat of the metronome for 3 full minutes. At the end of the 3 minutes, sit down on the bench immediately. Start the pulse count within the first 5 seconds and continue for 1 full minute. Do not count for 15 seconds and multiply by 4, because the heart rate will be higher than the actual minute heart rate. The 1-minute postexercise heart rate is the score for the test. Refer to the following chart for scoring.

### Postexercise 1-Minute Heart Rate (beats per minute)

| Fitness Category | 18–25 Yrs. | | 26–35 Yrs. | | 36–45 Yrs. | |
| | Men | Women | Men | Women | Men | Women |
|---|---|---|---|---|---|---|
| Excellent | 70–78* | 72–83 | 73–79 | 72–86 | 72–81 | 74–87 |
| Good | 82–88 | 88–97 | 83–88 | 91–97 | 86–94 | 93–101 |
| Above average | 91–97 | 100–106 | 91–97 | 103–110 | 98–102 | 104–109 |
| Average | 101–104 | 110–116 | 101–106 | 112–118 | 105–111 | 111–117 |
| Below average | 107–114 | 118–124 | 109–116 | 121–127 | 113–118 | 120–127 |
| Poor | 118–126 | 128–137 | 119–126 | 129–135 | 120–128 | 130–138 |
| Very poor | 131–164 | 141–155 | 130–164 | 141–154 | 132–168 | 143–152 |

*Count the pulse for 1 full minute after 3 minutes of stepping at 24 cycles/min. on a 12-inch bench.

# Assessment Activity 3-4

## Calculating Target Heart Rate

**Directions:**  Use the Karvonen formula to determine your target heart rate for exercise by filling in the following chart.

Karvonen formula: $THR = (HR_{max} - RHR)$
$\times\ TI\% + RHR$

*Key*

$THR$   – target heart rate
$HR_{max}$ = maximum heart rate ($HR_{max} = 220 - $ age)
$RHR$   = resting heart rate
$TI\%$   = training intensity

*Example*
- A 23-year-old man in good condition (0.75 training intensity from Table 3-3)
- $RHR = 66$ bpm (beats per minute)
- $HR_{max} = 206.9 - (0.67 \times$ Age)
  $= 206.9 - (0.67 \times 23)$
  $= 206.9 - 15.4$
  $= 191.5$ converted to 192 bpm

$THR = (192 - 66) \times 0.75 + 66$
  $= 126 \times 0.75 + 66$
  $= 160.5$ bpm

Your target heart rate is:
$HR_{max} = 206.9 - (0.67 \times$ age)
$THR = (HR_{max} - RHR) \times TI + RHR$
  $= ($ _____ - _____ $) \times$ _____ + _____
  $=$ _____ $\times$ _____ + _____
  $=$ _____ bpm

**Name** _____   **Date** _____   **Section** _____

# Assessment Activity 3-5

## Design an Exercise Program

**Directions:**   Design an exercise program for yourself. First, identify your goals (weight loss, health enhancement, improved level of physical fitness, stress reduction, etc.). Second, respond accordingly to each of the following five items.

1. Activity or activities: _____

2. Frequency of exercise: _____

3. Intensity of exercise: _____

4. Duration of exercise: _____

5. Activity schedule: Place the activity or activities in the following weekly calendar with the suggested amount of time devoted to each activity.

| Sunday | Monday | Tuesday | Wednesday | Thursday | Friday | Saturday |
|--------|--------|---------|-----------|----------|--------|----------|
|        |        |         |           |          |        |          |
|        |        |         |           |          |        |          |
|        |        |         |           |          |        |          |
|        |        |         |           |          |        |          |
|        |        |         |           |          |        |          |

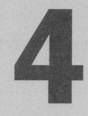
# Building Muscular Strength and Endurance

## ONLINE LEARNING CENTER

Log on to our Online Learning Center (OLC) for access to these additional resources:

- Chapter key term flashcards
- Learning objectives
- Additional goals for behavior change
- Concentration game
- Self-scoring chapter quizzes
- Additional lab activities

The OLC also offers Web links for study and exploration of wellness topics. Access these links through **www.mhhe.com/anspaugh8e.**

## GOALS FOR BEHAVIOR CHANGE

- Begin a strength-training program or improve the one in which you already participate.
- Supply your close family members with at least five health-related reasons they should participate in resistance training.
- Identify the parts of your body where you would like to make the greatest physical change and explain why.
- Identify some of the tasks or sports that you perform daily, weekly, or monthly that would be easier to do if you increased your strength.

## Objectives

After completing this chapter, you will be able to do the following:

- ✔ Explain the benefits of resistance training for older people.
- ✔ Define the different types of muscle contraction.
- ✔ Identify the various systems of dynamic and static exercise training.
- ✔ Describe the limitations of isometric exercise training.
- ✔ Explain the advantages and disadvantages of circuit resistance training.
- ✔ Define each of the principles of resistance training.
- ✔ Describe the short- and long-term effects of anabolic steroid use.
- ✔ Describe the health benefits of resistance training.
- ✔ Describe the progressive resistance technique that increases muscle endurance.

## [ Key Terms ]

anaerobic

atrophy

circuit resistance training (CRT)

concentric contraction

eccentric contraction

ergogenic aids

hypertrophy

isokinetic

isometric

isotonic

muscle dysmorphia

muscular endurance

muscular strength

repetitions

sarcopenia

sets

variable resistance

**E**vidence has been steadily mounting of the growing importance of muscular development for health enhancement, fitness, and aesthetic purposes.[1] The muscular system improves through resistive forms of exercises, such as weight training and calisthenics. Resistive exercises complement aerobic forms of exercise, because each uniquely contributes to health, physical fitness, and personal appearance.[2] Both types of exercise are required for a well-rounded conditioning program, and together they produce optimum results. However, best results are obtained by performing strength and endurance programs on separate days.[3]

Aerobic activities, which improve cardiorespiratory function and enhance health status in many ways, were presented in Chapter 3. Resistance exercises also contribute to physiological and psychological health. Many experts are convinced that resistance training is the only type of exercise capable of slowing, and possibly reversing, declines in muscle mass, bone density, and strength. Not long ago, these negative changes were considered to be the result of the aging process.[4] But today the evidence clearly indicates that a significant %age of age-related losses are the result of *disuse atrophy*.[5] Disuse atrophy explains the loss of muscle mass and strength because of a sedentary lifestyle personified by low-level muscle stimulation well below the threshold for developing and maintaining muscle mass.[6]

The body contains more than 600 muscles, and 65% of these are located above the waist.[7] All muscles, regardless of location, respond to the physiological law of use and disuse. "Use it or lose it" is an axiom that applies to all human beings during every phase of the life cycle. Americans tend to become more sedentary as they age. The declining stimulation results in a progressive shrinking and weakening of the muscles.

With few exceptions—notably cross-country skiing, rowing, and swimming—aerobic activities provide limited stimulation of upper body musculature. Sedentary living neglects the muscular system entirely and accelerates the loss of muscle tissue and body strength. The need for resistance training was illustrated in a study of runners during a 10-year period. Runners who did no resistance training suffered muscle **atrophy** in their upper bodies while maintaining muscle size in their legs.[8] Their arms, which received little stimulation from jogging, decreased in circumference.

Jogging is unable to stimulate the arms at or above the threshold needed for muscular development or maintenance, but the addition of resistive exercises can. This is an example of how the two types of training complement each other.

## The Health Benefits of Resistance Training

Irrefutable evidence proves that strength training produces unique health benefits for people of all ages as well as for those with various types of infirmities. The American College of Sports Medicine, the American Heart Association, and the surgeon general's *Report on Physical Activity and Health* have all proclaimed and strongly supported the need for strength training for enhancing health and for improving quality of life. Strength training increases muscle mass and decreases the fat content of the body. The implications for weight loss and management are enormous, because muscle tissue is more metabolically active than is fat tissue. This means that the body burns more calories under any condition, including rest.[9]

An improvement in strength reduces the exerciser's heart rate and blood pressure while he or she is lifting weights. The practical application of these responses is that there is less stress on the heart when people lift or move moderately heavy objects in everyday life.[10] Heavy resistance training and circuit weight training have the potential to produce a high enough volume of work to improve cardiorespiratory endurance by an average of 6%.[11]

Resistance training increases the strength and endurance of the antigravity muscles, improving posture and producing less stress on the lower back.[12] Stronger, more stable joints are better able to withstand physical stress or trauma.

Strength training also enables one to perform the functions of daily life with less effort. Stronger muscles allow people to perform functional tasks that become more difficult as people age, such as getting in and out of a car, in and out of a bathtub, or up from an easy chair and climbing stairs. Dynamic forms of resistance training have a high degree of transferability to everyday activities.[13,14]

An increase in leg strength helps those who have osteoarthritis (wear-and-tear arthritis) because stronger muscles absorb a greater share of the physical stress at joints. In effect, stronger muscles spare the joint structures from some of the weight-bearing activity. Rheumatologists (physicians who specialize in the diagnosis and treatment of arthritic conditions) often recommend weight training to their patients because it alleviates symptoms and strengthens the muscles, tendons, and ligaments that surround the joints.[15] Additionally, resistance exercises promote the secretion of synovial fluid, which lubricates the joints and adds to the joints' shock-absorbing qualities.[16]

An improvement in leg strength also leads to better balance and decreases the likelihood of falling, which reduces the chances that a fracture might occur.[17] Osteoporosis is a systemic disease characterized by the deterioration of the skeletal system. Bone mineral content decreases, so that the bones become fragile and susceptible to fracture.[18] Women are more prone to osteoporosis, but men are also affected as they age. People can protect the skeletal system by eating a nutritious diet and by participating regularly in weight-bearing and resistive exercise.[19] Resistive exercises are versatile, having the capacity to stress all of the joints and the bones that articulate with them, and they produce lateral forces that increase the thickness and density of bones, so they have the potential to prevent osteoporosis.[20]

The results brought about by resistance exercises allow people to live independently and with dignity as they age. Evidence indicates that Americans are living longer, and many will live with physical and functional limitations.[21] Illnesses occur with greater frequency and severity as we age, but much of the disability associated with aging is not due entirely to the aging process. Many authorities attribute at least 50% of these changes to disuse atrophy.[22] Our typically sedentary lifestyles, more prevalent among the aging population than among any other group of Americans, are responsible for a significant number of these illnesses. Those who stimulate their muscles regularly, regardless of their age, do not experience the type of physical deterioration observed in those who are physically inactive. Recent research indicates that physical inactivity is responsible for the majority of age-related muscle loss.[23,24] The loss of muscle from aging and inactivity is referred to as **sarcopenia**, which literally means "flesh or muscle loss."

Strength training also produces an impressive array of psychological and emotional benefits, which include improvements in self-esteem, self-confidence, and body image.[25] It helps improve the mood of mildly to moderately depressed individuals. Resistive exercise programs improve reaction time and may contribute to more restful sleep. Just the Facts: The Benefits of Resistance Training provides a summary of the positive outcomes that can be achieved through resistance training. Also see Wellness for a Lifetime: Strength Training for Older Adults (page 114).

Many cardiac patients participate in strength development exercise. Substantial benefits may be gained at minimal risk.[26] Improving upper and lower body strength allows cardiac patients to perform everyday lifting activities with less effort and greater movement efficiency. Also, strength training may have a positive impact on cardiorespiratory endurance, hypertension, blood fat levels, and psychological well-being, and it improves blood sugar and insulin control.[27,28]

## [ JUST THE ] FACTS
### The Benefits of Resistance Training

Resistance training produces the following positive results:

- Increases muscle mass and decreases fat mass
- Increases strength and muscle endurance
- Increases basal metabolic rate (BMR)
- Develops the antigravity muscles (abdominal, lower back, hips, front and back of the thighs, both calves)
- Increases bone density (resulting in less risk for bone fracture)
- Decreases the risk for low-back pain
- Improves dynamic balance (resulting in less risk of falling)
- Improves mobility, such as that necessary for walking and stair climbing
- Improves reaction time
- Contributes to more restful sleep
- Helps elevate the mood of mildly to moderately depressed people
- Improves body image, self-esteem, and self-confidence
- Improves the effectiveness of insulin in older adults
- Aids in weight loss and weight management
- May increase HDL cholesterol (the protective form)

## Anaerobic Exercise

Strength development exercises are **anaerobic.** *Anaerobic* literally means "without oxygen," and when applied to exercise, it refers to high-intensity physical activities in which oxygen demand is above the level that can be supplied during performance. Short-term supplies of fuel stored in the muscles provide the energy for anaerobic activities.[38] As a result, these can be sustained for only several seconds. Sprinting 100 yards, lifting a heavy weight, and running up two or three flights of stairs are some examples of anaerobic activities.

## Muscular Strength

**Muscular strength** is the maximum force that a muscle or muscle group can exert in a single contraction. It is best developed by some form of progressive resistance exercise, such as weight training with free weights (barbells and dumbbells) or single or multistation machine weights.

Muscular strength is developed best through high-intensity exercise. Lifting heavier loads a few times to

# Wellness for a Lifetime

## Strength Training for Older Adults

One of the realities of aging is muscle atrophy (decrease in size), resulting in a loss of strength, power, balance, and coordination. However, scientists have shown that a substantial amount of muscle loss is due to lack of appropriate physical activity rather than to the aging process. Engaging regularly in resistance exercises can build muscle, maintain muscle, and limit the loss of muscle tissue.

Inactive people can expect to lose approximately 25% of the force-generating capacity of muscle by age 65, and up to 40% over a lifetime.[29] The loss of muscle strength begins at approximately age 30 and is most pronounced after the age of 70.[30] The loss of leg strength is greater than the loss of arm strength for both sexes. Data from the ongoing Framingham Study showed that 40% of female subjects 55 to 64 years of age, 45% of female subjects 65 to 74 years of age, and 65% of female subjects 74 to 85 years of age were unable to lift 10 pounds. The loss of muscle strength is most pronounced after age 70.[31] Evidence clearly indicates that after 60 years of age, muscle strength decreases by a consistent rate of 1 to 2% per year for dynamic, isometric, and isokinetic contractions.[32]

Because of this limitation, everyday functions taken for granted by the young become physical challenges, including opening bottle caps and jar lids, carrying groceries, and climbing stairs. If muscle atrophy progresses unabated, walking without assistance becomes difficult if not impossible, and the likelihood of falling increases.[33,34,35]

The good news is that the muscles of older people respond to training in much the same way as the muscles of young adults. Older people may make greater gains because of their initial level of debility (weakness). Studies have shown that older neuromuscular systems are not only trainable but also show exceptional adaptations to training. For example, the strength gains in these studies ranged from 16 to 174%, and the increases in muscle size ranged from 7 to 62% for both male and female subjects between the ages of 60 and 98.[36] Also, power-training resistance programs featuring higher velocities and more powerful movements increased the maximal rate-of-force production in these older subjects and, as a result, might be more effective than strength training for improving physical function.[37]

---

fatigue produces larger gains than does lifting lighter loads many times to fatigue.[39] Weight trainers speak of the amount of work accomplished during the workout in terms of exercise repetitions and sets and in terms of the percentage of 1 repetition maximum (1 RM) for each exercise. A **repetition** is one complete lift of an exercise, beginning with the starting position, moving the weight through a full range of motion, and returning to the starting position. Doing this 10 times in a continuous fashion is referred to as 10 repetitions, or 10 reps, and these 10 reps represent 1 set of that exercise. Repeating the entire sequence 2 more times completes 3 sets of the exercise. One RM represents the heaviest load that can be lifted 1 time. Ten RM is a lighter load that can be lifted 10 times but not 11. In other words, maximum fatigue occurs on repetition number 10, thereby preventing repetition number 11.

Do not attempt to establish 1 RM by lifting a maximum load for any exercise because untrained musculoskeletal systems are susceptible to injury. However, 1 RM can be safely predicted in a reasonably accurate fashion without having to attempt a maximum load.[40] The predicted 1 RM can be calculated by the selection of a weight that produces fatigue with fewer than 10 repetitions. For example, a subject can perform a maximum of 8 repetitions with 140 pounds in the bench press. From the data, what is this subject's predicted 1 RM for the bench press? The formula is as follows:

$$1 \text{ RM} = \frac{\text{Weight lifted}}{(1.0278 - 0.0278R^*)}$$

*R is the number of repetitions performed.

$$= \frac{140 \text{ lbs.}}{1.0278 - 0.0278(8)}$$

$$= \frac{140}{1.0278 - 0.2224}$$

$$= \frac{140}{0.8054}$$

$$= 173.8, \text{ or } 174, \text{ lbs.}$$

Thus, 174 pounds is this subject's predicted 1 RM for the bench press exercise. One hundred forty pounds represents 80% of the 1 RM (40/174 = 0.80, or 80%). Eighty percent is more than a sufficient stimulus for developing strength and muscle hypertrophy (increase in muscle size). It is time consuming and not necessary to calculate 1RM for all weight training exercises. There is a quicker and much simpler way to determine one's starting weight. Research indicates that muscular strength, muscle mass, and to some extent muscle endurance may be developed simultaneously by selecting a weight that supplies enough resistance to perform a minimum of 8 repetitions but not more than 12 repetitions.[41] Such a weight will be the approximate equivalent of 60 to 80% of 1 RM without actually having to calculate it.

Each set in the program should be performed to muscle fatigue rather than complete failure. Muscle fatigue is exemplified by stopping the set when the exerciser realizes that he or she is unlikely to complete an additional repetition. Complete failure is characterized by straining as the lifter continues in his or her attempts to perform the lift until unable to move the weight through a full range of motion. Training to complete failure increases the probability of incurring an exercise-related injury, and/or it may produce severe delayed onset muscle soreness. Advanced weight trainers would select weights equal to 80 to 100% of 1 RM.

Children and adolescents (youth) should never lift maximum loads. In fact, resistive training for youth has been a controversial topic for decades. See Wellness for a Lifetime: Resistive Training for American Youth for a discussion of the efficacy and safety of resistance training for youth.

## Muscle Contraction and Resistance Training

Muscle contraction is either static or dynamic. *Static contractions* occur when muscles exert force but do not move (shorten or lengthen). *Dynamic contractions* involve muscle contractions that are either *concentric* (muscle shortening) or *eccentric* (muscle lengthening).[50] See Figure 4-1 for an illustration of each.

Some of the exercises commonly used to develop the major muscle groups of the body are shown in Figures 4-2 to 4-17. The anatomical charts in Figures 4-18 and 4-19 show the location of the muscles stressed in each exercise. These exercises are demonstrated on exercise machines and free weights, methods that are relatively equivalent and work the same muscle groups.

See Assessment Activity 4-1 for a method of determining your strength based on body weight and gender.

## Static Training (Isometrics)

**Isometric** contractions (in which muscle length is constant) occur when muscles produce tension but do not shorten because the resistance is beyond the contractile force that can be generated by the exercising muscles. Examples of isometric contractions are pushing against a wall, pushing sideways or upward against a door jamb, and loading a weight machine with poundage beyond one's capacity to lift. See Figure 4-20 for an illustration.

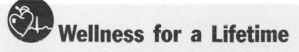

# Wellness for a Lifetime

## Resistive Training for American Youth

Evidence has been accumulating steadily over the last decade supporting resistive training for youth.[42] The American Academy of Pediatrics, the American College of Sports Medicine, the American Orthopedic Society, and the National Strength and Conditioning Association strongly support resistive training for youth. The key elements of these programs are competent and skillful supervision and properly designed training programs.[43]

Resistive training is significantly different from competitive bodybuilding, Olympic-style weight lifting, and power lifting. The term *youth* refers to boys and girls who are prepubertal and postpubertal youngsters up to the age of 18.

The prevailing opinion, prior to the 1990s, among scientists, educators, and clinicians was that resistance training could not produce strength gains in prepubertal children. The reason given was that children were too young to produce testosterone, the hormone that is primarily responsible for increasing muscle size and strength. But recent studies featuring higher training volumes and longer workouts for children and adolescents have shown that gains in strength are not only possible but probable.[44] Eight to 12 weeks of resistive training typically results in strength gains on the order of 30 to 50%. Percentage increases in strength among resistive-trained youth are similar to those made by resistive-trained adults.[45]

Since children are deficient in testosterone, other mechanisms for developing strength become primary. Strength gains in children appear to be mediated by the nervous system. Neural adaptations to strength training include the recruitment of more motor units (one nerve and all of the muscle fibers that it innervates), motor unit coordination, and other factors. Learning contributes to performance as one's skill level on each exercise improves.[46]

Muscle strength and endurance improve, but there are other benefits associated with resistive training, including an increase in bone mineral density, weight control, an improved cardiovascular risk profile, enhanced motor skills and sports performance, increased resistance to potential injuries from sports and recreational activities, and improved well-being.[47,48]

Resistive training programs for youth should adhere to the following guidelines. They should (1) be developed and supervised by qualified professionals; (2) focus on proper technique instead of the amount of weight lifted; (3) gradually increase resistance as strength improves; (4) range from 6 to 15 repetitions per exercise, depending on age, needs, and goals; and (5) be varied to keep it fresh and challenging.[49]

Resistance training is a safe and beneficial activity for youth of both sexes when the guidelines are followed.

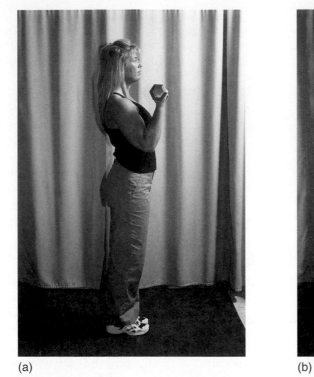
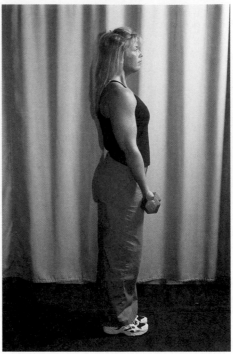

(a)                                    (b)

**FIGURE 4-1** Contractions

The two types of contractions: (a) a concentric contraction; (b) an eccentric contraction.

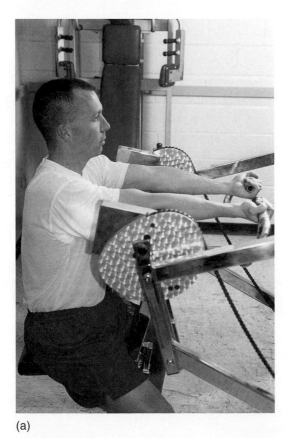
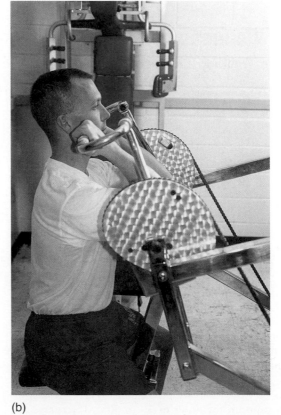

(a)                                    (b)

**FIGURE 4-2** Biceps Curl

(a) Start with your arms extended, palms up. (b) Flex both arms, slowly move the weight through a full range of motion, and return to the starting position. The prime mover is the biceps brachii.

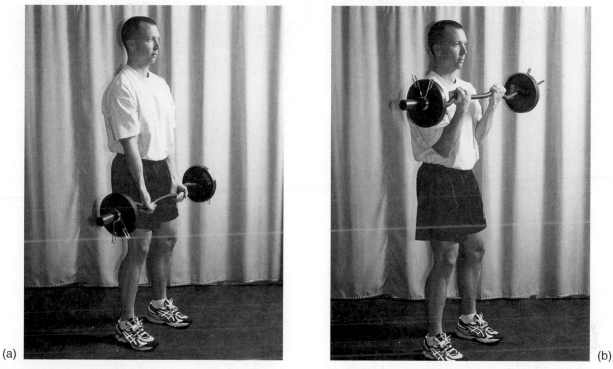

(a)                                                                (b)

**FIGURE 4-3** Biceps Curl (Free Weights)

(a) Start with the arms extended, palms facing forward. (b) Flex both arms and raise the weight through a full range of motion. This exercise is performed in the standing position so the performer's knees are slightly bent to prevent excessive strain on the low back. The prime movers are the biceps muscles.

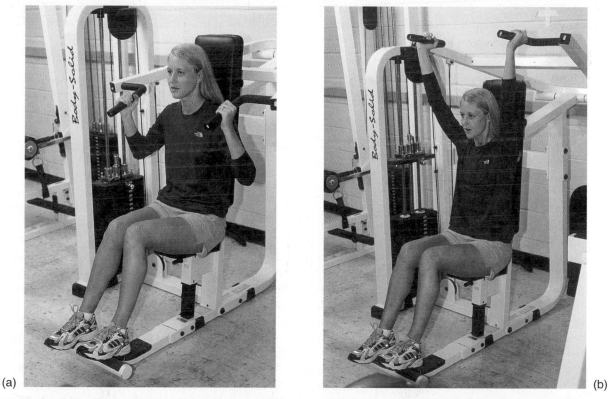

(a)                                                                (b)

**FIGURE 4-4** Overhead Press

(a) Sit upright with your hands approximately shoulder width apart. (b) Slowly press the bar upward until your arms are fully extended, and lower to the starting position. Avoid an excessive arch in your lower back. The prime movers are the triceps and deltoid muscles.

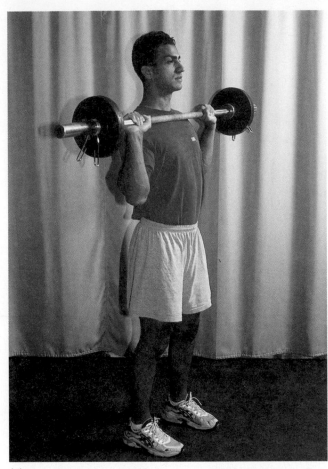
(a)

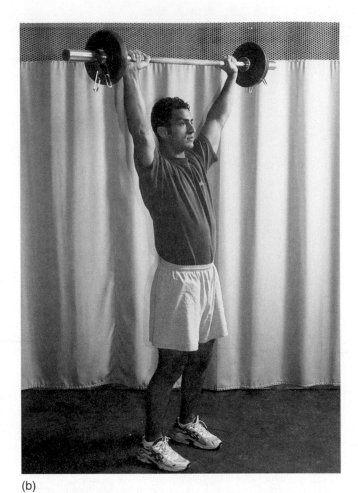
(b)

**FIGURE 4-5** Overhead Press (Free Weights)

(a) Hold the bar at shoulder height. (b) Press the bar upward until the arms are fully extended and then lower the weight to the starting position. The knees are slightly bent throughout the movement to prevent excess strain on the low back. The prime movers are the triceps and deltoids.

Optimal strength development from isometric contractions occurs with 5 to 10 sets of 6-second contractions at maximal or near-maximal force.[51]

Isometric exercises are effective for developing strength, but this approach has some important limitations. The most serious of these is a higher than expected rise in exercise arterial blood pressure and an increased workload on the heart throughout the entire contraction.[52] All-out straining isometric contractions should not be performed by people with heart and vascular disease. A second limitation is that strength developed isometrically is joint-angle specific. Maximum strength development occurs at the angle of contraction, with a training carryover of approximately 20° in either direction from that angle.[53] To develop strength throughout the muscle's range of motion, you must perform isometric contractions in at least three different points in the range of motion.

Because muscles cannot overcome the resistance in isometric training, measuring improvement is difficult,

constituting another limitation of this system.[54] Improvements in strength can be measured if exercisers have access to specialized equipment, such as dynamometers and tensiometers, that record the amount of force applied. Motivation for exercise is difficult to sustain without feedback.

Research indicates that isometric exercise systems are as effective as dynamic exercise systems for developing strength. The question is not which system is better but which system best satisfies the intended use for the newly acquired strength. The transferability of strength to occupational and leisure pursuits is relevant.

Strength developed in the muscles is highly specific to the manner in which the muscles are trained. Muscles trained isometrically perform best when stressed isometrically; muscles trained dynamically perform best when stressed dynamically. There is some transfer of isometric training to everyday life. Isometric muscle contractions are necessary for maintaining standing and sitting posture.[55] Carrying groceries, a baby, or any

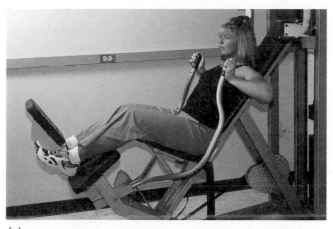
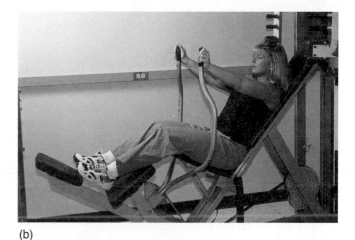

(a)                                                    (b)

**FIGURE 4-6** Bench Press

(a) Sit back with your knees bent and your feet flat on the bench to prevent arching your back. (b) Slowly press the bar forward, fully extending your arms, and return to the starting position. The prime movers are the pectoralis major, triceps, and deltoid muscles.

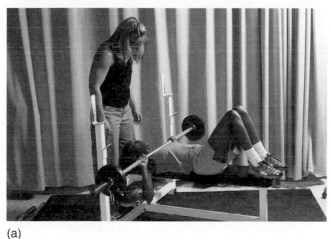
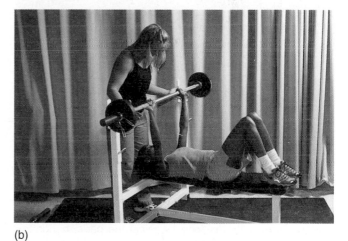

(a)                                                    (b)

**FIGURE 4-7** Bench Press (Free Weights)

(a) Lie on your back with knees bent and feet flat on the bench. (b) Press the bar overhead by completely extending your arms and return to the starting position. For safety, this exercise requires at least one spotter to assist the performer in returning the weight to the rack after the last repetition. The prime movers are the pectoralis major, triceps, and deltoids.

object in a fixed position or pushing and pulling objects requires isometric strength, but most movements are dynamic, and transfer is more widely applicable from dynamic systems of training.[56]

## Dynamic Exercise

Dynamic exercises include **isotonic** (equal tension), variable resistance, free-weight, and **isokinetic** (equal speed) exercises.

### Isotonic Training

Isotonic muscle contractions occur when muscles shorten and move the bones to which they are attached, resulting in movement around the joints. Isotonic move-

ments consist of concentric and eccentric muscle contractions. The **concentric contraction** occurs when a muscle shortens as it develops the tension to overcome an external resistance. The **eccentric contraction** occurs when the muscle lengthens and the weight (resistance) is slowly returned to the starting position. When muscles contract eccentrically, they are resisting the force of gravity as they lengthen, so that the weight is not allowed to free-fall. In general, muscles can produce about 30 to 40% more tension eccentrically than concentrically.[57] But no advantage exists for training programs that emphasize eccentric contractions. Research indicates that conventional isotonic programs develop as much strength and produce less of the delayed muscle soreness associated with eccentric contractions.

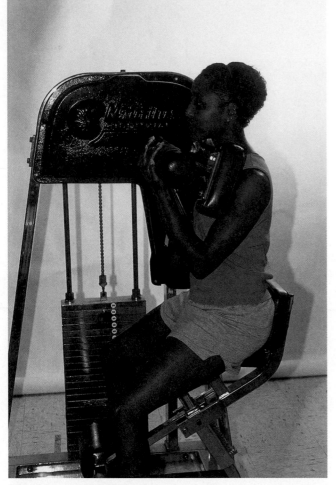
(a)

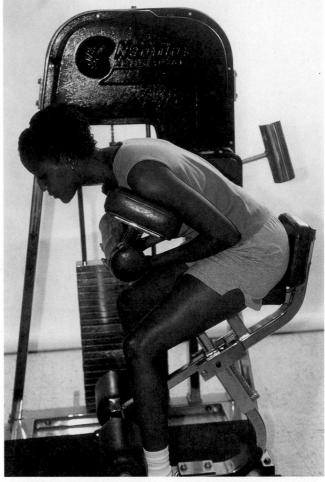
(b)

**FIGURE 4-8** Abdominal Crunch
(a) Sit upright with your chest against the pads, hands folded across your stomach or lightly placed on the front pads.
(b) Slowly press forward through a full range of motion, and return to the starting position. The prime mover is the rectus abdominis muscle.

Isotonic exercises produce delayed muscle soreness 24 to 48 hours after a workout.[58] Eccentric contractions cause microscopic damage to muscle fibers, their connective tissue, and the cell membranes.[59] Soreness occurs because the damaged tissues swell and apply pressure on the nerves. Delayed muscle soreness is more common among beginning exercisers, exercisers who attempt to overload too quickly, and those who change from one activity to another. Novice weight trainers should avoid intense exercise during the first 5 to 10 exercise sessions to minimize delayed-onset muscle soreness and to allow time for the musculoskeletal system to adapt to the training stimulus. But delayed-onset muscle soreness should not be completely avoided because the structural muscle damage that produces it and the subsequent healing process that occurs afterward are necessary to maximize the training response.[60] In other words, beginners should

exercise hard enough to cause some muscle soreness the day following the workout.

Stretching exercises, light workouts, or complete rest may be required to alleviate muscle soreness. Prevention is the best treatment. Prevention involves allowing enough time to adjust to a new routine (at least 1 month), overloading the muscles in small increments (not trying to do too much too fast), and exercising within capacity. Because muscle soreness may last 48 hours, those who use isotonic exercise systems are advised to exercise no more than every other day. This schedule ensures that the next bout of exercise will occur after soreness has abated and healing has occurred.

## Variable Resistance Training

**Variable resistance** exercise equipment was developed because isotonic exercises do not maximally stress mus-

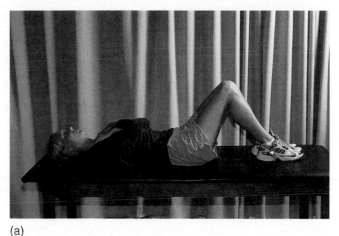

(a)

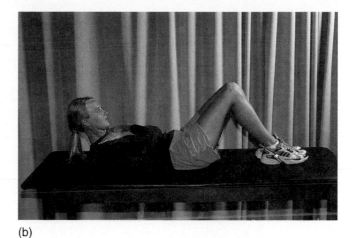

(b)

**FIGURE 4-9** Abdominal Crunch (Mat Exercise)

(a) Lie on your back (supine position), arms crossed over the chest, feet flat on the floor. (b) Lift your head and chest off the mat until your shoulder blades clear the mat. At this point, return to the starting position. The prime mover is the rectus abdominis.

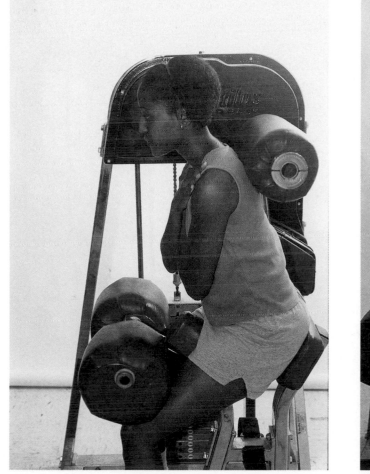

(a)

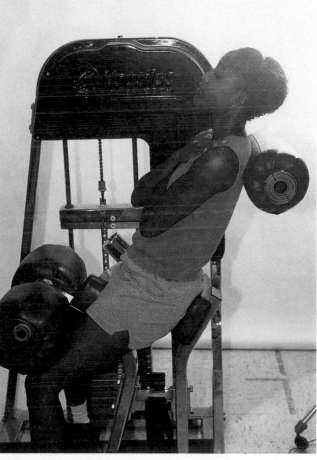

(b)

**FIGURE 4-10** Lower-Back Extension

(a) Place your thighs and back against the pads. (b) Slowly press backward until your back is fully extended, and return to the starting position. The prime movers are the erector spine and gluteus maximus muscles.

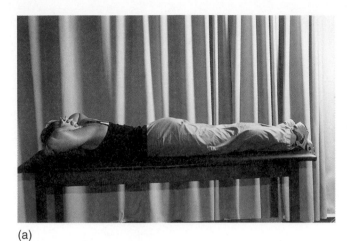

(a)

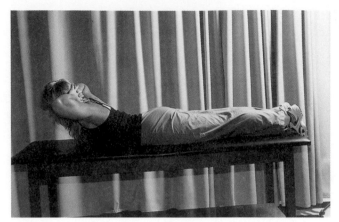

(b)

**FIGURE 4-11** Back Extension (Mat Exercise)

(a) Lie facedown (prone position) and clasp the hands together behind your head as shown. (b) Lift your upper torso off the mat. This should be uncomfortable but not painful. Do not hyperextend the spine. The prime movers are the erector spine and gluteus maximus.

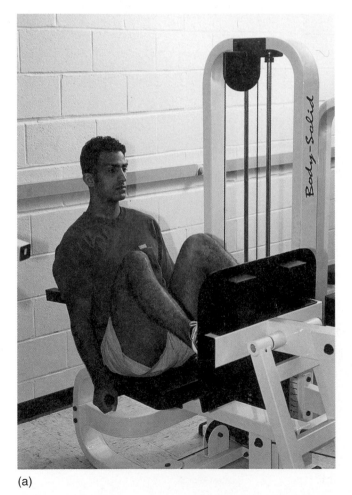

(a)

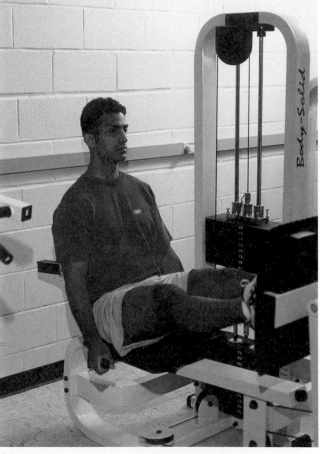

(b)

**FIGURE 4-12** Leg Press

(a) Adjust the seat so that your legs are bent at approximately 90°. (b) Slowly extend your legs fully, and return to the starting position. The prime movers are the quadriceps and gluteus maximus muscles.

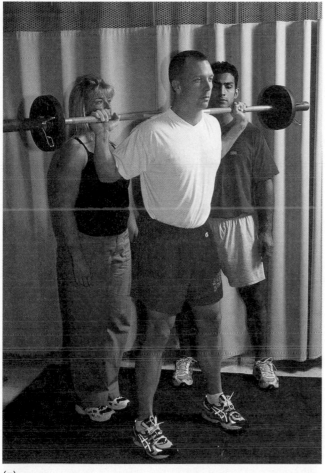
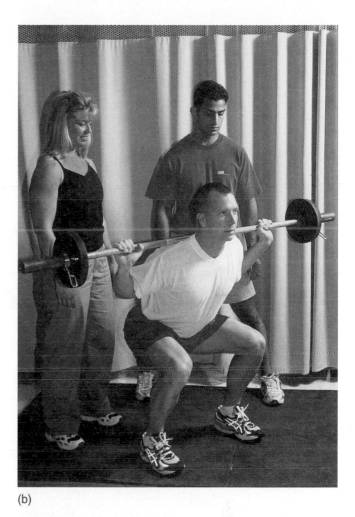

(a)                    (b)

**FIGURE 4-13** Half-Squat (Free Weights)

(a) Stand with the weight on your shoulders. (b) Squat down until your knees are bent at approximately 90° and return to the starting position. Keep your back straight throughout. There should be two spotters to place the weight on your shoulders at the start of the exercise and to remove it at the end. The prime movers are the quadriceps and gluteus maximus.

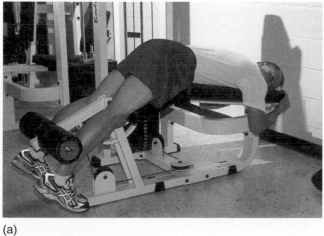
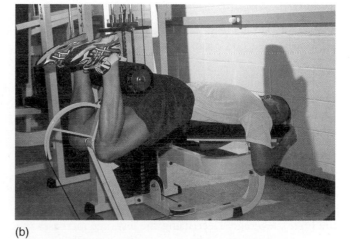

(a)                    (b)

**FIGURE 4-14** Hamstring Curl

(a) Lie facedown with your lower legs under the pads. (b) Curl the weight approximately 90°, and return to the starting position. The prime mover is the hamstring muscle group.

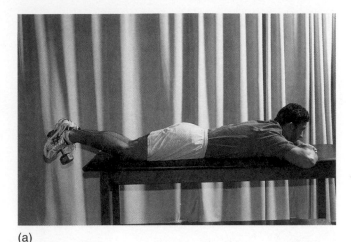

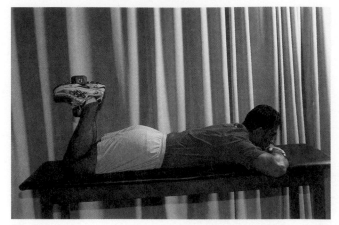

(a)

(b)

**FIGURE 4-15** Hamstring Curl (Free Weights)

(a) Lie in the prone position holding a dumbbell between your feet as shown. (b) Bend your knees to raise the dumbbell to the vertical position and return to the starting position. Ankle weights can be substituted for a dumbbell. The prime mover is the hamstring muscle group.

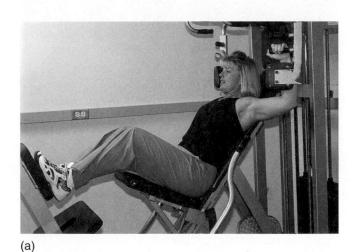

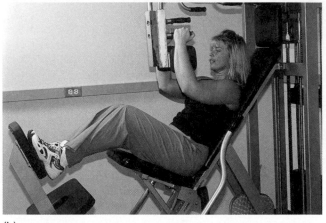

(a)

(b)

**FIGURE 4-16** Chest Press

(a) Keep your upper arms parallel to the floor, bend your elbows at 90°, and place your hands on the handles. (b) Slowly push the bars until your elbows are pointing forward, and return to the starting position. The prime movers are the pectoralis major and deltoid muscles.

cles throughout their full range of motion. The maximum weight lifted isotonically is limited to the weakest point in the musculoskeletal leverage system. The weight appears lighter at some points in the joint movement and heavier at others. In reality, the weight is constant and the human bony leverage system changes.

Variable resistance equipment is designed to provide maximum resistance through the full range of motion. Universal Gym equipment accomplishes this by altering the lifter's leverage. Decreasing the leverage increases the resistance at points in the movement where the muscles are strongest. Nautilus equipment uses a system of cams to decrease musculoskeletal leverage, which in turn increases lifting resistance. Variable resistance training challenges people to exert more force throughout the range of motion, which should result in greater returns. Whether variable resistance weight training is more effective than conventional weight training is yet to be resolved. Evidence indicates that it is as good and may be better, even though it varies the resistance imprecisely. However, variable resistance equipment does "provide a more consistent training stimulus through the range of motion but the applicability to real-movements is limited compared to free weights."[61]

### Free-Weight Training

Isotonic training with free weights continues to be an appropriate method of strength development. Free-

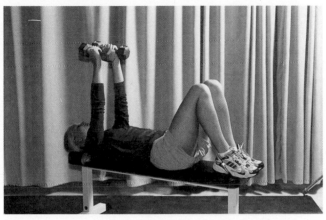
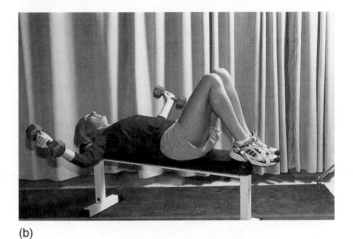

(a)                                                                    (b)

**FIGURE 4-17** Lateral Supine Raises (Free Weights)

(a) Lie on your back, arms extended upward with a dumbbell in each hand. (b) Lower the weights laterally until the upper arms are parallel to the floor. Maintain a slight bend in the elbows throughout the movement. Then raise your arms in the same arc to the starting position. The prime movers are the pectoralis major and deltoid muscles.

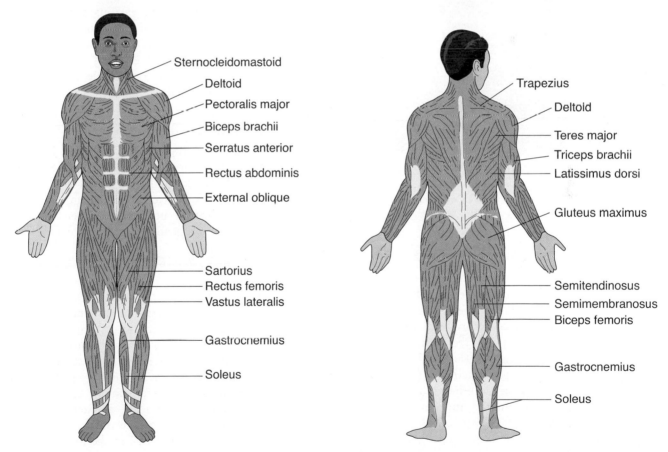

Sternocleidomastoid
Deltoid
Pectoralis major
Biceps brachii
Serratus anterior
Rectus abdominis
External oblique

Sartorius
Rectus femoris
Vastus lateralis

Gastrocnemius

Soleus

Trapezius
Deltoid
Teres major
Triceps brachii
Latissimus dorsi

Gluteus maximus

Semitendinosus
Semimembranosus
Biceps femoris

Gastrocnemius

Soleus

**FIGURE 4-18** Selected Muscles of the Body—Front View

**FIGURE 4-19** Selected Muscles of the Body—Rear View

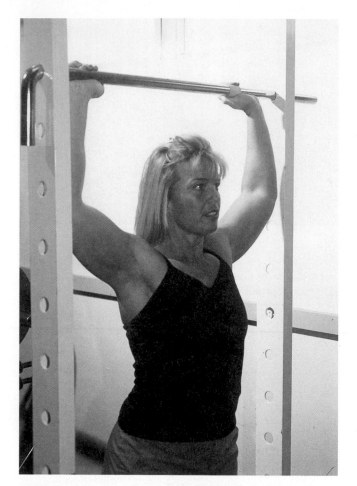

**FIGURE 4-20** Isometric Contraction

An isometric contraction is a static contraction against an immovable object.

weight training provides many advantages. For athletes, it yields some flexibility in strength development because the movements are not confined to a track. Exercises can be selected or improvised to simulate the movements required by specific sports, allowing the development of the muscles that will be used in competition.[62] Concurrently, ancillary musculature that plays a supporting or stabilizing role for the major muscles is also stimulated and developed.

For noncompetitors, free weights have several advantages. The equipment is inexpensive and versatile. A starter set of free weights typically costs less than $150. Free weights do not require much space, so the workout can occur in the home.

The main limitation of free-weight exercise is that this system does not provide maximum resistance throughout the full range of motion. A second limitation is the need for one or two spotters to assist with exercises such as the bench press and half-squats.[63]

## Isokinetic Training

Isokinetic resistance training involves dynamic movements performed on exercise devices that produce maximum resistance throughout the full range of motion. The movement speed is preselected by the exerciser and remains constant throughout the movement. Isokinetic exercise theoretically improves on traditional and variable resistance dynamic systems.[64] Isokinetic devices adjust the resistance to accommodate the force applied by the exerciser. The greater the application of force, the greater the resistance to movement supplied by the device while the speed of movement is held at a constant rate. Maximum force applied through the full range of motion is countered with maximum resistance at all joint angles. This activates the greatest number of motor units and may produce greater gains in strength than other dynamic systems of exercise.

Historically, muscle fibers have been classified according to fiber type. The various fiber types and their respective percentages are influenced by genetics and exercise habits. The fiber composition of skeletal muscles has a significant influence on both endurance and power events. For more on muscle fiber types, see Just the Facts: Muscle Fiber Types.

## Circuit Resistance Training

**Circuit resistance training (CRT)** is effective for people who wish to develop several fitness dimensions simultaneously. Muscular strength and endurance, changes in body composition, and improvement in cardiorespiratory endurance can be attained together. Endurance is the application of repeated muscular force against a submaximal resistance.

A circuit usually consists of 8 to 15 exercise stations. The weight selected for each exercise station should equal 40 to 60% of 1 RM.[70] The exerciser moves from one exercise station to the next with little or no rest (30 seconds maximum rest) and performs a 15- to 45-second set of 8 to 20 repetitions at each station.[71] The circuit is repeated two or three times for a total elapsed time of 30 to 50 minutes per workout. As fitness improves, overload can be applied by (1) increasing the amount of weight at each station, (2) increasing the amount of exercise time at each station (up to 45 seconds), (3) decreasing the amount of rest between stations, or (4) any combination of these.

The CRT system is challenging, versatile, and fun. Exercise stations can be rearranged, exercises that develop similar muscle groups can be substituted for each other, and the order in which the circuit is traversed can be changed. Because relatively light weights are used, the likelihood of injury is reduced. Circuits can be set up in small spaces. Machine weights are

## [ JUST THE FACTS ]

### Muscle Fiber Types

In humans, muscles fall into one of two fiber types: slow-twitch, or Type I (also referred to as slow oxidative), and fast-twitch, which consists of two subtypes, Type IIa and Type IIx. The Type II fibers are called fast-glycolytic fibers because they contract rapidly without the involvement of oxygen.

Each fiber type can be identified by its speed of contraction, its contractile force, and its rate of fatigue. Type I fibers are aerobic, contract more slowly than Type II fibers, and are resistant to fatigue. They are slow to fatigue because of their rich supply of capillaries, myoglobin content, and number of mitochondria and mitochondrial oxidative enzymes.[65] The capillary density of these fibers allows for a greater exchange of oxygen between the blood and muscle fibers. Myoglobin, a compound similar to hemoglobin, accepts oxygen from the blood and shuttles it to muscle mitochondria, where it is used in conjunction with oxidative enzymes to break down foodstuffs to form adenosine triphosphate (ATP). As a result, Type I fibers are well equipped for endurance work. ATP is the actual unit of energy used for muscle contraction.

Fast-twitch fibers contract more forcefully and more rapidly but fatigue more quickly than Type I fibers. Their tendency to tire easily is due to a small number of mitochondria combined with very limited amounts of myoglobin.

Type IIa fibers are "intermediate fibers," or fast-oxidative glycolytic fibers, that are capable of using oxygen. These fibers are adaptable to endurance training, and their oxidative capacity increases as a result. Endurance training converts Type IIx fibers to Type IIa fibers. However, the magnitude of change is approximately no more than a few percentage points.[66]

At this point, there appear to be no apparent age or sex differences in the distribution of muscle fiber type. The average male or female possesses 47 to 53% Type I fibers, while endurance athletes range from 70 to 80% Type I fibers.[67] In contrast, power athletes have 70 to 75% Type II fibers.[68] The aging process results in a selective loss of Type II fibers, with most of the loss occurring from the Type IIx fibers.[69]

The ratio of slow-twitch to fast-twitch muscle fibers can be determined by examining under a powerful microscope, muscle biopsies from selected sites in the body. The muscle composition of world-class aerobic athletes (distance runners, cyclists, cross-country skiers) is predominantly slow-twitch, whereas the muscle composition of the world-class power or anaerobic event athletes (shot-putters, sprinters, power and Olympic weight lifters) is primarily fast-twitch. Knowing the ratio of fiber type could be important for these competitors, but it is relatively unimportant when one exercises for health reasons. Health enthusiasts can participate in a variety of activities with some degree of success and satisfaction regardless of fiber type.

---

ideal for CRT because of the speed with which resistances can be changed, but free weights are adaptable to this system as well. The main limitation of CRT is that optimal gains in strength or cardiorespiratory endurance are difficult to achieve. Strength is most efficiently developed through lifting heavier weights combined with a substantial rest period between sets.[72] Cardiorespiratory endurance can best be achieved through rhythmic and continuous activities, such as jogging, cycling, cross-country skiing, and rowing, performed for a minimum of 20 minutes per workout. An example of a circuit is presented in Just the Facts: Circuit Resistance Training.

## Muscular Endurance

**Muscular endurance** is the application of repeated muscular force against a submaximal resistance. Inflating a tire with a bicycle pump, walking up five flights of stairs, lifting a weight 20 times, and doing 50 sit-ups are some examples of activities that develop muscular endurance. It is developed by many repetitions against resistances that are considerably less than maximum. Also, the rest periods between sets is purposely short, 90 seconds or less, as this is one of the requirements of resistance protocol that emphasizes improvement in muscular endurance.

Research has shown that the greatest effect on muscle endurance occurs with submaximal loads that can be lifted 20 or more times.[73] Endurance programs such as these may simultaneously build strength if the exercises are performed to failure (max fatigue).[74] The last four or five repetitions become a struggle and by the time the very last repetition is performed, all available motor units have been recruited and fatigued so no further repetitions can be accomplished even with exceptional effort.[75] As with other types of isotonic resistance training programs, muscle endurance exercises should be performed no more than every other day.

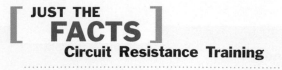

The following is an example of a circuit. You should warm up before CRT and finish the workout with a cooldown.

| | | |
|---|---|---|
| Station 1 | Leg presses or half-squats | 15–30 secs. |
| Station 2 | Bench presses | 15–30 secs. |
| Station 3 | Back hyperextensions | 15–30 secs. |
| Station 4 | Biceps curls | 15–30 secs. |
| Station 5 | Overhead presses | 15–30 secs. |
| Station 6 | Sit-ups or abdominal crunches | 15–30 secs. |
| Station 7 | Push-ups | 15–30 secs. |
| Station 8 | Lateral raises | 15–30 secs. |
| Station 9 | Hamstring curls | 15–30 secs. |
| Station 10 | Pull-ups | 15–30 secs. |

Isometric, or static, muscle endurance is the ability to sustain, or hold, a submaximal contraction for a time.[76] Examples are carrying objects, such as groceries and other packages; pushing or pulling objects, such as a lawn mower; and carrying children.

Assessment Activity 4-2 presents a method of determining your muscular endurance. Assessment Activity 4-3 measures abdominal muscle endurance, and Assessment Activity 4-4 measures muscular strength and endurance with calisthenics.

## Principles of Resistance Training

As with aerobic exercise, the FITT principle (frequency, intensity, time, and type of exercise) applies to resistance training as well. Also important are the principles of overload, progression, specificity, and variety. These principles were established over many years through research and experience. The current set of guidelines recommended for average healthy adults was published in 2002 by the American College of Sports Medicine (ACSM).[77]

Novice trainers should select loads (weights) that allow 8 to 12 repetitions maximum (RM). Intermediate and advanced trainers should use a wider loading range from 1 to 12 RM in a periodized fashion, gradually shifting emphasis to heavy loading (1 to 6 RM), with at least 3 minutes of rest between sets. Periodization is the introduction of variety into the resistance training program. Systematically adjusting the volume of work (repetitions and sets) and the intensity of work over a set period of time decreases the risk of incurring staleness.

It also helps maintain motivation. Other recommendations advanced by the ACSM include the following:

1. Repetitions should be performed at a moderate speed—that is, 1 to 2 seconds for concentric contraction, 1 to 2 seconds for eccentric contractions.
2. Frequency of training should be 2 or 3 days per week for novice and intermediate weight trainers and 4 or 5 days per week for advanced weight trainers.
3. Weight training for muscle endurance should feature light to moderate loads (40 to 60% of 1 RM), more than 15 repetitions per set, and less than 90 seconds' rest between sets.

### Frequency

*Frequency* refers to the number of training sessions per week. Dynamic resistance exercises (isotonic and isokinetic) should be performed every other day (7 training sessions every 2 weeks) or three times per week (6 training sessions every 2 weeks). Near-maximum gains in strength for novice weight trainers occur with these exercise frequencies.

Isometrics can be performed every day because muscle soreness does not result. However, for physiological and psychological reasons, you should designate 2 to 3 days of rest throughout the week. Evidence indicates that alternate-day isometric training is 80% as effective as daily training.[78] However, daily training using maximal voluntary isometric contractions produces the best results.

### Intensity

*Intensity* refers to the amount of weight used for a given exercise. It is probably the most important variable in resistance training, and it is the most important stimulus associated with the development of strength and muscle endurance.[79]

The intensity level for resistance exercise varies according to the training system used. Optimal strength development through isometrics involves maximal contractions, 5 to 10 sets with a total contraction time of 30 to 60 seconds. Optimal strength development through dynamic systems of exercise should include 3 to 5 sets of 4 RM to 6 RM per set, with at least 3 minutes' rest between sets, and this should be performed three times per week. If muscle endurance is the primary goal, the workout should consist of 3 to 5 sets of 15 RM to 25 RM per set, with less than 90 seconds' rest between sets, performed three times per week. For bodybuilding or increasing muscle size, the recommended loading is 6 to 12 RM—that is, the weight selected should be light enough to allow a minimum of 6 repetitions but heavy enough not to exceed 12 repetitions.[80] There should be 1 to 2 minutes' rest between sets, and the exercises should be performed at a moderate speed. Multiple sets are needed to maximize muscle hypertrophy. Hypertrophy is an increase in muscle size.

There is a preferred order of exercise associated with resistance training. Large muscle multiple-joint exercises (half-squat, bench press, etc.) should precede small muscle exercises (biceps curl, triceps extension, etc.) because research has shown that, by first exercising the larger muscles, the intensity of the workout can be increased.[81] The rationale supporting larger to smaller muscle groups is that exercises requiring the most muscle mass should be stressed while the exerciser is fresh. If the reverse order were followed, the smaller muscle groups would be fatigued, limiting their contribution to larger muscle exercises and thereby reducing the intensity of the workout.

## Time (Duration)

The duration, or length, of each exercise session is dependent on the number of exercises, repetitions, and sets; the amount of rest between sets; and the time available to the performer. Conventional resistance programs (3 sets, 10 to 12 exercises, 8 to 12 reps) take about 50 minutes. Serious bodybuilding requires 2 to 4 hours in advanced weight training systems, 6 days per week. Availability of time and individual goals will dictate the length of the workout. The length of the exercise session is consistent with the volume of work accomplished during the workout. The volume of work is dependent upon the number of sets, reps, and resistance (load). For example: volume = sets × reps × resistance. If the subject does 3 sets of an exercise at 10 reps each with a load of 75 pounds, the volume of work is calculated as follows:

$$Volume = 3 \times 10 \times 75$$
$$= 2,250 \text{ lbs.}$$

Changing any one of these factors will change the volume of work accomplished during the session.

## Overload and Progression

The principle behind strength increase is straightforward—the muscles must be subjected periodically to greater resistance as they adapt to the previous resistance. This overload principle applies to all muscles, regardless of the system of training.

Overload may be applied by progressively increasing the amount of weight lifted or the number of sets and repetitions performed or by decreasing rest time between sets. An increase in the number of repetitions leads primarily to increases in muscle endurance, an increase in the amount of weight lifted leads primarily

to an increase in muscle strength, and a decrease in rest time increases muscular and aerobic endurance.

The principle of progression relates to the application of overload. It dictates how much and when an increase in resistance, reps, or sets or a decrease in rest time should occur. The "two-for-two rule" is a general guideline for the application of progressive overload for resistance training.[82] For training loads (weight), the rule states that the load should be increased when exercisers can perform two additional repetitions beyond what they are accustomed to on two consecutive weight-training sessions. For example, an increase in training load is indicated when participants who have been performing 10 repetitions of an exercise progress to 12 repetitions on two consecutive training sessions. At this point, the load should be increased by 2 to 10%.

## Specificity

The principle of specificity reflects the body's response to exercise. The type of training dictates the type of muscle development. Training programs that emphasize high resistance and low repetitions increase muscle strength and size. The gains are the result of muscle **hypertrophy**, an increase in the diameter of muscle fibers, and the recruitment of more motor units.

Training programs that emphasize low resistance and a high number of repetitions develop muscle endurance. The adaptations are specific to the muscle actions involved, speed of muscular contraction, range of motion, muscle groups being trained, energy systems involved, and intensity and volume of training.[83]

The effectiveness of resistance training programs is based on the knowledgeable use of principles that guide such programs. However, other factors contribute to program effectiveness. These are found in Real-World Wellness: Other Important Considerations for Resistance Training (page 130).

## Variety

Variety is an important component of a resistance training program because muscles adapt and plateau in 3 to 4 months under the same training stimulus. This results in a significant reduction in program effectiveness that is characterized by diminished returns in muscle strength, size, and endurance. The program should be changed or varied every few months. Variation can occur by systematically manipulating sets, reps, rest, intensity, and volume of work; using free weights instead of machine weights and vice versa; and by employing different exercises for each body part. Variations of this type keep the program fresh and the motivation high.

## Real-World Wellness

### Other Important Considerations for Resistance Training

*In addition to the principles of resistance exercise, what factors should I consider to ensure the effectiveness and safety of my resistance training program?*

Here are some other important factors for novice weight trainers:

*Order of exercises.* Many people believe that large muscle exercises should precede small muscle exercises. This format allows one to train at a higher intensity level. Large muscle exercises, such as half-squats or leg presses, should be performed prior to hamstring curls; bench presses should precede tricep extensions. If small muscle group exercises precede large muscle exercises, fatigue (preexhaustion) is carried over to large muscle exercises, which limits their effectiveness.

Novice exercisers should not exercise the same muscles in consecutive exercises, because they are likely to be less tolerant to the preexhaustion phenomenon that occurs from the buildup of lactic acid resulting from the previous exercise.

*Rest intervals between sets.* The rest period depends on the goals of training. For example, if the goal is strength development, the rest period between sets should be 3 to 5 minutes. If bodybuilding Is the goal, the rest period should be 1 to 2 minutes. If circuit training is the system used, the rest period between exercises should be 15 to 30 seconds.

*Speed of movement.* For the general public, speed of movement should be relatively slow and controlled. It should take 2 to 3 seconds for the concentric contraction and the same amount of time for the eccentric contraction.

*Multiple sets versus single sets.* Although 1 set of each exercise performed 2 to 3 days per week increases strength, it is a minimal effort. Doing 2 to 3 sets three times per week is better.

*Breathing patterns.* Most important, never hold your breath during physical exertion because this produces an extraordinary rise in blood pressure. Breathe rhythmically during exertion. The suggested pattern of breathing during weight training is to exhale during concentric contractions, while muscles are shortening, and to inhale during eccentric contractions, while muscles are lengthening and returning weights to starting positions.

*Spotting.* Spotters are needed for certain exercises performed with free weights. These include multijoint exercises, in which weights must be returned to a rack on completion, and exercises during which weights need to be properly positioned. Half-squats and bench presses are examples of exercises requiring assistance.

*Safety.* The chances of sustaining an injury from resistance training are relatively small, but as with all physical activities, the chance exists. Safety is enhanced by using correct lifting techniques, making use of spotters, breathing properly, maintaining equipment in good working order, and wearing proper exercise clothing.

*Full range of motion.* To develop strength throughout the full range of motion, exercising muscles must produce force through complete flexion and extension. Be careful not to hyperextend or overextend, which can result in injury.

## Ergogenic Aids

**Ergogenic aids** are substances, techniques, or treatments that theoretically improve physical performance in addition to the effects of normal training. This discussion on ergogenic aids will be limited to a few of those reputed to accelerate muscle and strength development.

Many athletes and nonathletes take supplements of various types to accelerate muscle development. This short summary of a few of the many ergogenic aids suffices to show that some of these have performance-enhancing qualities, but many do not.

### Protein Supplementation

The adult requirement for protein is 0.8 gram (g) per kilogram (1 kg = 2.2 lbs.) of body weight. Research has shown that resistance training may push this requirement to 1.4 to 1.7 g/kg of body weight.[84] Values such as these are easily obtained with the typical American diet, particularly for active people, who tend to consume more calories than does the average adult. Protein in excess of these values has resulted in no further gains in strength, power, or muscle size.[85]

## Vitamins and Minerals

Physical performance is adversely affected by vitamin and mineral deficiencies. Those who have deficiencies can supplement their diets with the missing element or elements. However, the performance of well-nourished, physically active people is not improved through vitamin and mineral supplementation.

While vitamins do not furnish energy for muscle contraction, nor do they significantly contribute to body mass, they do provide functions that are crucial for normal energy metabolism, so it is important to obtain the daily requirement and then some. The antioxidant vitamins, such as C and E, may speed recovery from vigorous exercise. They also neutralize the free radicals (harmful elements that may damage cells; they are the product of oxidation) that are produced during high-intensity exercise.[86] Vitamins C and E and other substances with antioxidant properties mop up and neutralize free radicals, but in the process become "used up" themselves. Free radicals are implicated in the aging process and diseases such as cancer, atherosclerosis, rheumatoid arthritis, and macular degeneration. Keeping them controlled is very important, and since vigorous exercise produces them, antioxidant supplementation seems to be a good idea for very active people. But scientists recommend that antioxidants be obtained by eating fruits, vegetables, wholegrain breads, cereals, and vegetable oils rather than through supplements.[87] Also, there is evidence indicating that exercise training stimulates the body to increase its own production of antioxidants, thereby negating the need for supplements.[88] Scientists conclude that consuming foods rich in antioxidants is good for nutritional practice, but the evidence for or against supplements is not compelling.

## Creatine

Many, but not all, studies show that supplementing with creatine may enhance performance in short-term, high-intensity activities, such as resistance training. Creatine is a nitrogen-containing organic compound found in meat, poultry, and fish.[89] In addition to dietary creatine, the body synthesizes creatine in the liver, kidneys, and pancreas from nonessential amino acids. A third source is supplemental creatine monohydrate, which comes in powder, tablet, and liquid form. Creatine monohydrate supplementation increases skeletal muscle creatine content for most people. It is particularly advantageous for strict vegetarians, who eat no animal flesh and have low dietary levels as a result.[90] Creatine monohydrate supplementation promotes faster recovery from repetitive high-intensity exercises, so that users can perform a higher than normal volume of work.[91]

Evidence indicates that creatine supplementation is safe in the short term, but long-term data are lacking. It does not benefit the casual exerciser.[92]

## Ginseng

This herb has been used for centuries as a cure-all and an energizer. Theoretically, it improves physical performance by combating fatigue. In some animal studies, ginseng supplementation increased levels of free fatty acids in the blood while maintaining blood glucose level during exercise. Simultaneously, glycogen (stored sugar) values in the muscles were slightly higher.[93] This indicated that ginseng had a glycogen-sparing effect as the body selected the available fatty acids for fuel over glucose. Theoretically, this would improve endurance performance. However, studies with human subjects have not corroborated animal study results. In essence, research thus far on the relationship between ginseng and human physical performance indicates no improvement in oxygen utilization, aerobic performance, or exercise recovery rate.[94]

## Chromium Picolinate

Chromium is a micromineral that contributes to carbohydrate and fat metabolism. Chromium may improve insulin's effectiveness in blood glucose regulation.[95] Insulin has become an item of interest to those involved in sports and activities requiring muscle size, strength, and power because it decreases protein catabolism (breakdown of protein), increases protein synthesis (muscle building), and increases intramuscular availability of glucose.[96] When insulin is secreted into the blood, chromium is simultaneously released from the spleen, bones, and soft tissues. Chromium may facilitate the binding of insulin to cellular receptor sites, making it easier for the cells to receive glucose from the blood.

By itself, chromium is difficult to absorb. Chromium picolinate is a commercial preparation that is organic and somewhat more easily absorbed. Chromium deficiencies in the United States are rare.

The majority of available evidence to date indicates that chromium supplementation has little or no discernible effect on the development of muscle mass, fat loss, or exercise performance in humans.[97]

## Ubiquinone (Co-Q10)

Ubiquinone (Co-Q10) is a lipid found in the cell's mitochondria. It is an electron carrier that prevents oxidative damage to lipid tissues by donating electrons to free radicals (oxidants). Free radicals are rendered harmless when they receive an electron, so Co-Q10 functions as an antioxidant. Muscle concentrations of Co-Q10 decline with age, various disease states, and exercise.[98] As previously mentioned, physical activity generates free radicals, and physically active people should ensure an adequate intake of antioxidants through dietary and supplemental means, and this includes supplements of Co-Q10. Tissue concentrations were higher in physically active people but it did not seem to translate to improved aerobic performance in healthy people. However, there is evidence supporting improved physical performance on a treadmill in heart disease patients.[99] Co-Q10 is highly involved in the production of energy in nearly every cell of the body because it is an integral part of mitochondria (specialized organelles that produce ATP in the presence of oxygen and oxidative enzymes).[100] The mitochondria are responsible for generating about 95% of the energy extracted from the foods consumed.

## Conjugated Linoleic Acid (CLA)

Conjugated lenoleic acid (CLA) is found in beef, lamb, and dairy products.[101] It is a polyunsaturated fat that has strong antioxidant properties. Animal studies indicate that CLA may play a role in cancer prevention, cancer treatment, lowering cholesterol, reducing body fat, and increasing muscle mass. How do these results translate to humans? More than 30 clinical studies in human subjects showed that CLA might reduce the risk for colon, rectal, and breast cancer, but the evidence is weak.[102] The effect of CLS on fat loss is very small.[103] A possible adverse effect of CLA supplementation is that it may lower HDL cholesterol. HDLs protect the body from cardiovascular disease.

It is obvious from the paucity and conflicting current information that more and better research designs are needed to clarify the effects of CLA on human beings. These types of studies will probably not occur, because CLA is found in natural food sources that cannot be patented.

## Androstenedione (Andro)

Androstenedione (andro) is a precursor hormone to the male hormone testosterone. It is manufactured in the adrenal glands, which sit atop the kidneys.[104] Proponents of andro claim that it burns fat, builds muscle, and slows aging. Studies in males of all ages have shown that andro did not increase testosterone level and did not contribute to muscle mass or strength gains in weight training subjects.[105] Half of the subjects received andro, while the other half were given a look-alike placebo. Strength gains and increases in muscle mass were equal in both groups, indicating that the gains made were solely the result of the weight training program. The conclusion at this time is that andro does not seem to be effective. Furthermore, the health effects of long-term use are unknown. The

Anabolic Steroid and Control Act of 2004 classified andro as a controlled substance, thereby making its use as a performance-enhancing drug illegal.[106]

## Human Growth Hormone (hGH)

Human growth hormone (hGH) is secreted by the pituitary gland, which historically was referred to as the body's master gland because it secretes a number of hormones that affect other glands and organs.

Human growth hormone, in the recent past, had to be extracted from human cadavers. It was in short supply and expensive. Now it is made in laboratories, and it is still expensive, but limited supplies are no longer a problem. It is reputed to build skeletal mass, decrease fat mass, increase muscle mass, and shorten recovery from intense exercise.[107] Placebo-controlled studies do not support these claims in young, healthy, physically active subjects. However, subjects over the age of 60 who received human growth hormone had an increase in lean body mass, a decrease in fat mass, and an increase in bone density.[108]

The major medical problem associated with human growth hormone usage in adults is the risk of developing acromegaly. Acromegaly is a disorder that results in the growth and thickening of the bones of the brow, jaw, hands, and feet long after the skeleton's normal growth has ended. The internal organs also enlarge, and the victim suffers muscle and joint weakness and ultimately heart disease. Cardiomyopathy is a serious disease of the heart that involves inflammation and reduced heart muscle function. It is the most frequent cause of death from human growth hormone usage; diabetes and hypertension are other reported side effects. The past two decades have seen a rise in the use of human growth hormone as an ergogenic aid even though it has not proven to be effective for elite athletes.[109] The International Olympic Committee and other major sports governing bodies have banned this substance as a performance-enhancing aid.[110] Currently, there is not an effective test for discovering users of human growth hormones.

## Anabolic-Androgenic Steroids

Anabolic steroids are synthetic derivations of the male sex hormone testosterone. They have anabolic properties (develop muscle mass) and androgenic properties (develop secondary male sexual characteristics).[111] They build muscle mass and strength, and as a result, they improve physical appearance and physical performance.

Anabolic steroid use by nonathletes is on the rise. This is particularly true for young men. A national survey of male high school seniors revealed that 7% of them were using or had used steroids. One-third of them stated that they were not participating in high school sports, and more than 25% of these respondents stated that their primary motivation for using steroids was for improving physical appearance.[112] Surveys such as these, while helping to illustrate the scope of the problem, underestimate the actual numbers of users because many respondents are unwilling to admit their engagement in this type of behavior. Heavy steroid users are more likely than light users to take two or more steroids simultaneously and more apt to take these drugs by injection rather than in pill form. Injection as a method of delivery is highly characteristic of drugs that involve addiction.[113] The steroid "hook" is insidious and powerful, as evidenced by the number of people who continue to use steroids despite the danger to their health.

Although definitive evidence of the long-term effects of steroid use is not available, the potential for long-term harm is certainly real. Predicting how and when the effects of steroids will be manifested is impossible because people respond differently to these drugs as a result of differences in body chemistry. The steroid effect is complicated further by the fact that black market preparations contain additives, and some preparations are contaminated. The potential for harm is readily discernible; 80 to 90% of steroids used are purchased through the black market. Table 4-1 presents some of the known and possible effects of steroid use.

## TABLE 4-1   Overview of Anabolic Steroid Effects

**Effects Supported by Strong Evidence in Males and Females**

| | |
|---|---|
| Stunted growth when taken before puberty | Deepening of the voice (in women) |
| Coronary artery disease | Menstrual irregularities (in women) |
| Low HDL cholesterol | |
| Sterility, low sperm count (in men) | Development of facial and body hair (in women) |
| Liver tumors and liver disease | Decreased breast size (in women) |
| Death | Clitoris enlargement (in women) |
| Acne | |
| Water retention | Fetal damage (when taken during pregnancy) |
| Oily, thickened skin | |
| Male-pattern baldness (in women) | |

**Possible Effects in Males and Females**

| | |
|---|---|
| Diarrhea | Bone pains |
| Muscle cramps | Impotence (in men) |
| Breast development (in men) | Sexual problems |
| | High blood pressure |
| Aggressive behavior | Kidney disease |
| Headache | Depression |
| Nausea | |

Source: Adapted from Nieman, D. C. (2007). *Exercise testing and prescription*. New York: McGraw-Hill.

## Muscle Dysmorphic Disorder

**Muscle dysmorphia** (sometimes called bigorexia) is a subtype of body dysmorphia where people's perceptions of their bodies are distorted.[114] It is the opposite of anorexia nervosa in that the people with this condition obsess about being underdeveloped even though most of them are well muscled. As a result, they become preoccupied with and avid practitioners of weight training in an attempt to build more muscle and reduce body fat.[115] Attempting to meet these goals increases their susceptibility to the lure of anabolic androgenic steroids.

The constant preoccupation with their perceived underdeveloped bodies permeates all phases of their lives and can interfere with their occupations, social life, and family life. They hide their physiques under layers of loose clothing and avoid places, such as beaches and pools, where they might be seen without clothing.

Muscle dysmorphia occurs primarily to men, but the condition has been observed in some women.[116]

## Keeping a Daily Training Log

Beginning weight trainers should keep a daily log of their training activities. The advantages of keeping such a record far outweigh the minimal amount of bother, time, and effort required to make the entries during the workout. Each entry should be recorded during the rest period between sets.

The advantages of maintaining a daily training log include the following:

- You will always know which exercises you performed and the amount of weight used for each.

- You will always know the number of repetitions and sets that you performed of each exercise.

- The training log provides an objective account of your improvement. You can compare the amount of weight you are currently lifting with the amount at the beginning of your training.

- The training log provides an accurate history.

- The training log is a motivating device that provides objective feedback of performance improvement.

A sample training log is shown in Figure 4-21. A blank training log is given in Assessment Activity 4-5 for you to use to document your resistance training program. It will be helpful to make additional copies of this training log.

Name ___Cathy Smith___

Starting date ___Jan. 1, 2007___

Program objectives ___To gain strength and muscle definition___

| Exercise | Jan. 1 | | | Jan. 3 | | | Jan. 5 | | | Jan. 7 | | | Jan. 9 | | | Jan. 11 | | | Jan. 13 | | |
| --- | --- | --- | --- | --- | --- | --- | --- | --- | --- | --- | --- | --- | --- | --- | --- | --- | --- | --- | --- | --- | --- |
| | Resis. (lbs.) | Reps | Sets | Resis. (lbs.) | Reps | Sets | Resis. (lbs.) | Reps | Sets | Resis. (lbs.) | Reps | Sets | Resis. (lbs.) | Reps | Sets | Resis. (lbs.) | Reps | Sets | Resis. (lbs.) | Reps | Sets |
| 1. Bench press | 60 | 10 | 3 | | | | | | | | | | | | | | | | | | |
| 2. Biceps curl | 25 | 10 | 3 | | | | | | | | | | | | | | | | | | |
| 3. Back exten-sion | 80 | 10 | 3 | | | | | | | | | | | | | | | | | | |
| 4. Leg press | 150 | 10 | 3 | | | | | | | | | | | | | | | | | | |
| 5. Ham-string curl | 30 | 10 | 3 | | | | | | | | | | | | | | | | | | |
| 6. Chest press | 30 | 10 | 3 | | | | | | | | | | | | | | | | | | |
| 7. Abdom-inal crunch | — | 25 | 3 | | | | | | | | | | | | | | | | | | |
| 8. Over-head press | 35 | 10 | 3 | | | | | | | | | | | | | | | | | | |

**FIGURE 4-21** Sample Training Log

*Resistance* (abbreviated as Resis.) refers to the amount of weight (in pounds) lifted or pressed. *Reps* (for repetitions) is the number of times the weight is lifted or pressed. *Sets* are the groups of reps.

# Summary

- The physiological law of use and disuse applies to all human beings during all phases of the life cycle.
- The muscular systems of older adults are trainable and respond to resistance training with an increase in strength and muscle size.
- Muscular strength is the maximum force that a muscle or muscle group can exert in a single contraction.
- Dynamic exercises consist of concentric and eccentric muscle contractions.
- Isotonic exercises are dynamic in that muscles shorten and lengthen, producing movement around a joint.
- Variable resistance exercise equipment is designed to provide maximum resistance throughout the full range of motion.
- Circuit resistance training is a versatile system that allows a person to develop several fitness dimensions simultaneously.
- The principles of exercise—intensity, duration, frequency, overload and progression, specificity, and variation—apply to resistance training. These can be manipulated to meet all muscle development objectives.
- Muscle fiber types are influenced by genetics and exercise habits.
- The suggested breathing pattern during resistive exercises is to exhale during the concentric contraction and inhale during the eccentric contraction.
- Many studies have shown that creatine supplementation may enhance performance in short-term, high-intensity activities.
- Anabolic steroids are performance-enhancing drugs that are harmful and illegal.
- Research in the last decade has shown that resistance training contributes to wellness in a variety of ways.
- Muscle endurance is the ability to apply repeated muscular force.

# Review Questions

1. Define *muscular strength* and *muscular endurance*.
2. What are the differences among isometric, isotonic, isokinetic, and variable resistance exercises?
3. What are concentric and eccentric contractions?
4. What are the health benefits of participating in resistance exercise?
5. Name and define the principles of conditioning as they relate to resistance training.
6. What are the health consequences and physical performance benefits of steroid use?

# References

1. American College of Sports Medicine. (ACSM). (2010). *ACSM's guidelines for exercise testing and prescription* (8th ed.). Philadelphia: Wolters Kluwer/Lippincott Williams and Wilkins.
2. Ibid.
3. Ibid.
4. Nieman, D. C. (2007). *Exercise testing and prescription* (6th ed.). Boston: McGraw-Hill.
5. ACSM (2010).
6. Powers, S. K., & E. T. Howley. (2009). *Exercise physiology* (7th ed.). Boston: McGraw-Hill.
7. Frontera, W., & J. Bean. (2005). *Strength and power training*. Boston: Harvard Health Publications.
8. ACSM (2010).
9. Wilmore, J. H., D. L. Costill, & W. L. Kenney. (2008). *Physiology of sport and exercise* (4th ed.). Champaign, IL: Human Kinetics.
10. Editors. (2009, October). Get stronger, thrive longer. *Consumer Reports on Health*, 21(10), 8.
11. ACSM (2010).
12. Editors (2009, October).
13. Kraemer, W. J. (2010). Musculoskeletal exercise prescription. In *ACSM's resource manual* (6th ed.), edited by J. K. Ehrman. Philadelphia: Wolters Kluwer/Lippincott Williams and Wilkins.
14. ACSM (2010).
15. Kramer, W. J. (2010). Adaptations to resistance training. In *ACSM's Resource Manual* (6th ed.), edited by J. K. Ehrman. Philadelphia: Wolters Kluwer/Lippincott Williams and Wilkins.
16. Ibid.
17. Ibid.
18. Ratamess, N. A. (2008). Adaptations to anaerobic training programs. In *Essentials of strength training and conditioning* (3rd ed.), edited by T. R. Baechle & R. W. Earle. Champaign, IL: Human Kinetics.
19. Powers & Howley (2009).
20. Nieman (2007).
21. Ibid.
22. Powers & Howley (2009).
23. Editors. (2009, July). Time to put some muscle into it. *Harvard Health Letter*, 34(9), 4.
24. Kraemer (2010).
25. Nieman (2007).
26. ACSM (2010).
27. Kraemer (2010).
28. Editors. (2009, July). Pump it up: 10 strength training tips for bones, balance, weight control. *Environmental Nutrition*, 32(7), 3.
29. Graves, B. S., M. Whitehurst, & B. W. Findley. (2006). Physiologic effects of aging and deconditioning. In *ACSM's resource manual* (5th ed.), edited by L. M. Kaminsky. Philadelphia: Lippincott Williams and Wilkins.
30. Kraemer (2010).
31. Nieman (2007).
32. Humphries, B., E. L. Dugan, & T. L. A. Doyle. (2006). Muscular fitness. In *ACSM's resource manual* (5th ed.), edited by L. M. Kaminsky. Philadelphia: Lippincott Williams and Wilkins.
33. Kraemer (2010).
34. ACSM (2010).
35. Faigenbaum, A. D. (2008). Age and sex related differences and their implication for resistance exercise. In *Essentials of strength training and conditioning* (3rd ed.), edited by T. R. Baechle & R. W. Earle. Champaign, IL: Human Kinetics.
36. Evetovich, T. and K. Ehersole. 2006. "Adaptations to Resistance Training." In *ACSMs Resource Manual* (5th ed.) edited by L. M. Kaminsky.

Philadelphia: Lippincott Williams and Wilkins.

37. Faigenbaum (2008).
38. Ratamess (2008).
39. Kraemer (2010).
40. Brzycki, M. (2004, July). What's a good formula for estimating a one repetition maximum? *Fitness Management, 20*(8), 50.
41. ACSM (2010).
42. Kraemer (2010).
43. Faigenbaum (2008).
44. Ibid.
45. Ibid.
46. Coe, D. P., & M. A. Fiatarone-Singh. (2010). Exercise prescription in special populations: Women, pregnancy, children and the elderly. In *ACSM's Resource Manual* (6th ed.), edited by J. K. Ehrman. Philadelphia: Wolters Kluwer/Lippincott Williams and Wilkins.
47. Ibid.
48. Faigenbaum (2008).
49. Ibid.
50. Kraemer (2010).
51. Nieman (2007).
52. Evetovich (2006).
53. Ibid.
54. Powers & Howley (2009).
55. Ibid.
56. Nieman (2007).
57. Ibid.
58. Wilmore et al. (2008).
59. Ibid.
60. Ibid.
61. Kraemer (2010).
62. Wilmore et al. (2008).
63. Ibid.
64. Nieman (2007).
65. Wilmore et al. (2008).
66. Nieman (2007).
67. Powers & Howley (2009).
68. Ibid.
69. Nieman (2007).
70. Ibid.
71. Kravitz, L. (2006). Applied exercise programming. In *ACSM's resource manual* (5th ed.), edited by L. M. Kaminsky. Philadelphia: Lippincott Williams and Wilkins.
72. ACSM (2010).
73. Kraemer, W. J., & J. A. Bush. (2001). Factors affecting the acute neuromuscular responses to resistance exercise. In *ACSM's resource manual* (4th ed.), edited J. L. Roitman. Philadelphia: Lippincott Williams and Wilkins.
74. American College of Sports Medicine. (2006). *ACSM's guidelines for exercise testing and prescription* (7th ed.). Philadelphia: Lippincott Williams and Wilkins.
75. Yessis, M. (2005, June). Defying strength training conviction. *Fitness Management, 21*(7), 40.
76. Nieman (2007).
77. Kraemer, W. J., et al. (2002). Progression models in resistance training for healthy adults—ACSM position stand. *Medicine and Science in Sports and Exercise, 34*(2), 364.
78. Nieman (2007).
79. ACSM (2010).
80. Kraemer et al. (2002).
81. Kraemer (2010).
82. Weir, J. P., & J. T. Cramer. (2006). Principles of musculoskeletal exercise programming. In *ACSM's resource manual* (5th ed.), edited by L. M. Kaminsky. Philadelphia: Lippincott Williams and Wilkins.
83. Kraemer (2010).
84. Pasiakos, S. M., & N. R. Rodriquez. (2010). Nutrition. In *ACSM's resource manual* (6th ed.), edited by J. K. Ehrman. Philadelphia: Wolters Kluwer/Lippincott Williams and Wilkins.
85. Volpe, S. L. (2006). Weight management. In *ACSM's resource manual* (5th ed.), edited by L. M. Kaminsky. Philadelphia: Lippincott Williams and Wilkins.
86. Nieman (2007).
87. Byrd-Bredbenner, C., et al. (2009). *Wardlaw's perspectives in nutrition.* New York: McGraw-Hill.
88. Powers & Howley (2009).
89. Nieman (2007).
90. Byrd-Bredbenner (2009).
91. Powers & Howley (2009).
92. Ibid.
93. Gammeren, D. V. (2001). Endurance performance. In *Sport supplements,* edited by J. Antonio & J. R. Stout. Philadelphia: Lippincott Williams and Wilkins.
94. California State University. (2010, February 23). Sports medicine. Retrieved from www.csulb.edu/divisions/students/hrc/health topics/sports medicine.htm.
95. Office of Dietary Supplements, National Institutes of Health. (2006, September 14). Dietary supplement fact sheet: Chromium. Bethesda, MD. Retrieved from http://ods.od.nih.gov.
96. Earnest, C. P., & C. Street. (2001). Skeletal muscle mass, strength, and speed. In *Sport supplements,* edited by J. Antonio & J. R. Stout. Philadelphia: Lippincott Williams and Wilkins.
97. California State University (2010, February 23).
98. Editors. (2006, September 15). Coenzyme Q10. Mayo Clinic.com, Tools for Healthier Lives. Retrieved from www.mayoclinic.com/health/coenzyme-q10/NS_patient_coenzymeq10.
99. California State University (2010, February 23).
100. Coenzyme Q10. (2010, February 22). *Wikipedia.* Retrieved from http://en.wikipedia.org/wiki/Coenzyme Q10.
101. Memorial Sloan-Kettering Cancer Center. (2010, February 24). Conjugated linoleic acid. Retrieved from http://www.mskcc.org/mskcc/html/69191.cfm.
102. Conjugated linoleic acid. (2010, February 24). *Wikipedia.* Retrieved from http://en.wikipedia.org/wiki/Conjugated_linoleic_acid.
103. Editorial Staff. (2010, February 24). Conjugated linoleic acid overview information, *Web MD.* Retrieved from www.webmd.com/vitamins-supplements/ingredientmono-826-co. . .tivelngredientName=CONJUGATED+LINOLEIC+ACID&SOURCE=2&print=true
104. Wilmore et al. (2008).
105. Hoffman, J. R., & R. R. Stour. (2008). Performance enhancing substances. In *Essentials of strength training and conditioning* (3rd ed.), edited by T. R. Baechle & R. W. Earle. Champaign, IL: Haman Kinetics.
106. Ibid.
107. Nieman (2010).
108. Rudman, D., et al. (1990). Effects of human growth hormone in men over 60 years old. *New England Journal of Medicine, 323,* 1.
109. Hoffman & Stour (2008).
110. Neiman (2007).
111. Hoffman & Stour (2008).
112. Ibid.
113. Neiman (2007).
114. Hoffman & Stour (2008).
115. Ibid.
116. Muscle dysmorphia. (2010, February 16). *Wikipedia.* Retrieved from www.en.wikipedia.org/wiki/Muscle dysmorphia.

# Suggested Readings

Editors. (2009, July). Pump it up: 10 strength training tips for bones, balance, weight control. *Environmental Nutrition*, 32(7), 3.

This article offers a number of reasons why weight training should be a part of an exercise program, most of which revolve around health enhancement. Also, 10 tips for novices that will increase their enjoyment and the probability of constructing a successful program are offered.

Editors. (2009, July). Time to put some muscle into it. *Harvard Health Letter*, 34(9), 4.

This article discusses the reasons for including strength training in an exercise program. One of the major benefits is that strength training is the best way to stave off the muscle loss that occurs with age. This article advocates the inclusion of training for muscle power as well as strength and provides examples of two simple power exercises that can be included in a starter program.

Editorial Staff. (2009, October). Get stronger, thrive longer. *Consumer Reports* on Health, 21(10), 8.

The jist of this article is that two 15-minute strength-training workouts per week can provide many health benefits. The authors discuss several health benefits that derive from research evidence. A streamlined full-body workout is presented with illustrations of the exercises that are supported.

Standley, L. J. (2010, February 16). The muscular system. Retrieved from www.drstandley.com/bodysystems muscular.shtml.

This article covers the muscular system for the layperson. It discusses the three types of muscle—skeletal, smooth, and cardiac. Each type of muscle is illustrated and defined, and its function in the body is discussed. Basic principles of muscle contraction are also discussed.

Mac B. (2010, February 22). Weight training. Retrieved from www.brainmac.co.uk/weight.htm.

This article is a primer on weight training. It covers basic muscle physiology and defines muscle hypertrophy, endurance, and power. It also covers repetitions, sets, resistance, and rest intervals between sets and between workouts. Different training systems (pyramid system, super sets) are explained. And finally, the selection of exercises that comprise the program are discussed, with examples of various exercises that are available.

**Name** _____   **Date** _____   **Section** _____

# Assessment Activity 4-1

## Calculation of Strength (Selected Muscle Groups)

**Directions:** The calculation of strength by this method is expressed as the ratio of strength to body weight. The amount of weight accomplished for each lift is converted to a proportion of your body weight and is determined in the following manner:

1. Find your 1 RM for each of the following exercises: biceps curl (two arm), overhead press, bench press, half-squat or leg press, and hamstring curl.

2. Divide your 1 RM for each exercise by your body weight. For example, a 130-lb. woman performs a 1 RM bench press of 80 lbs. Her score is $80 \div 130 = 0.61$. Look at the chart for an interpretation of her score. Look under the Bench Press column and note that her score of 0.61 is in the average category. In this example, the woman has the following results on the five lifts: biceps curl = 0.28 (fair), overhead press = 0.26 (fair), bench press = 0.61 (average), half-squat or leg press = 1.35 (good), and hamstring curl = 0.52 (good). These data are plotted in the first strength profile chart.

3. When you have computed a score for each of your lifts, turn to the strength profile charts. Plot your data in the blank chart provided.

4. Refer to Figures 4-1 through 4-15 for a refresher on how to do these exercises.

### Strength/Body Weight Ratio

**Women**

| Biceps Curl | Overhead Press | Bench Press | Half-Squat or Leg Press | Hamstring Curl | Strength Category |
|---|---|---|---|---|---|
| 0.45 and above | 0.50 and above | 0.85 and above | 1.45 and above | 0.55 and above | Excellent |
| 0.38–0.44 | 0.42–0.49 | 0.70–0.84 | 1.30–1.44 | 0.50–0.54 | Good |
| 0.32–0.37 | 0.32–0.41 | 0.60–0.69 | 1.00–1.29 | 0.40–0.49 | Average |
| 0.25–0.31 | 0.25–0.31 | 0.50–0.59 | 0.80–0.99 | 0.30–0.39 | Fair |
| 0.24 and below | 0.24 and below | 0.49 and below | 0.79 and below | 0.29 and below | Poor |

**Men**

| Biceps Curl | Overhead Press | Bench Press | Half-Squat or Leg Press | Hamstring Curl | Strength Category |
|---|---|---|---|---|---|
| 0.65 and above | 1.0 and above | 1.30 and above | 1.85 and above | 0.65 and above | Excellent |
| 0.55–0.64 | 0.90–0.99 | 1.15–1.29 | 1.65–1.84 | 0.55–0.64 | Good |
| 0.45–0.54 | 0.75–0.89 | 1.00–1.14 | 1.30–1.64 | 0.45–0.54 | Average |
| 0.35–0.44 | 0.60–0.74 | 0.85–0.99 | 1.00–1.29 | 0.35–0.44 | Fair |
| 0.34 and below | 0.59 and below | 0.84 and below | Less than 1.0 | 0.34 and below | Poor |

## Strength Profile Charts

**Example**

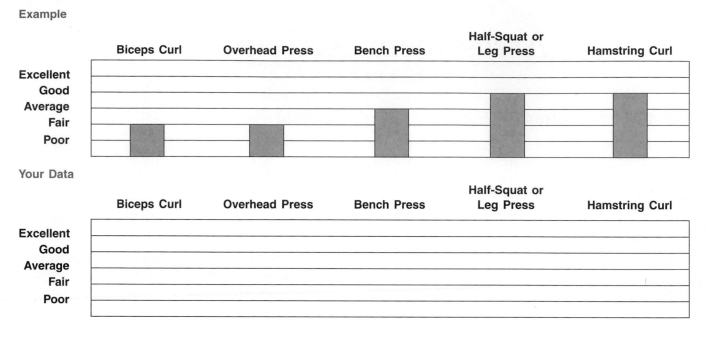

**Your Data**

|  | Biceps Curl | Overhead Press | Bench Press | Half-Squat or Leg Press | Hamstring Curl |
|---|---|---|---|---|---|
| **Excellent** | | | | | |
| **Good** | | | | | |
| **Average** | | | | | |
| **Fair** | | | | | |
| **Poor** | | | | | |

**Name** _____   **Date** _____   **Section** _____

# Assessment Activity 4-2

## Muscular Endurance

**Directions:** Through trial and error, select a weight that you can use while performing 20 RM for each of the following exercises: bench press, leg extension or half-squat, biceps curl, and hamstring curl. For example, a male subject weighing 150 lbs. can perform 20 RM of 100 lbs. in the bench press. The score for this exercise is computed as follows:

$$\frac{100 \text{ lbs.}}{150 \text{ lbs.}} = 0.67, \text{ or } 67\%$$

Now look at the chart under Bench Press and observe that a score of 67% is average. Perform each of the four exercises (20 RM) and calculate the muscle endurance scores following the example.

### Muscle Endurance: Body Weight Ratio 20 RM

**Men**

| Bench Press | Leg Extension or Half-Squat | Biceps Curl | Hamstring Curl | Strength Category |
|---|---|---|---|---|
| ≥ 76%* | ≥ 166% | ≥ 50% | ≥ 40% | Excellent |
| 70–75 | 150–165 | 43–49 | 33–39 | Good |
| 60–69 | 133–149 | 37–42 | 27–32 | Average |
| 50–59 | 116–132 | 30–36 | 20–26 | Fair |
| < 50** | < 116 | < 30 | < 20 | Poor |

**Women**

| Bench Press | Leg Extension or Half-Squat | Biceps Curl | Hamstring Curl | Strength Category |
|---|---|---|---|---|
| ≥ 50% | ≥ 115% | ≥ 32% | ≥ 38% | Excellent |
| 42–49 | 100–114 | 23–31 | 31–37 | Good |
| 35–41 | 88–99 | 15–22 | 23–30 | Average |
| 27–34 | 77–87 | 12–14 | 15–22 | Fair |
| < 27 | < 77 | < 12 | < 15 | Poor |

\* ≥ equal to or greater than

\*\* < less than

**Name** _____   **Date** _____   **Section** _____

# Assessment Activity 4-3

## Abdominal Muscular Endurance—the Canadian Trunk Strength Test

**Directions:** The Canadian trunk strength test is an alternative to the conventional sit-up test to measure abdominal muscular endurance. It is not necessary or desirable to raise the trunk more than 30°. Sit-ups beyond 30° cause the abdomen to contract isometrically, so the hip flexors supply the power to raise the trunk above this level. The Canadian trunk strength test is performed in the following manner:

1. Lie on your back with knees bent 90°.

2. Extend your arms so that the fingertips of both hands touch a strip of tape perpendicular to the body on each side.

3. Place two additional strips of tape parallel to the first two strips, 8 cm apart.

4. Curl up, sliding your fingertips along the mat until they touch the second set of tape strips, and then return to the starting position.

5. The curl-up is slow, controlled, and continuous with a cadence of 20 curl-ups/min. (3 secs./curl-up).

6. A metronome provides the speed of movement. It is set at 40 beats/min. (curl up on one beat, down on the second).

7. Perform as many curl-ups as you can, up to a maximum of 75 without missing a beat. See Figure 4-22 for a demonstration of the Canadian trunk strength test and then look at the chart for an interpretation of your score.

### Standards for the Canadian Trunk Strength Test

| | Number Completed | | | | | |
| --- | --- | --- | --- | --- | --- | --- |
| | Men—Age | | | Women—Age | | |
| **Strength Category** | **< 35** | **35–44** | **> 45** | **< 35** | **35–44** | **> 45** |
| Excellent | 60 | 50 | 40 | 50 | 40 | 30 |
| Good | 45 | 40 | 25 | 40 | 25 | 15 |
| Marginal | 30 | 25 | 15 | 25 | 15 | 10 |
| Needs work | 15 | 10 | 5 | 10 | 6 | 4 |

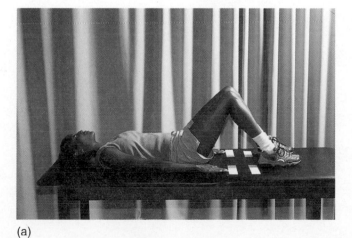

(a)

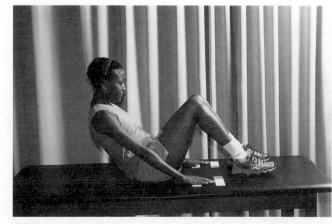

(b)

**FIGURE 4-22** Canadian Trunk Strength Test

**Name** _____   **Date** _____   **Section** _____

# Assessment Activity 4-4

## Assessing Muscular Strength and Endurance with Selected Calisthenic Exercises

**Directions:**  The tests making up this assessment require minimal equipment and are easy to administer.

*Chin-ups:* Grasp an overhead horizontal bar, hands shoulder-width apart, palms facing forward. On the upstroke, your chin must go above the bar and your arms must extend fully on the downstroke. Your legs must remain extended throughout the exercise and should not be used to thrust your body upward (Figure 4-23).

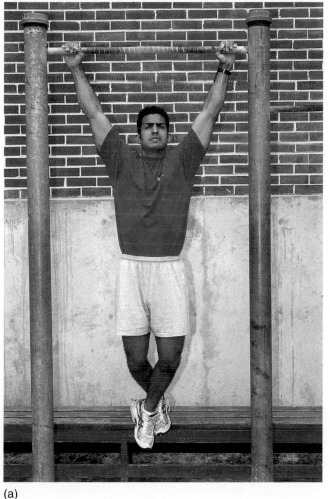

(a)

(b)

**FIGURE 4-23** Chin-Ups

*Flexed-arm hang:* Perform this exercise if you cannot do chin-ups. Have someone assist you to the exercise position with your chin above the bar, palms facing away from your body. A stopwatch is started as soon as you assume this position and is stopped if you tilt your head back to keep your chin above the bar, if your chin touches the bar, or if your chin drops below the bar. Record the time to the nearest whole second (Figure 4-24).

*Push-ups:* Assume a prone position (face down) with your arms extended, hands on the floor under your shoulders. Keep your back and legs straight and your feet together. The person counting the push-ups should place a fist under your chest. Bend your elbows, lowering your chest until contact is made with the counter's fist, and then return to the starting position by straightening your arms. Repeat as many times as possible without resting to a maximum score of 46 push-ups (Figure 4-25).

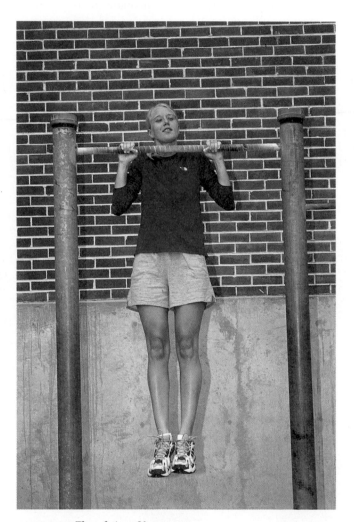

**FIGURE 4-24** Flexed-Arm Hang

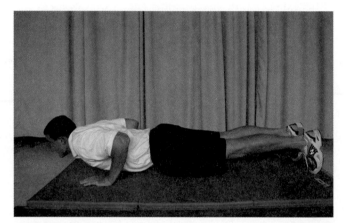

(a)

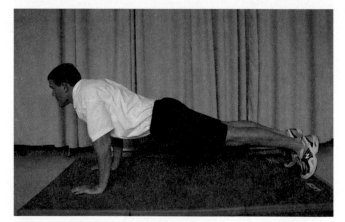

(b)

**FIGURE 4-25** Push-Ups

*Modified push-ups:*   Perform this exercise if you cannot do the standard push-up. The modified version is performed in the same manner as the standard push up, except that you support your body weight with your hands and knees. Do as many as you can without rest to a maximum of 24 (Figure 4-26).

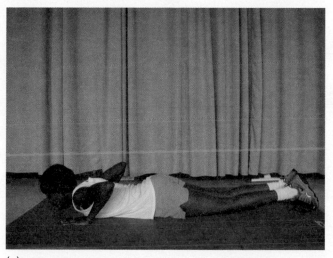

(a)

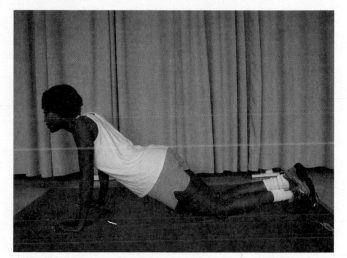

(b)

**FIGURE 4-26** Modified Push-Ups

## Muscular Strength and Endurance Standards

| Chin-Ups | Flexed-Arm Hang (secs.) | Push-Ups | Modified Push-Ups | Strength Category |
|---|---|---|---|---|
| 20 or more | 30 or more | 40 or more | 24 or more | Excellent |
| 15–19 | 24–29 | 32–39 | 14–23 | Good |
| 10–14 | 15–23 | 27–31 | 8–13 | Average |
| 6–9 | 9–14 | 20–26 | 2–7 | Fair |
| 5 or less | 8 or less | 19 or less | 1 or less | Poor |

**Name** _____ **Date** _____ **Section** _____

# Assessment Activity 4-5

## Resistance Training Log

**Directions:** Keep a record of your resistance fitness activities on the form provided. Make copies of this form for repeated uses.

**Daily Training Log**

Name _____

Program objectives _____ Starting date _____

| Exercise | Date: | | | Date: | | | Date: | | | Date: | | | Date: | | | Date: | | |
|---|---|---|---|---|---|---|---|---|---|---|---|---|---|---|---|---|---|---|
| | Resis.* (lbs.) | Reps | Sets | Resis. (lbs.) | Reps | Sets | Resis. (lbs.) | Reps | Sets | Resis. (lbs.) | Reps | Sets | Resis. (lbs.) | Reps | Sets | Resis. (lbs.) | Reps | Sets |
| | | | | | | | | | | | | | | | | | | |
| | | | | | | | | | | | | | | | | | | |
| | | | | | | | | | | | | | | | | | | |
| | | | | | | | | | | | | | | | | | | |
| | | | | | | | | | | | | | | | | | | |
| | | | | | | | | | | | | | | | | | | |
| | | | | | | | | | | | | | | | | | | |
| | | | | | | | | | | | | | | | | | | |

*Resis., resistance; reps, repetitions

# Improving Flexibility

 **ONLINE LEARNING CENTER**

Log on to our Online Learning Center (OLC) for access to these additional resources:

- Chapter key term flashcards
- Learning objectives
- Additional goals for behavior change
- Concentration game
- Self-scoring chapter quizzes
- Additional lab activities

The OLC also offers Web links for study and exploration of wellness topics. Access these links through **www.mhhe.com/anspaugh8e.**

**GOALS FOR BEHAVIOR CHANGE**

- Begin participating regularly in a stretching program to improve flexibility.
- Identify some of the tasks or sports that you perform regularly for which being more flexible would be helpful.
- Practice correct lifting techniques when moving heavy objects.
- Modify your work or study area to lower the risk for neck and back pain.
- Try two safe ergogenic aids and analyze their effectiveness.

## Objectives

After completing this chapter, you will be able to do the following:

✔ Define *flexibility*.
✔ Identify factors affecting flexibility.
✔ Distinguish among static, ballistic, and proprioceptive neuromuscular facilitation stretching.
✔ Assess and prescribe a personal flexibility program.
✔ Discuss the high incidence of neck pain, upper-back pain, and lower-back pain in the United States.
✔ Demonstrate proper lifting techniques for prevention of lower-back injury.

**[ Key Terms ]**

| | |
|---|---|
| agonist | proprioceptive |
| antagonist | neuromuscular |
| ballistic stretching | facilitation (PNF) |
| flexibility | proprioceptor |
| Golgi tendon organ | repetitive strain injury |
| goniometer | static stretching |
| Pilates | stretch reflex |

**M**usculoskeletal conditioning includes exercises that increase muscle strength and endurance, and exercises that improve flexibility. This chapter examines the relationship between flexibility and wellness, identifies and illustrates safe and effective stretching exercises, discusses types of stretching and stretching techniques, and presents guidelines for developing a sound flexibility program.

## Flexibility and Wellness

**Flexibility** programs are planned, deliberate, and regularly performed sets of exercises designed to progressively increase the range of motion of a joint or series of joints.[1] Flexibility may be defined and measured statically or dynamically. For the purpose of this text, it will be defined statically as the range of motion of a single joint or a series of joints.[2] The joints are surrounded by connective tissues consisting of muscles, tendons, and ligaments. The tendons connect muscles to bones and the ligaments connect bones to bones.[3] These structures respond to stretching exercises, which result in the development of a greater range of motion (ROM). Athletes involved in sports that require greater than average flexibility devote much training time to improving this component of physical fitness. For instance, martial arts participants, ballet dancers, and gymnasts demonstrate an extraordinary range of motion well beyond the capacity of most people. Flexibility is an important component of health-related physical fitness but one that is often neglected even though it requires a minimal investment in time, effort, and equipment.

Factors that limit joint movement include (1) the bony structure of the joints (the skeleton is established by heredity, but it can be harmed by trauma, disease, calcium deposits, etc.); (2) the amount of tissue (muscle and fat) around and adjacent to the joint; (3) the elasticity of muscles, tendons, and ligaments; and (4) the skin (scar tissue from surgery or a laceration over a joint may limit movement).[4] Other factors that influence flexibility are age, gender, and level and type of physical activity. Young people are more flexible than adults because tendons lose their elasticity with age. Preschool-age children are very flexible due to limited bony calcification—that is, the ends of the long bones have yet to ossify (the conversion of cartilage to bone). Peak flexibility occurs between 15 and 18 years of age and begins to decline by the mid-20s.[5] Inactivity may play a greater role than the aging process in the loss of flexibility because muscles and other soft tissues lose elasticity when not used. Also, aging is often accompanied by conditions, such as arthritis, that compromise range of motion. Older people develop fibrous connective tissue that replaces deteriorating muscle fibers in a

**[ JUST THE ]**
# FACTS
### Benefits of Flexibility Training

Here are some of the claims made in support of flexibility training:

• Reduction of stress and tension

• Muscle relaxation

• Improved fitness, posture, and symmetry

• Relief of muscle cramps

• Relief of muscle soreness

• Prevention of injury

• Reduced frequency of injury

• Return to full range of motion after an injury

process referred to as fibrosis. Stretching exercises can slow the fibrotic process or restore some of the lost flexibility when older individuals engage in flexibility exercises. Active individuals are usually more flexible than inactive people.[6] Women tend to be more flexible than men because the hormones that permit women's tissue to stretch during the childbirth process facilitate all body stretching.[7] The range of motion for most movements begins to decline in the mid-20s for men and women. Flexibility improves for males between the ages of 6 and 10 and begins to decline during adolescence and early adulthood, while flexibility for females improves throughout adolescence and reaches a peak between the ages of 25 and 29.[8] (Complete Assessment Activities 5-1 through 5-4 at the end of this chapter to determine your flexibility.)

Joint flexibility is important for several reasons. Inflexible muscles around the joints limit range of movement, eventually inhibiting activities of daily life. This phenomenon is most frequently seen in older people who have difficulty reaching down to tie their shoes or bending over to get a drink of water from a fountain. Lack of flexibility in the shoulders can affect the performance of normal daily activities, such as changing an overhead lightbulb or removing a can of vegetables from a cupboard.[9] Tight muscles may also contribute to joint deterioration by subjecting the bones to excessive pressure, causing pain and abnormalities in joint lubrication. One of the consequences of aging, particularly when it is accompanied by inactivity, is dehydration. Dehydration contributes to the development of adhesions that are characterized by the abnormal union of connective tissues resulting in stiff joints.[10] Stretching exercises stimulate the production or retention of lubricating fluid between the connective tissues, reduce the risk for adhesion formation, and maintain joint mobility. Regular flexibility exercises can improve

# Nurturing Your Spirituality

## The Ancient Arts of Tai Chi and Yoga

Medical health care training and delivery have been gradually adopting a more holistic view of treating patients. This holistic view recognizes the role of spirituality in the healing process. Johns Hopkins Medical School currently offers an elective course for its medical students on spirituality and healing.[14] The National Institutes of Health has awarded grants to a small number of medical schools to develop and promote courses on this subject.

At the same time that spirituality is making a medical comeback, Americans are searching for ways to alleviate stress, promote relaxation, and enhance health. Two physical arts that blend spirituality and health, tai chi and yoga, are gaining popularity.

Tai chi originated as a self-defense art, but it has evolved into a religious ritual, a relaxation technique, and an exercise program for people of all ages, including the elderly. Tai chi features slow, balanced, low-impact movements that may reduce stress and improve flexibility, balance, and strength.[15] It requires concentration, controlled breathing, and balance while body weight is shifted as a person transitions from one movement to another. It is often referred to as *movement meditation* because it promotes muscle relaxation through movement.[16]

The potential benefits of tai chi include the following:

- Improved flexibility[17]
- Physical therapy, because it may assist in recovery from injury
- Improved balance and coordination
- Improved strength, particularly of the lower body (buttocks, thighs, and calves)
- Improved posture
- Increased ability to relax
- Possible slight reduction in the resting blood pressure

It takes years to become adept at tai chi, but several movements and positions can be learned with a few weeks of instruction.

Yoga originated in India about 6,000 years ago. There are several types, but hatha yoga seems to be most popular among Americans. Hatha yoga features a system of exercises that promote physical fitness and mental well-being.[18]

Yoga is a Sanskrit word that means "union." Its practitioners strive for total union in experience, a union of physical, mental, and spiritual states. Achieving this union results in a calm, relaxed, tranquil attitude.

Research indicates that yoga's meditative characteristics may prevent or at least decrease the severity of psychosomatic illness. Psychosomatic illnesses are mind-body maladies. They are caused by negative mental states and attitudes that produce changes in body physiology that result in disease. Some common psychosomatic diseases are tension headaches, ulcers, asthma, stress, essential hypertension, impotence, back pain, and menstrual problems.[19]

Master practitioners can, at will, influence body responses controlled by the autonomic nervous system, such as breathing rate, heart rate, and blood pressure. But it takes years of practice to achieve this level of control.

The exercises and body positions featured in yoga promote mobility and flexibility, but some of these positions are potentially unsafe. It is important to learn from an experienced instructor to minimize mistakes.

Practiced regularly, yoga may lower resting blood pressure, relieve mild depression, and contribute to strength and balance. Anecdotal evidence (evidence that comes from personal reports) also indicates that practitioners experience more energy and feel calmer and more focused than nonpractitioners.[20]

---

body posture. Flexibility exercises following aerobic activity reduce muscle soreness.[11]

According to the American College of Sports Medicine (ACSM), stretching exercises may prevent injuries.[12] The supporting data come primarily from observational studies, which are not as definitive as randomized, controlled clinical trials. Studies with larger samples and better controls indicate little relationship between stretching and the risk for injury. Even though scientific evidence does not strongly support flexibility training for injury prevention, sports medicine specialists advocate its use.[13] Based on the available evidence as well as experience, flexibility exercises help

maintain a full range of joint motion. While this is true, people who are at the extremes of flexibility from inflexible to extremely flexible seem to be more susceptible to joint injury due to less stable joints.[21] Also, extreme flexibility appears to be detrimental to performance in running and weight lifting because tight muscles perform more efficiently in these activities.[22]

Maintenance of flexibility is most important for the prevention of lower-back pain.[23] For example, a sedentary lifestyle characterized by sitting for long periods leads to a loss of flexibility and increases the likelihood of lower-back injury. Flexibility of the hamstring muscles (a group of muscles in the back of the thighs) and the lower-back muscles contributes to good posture. Posture is also improved by the development of strong abdominal muscles and the maintenance of normal body weight. Extra body weight, particularly that which accumulates around the abdominal area, throws the body out of balance and applies a forward force on the lower (lumbar) spinal area, which places extra stress on the lower back.[24]

Good posture and core body strength (strong abdominal and strong back muscles) are the foundation of a healthy back. A system of exercise that emphasizes proper posture and core strength was developed in the early 20th century by Joseph Pilates.[25] Today, the system is simply known as **Pilates**, and it has become very popular with the general public, fitness leaders, and physical therapists.[26] Pilates developed more than 500 exercises that emphasize torso strength and proper breathing. These exercises are performed with precision, under control, and with good form.

The program is based on six principles:

1. stabilization—movement is initiated from a stable source
2. control—all movements are controlled actions
3. flow—movements are flowing as opposed to sudden and sharp
4. concentration—heightened awareness and focus on the body
5. breathing—optimal intake of oxygen with improved circulation

6. full range of motion—for the possible reduction of chronic injuries

Pilates exercise systems are taught in one of two formats:

1. group mat classes without equipment, or
2. using Pilates specialized equipment to perform the exercises

The benefits received (healthy spine and torso) from Pilates training, as related to the six basic principles, are perceived as potential by the scientific community because there are not scientific studies to support or refute them.[27] The best advice at this point is that people who enjoy and believe in the Pilates system should continue to participate.

The benefits of flexibility training are summarized in Just the Facts: Benefits of Flexibility Training. See also Nurturing Your Spirituality: The Ancient Arts of Tai Chi and Yoga on page 153.

## Developing a Flexibility Program

Flexibility can be improved by exercises that promote the elasticity of the soft tissues. Figures 5-1 through 5-8 demonstrate exercises that can maintain and improve the flexibility of the major body sites. These 10-minute exercises can be done every day, both before and after exercise, and on days of rest from exercise.

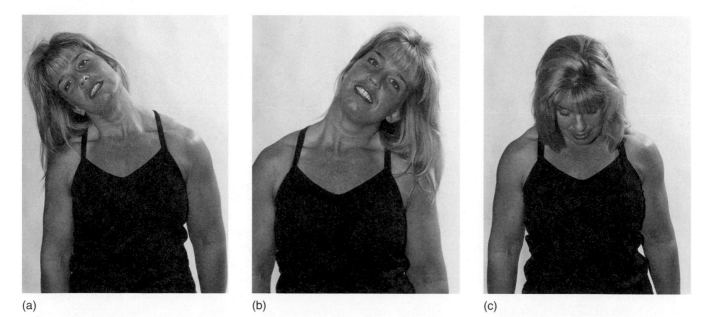

(a)                (b)                (c)

**FIGURE 5-1** Neck Stretches

Slowly bend your neck from side to side and to the front. Do not do head circles, because these require hyperextension (excessive extension) of the cervical (neck) area of the spinal column, which produces potentially harmful compression of the intervertebral disks.

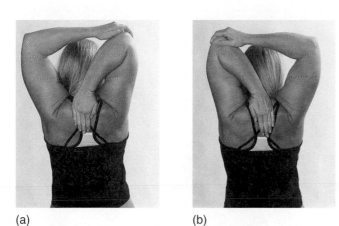

(a)                              (b)

**FIGURE 5-2** Shoulder Stretch
(a) Gently pull your right arm behind your head and hold for 15 to 30 seconds. (b) Repeat with the other arm.

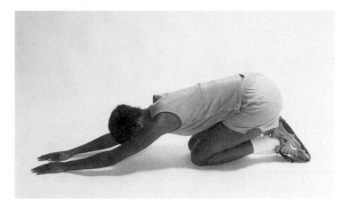

**FIGURE 5-3** Chest and Shoulder Stretch
Stretch your arms to full extension with both palms on the floor and press your chest down to the floor. Hold 15 to 30 seconds and slowly release.

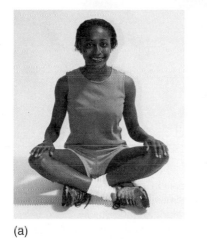

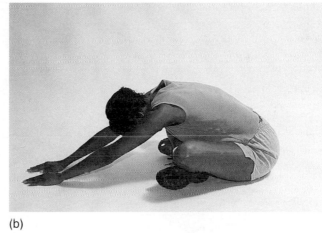

(a)                              (b)

**FIGURE 5-4** Back Stretch
(a) Cross your legs and lean forward, extending your arms to the front. (b) Hold for 15 to 30 seconds and slowly release.

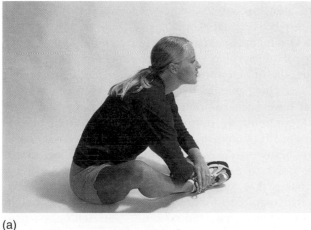

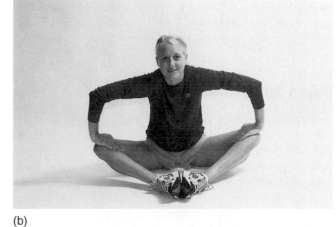

(a)                              (b)

**FIGURE 5-5** Groin Stretch
(a) Place the soles of your feet together and lean forward. Hold 15 to 30 seconds. (b) Variation: Push down gently on both knees and hold for 15 to 30 seconds.

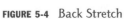

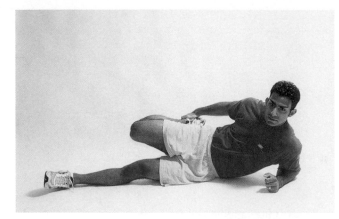

**FIGURE 5-6**  Quadriceps Stretch

Lie on your side as shown. Bend the knee of your top leg, grasp your ankle with your free hand, and slowly pull your heel toward your buttocks until you feel the stretch in the muscles in the front of your thigh. Hold 15 to 30 seconds, roll over to the other side, and repeat with your other leg.

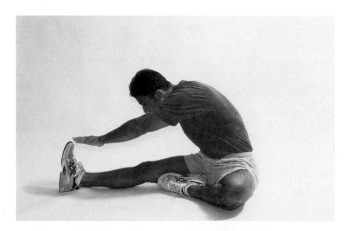

**FIGURE 5-7**  Hamstring Stretch

Place the sole of your left foot against the thigh of your extended right leg. Lean forward without bending the knee of your extended leg. Hold for 15 to 30 seconds and repeat with your other leg.

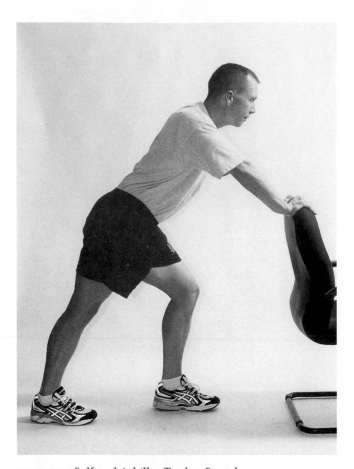

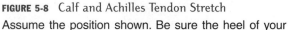

**FIGURE 5-8**  Calf and Achilles Tendon Stretch

Assume the position shown. Be sure the heel of your extended leg remains in contact with the floor and both feet are pointed straight ahead. Slowly move your hips forward until you feel the stretch in the calf of your extended leg. Hold 15 to 30 seconds and repeat with your other leg.

## When to Stretch

Stretching exercises can be included in the warm-up prior to exercise and in the cooldown following exercise and done on nonexercise days. Stretching prior to working out should occur only after the muscles have been warmed up with 5 to 10 minutes of such cardiovascular activities as brisk walking, slow jogging, stationary bike riding, or similar activity.[28,29] A gradual warm-up increases heart rate slowly and raises the temperature of muscles, tendons, and ligaments by increasing blood flow to these structures. Stretching after a warm-up is safer and more productive than stretching

before: Stretching cold muscles increases the probability of incurring a soft tissue injury.[30] Warm up prior to stretching for approximately 10 minutes on the days of rest between workouts.

The highest payback from stretching comes at the end of an aerobic or resistive workout. During this time, the muscles are thoroughly warmed and capable of stretching maximally and safely. Also, the muscles that have been contracting and shortening vigorously and continuously during the workout should be systematically stretched and lengthened after the workout.[31] However, there is emerging evidence that stretching prior to exercise may be counterproductive for activities that require strength, power, and speed such as that required for sprinting, vertical jumping, weight lifting, shuttle run, and so on.[32,33] Stretching, particularly static stretching, lengthens the contractile units of muscles and consequently reduces their ability to produce force, at least temporarily. Some evidence indicates that performance decrements may last as long as

60 minutes. Based on the evidence at hand, it would be best to warm up (as described in Chapter 3) prior to activities that require strength, power, and speed, and to stretch after such activities.

## Types of Stretching

Muscles must contract for movement to occur. The contracting muscles are called **agonists** and are the prime movers. For an agonist to contract, shorten, and produce movement, a reciprocal lengthening of its **antagonist** must occur. For example, when the biceps muscle of the upper arm contracts, its opposite, the triceps muscle, must relax and lengthen. In this case, the biceps is the agonist and the triceps is the antagonist, but the triceps becomes the agonist for movements that require it to contract, making the biceps the antagonist. Understanding these concepts is necessary to understanding stretching techniques.

**Static stretching** involves slowly moving to desired positions, holding them for 15 to 30 seconds, and then slowly releasing them. This method of stretching does not activate the **stretch reflex** (automatic or reflexive contraction of a muscle being stretched), so the muscle is essentially stretched without opposition.

The stretch reflex consists of two **proprioceptors,** sensory organs found in muscles, joints, and tendons that provide information regarding body movement and position. These proprioceptors are the muscle spindle and the **Golgi tendon organ.**[34] The muscle spindle is a receptor sensitive to changes in muscle length. The Golgi tendon organ is a receptor that is also sensitive to changes in muscle length but additionally responds to increases in muscle tension.[35]

Stretching the muscles also stretches their muscle spindles, which send a volley of sensory impulses, informing the central nervous system (CNS) that the muscles are being subjected to stretch. Impulses are sent back to the muscles, which cause them to contract reflexively, thus resisting the stretch. But if a muscle is stretched statically and the position is held for at least 6 seconds, the Golgi tendon organ responds to the change in length and tension by sending a volley of signals of its own to the CNS. Unlike the signals from the muscle spindle, those initiated by the Golgi tendon organ cause the antagonist muscle (the muscle being stretched) to relax reflexively. This protective mechanism allows the muscle to stretch through relaxation as the Golgi tendon organ nullifies or overrides the signals of the muscle spindle. Thus, stretching positions held for at least 6 seconds and preferably for 15 to 30 seconds allow muscles to lengthen and stretch with minimal chance of injury.[36]

Static stretching should produce a feeling of mild discomfort but not pain. Static stretching (see Figures 5-1 to 5-8) results in little or no muscle soreness, has a low incidence of injury, requires little energy, and can be done alone. For these reasons, static stretching is the preferred system for increasing flexibility.

The following guidelines should be followed for safe and effective static stretching:[37]

- Warm up for a few minutes before stretching by walking, jogging slowly, doing light calisthenics, or doing a similar activity.
- Stretch to the point of mild discomfort.
- Do not stretch to the point of pain.
- Hold each stretch for 15 to 30 seconds minimum.
- Do not hold your breath during a stretch; breathe rhythmically and continuously.
- Move slowly from position to position.
- Perform each stretch at least four times.
- Stretch after the workout; this produces the greatest benefit because the muscles are warm and more amenable to stretching.
- Perform stretching exercises five or six times per week.

Deliberate attempts to improve flexibility should occur throughout the life cycle. See Wellness for a Lifetime: Flexibility Guidelines for Children and Older Adults on page 158 for more specific information.

**Proprioceptive neuromuscular facilitation (PNF)** is another effective and acceptable stretching technique. It is more complex than most methods of stretching, but it is the most effective.[38,39,40] By combining slow, passive movements (the force for passive movement is supplied by a partner) with maximal voluntary isometric contractions, you can bypass the stretch reflex stimulation that accompanies changes in muscle and tendon length.

All variations of PNF stretching require a partner and some combination of passive stretching and isometric contractions. Two of the common PNF methods, contract-relax (CR) and slow reversal-hold-relax (SRHR), are presented in Figures 5-9 and 5-10 (page 158). For comparison, both figures exemplify stretching the hamstring group (muscles in the back of the thigh). The hamstrings are the antagonist muscle group, and the quadriceps muscles (muscles in the front of the thigh) are the agonists. For example, the CR method is performed as follows (Figure 5-9):

1. A partner gently pushes the upraised leg in the direction of arrow A. This movement passively stretches the antagonist (hamstrings).
2. The subject follows this with a 6-second maximal contraction of the agonist (quadriceps).
3. This is followed by another passive stretch of the hamstrings.

This is repeated twice, with a few seconds of rest between sequences.

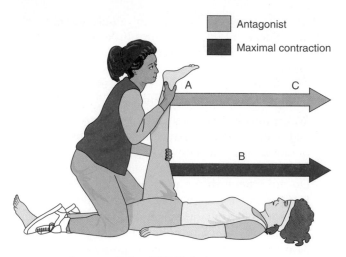

**FIGURE 5-9** Contract-Relax (CR) Technique

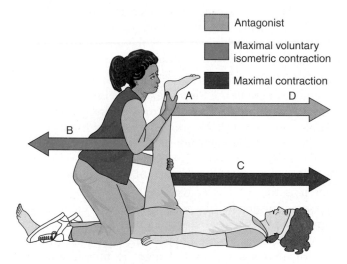

**FIGURE 5-10** Slow Reversal-Hold-Relax (SRHR) Technique

The SRHR method is performed in the following manner (Figure 5-10):

1. A partner gently pushes the upraised leg in the direction of arrow A.
2. The subject then performs a 6-second maximal voluntary isometric contraction (MVIC) of the antagonists (hamstrings) against resistance supplied by the partner.
3. The subject follows this with a 6-second maximal contraction of the agonists (quadriceps).
4. This is followed by another passive stretch of the hamstrings.

This sequence is repeated twice, with a few seconds of rest between exercises.

Although PNF appears to be the most effective stretching method for enhancing flexibility, it has some limitations. It requires a partner; it produces more pain and muscle stiffness; it requires more time; and it increases the risk for injury, particularly when used by novices.[45,46]

**Ballistic stretching** uses dynamic movements or repetitive bouncing motions to stretch muscles. Each time a muscle is stretched in this manner, the muscle spindle (one of two receptors that make up the stretch reflex) located in that muscle is also stretched. It responds by sending a volley of signals to the central nervous system that order the muscle to contract, thus resisting the stretch. This not only is counterproductive—the muscle is forced to pull against itself—but also can lead to injury because the elastic limits of the muscle may be exceeded. Ballistic stretching is not recommended for flexibility development for the general public.[47] Many competitive athletes—performers participating in track and field, gymnastics, martial arts, dancing, and so on—use ballistic stretching to improve sport-specific flexibility.[48] Years of training using ballistic stretching enables these athletes to adapt and withstand the rigors of such training in relative safety.

## Wellness for a Lifetime
### Flexibility Guidelines for Children and Older Adults

Evidence indicates that flexibility can be increased in healthy older adults who participate in aerobic activities supplemented with stretching exercises.[41,42] Physical activities, such as walking and aerobic dance, coupled with stretching exercises increase the range of motion of older adults.[43]

Recommendations for improving the flexibility of children are somewhat different. Because children are more flexible than adults, 5- to 9-year-olds need less time devoted to flexibility exercises than do older adults.[44] However, some formal stretching is required, and activities such as tumbling and climbing are suggested. For older

children, ages 10 through 12, the amount of time spent on improving flexibility should be greater than that of younger children but less than that of adults. Children, especially some boys, may begin to lose flexibility at this early age, so regular stretching exercises and physical activities, such as tumbling, that promote flexibility are recommended.

It is important to establish the habit of regularly stretching the muscles, tendons, and joints throughout one's lifetime. Stretching becomes even more important as we become older.

## Flexibility Assessment

Measuring flexibility is rather difficult, and several instruments have been developed for this purpose. Probably the most widely used device is the **goniometer**. This is a protractor-like device that measures the range of motion of a specific joint. This method is an accurate means of assessing flexibility.[49] However, for the average person, assessing flexibility by using a goniometer is not practical.

Several tests are suitable for measuring flexibility when more sophisticated means cannot be used. (The directions and norms for these tests are provided in the assessment activities.) You should warm up and follow the rules for general stretching before taking the assessments.

## Preventing Back and Neck Pain

All people experience tense muscles and muscle soreness in various parts of the body on an occasional basis. The neck, shoulder, and back are particularly susceptible to the types of pressures that cause pain. Sedentary lifestyles contribute to back pain; unfortunately, 70% of Americans are sedentary or marginally active. Also contributing to neck and back pain are occupations that require workers to stand for long periods or to spend a significant amount of time sitting behind a desk, in front of a computer, or behind the wheel of an automobile. See Just the Facts: Neck Pain for more on neck pain.

According to the U.S. Department of Labor, Occupational Safety and Health Administration (OSHA), **repetitive strain injuries** are the nation's most common and costly occupational health problem affecting millions of American workers and costing more than $100 billion annually.[50] Repetitive strain injuries occur when repeated stress is placed on some part of the body such as the hand, wrist, or neck. According to the U.S. Bureau of Labor Statistics, nearly 65% of all occupational illnesses were the results of exposure to repeated trauma to the upper body (wrist, elbow, or shoulder).[51] Carpal tunnel syndrome, which is the leading type of repetitive strain injury, affects more than 8 million Americans and is responsible for more days of lost work than any of the other work-related injuries.

Typing or key entry; repetitive use of tools; the repetitive placing, grasping, or moving of objects other than tools; athletic endeavors such as tennis and basketball; and the arts, such as dance or playing certain musical instruments, result in such injury.[52] Musculoskeletal problems are highly associated with these work-related physical tasks when the level of exposure is high. Performing unaccustomed physical work or engaging in unfamiliar sports also produces stress on

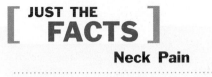

**[ JUST THE FACTS ]**
### Neck Pain

There are more than 70 million visits to physicians and other health care professionals for neck and back pain every year.[53] Approximately 10 to 15% of the population experience neck pain at any given time.[54] Most cases are transitory annoyances that usually resolve themselves in about 7 days. Normally, visiting a physician is unnecessary unless neck pain lasts longer than 2 weeks or is accompanied by any of the following signs and symptoms:[55]

1. Severely restricted movement on turning the head left or right or an inability to touch the chin to the chest
2. Headaches, fever, weight loss
3. Pain that worsens at night
4. No relief from rest or painkilling medications
5. Pain, numbness, or tingling sensations in the fingers, arms, or legs
6. Difficulty walking, clumsiness, or weakness
7. Problems with the bladder or bowels or sexual dysfunction

Neck pain can be prevented by practicing simple lifestyle behaviors.[56] Most neck pain occurs from poor posture and the wear and tear of aging. Posture can be improved by stretching the abdominal and low-back muscles as well as stretching hips and hamstring muscles. Better posture will center the head over the spine and keep it in proper alignment. Here are some other lifestyle behaviors that may contribute to reducing neck pain:

1. Gently stretch the neck from side to side and in as many directions as pain allows.
2. Take frequent breaks if you sit in front of a computer for long periods of time, or if you are on a long drive.
3. If you work at a computer, make sure the screen is at eye level.
4. Stretch frequently.
5. Use over-the-counter pain relievers such as aspirin, ibuprofen, or Aleve.
6. Alternate the application of heat and cold therapy.

the back and neck. Activities that require repetitive overhead reaching or extended sitting at a computer may produce pain and discomfort in the back, shoulders, and neck. The exercises in Figures 5-1 through 5-4, coupled with a few minutes of moving about, may prevent or alleviate pain in these areas of the body.

These problems can be significantly lessened if (1) employers ergonomically design the layout of workstations, job methods, tools, and materials to reduce

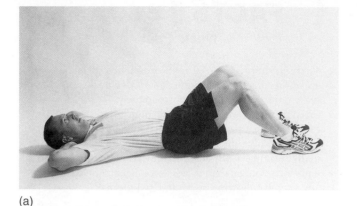

(a)

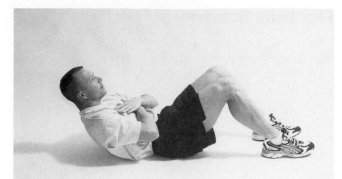

(b)

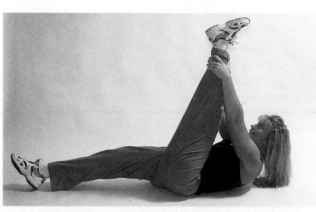

(c)

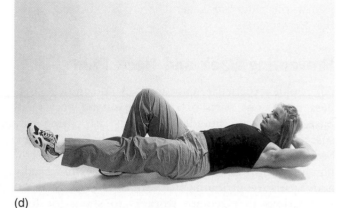

(d)

**FIGURE 5-11**  Maintaining a Healthy Back

(a) To develop the abdominal muscles, lie on your back in the position shown, and contract your abdominal muscles to force the lower back against the floor. Hold for 6 to 10 seconds. Relax and repeat 5 to 10 times.

(b) To develop the abdominal muscles, lie on your back, cross your arms over your chest, and raise your shoulder blades off the floor as shown. Return to the starting position. Repeat 5 times and work up to 25.

(c) To stretch the hamstrings, hips, and buttocks, raise one leg and extend the other. Reach up and grasp the upright leg below the calf. Alternate legs and work up to 20 repetitions with each.

(d) To develop lower abdominal muscles, keep one leg bent with that foot flat on the floor. Raise the extended leg about 6 inches off the floor, and return to the starting position. Do 10 reps and repeat with the other leg. Work up to 25 reps.

exposure to the physical factors related to performing repetitive tasks; and (2) employees become aerobically fit and engage in activities to promote muscle strength and joint flexibility.

The lower back consists of five lumbar bones, six shock-absorbing disks, the spinal cord, nerves, muscles, and ligaments. Lower-back pain affects 80 to 90% of American adults at some point in their lives. It is the fifth most common reason for visiting their primary care physicians, even though 90% of people affected recover within a month.[57]

The high incidence of lower-back pain is caused by the following: excess body weight, weak abdominal muscles, weak and inflexible back muscles, weak and inflexible hamstring muscles, poor posture, cigarette smoking, the lifting of objects incorrectly, work- or sports-related injuries, and diseases such as osteoarthritis and osteoporosis.[58]

Excess body weight, especially that which is stored in the abdominal region, stresses the lower back by pulling the spinal column forward. This causes an excessive amount of arch in the lower back, which results in poor alignment of the spine. As a result, obese people are more susceptible to lower-back problems than are normal-weight people.[59]

Weak abdominal muscles, weak and inflexible back muscles, and tight hamstring muscles distort upright posture and tilt the pelvis forward, which increases stress on the lower back.[60] Strong abdominal muscles may account for up to 40% of torso support.[61] Figure 5-11 illustrates exercises that stretch the lower back and develop the abdominal muscles.

Smokers have a higher incidence of lower-back pain than do nonsmokers. Smoking appears to increase degenerative changes in the spine. Smoking also prolongs lower-back pain and hampers the healing process

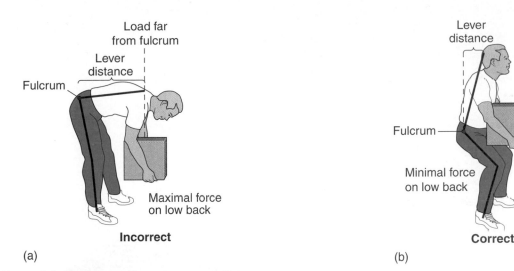

Load far
from fulcrum

Lever
distance

Fulcrum

Maximal force
on low back

**Incorrect**

(a)

Lever
distance

Fulcrum

Minimal force
on low back

**Correct**

(b)

**FIGURE 5-12**   How to Lift Objects

(a) Lifting an object from the floor with straight legs and a bent back places significant stress on the lower back, increasing the likelihood of injury. Notice the distance between the box being lifted and the body of the lifter. (b) Lifting an object from the floor with bent legs and a straight back allows the lifter to keep the box close to the body, which places the majority of stress on the legs rather than on the lower back.

by reducing the oxygen supply to the affected areas of the back. This occurs because the carbon monoxide in cigarette smoke attaches readily to hemoglobin, crowding out oxygen.[62]

Figure 5-12 demonstrates correct and incorrect ways to lift a weight from the floor. Lifting correctly substantially lowers the risk of sustaining a lower-back injury. Employ the following principles when lifting objects:[63]

1. Stand squarely in front of and close to the object to be lifted.
2. Bend from the knees as opposed to the waist, and squat down as far as is comfortable.
3. Tighten the abdominal muscles and keep the buttocks tucked in.
4. Lift with the legs, not the lower back.
5. Don't raise a heavy object higher than the waist, and keep a light load below shoulder level.
6. Keep the object close to the body throughout the lift.
7. If you need to turn to set the object down, don't twist from the waist. Instead, turn your entire body, feet, hips, and shoulders, and then set the object down.
8. Do not attempt to lift objects that are excessively heavy unless help is available.

See Just the Facts: Tips for Preventing and Treating Back and Neck Pain.

# [ JUST THE ] FACTS

## Tips for Preventing and Treating Back and Neck Pain

The following behaviors may help alleviate or prevent back and neck pain:

- If you sit, stand, or work in one place for extended periods, periodically walk around for a few minutes and do some simple stretching exercises.

- If your job requires long periods of standing, you can reduce the stress on your lower back by placing one foot and then the other on a small stool for a few minutes at a time. This rounds the spine and reduces lower-back stress. You can also shift your weight from one foot to the other.

- If you drive for long periods, sit comfortably and make sure you can easily reach the dash, pedals,

and steering wheel. You can also try placing a small pillow behind your lower back. Also, stop the vehicle every 2 to 3 hours to take a short stretch break.

- Exercise regularly to develop the abdominal muscles and to stretch the back muscles.

- Stretch the back muscles and hamstrings at least three times per week.

- Maintain a healthy body weight.

- Bend at the knees while lifting objects, so that your legs do most of the work.

- Do not smoke cigarettes, because they contribute to the degeneration of the spine.

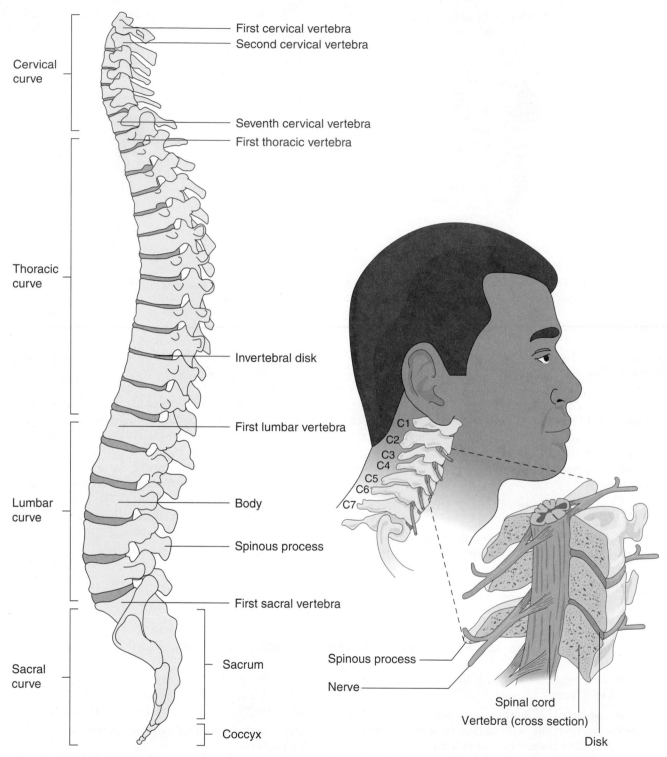

**FIGURE 5-13** The Vertebral Column

(a) The complete column viewed from the left side. Note that the vertebrae of the sacrum are fused into one bone, and those of the coccyx have also fused into one bone. (b) The vertebrae of the cervical curve from the right side.

The spinal column consists of 33 bones (the vertebrae) and represents the only bony connection between the upper and lower halves of the body. Although humans are born with 33 separate vertebrae, by adulthood 5 vertebrae of the sacrum have fused into 1 bone, and the 4 vertebrae of the coccyx have fused into 1 bone, leaving a total of 24 vertebral bones.[64] See Figure 5-13, which illustrates the shape and bony structure of the vertebral column.

Located between the bones of the spine are rings of tough, fibrous tissue—the disks, which act as shock absorbers, keeping the vertebrae from rubbing against each other. The spinal column is S-shaped and consists of naturally occurring curves. When these curves are balanced, the body weight is evenly distributed, and movement occurs fluidly, and the vertebral column is 16 times stronger than if it were straight.[65] Misalignment in these regions applies substantial stress to the concave, or inner, side of the curves. The more pronounced the curves, the greater the stress because of the uneven distribution of weight on the bones and disks.

Approximately 90% of all back problems occur in the lumbar region (lower back) of the spine because that region carries the weight of the torso (the trunk of the human body). The lower back is most vulnerable to strains, as well as other problems, because it is subjected to the greatest amount of physical stress.[66] Fatigue causes the pelvis to tilt forward when a person is standing, increasing stress on the spinal column and its supporting structures. Wearing high-heeled shoes does the same thing.

## Summary

- Flexibility refers to the range of motion at a joint or series of joints and is specific to each joint.
- Factors that influence flexibility of a joint are the bony structure, the amount of tissue at the joint, the skin, and the elasticity of the muscles, tendons, and ligaments at the joint.
- Flexibility is influenced by age, gender, and physical activity.
- The maintenance of flexibility of the hamstrings and lower-back muscles is important in the prevention of lower-back pain.
- Normal body weight and good posture are also necessary for a healthy back.
- Ballistic stretching is counterproductive to improving joint elasticity and may contribute to injury.
- Static stretching is the recommended type of exercise. Stretches should be held for 15 to 30 seconds and repeated at least three times.
- Stretching should not be painful, only mildly uncomfortable.
- Stretching exercises can be performed daily.
- Proprioceptive neuromuscular facilitation is the most effective but most difficult form of stretching.
- Proprioceptive neuromuscular facilitation combines passive movement with isometric contractions.
- The goniometer is the most widely used device to measure flexibility.
- Lower-back pain is one of the most common reasons for visiting a physician.
- Factors associated with lower-back and neck pain include excess weight; poor posture; inactivity; fatigue; weak abdominal muscles; the wearing of high heels; stress; cigarette smoking; weak, inflexible back and hamstring muscles; incorrect lifting; work or sports injuries; and disease.

## Review Questions

1. Explain why flexibility is such an important component of health-related fitness.
2. Discuss the steps to take when developing a flexibility program.
3. What concepts are necessary to understand about stretching?
4. Distinguish among static, ballistic, and PNF stretching.
5. Discuss the guidelines that should be followed for safe and effective stretching.
6. What factors are associated with lower-back and neck problems?
7. Describe the proper lifting technique for preventing back injury.
8. Discuss the role of repetitive movements in the development of upper-back and neck pain.
9. What can an employer and an employee do to reduce the potential for repetitive motion injuries?

## References

1. Nieman, D. C. 2007 *Exercise testing and prescription* (6th ed.). Boston: McGraw-Hill.
2. American College of Sports Medicine (ACSM). (2010). *ACSM's guidelines for exercise testing and prescription* (8th ed.). Philadelphia: Wolters Kluwer/Lippincott Williams and Wilkins.
3. Nieman (2007).
4. Jeffreys, I. (2008). Warm-up and stretching. In *Essentials of strength training and conditioning* (3rd ed.), edited by T. R. Baechle & R. W. Earle. Champaign, IL: Human Kinetics.
5. Ibid.
6. Ibid.
7. Ibid.
8. Wells, G. D. (2007). Flexibility for health and performance. Retrieved from www.per4m.ca.
9. Knudson, D. V., P. Magnusson, & M. McHugh. (2000, June). Current issues in flexibility fitness. *PCPFS Research Digest*, 3(10), 1.
10. Daniels, C. (2010, June 22). Computer ergonomics-osteoarthritis. Retrieved from www.klis.com/computers&health/#Osteoarthritis.
11. Nieman (2007).
12. ACSM (2010).
13. Nieman (2007).
14. Johns Hopkins University. (1998). Can religion be good medicine? *The Johns Hopkins Medical Letter*, 10(9), 3.
15. Harvard Medical School. (2009, May). The health benefits of tai chi. *Harvard Medical Publications*. Retrieved from www.health.harvard.edu/newsletters/Havard_Woman_Health_Watch/2009/May/The health benefits of tai chi.
16. Ibid.
17. Ibid.

18. Mayo Clinic Staff. (2010, January 16). Yoga: Tap into the many benefits of yoga. Mayo Clinic. Retrieved from www.mayoclinic.com/health/yoga/cmooоо4/METHOD=print.
19. WebMD. (2008, August 12). The health benefits of yoga. Retrieved from www.webmd.com/balance/the health-benefits-of-yoga.
20. Ibid.
21. Powers, S. K., & E. Howley. (2009). *Exercise physiology* (7th ed.). Boston: McGraw-Hill.
22. Ibid.
23. Nieman (2007).
24. Ibid.
25. Staff. (2010, March 1). Pilates. Retrieved from http://en.wikipedia.org/wiki/pilates.
26. Ibid.
27. Ibid.
28. ACSM (2010).
29. Spring, T., B. Franklin, & A. dejong. (2010). Muscular fitness and assessment. In *ACSM's Resource Manual* (6th ed.), edited by J. K Ehrman. Philadelphia: Wolters Kluwer/Lippincott Williams and Wilkins.
30. Nieman (2007).
31. Spring et al. (2010).
32. Ibid.
33. ACSM (2010).
34. Jeffreys (2008).
35. Ibid.
36. Powers & Howley (2009).
37. ACSM (2010).
38. Powers & Howley (2009).
39. Jeffreys (2008).
40. Spring et al. (2010).
41. Jeffreys (2008).
42. Nieman (2007).
43. Graves, B. S., M. Whitehurst, & P. L. Jacobs. (2010). Lifespan effects of aging and deconditioning. In *ACSM's resource manual* (6th ed.), edited by J. K. Ehrman. Philadelphia: Wolters Kluwer/Lippincott Williams and Wilkins.
44. Hale, B. S., & Franks, B. D. (2001). *Get fit: A handbook for youth ages 6–17.* Washington, DC: The President's Council on Physical Fitness and Sports.
45. Nieman (2007).
46. Jeffreys (2008).
47. Powers & Howley (2009).
48. Walker, B. (2006, September 26). Warm-up activities and stretching exercise. Retrieved from www.thestretchinghandbook.com/archives/warm-up.htm.
49. Spring et al. (2010).
50. Epinions.com. (2006, June 8). Repetitive strain injury. Retrieved from www.epinions.com/content 4762935428.
51. RSI-Therapy.com. (2006, October 2). *RSI statistics.* Retrieved from www.rsi-therapy.com/statistics.htm.
52. WebMD Staff. (2010, March 3). Repetitive strain injury. Retrieved from www.eecs.umich.edu/~cscott/rsi.html.
53. Editors. (2004, September). Save your neck. *Body and Soul,* 26.
54. Kostiuk, J. P., & S. Margolis. (2004). *Back pain and osteoporosis–The Johns Hopkins white papers.* Baltimore: Johns Hopkins Medicine.
55. Ibid.
56. Mayo Clinic Staff. (2010, February 17). Neck pain–Lifestyle and home remedies. Retrieved from www.mayoclinic.com/health/neck-pain/D500542/DESECTION=lifestyle%2Dand%2Dhome%2Dremedies.
57. Parkinson, G. (2006). Low back pain. Edited by J. N. Katz. Boston: Harvard Health Publications.
58. National Institute of Neurological Disorders and Stroke. (2009, December 21). Low back pain fact sheet. Retrieved from www.ninds.nih.gov/disorders/backpain/detail backpain.htm.
59. WebMD. (2008, February 6). Low back pain–Prevention. Retrieved from www.webmd.com/back-pain/tc/low-back-pain-prevention.
60. Neiman (2007).
61. Transversus abdominis muscle. (2010, June 22). *Wikipedia.* Retrieved from http://en.wikipedia.org/wiki/Transversus_abdominus_muscle.
62. WebMD (2008, February 6).
63. Neiman (2007).
64. National Institute of Neurological Disorders and Stroke. (2009, December 21).
65. National Association for Fitness Certification. (2006, September 26).
66. National Institute of Neurological Disorders and Stroke. (2009, December 21).

# Suggested Readings

American Academy of Orthopedic Surgeons. (2010, March 5). Warm up, cool down and be flexible. Retrieved from http://orthoinfo.aaos.org/topic.cfm?topic=a00310.

This article describes the importance of warming up and cooling down and provides instructions on what is involved in both. Ten stretching exercises for adults are presented, described, and illustrated. These exercises are recommended by the American Academy of Orthopedic Surgeons. Lastly, guidelines for static stretching are provided.

American Heart Association. (2009, January 22). Stretching and flexibility exercises. Retrieved from www.americanheart.org/presenter.jhtm/?identifier=3048117.

This article discusses, illustrates, and describes seven basic stretching exercises that adults should perform. The illustration and descriptions of each exercise are presented in a clear and precise manner.

My Fit Health and Fitness. (2010, March 5). Stretches and flexibility exercises. Retrieved from www.myfit.ca/exercise-database/stretches.asp?exercises=flexibility.

Flexibility is defined and two types of stretching—static and ballistic—are discussed. Eighteen static stretching exercises are illustrated and described. Performing this program would stretch the major muscles of the body. The answer to when people should stretch is also provided.

Sports Fitness Advisor. (2010, March 5). Flexibility exercises. Retrieved from www.sport-fitness-advisor.com/flexibility-exercises.html.

This article defines static and dynamic stretching. Eight static stretches for the major muscle groups and joints are described and illustrated. Finally, guidelines for stretching are presented.

Waehner, P. (2007, August 23). Exercise for beginners Flexibility. Retrieved from http://exercise.about.com/cs/exbeginners/a/legflexibility.htm.

This article provides clear and concise instructions for beginners who are about to start an exercise program. The article focuses on flexibility and offers reasons for including stretching exercises in the program. Also covered are instructions on how to stretch.

Name _____   Date _____   Section _____

# Assessment Activity 5-1

## Sit-and-Reach Test

The sit-and-reach test is used to measure hip flexor, lower-back, and hamstring flexibility. It is measured with a testing box, which can be purchased or built. The box should be 12 inches high and have an overlap in front, so that negative (minus) readings can be obtained when subjects are unable to reach their feet (the footline). For simplicity and standardization purposes, the footline is given a value of 0, and plus and minus readings are given in inches.

**Directions:**

1. Warm up for 3 to 5 minutes before taking this test.

2. After warming up, remove your shoes and sit with both feet flat against the end board of the box, with your legs fully extended and your knees locked.

3. Extend your arms forward as shown in the photo, one hand on top of the other with your fingertips perfectly even.

4. Bend forward from the waist as far as possible while sliding your hands along the scale.

5. Hold the maximum stretch for at least 1 second.

6. Perform three trials: The final score is the best of the three.

7. Lock your knees during all trials.

8. Use the following sit-and-reach test standards to interpret your score.

Trial 1: _____ inches

Trial 2: _____ inches

Trial 3: _____ inches

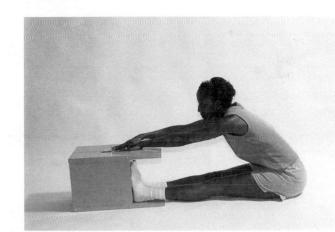

## Sit-and-Reach Test Standards

| Classification | Distance Reached in Inches (Footline at 0) |
|---|---|
| Excellent | ≥ 7* |
| Good | 4.0–6.9 |
| Average | 0–3.9 |
| Fair | −3.0−−0.25 |
| Poor | ≤ −3.1** |

*≥ greater than or equal to

** ≤ less than or equal to

**Name** _____   **Date** _____   **Section** _____

# Assessment Activity 5-2

## Shoulder Flexion Test

**Directions:** The objective of the shoulder flexion test is to measure the deltoids and shoulder girdle. A measuring scale and straightedge are needed to perform this assessment. Begin by assuming a prone position with your arms fully extended. Your chin should remain in contact with the floor throughout the exercise. Grasp the straightedge with both hands and raise it as high as possible from the floor. The distance from the floor to the straightedge is measured as the height in inches. Repeat this assessment three times and record the best number in inches as the final score. See the following chart for your classification.

Trial 1: _____ inches

Trial 2: _____ inches

Trial 3: _____ inches

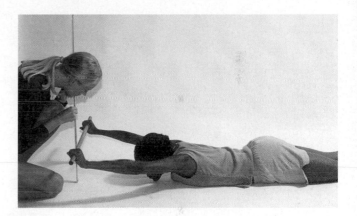

### Shoulder Flexion Test Standard*

| Classification | Men | Women |
|---|---|---|
| Excellent | 26 or above | 27 or above |
| Good | 23–25 | 24–26 |
| Average | 18–22 | 19–23 |
| Fair | 13–17 | 14–18 |
| Poor | 12 or below | 13 or below |

*All scores are in inches. Use the best of three trials as the score.

**Name** _____   **Date** _____   **Section** _____

# Assessment Activity 5-3

## Sling Test

**Directions:** The purpose of this test is to determine the length and flexibility of your sling muscles (the extensor muscles of the back). If you have back problems or have had back surgery, consult a physician before attempting this test. This is a test and not an exercise, so it should not be used to increase flexibility.

Begin by lying on your back on the floor and bending both knees. Pull your right leg to your chest by tightly holding your knee with both hands. Straighten out your left leg and push it to the floor without letting your right leg move away from your chest.

A tester uses a ruler to measure the distance between the floor and back of the knee. Reverse your leg position and measure.

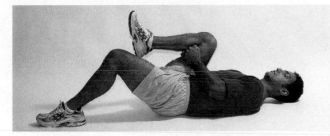

## Sling Test Standards

| Classification | | Standard |
|---|---|---|
| Excellent | 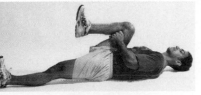 | Able to hold one leg firmly against the chest with the other leg flat against the floor |
| Average | 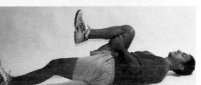 | Able to hold one knee against the chest while the other knee is bent 2 to 4 inches off the floor |
| Fair | 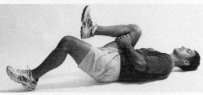 | Able to hold the knee firmly against the chest while the other leg is 4 to 8 inches off the floor |
| Poor | 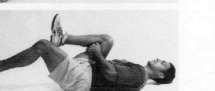 | Unable to pull one leg firmly against the chest without pain or discomfort and/or raising the other leg off the floor significantly (more than 8 inches) |

Name _____   Date _____   Section _____

# Assessment Activity 5-4

## Trunk Extension

**Directions:** The purpose of this assessment is to measure the flexibility of the abdominal and hip flexor muscles. Begin the test by lying face down on the floor. Have a partner hold your legs as shown. Grasp your hands in the lower-back area, breathe in, lift your upper body as high off the floor as possible, and hold. A tester measures the distance between the floor and your chin. Repeat this two more times and record your best score. See the following chart for your classification.

Trial 1: _____ inches

Trial 2: _____ inches

Trial 3: _____ inches

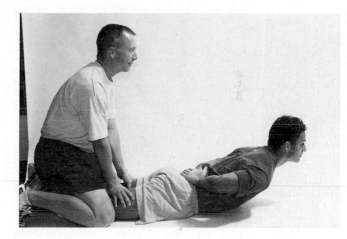

## Trunk Extension Assessment Standards*

| Classification | Men | Women |
| --- | --- | --- |
| Excellent | 22 | 24 |
| Good | 19–21 | 20–23 |
| Average | 17–18 | 18–19 |
| Poor | 16 | 17 |

*Scores are in inches.

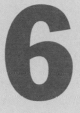
# Forming a Plan for Good Nutrition

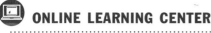

## ONLINE LEARNING CENTER

Log on to our Online Learning Center (OLC) for access to these additional resources:

- Chapter key term flashcards
- Learning objectives
- Additional goals for behavior change
- Concentration game
- Self-scoring chapter quizzes
- Additional lab activities

The OLC also offers Web links for study and exploration of wellness topics. Access these links through **www.mhhe.com/anspaugh8e**.

## GOALS FOR BEHAVIOR CHANGE

- Decrease or increase your intake of the energy nutrients to meet dietary recommendations.
- Craft a nutrition profile that identifies your intake of essential nutrients and highlights your dietary strengths and shortcomings.
- Formulate a plan for implementing the Dietary Guidelines for Americans that addresses your dietary shortcomings.
- Identify and practice specific strategies for improving your diet.

## Objectives

After completing this chapter, you will be able to do the following:

✔ Describe the functions and purposes of the essential nutrients.

✔ Discuss ways to apply the *Dietary Guidelines for Americans*.

✔ Explain the role of nutrients that are not classified as essential, such as fiber, phytochemicals, and botanicals, but that are thought to have unique health benefits.

✔ Determine your RDA for protein, carbohydrates, fat, and saturated fat.

## [ Key Terms ]

| | | |
|---|---|---|
| amino acids | enhanced food | monounsaturated fat |
| antioxidants | essential nutrients | MyPyramid.gov |
| botanicals (phytomedicinals) | folate | natural |
| | foodborne illness | nutrient-dense foods |
| calorie | free radicals | phytochemicals |
| carbohydrate loading (glycogen loading) | functional fiber | phytomedicinals |
| | functional foods | polyunsaturated fat |
| complex carbohydrates | Glycemic Index (GI) | Recommended Dietary Allowances (RDAs) |
| Daily Values (DVs) | Glycemic Load (GL) | |
| dietary fiber | hydrogenation | saturated fat |
| *Dietary Guidelines for Americans* | insoluble fiber | soluble fiber |
| | legumes | trans fatty acids |
| Dietary Reference Intakes (DRIs) | macronutrients | vitamins |
| | micronutrients | vitamin supplements |
| discretionary calories | minerals | water intoxication |

**N**utrition has captured the interest of Americans perhaps more than any other topic related to fitness and wellness. Whether concerning antioxidants or phytochemicals, homocysteine or cholesterol, omega-3 fatty acids or trans fatty acids, HDLs or LDLs, low-fat or low-carb, nutrition issues make headlines in both scientific journals and popular magazines, and everybody seems to be an expert. So much is written by so many people that it is difficult to know what and whom to believe.

This chapter presents basic concepts of the science of *nutrition,* the study of nutrients and the way the body processes them, to guide you through the maze of nutrition information. The concepts presented here are within the framework of the *Dietary Guidelines for Americans,* which is updated every five years, and should provide you with a basis for sound nutritional planning.

## Nutrition and Health

The relationship between nutrition and health has changed dramatically during the last 50 years. The deficiency diseases of the past, such as scurvy and rickets, have been replaced by diseases caused by poor diets and physically inactive lifestyles. Poor diet contributes substantially to the burden of preventable illness and premature death and is associated with 4 of the 10 leading causes of death. Cardiovascular disease, stroke, Type 2 diabetes mellitus, and some cancers have

long been connected to nutrition.[1,2] Likewise, sedentary lifestyles have been associated with the same conditions (see Just the Facts: Health Conditions Associated with Poor Diet and Physical Inactivity). Moreover, sedentary lifestyles and a poor diet that is associated with excess calories are the most important factors related to overweight and obesity, the epidemic of the 21st century.[3]

While the hallmark of the American diet is excessive calories, sodium, sugar, fat, and saturated fat), the low intake of some foods and nutrients causes concern. Here are a few examples:

- 66% of American adults don't consume the recommended daily amount of vitamin D.[5]
- Women consume 13 grams of fiber per day; men consume 17 grams per day. Both are at least 10 grams short of dietary recommendations for women and men, respectively.[6]
- 84% of adults do not consume the recommended 2 to 4 servings of fruit each day.[7]
- 70% of adults do not consume the recommended 3 to 5 servings of vegetables each day.[8]
- 17% of Americans are vitamin C deficient.[9]
- Iron deficiency is the most common trace mineral deficiency worldwide. In the United States, 3.3 million women of childbearing age have iron deficiency anemia.[10,11]
- Americans of all ages don't consume foods that provide sufficient quantities of folic acid, magnesium, vitamin A, folate, and potassium.[12]

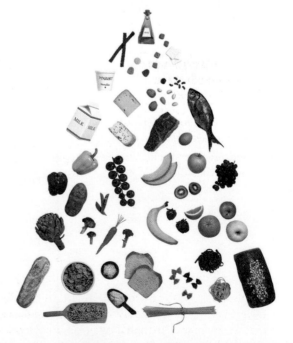

Eating a variety of foods is the best way to ensure that your diet is nutritionally balanced. Have you tried an unfamiliar food lately?

## [ JUST THE FACTS ]
### Sorting Through Nutrition Acronyms

Nutrition acronyms abound with more than a dozen that are used to communicate important aspects of nutrition. Some of them refer to information intended for the general public while others communicate information important to health professionals and researchers. Five acronyms used throughout this text and included in some of your nutrition assessments are as follows.

**Dietary Reference Intakes (DRI):** DRI represents the umbrella term under which all of the other terms fall, including RDAs, AIs, ULs, and DVs.

**Recommended Dietary Allowance (RDA):** RDA represents the nutrient intake that is sufficient to meet the needs of nearly all healthy people in an age and gender group. If an RDA is set for a particular nutrient, aim for this intake. Consistently falling short of this intake increases the chances of developing nutrition-related problems.

**Adequate Intake (AI):** An RDA for a nutrient can be set only if there is sufficient information on the need for that nutrient. Presently, there is not enough information on some nutrients, such as calcium, vitamin D, copper, biotin, fiber, and essential fatty acids, to set such a precise standard. For these and other nutrients, the DRIs include a category called Adequate Intake (AI). AIs provide benchmarks that indicate an adequate level of a nutrient. However, an AI designation means that a consensus opinion has not yet emerged from the scientific community to establish a definitive recommendation. If an RDA is not set for a nutrient, aim for this intake.

**Tolerable Upper Intake Levels (UL):** ULs represent the safe upper limit of a nutrient from total intake of food including dietary intake, fortified food, and supplements to avoid the possibility of adverse health effects. ULs are not intake goals. Rather, to avoid toxicity and other nutrition-related problems, dietary intake should be below ULs.

**Daily Values (DVs):** DVs are nutrient standards used on food labels. Since RDAs and AIs are gender and age specific, there are too many categories to be used on a food label. DVs serve as a condensed system for allowing consumers to compare their intake of vitamins, minerals, protein, and other dietary components such as cholesterol, fiber, and carbohydrates to recommended intakes. DVs are set at or close to the highest RDA or AI standard presented in the various age and gender categories for a specific nutrient.

Sources: Byrd-Bredbenner, G. Moe, D. Beshgetoor, & J. Berning. (2009). *Wardlaw's perspectives in nutrition* (8th ed.). New York: McGraw-Hill.
Wardlaw, G., & A. Smith. (2011). *Comtemporary nutrition* (8th ed.). New York: McGraw-Hill.

Fortunately, improving your diet is not difficult. You don't have to give up your favorite foods to achieve a healthy diet. For many people, cutting back on less healthful foods and making small dietary changes may profoundly affect health and wellness. It is never too late to benefit from dietary improvements. The easy availability of many healthy options makes dietary improvement a realistic goal for most Americans.

## Essential Nutrients

Food is made up of six classes of nutrients, including carbohydrates, fat, protein, vitamins, minerals, and water.

The standard for expressing the recommended intake of nutrients is called **Dietary Reference Intakes (DRIs).** DRIs serve as the framework for nutrition (see Just the Facts: Sorting Through Nutrition Acronyms). The energy-yielding nutrients (carbohydrates, fat, and protein) are called **macronutrients** because they are required by the body in larger amounts than are vitamins and minerals, referred to as **micronutrients.** These nutrients are called **essential nutrients** because they cannot be made by the body and, therefore, must be supplied through the diet. (See Table 6-1 on page 176.) Some experts list fiber as a seventh nutrient, although technically some fibers are carbohydrates and are usually listed with the carbohydrates. Carbohydrates, fat, and protein are called *energy nutrients* because they provide energy (calories) to the body to regulate chemical processes. Water and fiber are nonnutrients and are part of a healthy diet.

## Calories

Food energy is expressed in kilocalories. A kilocalorie equals 1,000 calories of heat energy. A **calorie** is the amount of heat required to raise the temperature of a gram of water by 1°C. Common reference to kilocalories usually excludes the prefix *kilo*, mainly for convenience. A gram of carbohydrates provides 4 calories (kilocalories) of energy, a gram of protein also provides

**TABLE 6-1** Daily Values of Selected Essential Nutrients for People over 4 Years of Age

| Nutrient | Unit of Measurement | Daily Value |
|---|---|---|
| Fat† | Gram | < 65 – < 107 / (30% kcal) |
| Saturated fatty acids† | Gram | < 20 – < 36 / (10% kcal) |
| Protein† | Gram | 50–80 (10% kcal) |
| Cholesterol‡ | Milligram | < 300 |
| Carbohydrate† | Gram | 300–480 (60% kcal) |
| Fiber | Gram | 25–37 (11.5 g/1,000 kcal) |
| Biotin | Milligram | 0.3 |
| Calcium | Milligram | 1,000 |
| Chloride | Milligram | 3,400 |
| Chromium | Microgram | 120 |
| Copper | Milligram | 2 |
| Folate | Microgram | 400 |
| Iodine | Microgram | 150 |
| Iron | Milligram | 18 |
| Magnesium | Milligram | 400 |
| Manganese | Milligram | 2 |
| Molybdenum | Microgram | 25 |
| Niacin | Milligram | 20 |
| Pantothenic acid | Milligram | 10 |
| Phosphorus | Milligram | 1,000 |
| Potassium | Milligram | 3,500 |
| Riboflavin | Milligram | 1.7 |
| Selenium | Microgram | 70 |
| Sodium | Milligram | < 2,400 |
| Thiamin | Milligram | 1.5 |
| Vitamin A | Retinol Equivalents | 1,000 |
| Vitamin B12 | Microgram | 6 |
| Vitamin B6 | Milligram | 2 |
| Vitamin C | Milligram | 60 |
| Vitamin D | International Units | 400 |
| Vitamin E | International Units | 30 |
| Vitamin K | Microgram | 80 |
| Zinc | Milligram | 15 |

Daily Values (DVs) were established as a condensed system for presenting generic standards on food labels. These standards are applicable to ages 4 years old through adulthood. DVs are set at or close to the highest RDA, DRI, and/or AI standard seen in the various age and gender categories for a specific nutrient. While DVs are not to be confused with RDAs, they allow consumers to compare their intake to desirable or maximum intakes. The DVs on food package labels have yet to be updated to reflect the current state of knowledge. For example, the DRI for vitamin C was recently increased to 90 mg for adults and 120 mg for women during lactation but remains at 60 mg on food labels.

† No RDA has been set for these nutrients except protein. Cholesterol is not classified as an essential nutrient because the body makes it on its own. The values listed are based on a 2,000-calorie diet, with a caloric distribution of 30% from fat (one-third of this total from saturated fat), 60% from carbohydrate, and 10% from protein.

‡ Based on recommendations of federal agencies.

Source: Byrd-Bredbenner, G., G. Moe, D. Beshgetoor, & J. Berning. (2009). *Wardlaw's perspectives in nutrition* (8th ed.). New York: McGraw-Hill.

4 calories, a gram of fat provides 9 calories, and a gram of alcohol (not an essential nutrient) provides 7 calories. These values can be used to estimate the source of calories of a food (see Just the Facts: Estimating Calorie Source).

The recommended diet for Americans emphasizes complex carbohydrates as the main source of energy. Between 45 and 65% of calories should come from car-bohydrates, with no more than 10 to 25% from added sugar. No more than 20 to 35% of calories should come from fat; 10 to 35% of calories should come from pro-tein.[13] The typical American diet, however, is still high in fat calories and low in complex, whole-grain carbohydrate calories. You can tell how your calorie sources compare with dietary recommendations by completing Assessment Activities 6-3 and 6-4.

## [ JUST THE FACTS ]

### Estimating Calorie Source

Carbohydrates, fats, and protein yield 4, 9, and 4 calories per gram, respectively. These values can be used to estimate the percent of calories by energy source of a food. For example, a turkey sandwich on white bread yields 24 grams of protein, 14 grams of fat, and 29 grams of carbohydrate. Column 2 times column 3 produces the

number of calories for each energy source. Total calories in a turkey sandwich equal 338. Percent protein is determined by dividing protein calories by total calories. Repeat the procedure for carbohydrates and fat. Conclusion: 28% of the calories in a turkey sandwich come from protein, 34% from carbohydrates, and 38% from fat.

| (1) Energy Source | (2) Calories/gram | (3) Turkey Sandwich | (4) Calories | (5) % |
|---|---|---|---|---|
| Protein | 4 | 24 grams | 96 | 28 |
| Fat | 9 | 14 grams | 126 | 38 |
| Carbohydrate | 4 | 29 grams | 116 | 34 |
| **Total** | | | **338** | **100** |

## Carbohydrates

There are three types of carbohydrates: sugars, starches, and fiber. Sugar and starches provide 4 calories per gram. Fiber refers to the substances in food that resist digestion. Fiber has no calorie value because it's not absorbed. Most of the carbohydrates are plant based. Grains, vegetables, fruits, and legumes are examples. The simplest form of carbohydrates is sugar, also called *monosaccharide*. Monosaccharides include glucose and fructose (fruit sugar). Fructose is the sweetest of simple sugars. Disaccharides are double sugars, meaning that they are pairs of chemically linked monosaccharides. In this group of sugars are sucrose, or table sugar; lactose, or milk sugar; and maltose, or malt sugar.

Starches, also called *polysaccharides,* are **complex carbohydrates.** Whole-grain, high-fiber starches are the preferred source of carbohydrates. A diet high in starch is likely to be lower in fat, especially saturated fat and cholesterol; lower in calories; and higher in fiber. An added benefit of starch consumption over simple sugar consumption is that it helps the body maintain a normal blood sugar level through a slower, more even rate of digestion and glucose absorption. It takes 1 to 4 hours for the body to digest starch. This is one reason athletes involved in endurance activities, such as marathons, load up on complex carbohydrates before competition.

All carbohydrates are broken down in the intestine and converted in the liver into glucose. Glucose is blood sugar carried to cells, where it is used for energy. Glucose in excess of the body's need for energy is stored in limited amounts as glycogen in the muscles and the liver for future use; when glycogen stores are satisfied, glucose is converted to fat.

Many weight-conscious people mistakenly avoid starches, thinking that they are high in calories. Starch

foods are often made fattening when they are prepared. For example, a baked potato without additives yields a modest 90 calories. Adding fat in the form of butter, sour cream, margarine, or cheese adds substantially to the calories of a potato.

### Recommended Carbohydrate Intake

Between 45 and 65% of the calories in your diet should come from carbohydrates. For 1,500 calories, that translates into 169 to 244 grams of carbohydrates a day (see Just the Facts: Converting Carbohydrate Calories to Carbohydrate Grams). On the surface, it may appear that 169 to 244 grams of carbohydrates are excessive when considering that people on low-carbohydrate diets often consume less than 100 grams. This is a misconception. From the perspective of good nutrition, carbohydrates should be the primary source of energy because they are a major source of vitamins, minerals, fiber, and other nutrients good for health.

Vegetables, fruits, and grain products are high in carbohydrates. They are low in fat, depending on how they are prepared and what is added to them at the table. Meat and animal products are low in carbohydrates, with the exception of lactose (milk sugar) in dairy products. Most Americans eat fewer than the recommended servings of fruits, vegetables, and whole-grain foods.[14,15] An estimate of your carbohydrate intake can be determined by completing Assessment Activity 6-1.

There are important differences among carbohydrates. Foods that contain simple carbohydrates or refined grains, such as white bread, white rice, potatoes, sweetened soft drinks, candies, and sweets, are usually low in nutrients and high in simple sugar, and

[ JUST THE
**FACTS** ]
## Converting Carbohydrate Calories to Carbohydrate Grams

If you are on a 1,500-calorie diet, approximately how many carbohydrate calories and carbohydrate grams are recommended?

### Solution

1. Multiply total calories times the recommended 45% to 65%.
   a. $1,500 \times 0.45 = 675$ carbohydrate calories
   b. $1,500 \times 0.65 = 975$ carbohydrate calories
2. Divide carbohydrate calories by 4 (carbohydrates produce 4 calories/gram).
   a. $675 \div 4 = 169$ grams of carbohydrates
   b. $975 \div 4 = 244$ grams of carbohydrates

**Conclusion:** Between 169 and 244 grams of carbohydrates are recommended for a healthy person on a 1,500-calorie diet.

---

because they are quickly and easily digested they cause a surge in blood sugar levels and then rebound with a dramatic drop in blood sugar a few hours later. Sweetened soft drinks are a good example of foods that contribute to the escalating blood sugar levels of Americans. Americans get about 21% of their calories from beverages; most of them come from soft drinks with little or no nutrient value.[16] Refined grains and simple sugars including those in sweetened soft drinks are the carbohydrates that should be consumed in limited amounts. On the other hand, complex carbohydrate foods are loaded with nutrients and fiber, are digested slowly, and are associated with consistent blood sugar levels. These are the carbohydrates that should be emphasized in the diet.

Easy ways to add whole-grain, high-fiber carbohydrates include switching from white rice to brown rice, opting for whole-grain breads, snacking on dried fruit, and using legumes as a base for soups. Complex carbohydrates, such as whole-grain bread, cereal, rice, and oats, along with fruits and vegetables, form the foundation of a nutritious diet.

## Protein

Protein is different from carbohydrates and fats in that it contains nitrogen as well as carbon, hydrogen, and oxygen. Because of their unique chemical structures, proteins contain the basic materials that help the body form muscles, bones, cartilage, skin, antibodies, some hormones, and all enzymes. Protein is also an energy nutrient, yielding 4 calories per gram. As a source of energy, however, protein is inefficient because it must

first be processed by the liver and kidneys. Proteins generally directly supply little of the energy the body uses, except during prolonged exercise.[17]

The building blocks of protein are chemical structures called **amino acids**. There are approximately 20 amino acids: 11 can be produced in the body, and 9 must be supplied by the diet.[18] The latter are called *essential amino acids*. A *complete protein* is one that contains all the essential amino acids. A *high-quality protein* is a complete protein that contains the essential amino acids in amounts proportional to the body's need for them. Meat, fish, poultry, eggs, milk, and cheese are examples of high-quality, complete protein sources. Water-packed canned tuna is the most protein-dense food, with 87% of its calories as protein.[19]

An *incomplete protein* does not contain all the essential amino acids in the proportions needed by the body. Generally, plant protein sources are incomplete. This has important implications for *vegans,* people who limit their diets to plant sources, because protein synthesis operates on the all-or-none principle. That is, the body cannot make partial proteins, only complete ones. If an amino acid is supplied by one source in a smaller amount than is needed, the total amount of protein made from the other amino acids will be limited. It is necessary to combine protein sources from cereal and grains with legumes to obtain all essential amino acids from plant sources. The practice of combining amino acids from various plant sources is called *protein complementing.*

One plant protein source unique among sources of amino acids is **legumes**. Legumes come from plants with seed pods that split on two sides when ripe, such as black-eyed peas; chickpeas (garbanzo beans); lentils; soybeans; and black, red, white, navy, and kidney beans. Some nuts, such as peanuts, are also legumes. Legumes are high in fiber and minerals and a nutritionally dense food (see Table 6-2).

A legume that is singled out in the health literature because it contains all of the essential amino acids is soybean. In addition to being a complete protein, soybeans are good sources of folate, omega-6 fatty acids, minerals (such as iron), phytochemicals, and fiber and are low in saturated fat. Soybean products are available in a variety of foods. Examples include tofu, soy milk, soy nuts, soy chips, soy fruit bars, and soy powder, which can be mixed into dairy foods such as ice cream, milk shakes, yogurt, cheese, and butter; scrambled into eggs; mixed into soups, stews, and dips; blended in mashed potatoes; and baked into bread.[20-23]

Nuts are another good plant source of protein. Nuts also contain vitamin E, magnesium, potassium, folate, vitamin B6, niacin, copper, zinc, fiber, phytochemicals, and isoflavones. They are high in fat but

**TABLE 6-2**  Comparison of Selected Legumes

| Serving/1 Cup | Calories | Protein (grams) | Fat (grams) | Iron (milligrams)* | Fiber (grams) |
|---|---|---|---|---|---|
| Soybeans, dry | 274 | 68 | 37 | 29 | 17 |
| Lentils, dry | 649 | 54 | 2 | 17 | 59 |
| Kidney beans | 208 | 14 | 0 | 3 | 8 |
| Black beans | 200 | 14 | 0 | 4 | 14 |
| Chickpeas | 448 | 28 | 2 | 2 | 22 |
| Peanuts, raw | 832 | 38 | 72 | 6 | 14 |

*Rounded to nearest whole number.

almost all of that fat is unsaturated. Because they are high in calories, they must be consumed with an eye for serving size. An ounce of nuts (an amount that fits in the palm of the hand) provides about 160 to 190 calories.[24] Consumed in moderation, and in the place of other foods rather than in addition to other foods, nuts can contribute to a healthy diet.

## Recommended Protein Intake

For most people, the Recommended Dietary Allowance of protein is 0.36 gram per pound of body weight, or 54 grams for a 150-pound person and 72 grams for a 200-pound person. Growing children, pregnant or lactating women, and people recovering from illness require additional protein. You can estimate your protein intake by completing Assessment Activity 6-1.

Exercise and other physical activities can change the body's need for protein (nutrition needs associated with physical activity are discussed separately in this chapter), but enough protein is usually already consumed. When more protein is consumed than is needed by the body, it is converted into energy or stored as fat. High protein intake may cause the body to excrete calcium and put excessive strain on the kidneys to excrete into the urine the excess nitrogen supplied by the protein.[25] Although the kidneys of most healthy people can handle nitrogen excess easily, diseased kidneys have more difficulty. This is why people with kidney failure are placed on low-protein diets and why people who go on high-protein diets to lose weight (see Chapter 8) are encouraged to drink large quantities of water to flush the kidneys.

## Fat

Fats are oils, sterols (such as cholesterol), waxes, and other substances that are not water-soluble. Fat is an essential component of all cells. Fats help synthesize and repair vital cell transport and absorb fat-soluble vitamins. Fat stored as adipose tissue provides insulation and a ready source of energy. As an energy source, fat yields 9 calories per gram.

### Basic Fat Facts

Fat, also called *lipid*, is a compound made by chemically bonding fatty acids to glycerol to form glycerides. When three fatty acids are hooked to glycerol, the fat compound is a triglyceride. Almost 95% of fat stored in the body is a triglyceride, with the remaining 5% consisting of other glycerides and cholesterol. Scientific literature usually refers to triglycerides when it discusses fat. High triglyceride levels are common in the United States and are associated with increased risk of heart attack or stroke.[26] As an energy nutrient, fat yields 9 calories per gram regardless of its chemical makeup.

Chemically, fats are chains of carbon atoms strung together with hydrogen atoms. If a fat is a **saturated fat,** the carbon chain carries all the hydrogen atoms it can. If it is an unsaturated fat, there is room in the carbon chain for more hydrogen. If the fat is a **monounsaturated fat,** there is room for two hydrogen atoms. If the fat is a **polyunsaturated fat,** there is room for four hydrogen atoms. If it is highly polyunsaturated, there is room for many more hydrogen atoms. Manufacturers are required to list the types of fat by serving size on a food package label. (See Table 6-3 on page 180.)

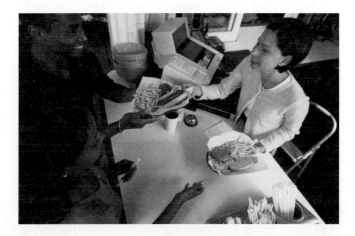

Even if your weight is healthy, too many high-fat take-out dinners may mean too few fruits and vegetables.

**TABLE 6-3** Fat Content of Selected Foods

| Food | Fat/(g) | Percentage of Total Calories from Fat* | | | |
|---|---|---|---|---|---|
| | | Total** | Saturated | Monounsaturated | Polyunsaturated |
| Egg, whole, raw | 5.01 | 64 | 19 | 25 | 8 |
| Butter (pat) | 11.4 | 100 | 67 | 31 | 4 |
| Margarine, regular, hard (stick) | 91.0 | 100 | 20 | 45 | 32 |
| Cheese, cream (1 ounce) | 9.9 | 90 | 57 | 25 | 3 |
| Cheese, cheddar (1 cup) | 37.5 | 74 | 47 | 20 | 2 |
| Cheese, cottage (1 cup) | 10.1 | 39 | 25 | 11 | 1 |
| Milk, whole (1 cup) | 8.2 | 49 | 30 | 14 | 2 |
| Milk, skim (1 cup) | 1.0 | 6 | 4 | 1 | Trace*** |
| Frankfurter (2 ounces) | 16.6 | 82 | 33 | 40 | 3 |
| Bologna, pork (slice) | 4.6 | 72 | 26 | 36 | 8 |
| Flounder, baked (0.8 ounce) | 1.9 | 9 | Trace | Trace | Trace |
| Fish sticks (1 ounce) | 3.4 | 39 | 10 | 18 | 10 |
| Tuna, canned, oil-packed (3 ounces) | 6.9 | 38 | 8 | 10 | 17 |
| Tuna, canned, water-packed (3 ounces) | 2.1 | 7 | Trace | Trace | Trace |
| Ground beef (3 ounces) | 19.2 | 65 | 25 | 28 | 3 |
| Steak, broiled, sirloin (2 ounces) | 4.89 | 56 | 24 | 26 | 2 |
| Pork chop, broiled (3 ounces) | 22.3 | 62 | 23 | 29 | 7 |
| Chicken breast, fried, flour-coated (7 ounces) | 17.4 | 36 | 10 | 14 | 8 |
| Beans, navy (1 cup) | 2.1 | 4 | Trace | Trace | 3 |
| Potato (baked) | 0.06 | 1 | Trace | Trace | 4 |
| Potato chips (1.5 ounces) | 13.0 | 61 | 16 | 11 | 31 |
| Ice cream, vanilla, regular (1 cup) | 22.5 | 48 | 28 | 14 | 2 |
| Apple (raw, unpeeled) | 0.5 | 6 | 1 | Trace | 2 |
| Danish pastry | 13.6 | 50 | 14 | 29 | 4 |

*Rounded off to the nearest whole number.

**Includes undifferentiated fats.

***Trace, less than 0.9% of fat.

There are two main types of polyunsaturated (poly) fats: omega-6 and omega-3. The omega-6s make up 90% of poly fats in the American diet and come primarily from plant oils, such as soybean, corn, sunflower, and safflower oils, as well as from nuts and seeds. Omega-6 provides linoleic acid, an essential fatty acid. The omega-3s come primarily from seafood and provide linolenic acid, another essential fatty acid. The consumption of omega-6s and omega-3s is associated with health benefits.[27–29]

Many people mistakenly assume that the word *polyunsaturated* on a food label means that the fat in the food is not saturated, but because of food-processing techniques, this assumption may be incorrect. If the words *hydrogenated* or *partially hydrogenated* are on the food label, the food contains varying amounts of saturated fat. Because fats are less stable, they are prone to spoilage. Consequently, for many foods, manufacturers use a chemical process called **hydrogenation,** in which hydrogen atoms are added to the unsaturated or polyunsaturated fats to make them more saturated and more resistant to spoilage. This process of hydrogenat-

ing food yields a new type of fat, not found in nature, called **trans fatty acids.** Trans fatty acids are saturated fats commonly found in margarine, fried fast foods, cookies, cakes, and many other foods made with shortening. Some scientists believe that trans fatty acids, even those originating from a polyunsaturated food source, are as detrimental to health as saturated animal fat. High intake of these fats increases the risk of coronary heart disease, stroke, and Type 2 diabetes and therefore should be kept to a minimum. Trans fats are one of the unhealthiest fats in the American diet and in some cities are banned in restaurants.[30] Fortunately, consumers can avoid trans fat by checking food labels. In doing so, be aware of sources of hidden trans fats[31] (see Just the Facts: Where Are Hidden Trans Fats?).

Saturated and unsaturated fats can be differentiated by their appearance. Saturated fat is typically solid at room temperature. Lard, fat marbled in meat, and hardened grease from a skillet are good examples. Polyunsaturated fats are usually liquid at room temperature. Examples are safflower and corn oils. Solid vegetable shortenings are partially hydrogenated and have a soft consistency. Coconut oil, palm kernel oil, and palm oil are exceptions. They are vegetable oils and are liquid at room temperature, but they are among the most saturated of fats.

Fish oils are among the most unsaturated fats available. They are roughly twice as unsaturated as vegetable oils. They do not harden, even at low temperatures. Their unsaturation has created special interest in relation to heart disease. Fatty acids in cold-water seafood—such as salmon, mackerel, sardines, herring, anchovies, whitefish, bluefish, swordfish, rainbow trout, striped bass, Pacific oysters, and squid—consist of omega-3 fatty acids, thought to be effective in lowering cholesterol and triglyceride levels and reducing clot-forming rates, thereby reducing the risk for heart disease. Health experts believe omega-3s offer such protection against heart disease that two servings a week are recommended.[32]

### Cholesterol

*Cholesterol*, a waxy substance that is technically a steroid alcohol found only in animal foods, is probably the most researched blood lipid. High levels of cholesterol are usually included among the major risk factors for cardiovascular disease. (For information on cholesterol, see Chapter 2.)

### Recommended Fat Intake

To many people, *fat* has negative connotations and is viewed almost as a toxin, but as stated earlier, fat is an essential nutrient. Experts recommend a diet that includes a total fat intake of 20 to 35% of total calories. No more than 10% of fat calories should come from saturated fats. Keep trans fatty acid consumption as low as possible.[33–35] Most fat should come from polyunsaturated and monounsaturated fats. Good sources of these fats are olive, canola, safflower, sunflower, and corn oils, as well as almonds, walnuts, avocados, and fish.[36] Fatty fish, such as salmon, sardines, trout, herring, bluefin tuna, albacore tuna, and mackerel, should be consumed at least twice a week to provide omega-3 fatty acids.[37] Plant sources of omega-3 fatty acids include soybeans, walnuts, flaxseed, and canola seeds.[38]

The advice to consume no more than 20 to 35% of calories as fat does not apply to children. During the early stages of development, fat is critical to the development of the brain, spine, and central nervous system, so the fat intake of infants and toddlers below the age of 2 should not be greatly restricted. Total fat intake for babies should comprise 40 to 55% of calories. Fat intake should be reduced gradually for children 2 to 5 years old until their fat intake makes up 30 to 35% of their total calories.[39]

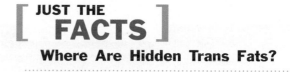

## [ JUST THE FACTS ]
### Where Are Hidden Trans Fats?

Baked goods including breads, cakes, cookies, doughnuts, crackers, and pies are the major source of trans fats. Trans fats are also found in many other common foods.

| Percentage of Trans Fats | Food Source* |
|---|---|
| 51% | in baked goods |
| 22% | in margarines |
| 10% | in fried potatoes |
| 6% | in potato chips, corn chips, popcorn |
| 5% | in shortening |
| 4% | in salad dressings |
| *1%* | *in breakfast cereals* |

*Total is not 100% due to rounding.

Source: Editor. (2009). Americans only vaguely aware where to find trans fats; Do you know? *Environmental Nutrition, 32*(5), 3.

Most Americans have an excessive fat intake and are challenged to make changes in both the amount and type of fat eaten. In trying to lower fat intake, people should not reduce fat calories to less than 15% of total calories without the supervision of a physician.[40] When fat makes up less than 15% of calories, carbohydrate intake increases and the result is an increase in blood triglyceride levels, which is not a healthful change. It is difficult to eat a balanced diet that contains less than 15% fat.[41] Table 6-4 presents a quick reference of maximum fat intake for selected caloric intakes. Figure 6-1 compares the saturated, monounsaturated, and polyunsaturated content of dietary fats. You can estimate your personal maximum fat intake by completing Assessment Activity 6-2. You can also learn how fatty your eating habits are by completing Assessment Activity 6-4.

### Vitamins

**Vitamins** are organic compounds (they contain carbon) that are necessary in small amounts for good health. The body can break vitamins down, but it cannot produce them, so vitamins have to be supplied in the diet. Unlike carbohydrates, fats, and proteins, vitamins yield no energy. Instead, some serve as catalysts that enable energy nutrients to be digested, absorbed, and metabolized. Some vitamins also interact with minerals. For example, vitamin C facilitates iron absorption, vitamin D improves calcium absorption, and thiamin requires the mineral magnesium to function efficiently.

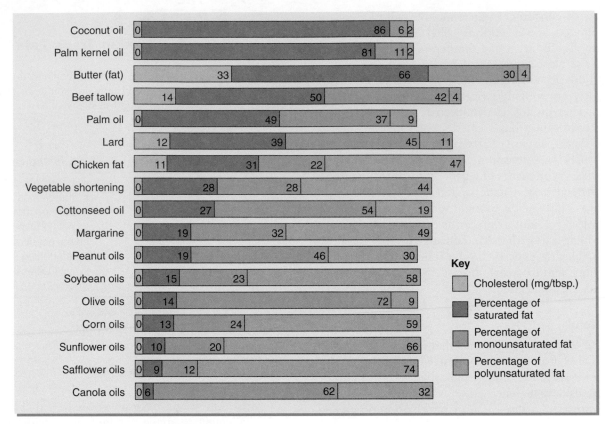

**FIGURE 6-1** Comparison of Dietary Fats

Vitamins are either water-soluble or fat-soluble (see Table 6-5). Water-soluble vitamins include vitamin C and vitamin B complex. They are present in the watery components of food, distributed in the fluid components of the body, excreted in the urine, needed in frequent small doses, and unlikely to be toxic except when taken in megadoses (very large quantities).

Fat-soluble vitamins include vitamins A, D, E, and K and are found in the fat and oily parts of food. Because they cannot be dissolved and absorbed in the bloodstream, these vitamins must be absorbed into the lymph with fat and transported in lipoproteins. When consumed in excess of the body's need, fat-soluble vitamins are stored in the liver and fat cells. Their storage makes it possible for a person to survive for months or years without consuming them. At least three of the fat-soluble vitamins (A, D, and K) may even accumulate to toxic levels. Megadoses of these vitamins should be avoided.

In preparing food for consumption, remember that vitamin content is easily compromised. Improper storage; excessive cooking; and exposure to heat, light, and air may reduce the vitamin content in food. Water-soluble vitamins are especially vulnerable to damage and loss depending on cooking method. Fat-soluble vitamins, on the other hand, generally are less likely to be compromised by cooking methods.[42]

**TABLE 6-4**  Maximum Fat, Saturated Fat, and Trans Fatty Acid Grams for Selected Caloric Intakes*

| Daily Caloric Intake | Total Fat Grams per Day | | Total Saturated Fat Grams per Day** | |
|---|---|---|---|---|
| | 35% Level | 20% Level | 10% Level | 7% Level |
| 1,000 | 39 | 22 | 11 | 8 |
| 1,500 | 58 | 33 | 17 | 12 |
| 2,000 | 78 | 44 | 22 | 16 |
| 2,500 | 97 | 56 | 28 | 19 |
| 3,000 | 117 | 67 | 33 | 23 |

*If a person on a 1,500-calorie diet wants to restrict fat intake to no more than 20% of calories, the limit is 33 grams (1,500 × 0.20 = 300 total fat calories; 300 ÷ 9 = 33). Saturated fat intake at the 7% level is restricted to 12 grams (1,500 × 0.07 = 105 saturated fat calories; 105 ÷ 9 = 12).

**Trans fat is not shown in saturated fat. It should be avoided as much as possible.

**TABLE 6-5** Vitamins: Food Sources and Wellness Benefits

| Vitamins | Food Sources | Wellness Benefits |
|---|---|---|
| **Fat-Soluble Vitamins** | | |
| 1. Vitamin A | Liver, carrots, eggs, tomatoes, dark green and yellow-orange vegetables and some fruits | Healthy skin and mucous membranes, improved night vision, defense against infections, antioxidant benefits (from carotenoids) |
| 2. Vitamin D | Fish oils and fortified milk, exposure to sunlight | Maintenance of blood levels of calcium and phosphorus, promotion of strong bones and teeth, possible reduction of risk for osteoporosis |
| 3. Vitamin E | Plant oils (corn, soybean, safflower, etc.), nuts, seeds | Formation of red blood cells, use of vitamin K, antioxidant benefits |
| 4. Vitamin K | Green vegetables, liver | Promotion of blood clotting, contribution to bone metabolism |
| **Water-Soluble Vitamins** | | |
| 5. Vitamin C (ascorbic acid) | Citrus fruits, green vegetables | Promotion of healthy gums and teeth, iron absorption; maintenance of normal connective tissues, help in wound healing, antioxidant benefits |
| **Vitamin B Complex** | | |
| 6. Thiamine ($B_1$) | Whole grains, legumes, liver, nuts | Carbohydrate metabolism, nerve function |
| 7. Riboflavin ($B_2$) | Dairy products, liver, enriched grains, spinach | Energy metabolism, production of red blood cells, improved health of skin and eyes |
| 8. Niacin | Nuts, grains, meat, fish, mushrooms | Energy metabolism, fat synthesis, fat breakdown, lowering of cholesterol (when prescribed in large doses) |
| 9. Pyridoxine ($B_6$) | Whole grains, meat, beans, nuts, fish, liver | Protein metabolism, possible immunity boost in the elderly, homocysteine metabolism |
| 10. Pantothenic acid | Whole grains, dried beans, eggs, milk, liver | Energy metabolism, fat synthesis, production of essential body chemicals |
| 11. Vitamin $B_{12}$ | Animal foods, dairy products, seafood | Folate metabolism, nerve function, formation of red blood cells, homocysteine metabolism |
| 12. Biotin | Cheese, egg yolks, mushrooms, grains | Glucose production, fat synthesis |
| 13. Folate $B_9$ (folic acid) | Green, leafy vegetables; liver, beans; grains; citrus fruits | DNA synthesis and protein metabolism, reduction of risk for certain birth defects, homocysteine metabolism |

## Antioxidant Vitamins

Three vitamins (vitamins C and E and plant pigments known as carotenoids) are classified as **antioxidants**—protective substances that help neutralize the activity of free radicals. **Free radicals**, also called oxidants, are naturally produced chemicals that arise from normal cell activity. Whenever the body uses oxygen or is exposed to a toxin, such as cigarette smoke, it forms free radicals. Some production of free radicals is essential to health and occurs naturally such as in breathing. The body cannot convert air and food into energy without producing free radicals. They also help the immune system fight off cancer cells and defend itself against infection.[43] However, when the production of free radicals is disproportional to the body's need for them, they may damage cells throughout the body. They may damage a cell's DNA in ways that lead to cancer, interact with cholesterol in the bloodstream and form oxidized LDL (see Chapter 2), cause cataracts and rheumatoid arthritis, and be a factor in the physiological changes

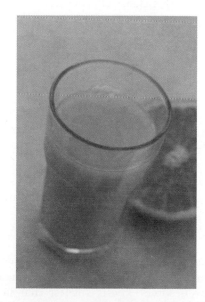

Antioxidant vitamins from foods such as citrus fruits may help protect young and old alike from heart disease and cancer.

associated with the aging process. Excess free radical production is thought to contribute to many diseases.[44,45] Anything that interferes with the destructive effects of free radicals offers a health advantage.

Foods can supply nutrients with antioxidant properties. Vitamins C and E, the mineral selenium, and the carotenoids (including beta-carotene) are well-known antioxidants. A common cooking practice illustrates this antioxidant effect. Some foods, such as bananas, peaches, apples, and potatoes, quickly turn brown when exposed to air. However, when such foods are dipped in lemon or orange juice, the vitamin C in the juice acts as an antioxidant and prevents browning.

Each antioxidant serves a different purpose, but all of them work closely together. For example, vitamin C helps regenerate vitamin E once it has become oxidized.[46] This illustrates the importance of a diet that supplies sufficient amounts of all of the antioxidants rather than focusing exclusively on one.

Should Americans take supplements of antioxidant vitamins? Information from the research community is inconclusive. The prevailing attitude in the medical community is that people do not need to take antioxidant supplements. This is not to say that antioxidants are not needed, just not in pill form. The preferred way to get antioxidants is from food. The daily consumption of 2 cups of fruit and 2.5 cups of vegetables (9 servings of fruits and vegetables), as the dietary guidelines recommend, satisfies the body's need for antioxidants and the thousands of other nutrients found in plant foods.[47–50] Emphasize dark green vegetables and orange, red, and yellow fruits and vegetables. Dark-pigmented fruits and vegetables are excellent sources of antioxidant vitamins and many other nutrients. Consume them together. It is possible that the beneficial effects of antioxidants occur when they are eaten in combination with each other. Don't take supplements of the antioxidant selenium. The difference between an adequate and a toxic dose of selenium is very small.[51]

## Vitamin C

Vitamin C, also called *ascorbic acid,* is essential to the formation of collagen, a protein used to form all the connective tissues of your body. It is required in the breakdown and absorption of some amino acids and other minerals (such as iron) and in the formation of some hormones. It may also help the immune system prevent infections.

Contrary to popular opinion, vitamin C does not prevent the common cold. Scientifically controlled studies reveal no difference in the incidence of colds among vitamin C users and nonusers. On a positive note, however, some experts suggest that large doses (up to about 1,000 mg/day) may have small effects on the duration and severity of cold symptoms.[52]

The RDA of vitamin C is 90 mg for men and 75 mg for women. Smokers need an additional 35 mg.[53] The Tolerable Upper Limit is 2,000 mg. That much, however, might also cause diarrhea and kidney stones in susceptible people.[54,55] Good food sources of vitamin C include broccoli, cantaloupe, citrus, peppers, potatoes, strawberries, apricots, kiwifruit, cauliflower, Brussels sprouts, and tomatoes.

Megadoses (over 2,000 mg) of vitamin C offer little benefit to the body and may be harmful. As a water-soluble vitamin, vitamin C doses in excess of the body's requirement are excreted through the kidneys. In other words, the body can absorb only so much. For those who absorb excess iron, supplements of vitamin C could be dangerous.[56] Large intakes may also produce errors in the results of some diagnostic tests (such as the hemoccult test, which tests for blood in the intestines).[57]

## Carotenoids

More than 600 carotenoids are found in nature. They give fruits and vegetables their yellow, orange, and red colors. They're also abundant in dark green vegetables. Three of the major carotenoids (alpha-carotene, beta-carotene, and beta-cryptoxanthin) can be converted by the body into vitamin A and are referred to as *provitamin A.* Until recently, beta-carotene was thought to offer the most health-protecting antioxidant effect. However, after studies showed that the incidence of lung cancer increased in smokers who took beta-carotene supplements, researchers concluded that beta-carotene is not the main protector.

One carotenoid currently being studied for its antioxidant potency is lycopene, the predominant carotenoid in the blood and in the prostate gland in males. It cannot be converted to vitamin A, but it has twice the antioxidant potency of beta-carotene. Benefits attributed to lycopene are a reduced risk for some cancers, especially those of the digestive tract and the prostate. The best source of lycopene is tomatoes.

Currently, carotenoid supplements, including beta-carotene and lycopene, are not recommended. Carotenoids interact with one another, and supplemental doses of one carotenoid may impair the absorption of others. Instead, eat a variety of vegetables and fruits to get a mix of carotenoids. Emphasize fruits and vegetables that are mostly yellow-orange, red, or dark green. It is likely that carotenoids are more beneficial to health when they are consumed together from food than when packaged separately, as in a supplement.

## Vitamin D

Vitamin D is an essential nutrient associated with aiding the immune system in preventing or slowing down inflammation, cancer, osteoarthritis, cardiovascular disease, periodontal disease, diabetes, risk of injuries from falls caused by loss of strength and balance, and overall death risk.[58–66] It is also required to maintain the body's calcium stores. In the absence of vitamin D, calcium cannot be absorbed.

Vitamin D is called the sunshine vitamin because the sun's ultraviolet rays cause a chemical in the skin to be converted to vitamin D. Exposure of the arms and legs to the sun for 5 to 15 minutes two or three times a week between 10:00 a.m. and 3 p.m. without sunscreen will satisfy the vitamin D requirement of most fair-skinned people during the summer months. If you're overweight, dark-skinned, or live in the northern half of the United States, a vitamin D supplement may be required.[67,68]

Seventy-five percent of Americans don't get enough vitamin D, and vitamin D deficiency is on the increase.[69] Although deficiencies are common, they may go unnoticed. Consequently, vitamin D deficiencies are often referred to as the "hidden epidemic."

Recommended intake of vitamin D is 400 IU. Food sources include fatty fish, fortified soy, fortified orange juice, and fortified cereals. Milk is also fortified with vitamin D and a good source of the nutrient. Many experts believe the current recommendation of 400 IU does not address the vitamin D deficiency epidemic and suggest that doubling vitamin D intake to 800 to 1,000 IU would improve vitamin D status and improve the overall health of Americans.[70,71] Many people should consider taking a vitamin D supplement of 400 to 1,000 IU because of the difficulty in getting this nutrient in their diet.[72–74] In shopping for a vitamin D supplement, choose one that contains vitamin $D_3$, which may be more potent than $D_2$.[75] Also, if you are supplementing your diet with extra calcium, don't overlook the body's need for vitamin D.

### Vitamin E

Vitamin E is a fat-soluble vitamin; it plays a role in the formation of red blood cells and maintenance of nervous tissues, and it aids in the absorption of vitamin A. Claims that vitamin E improves the skin, heals scars, prevents stretch marks, slows the aging process, and increases fertility are more folklore than fact.

Vitamin E, once considered the most promising of the antioxidant vitamins, has grown out of favor as a nutrient that is needed in supplemental doses. The results of hundreds of studies reveal surprising increases in all-cause mortality, rather than decreases, when comparing subjects taking vitamin E supplements with subjects taking placebos.[76] That is, vitamin E users had a greater chance of dying from all causes than users taking the placebo. Vitamin E users were no healthier in terms of reduced cancer incidence and

death from heart attack or stroke than those who didn't take vitamin E supplements. While the jury is still out on other possible benefits of vitamin E, the popular opinion among scientists is that the evidence does not warrant consumption of this nutrient in supplemental doses.[77]

The RDA of vitamin E is 15 mg (22 International Units, or IU). The Tolerable Upper Limit is 1,000 mg. Food sources include nuts, vegetable oils, and fortified cereals.

### Folate, Vitamin $B_6$, Vitamin $B_{12}$

Folate is a part of the vitamin B complex and combines with vitamins $B_6$ and $B_{12}$ to form parts of DNA and RNA and to make heme, the iron-containing protein in red blood cells (see Just the Facts: The Many Names of Vitamin B Complex). These three also assist in the metabolism of amino acids. The term **folate** refers to the natural form of the vitamin found in foods. *Folic acid* refers to the synthetic form of the vitamin found in supplements and fortified food.[78] Folic acid is about twice as potent as folate. Vitamins $B_6$ and $B_{12}$ are plentiful in foods, and deficiencies are unlikely to occur in a well-balanced diet. Good food sources are meat products, dairy products, and eggs. Nonmeat sources include spinach, whole-wheat bread, and breakfast cereals. Strict vegetarians who avoid all animal-based products

[ **JUST THE** ]
# FACTS
## The Many Names of Vitamin B Complex

Vitamin B complex is not a single vitamin, instead, it is an umbrella term that refers to 8 vitamins. They are listed below along with their other names.

Vitamin $B_1$    (thiamine)

Vitamin $B_2$    (riboflavin)

Vitamin $B_3$    (niacin plus niacinamide)

Vitamin $B_5$    (pantothenic acid)

Vitamin $B_6$    (pyridoxine, pyridoxal, and pyridoxamine)

Vitamin $B_7$    (biotin or vitamin H)

Vitamin $B_9$    (folate, in foods, or folic acid, in supplements

Vitamin $B_{12}$    (cobalamin)

Source: Tufts Media. (2009). The ABCs of Bs. *Tufts University Health and Nutrition Letter, 27*(5), 6.

may not get enough of these vitamins, especially $B_{12}$, and therefore may require supplementation.[79] Because the ability to absorb $B_{12}$ often diminishes with age, adults over 65 may also need a supplement.[80]

Folate, as its name implies, is found in foliage—leafy vegetables, such as lettuce and spinach. It is also found in citrus fruits, whole-grain bread, fortified cereals, and liver. Of the three B vitamins mentioned here, folate is the one in which Americans are most likely to fall short.

Because folate has been associated with a reduction in the chances of neurological birth defects, such as spina bifida, a woman planning a pregnancy may be advised by her physician to eat foods rich in folate and possibly to take a supplement.[81] In an effort to reduce the incidence of these birth defects, food fortification guidelines require food manufacturers to fortify certain grain products, such as flour, bread, cornmeal, pasta products, rice, and other cereal grain products, with folic acid.[82]

Folate is a nutrient of particular interest because of its relationship to homocysteine. Homocysteine is an amino acid that is linked to an increased risk of heart disease: the higher the homocysteine level, the greater the risk of developing heart disease. High homocysteine levels are associated with low levels of folate, $B_6$, and $B_{12}$, which work together to break down homocysteine into harmless components. When folate intake is increased, homocysteine levels go down. Therefore, theoretically, it would seem that an increased intake of folate, $B_6$, and $B_{12}$ would result in fewer heart attacks. So far, this finding has not been confirmed in major studies. High doses of these B vitamins do lower homocysteine levels but not the incidence of heart attack and stroke. A possible explanation for these contradictory findings is that high homocysteine levels may be an indicator of heart disease but not the actual cause.[83,84]

Regardless of the uncertainty about the homocysteine and heart disease connection, folate is an essential nutrient and must be included in the diet. The RDA of folate is 400 micrograms (mcg) and is easily achievable in the diet. Multivitamin supplements usually have 400 mcg of folic acid. Megadoses of folate should be avoided to prevent the possibility of a false negative for anemia (too few blood cells) caused by a vitamin $B_{12}$ deficiency.[85] If you take folate supplements, tell your physician, so that the appropriate tests can be ordered.

## Vitamin Supplements

Advertisements proclaim that vitamins provide energy, promote wellness, and prevent disease and that taking more results in more energy and better health. Consequently, most American adults take one or more **vitamin supplements** in multiple and single doses, in both natural and synthetic forms.[86] Vitamins do facilitate energy release from carbohydrates, fats, and proteins, but they do not provide energy. It is not possible to survive on water and vitamins.

Should you take a vitamin supplement? With the exceptions noted below, there is little health benefit from supplements of B vitamins, vitamin C, vitamin E, or multivitamins. This is the prevailing opinion of experts and is supported by the results of a large-scale study involving more than 160,000 women over a period of 8 years. Researchers could find no evidence that supplements reduced the incidence of cancer, cardiovascular disease, or death from any cause.[87,88,89] Past recommendations that justified vitamin supplements as a precaution against poor nutrition are not supported by findings in recent studies. Regardless, some experts still endorse taking a multivitamin because it is a low-risk strategy for good nutrition and many people don't eat enough nutritious whole foods to meet nutrient needs.[90,91] If you take a supplement, consume it with food. Food facilitates the absorption and interaction of nutrients in a multivitamin supplement.

Although healthy people don't need vitamin supplements if they are eating a balanced diet, there are several situations[92–95] in which a vitamin or mineral supplement may be called for:

*If you are age 50 or older,* you may need supplements of vitamins $B_6$, $B_{12}$, and D because of the difficulty in absorbing these vitamins with advancing age. Women, especially those not taking estrogen, may require more calcium and vitamin D to protect against osteoporosis.

*If you are dieting,* consuming fewer than 1,000 calories a day, you may benefit from a vitamin and mineral supplement.

*If you have a chronic illness, such as cancer or AIDS, or a disease of the digestive tract,* it may interfere with normal digestion and absorption of nutrients and justify your use of vitamin and mineral supplements.

*If you smoke,* you may need vitamin C supplements.

*If you drink excessive alcohol,* you may suffer from poor nutrition and the alcohol may interfere with the absorption and metabolism of vitamins.

*If you are pregnant and lactating (breast-feeding),* supplements of folic acid, iron, and calcium may be recommended for you.

*If you are a vegetarian,* you may need additional vitamin $B_{12}$. Calcium and vitamin D supplements may also be warranted if your milk intake and sun exposure are limited.

## Minerals

**Minerals** are simple but important nutrients. They are simple in that they are not composed of organic matter and therefore do not have the properties of living organisms. Chemically, inorganic substances lack compounds containing hydrocarbon groups. As inorganic compounds, they lack the complexity of vitamins, but they fulfill a variety of functions. For example, sodium and potassium affect shifts in body fluids, calcium and phosphorus contribute to the body's structure, iron is the core of hemoglobin (an oxygen-carrying compound in the blood), and iodine facilitates production of thyroxine (a hormone that influences metabolic rate).

There are 20 to 30 important nutritional minerals. Minerals should be consumed in smaller amounts than amounts of energy nutrients and water. Minerals present in the body and required in large amounts (more than 100 mg, or 0.02 teaspoon, per day) are called *major minerals* or *macrominerals*. They include, in descending order of prominence, calcium, phosphorus, potassium, sulfur, sodium, chloride, and magnesium. Major minerals contribute 60 to 80% of inorganic material in the human body.

Minerals required in small amounts (less than 100 mg per day) are called *trace minerals* or *microminerals*. There are more than a dozen trace minerals, the best known being iron, zinc, and iodine (see Just the Facts: Minerals).

Some minerals are similar to water-soluble vitamins in that they are readily excreted by the kidneys, do not accumulate in the body, and rarely become toxic. Others are like fat-soluble vitamins in that they are stored and are toxic if taken in excess.

Minerals are different from vitamins; they are indestructible and require no special handling during food preparation. The only precautions that need to be taken are to avoid soaking minerals out of food and throwing them away in cooking water.

Major minerals are abundant in the diet; therefore, deficiencies are highly unlikely, especially if a variety of foods are included. If a deficiency in major minerals does occur, it is most likely to be a calcium deficiency, especially among women.[96] Average daily calcium intake for women of all ages is 600 to 800 mg, far short of the recommended adequate intake of 1,000 to 1,200 mg. For men the daily intake of calcium averages 800 to 1,100 mg.[97] The following are some tips for increasing your calcium intake:

- Try to consume as much calcium as possible from food. Yogurt, cheese, skim milk, and low-fat dairy products are excellent sources of calcium and are fortified with vitamin D. Nondairy sources include fortified ready-to-eat cereals, soy beverages, sardines, salmon, collards, turnip greens, and dried beans.[98]

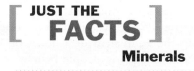

### JUST THE FACTS
#### Minerals

The following are some basic facts about minerals.

#### Major (Macro) Minerals

*Types:* calcium, phosphorus, potassium, sulfur, sodium chloride, and magnesium

#### Trace (Micro) Minerals

*Types:* iron, iodine, zinc, selenium, manganese, copper, molybdenum, cobalt, chromium, fluorine, silicon, vanadium, nickel, tin, cadmium

#### Minerals of Special Concern*

##### Calcium

*Wellness benefits:* contributes to bone and tooth formation, general body growth, maintenance of good muscle tone, nerve function, cell membrane function, and regulation of normal heartbeat

*Food sources:* dairy products, dark green vegetables, dried beans, shellfish

*Deficiency signs and symptoms:* bone pain and fractures, muscle cramps, osteoporosis

##### Iron

*Wellness benefits:* facilitates oxygen and carbon dioxide transport, formation of red blood cells, production of antibodies, synthesis of collagen, use of energy

*Food sources:* red meat (lean); seafood; eggs; dried beans; nuts; grains; green, leafy vegetables

*Deficiency signs and symptoms:* fatigue, weakness

##### Sodium**

*Wellness benefits:* maintains proper acid–base balance and body fluid regulation, aids in formation of digestive secretions, assists in nerve transmission

*Food sources:* processed foods, meats, table salt

*Deficiency signs and symptoms:* restlessness, fatigue, diminished strength. Deficiency is rare in the United States.

*Calcium and iron are of special concern because deficiencies are likely to exist, especially among women and children.

**Sodium is of concern because of the potential for overconsumption.

- Use calcium supplements to compensate for a calcium shortfall. Getting enough calcium from food requires consuming the equivalent of a quart of milk per day. As a result, many people benefit from an over-the-counter calcium supplement.
- Calcium is best absorbed in doses of 500 mg or less, taken with meals.[99] The most common type of calcium supplement is calcium carbonate, available in common antacids.[100]
- Take calcium supplements with or just after meals. Calcium is best dissolved and absorbed in stomach acids secreted during mealtime.[101]
- Look for calcium-fortified foods. A cup of calcium-fortified orange juice, for example, contains about the same amount of calcium as a cup of milk and is absorbed more easily.
- Get the recommended intake of vitamin D. Vitamin D is necessary for the body to absorb calcium.
- If you're taking other supplements or medicines, check with your physician or pharmacist. Calcium can interfere with the absorption of iron, zinc, and certain medicines.

Of the various trace minerals, iron is of concern to nutritionists because certain groups are at risk of having low iron levels. These include young children and early teens; menstruating women; and people with conditions that cause internal bleeding, such as ulcers or intestinal diseases.[102]

Iron deficiency in the diet is responsible for the most prevalent form of anemia.[103] Iron deficiency hampers the body's ability to produce hemoglobin, a substance needed to carry oxygen in the blood. A lack of hemoglobin can cause fatigue and weakness and can even affect behavior and intellectual function. Proper infant feeding through the use of iron-fortified milk or breast-feeding is the best safeguard against iron deficiency in infants. Among adolescents and adults, iron intake can be improved by increasing consumption of iron-rich foods, such as lean red meats, fish, certain kinds of beans, dried fruits, iron-enriched cereals and whole-grain products, and foods cooked in a cast-iron skillet. For some people, especially premenopausal women with inconsistent diets, iron supplements may be justified. In addition, consuming foods that contain vitamin C enhances the body's ability to absorb iron.

Iron deficiency is rare among healthy men and postmenopausal women. Even strict vegetarians can get iron in sufficient amounts by consuming legumes, dark green leafy vegetables, and fortified breads and cereals. However, it is possible to get too much iron. Some studies report that high iron levels may be linked to heart disease, but the jury is still out on this issue. Also, some people have a rare genetic disorder called *hemochromatosis,* which permits an unhealthy buildup of iron. Iron overload may cause liver cancer, heart disease, diabetes, sterility, or other complications.

Selenium is another trace mineral that may offer unique health benefits. It is an antioxidant associated with a reduced risk for arthritis and various cancers.[104] Because the results of studies of selenium as an anticancer nutrient are mixed, experts do not recommend selenium supplements at this time. Human studies are under way to determine if the health benefits of extra selenium intake can be confirmed. Fish, meats, eggs, and shellfish are good animal sources of selenium. Grains and seeds grown in soils containing selenium are good plant sources. Most adults get enough selenium in their diet. Excess selenium can be toxic. Daily intakes that exceed 400 mcg can cause toxicity if taken for many months.[105]

## Water

Water performs many functions. It is vital to digestion and metabolism because it acts as a medium for chemical reactions in the body. It carries oxygen and nutrients to the cells through blood, regulates body temperature through perspiration, and lubricates the joints. It removes waste through sweat and urine, protects a fetus, and assists in respiration by moistening the lungs to facilitate intake of oxygen and excretion of carbon dioxide. It is a vital component of the body's tissues and organs. For example, muscles are 75% water, as is the brain, and blood is composed of 92% water.[106] It also provides satiety, thus serving as a deterrent to the overconsumption of food.

Although most water intake comes from beverages, solid foods also make a significant contribution. Many fruits and vegetables are more than 80% water.[107]

How much water do you need? The Adequate Intake for water consumption is 15 cups for adult men and 11 cups for adult women[108] and is based on total water intake from foods and beverages, including milk, juice, and tap or bottled water (see Just the Facts: Bottled Water Comes with Many Names). Water in caffeinated beverages such as coffee, tea, and colas counts toward total water intake even though caffeine may have a diuretic effect on some people.[109,110] Most people can meet their water needs by drinking when they are thirsty.[111] It's important to remember that thirst is an early sign of your body needing more fluids, not a late sign.[112] The thirst mechanism may not be a reliable indicator during illness and exercise. Hydration guidelines related to exercise are presented in Chapter 3. One way to monitor water intake is to check the color and odor of urine. Dark yellow instead of pale urine is a sign of insufficient water intake, as is urine with a very strong

## [ JUST THE FACTS ]

### Bottled Water Comes with Many Names

If you don't like your water from the tap, you can buy purified water, spring water, mineral water, distilled water, and drinking water by the bottle, six pack, or case. Are there differences among the various types of bottled water? There are, but you almost need a dictionary to sort the differences. The following is a brief description of the common types of bottled water.[115]

- *Distilled water* comes from the stream of public water that has been boiled.

- *Drinking water* is public or municipal water, such as tap water. If the water comes directly from the tap without any treatment, the label has to identify the public source it comes from. If the water has been treated, no disclosure is required.

- *Mineral water* is spring water that naturally contains at least 250 milligrams of dissolved minerals (such as magnesium and calcium) per liter.

- *Purified water* has been treated with distillation, ion exchange, reverse osmosis, or a similar process.

- *Sparkling water* is spring water that contains carbon dioxide gas (as in cola beverages).

- *Spring water* comes from underground formations beneath the earth's surface. It makes up most of the bottled water sold in the United States. Theoretically, spring water is protected from pollution.

odor[113]—understanding, at the same time, that medicines and vitamin supplements can cause dark urine (see Real-World Wellness: How Can You Tell If You're Getting Enough Water?).

Under normal circumstances, too much water cannot be consumed because the body is efficient at getting rid of what it does not need. **Water intoxication,** the consumption of more water than the kidneys can excrete, is possible, though rare. It can lead to serious side effects, such as headache, blurred vision, cramps, convulsions, and possibly death. An excessive amount would have to approach many quarts each day. Very few people are at risk of drinking too much water.[114]

## Other Nutrients with Unique Health Benefits

In addition to the six classes of essential nutrients, many other substances in food contribute to health. Interest in these substances has sparked interest in enriched food, fortified food, functional food, nutraceuticals, botanicals, herbs, and fiber (see Just the Facts: Enhanced Foods). Many of these substances promote health and prevent illness; many more fall far short of their claims. New discoveries and recent developments in these areas have outpaced the scientific community's ability to monitor, test, and confirm various claims. Until these claims can be validated, the public should assume an attitude of skepticism. While many of the chemical compounds in food promise to promote health, taken indiscriminately they may do more harm than good. The exception is fiber, for which most claims are backed by years of solid evidence.

### Real-World Wellness

#### How Can You Tell If You're Getting Enough Water?

*Experts say that thirst is a good indicator of when and how much water to drink. But what if I'm a heavy sweater and lose an inordinate amount of water? How can I be sure that I'm properly hydrated?*

One of the times the thirst mechanism is not a reliable indicator of the need for water is during strenuous physical exertion. The following guidelines will help you determine whether to increase your fluid intake:[116]

- Weigh yourself before and after a workout. This will provide a gauge for determining how much water was lost during exercise and how much to replace.

- Drink 2.5 to 3 cups of fluids per pound of weight loss. This is especially important when weight loss approaches 2% of body weight. For example, someone who weighs 200 pounds and loses 4 pounds (2%) during a workout should consume 10 to 12 cups of fluids to be sufficiently hydrated (2.5 × 4 = 10 cups; 3 × 4 = 12 cups).

- Check the color of your urine. If it is dark and has a strong odor, you probably need more water.

### Phytochemicals, Phytonutrients

**Phytochemicals,** also called phytonutrients, are plant chemicals that exist naturally in all plant foods. Chemically, they are not vitamins, minerals, fiber, or any of

## [ JUST THE FACTS ]
### Enhanced Foods

The term **enhanced foods** refers to foods that have been modified and or supplemented for the purpose of achieving or facilitating a health benefit. As an umbrella term, *enhanced foods* includes enriched food, fortified food, functional food, nutraceuticals, and genetically modified food.[117]

*Enriched food.* Food that has been supplemented with naturally occurring nutrients often lost or compromised during processing. The addition of the vitamins thiamin, niacin, riboflavin, and folate and the mineral iron to bread is an example.

*Fortified food.* Food that has been supplemented with nutrients in excess of what was originally in the food or were not present. Three examples include milk fortified with vitamin D, orange juice fortified with calcium, and breakfast cereals fortified with 100% of the RDA for certain vitamins and minerals.

*Functional food.* The American Dietetic Association defines functional foods as whole foods and fortified, enriched, or enhanced foods that have a potentially beneficial effect on health.[118] Foods ranging from nuts to energy bars fall in this category. Unmodified whole foods, such as fruits and vegetables, are the simplest form of functional food in that they contain substances good for health beyond vitamins and minerals.[119] Tomatoes, for example, are good sources of vitamins and minerals and a substance called lycopene that may help prevent some forms of cancer. Another form of functional food is foods that have been modified, fortified, enriched, or enhanced. Orange juice, for example, is a known source of vitamin C and many other nutrients. If it has been fortified with calcium, it provides an added health benefit. Tomatoes and calcium-fortified orange juice, therefore, can be called functional foods.

*Nutraceuticals.* Functional foods that have been modified to produce druglike effects. Fruit juice with added herbs, such as ginkgo biloba or echinacea, is an example. When foods are consumed primarily for their medicinal value, they are viewed as nutraceuticals.

*Genetically modified food.* Food that has been altered at the genetic level to improve health benefits or to make it hardier.

the energy nutrients. Rather, they are the hundreds of thousands of active compounds found in small amounts in vegetables and fruits. Although phytochemicals have not been traditionally classified as essential nutrients, scientists believe that they might play an important role in preventing various diseases.

There is a great deal of excitement in nutrition and food sciences about the potential of phytochemicals in health promotion. The reported health benefits of several phytochemicals are highlighted in Table 6-6. As scientists continue to isolate, identify, and study specific plant chemicals, it is likely that the place of such chemicals in disease prevention will become more important.

## Botanicals (Phytomedicinals) (Herbs)

Plants used medically are technically called **botanicals** or **phytomedicinals**. The popular literature usually refers to them as *herbs*. Herbs number in the thousands; however, few are backed by well-conducted research studies similar to those used to test over-the-counter drugs in the United States. Herbs, however, are not regulated as drugs; instead, they are classified as dietary supplements. There is considerable debate about their effectiveness and safety. Consequently, some experts refer to the dietary supplement industry as the "Wild West." The names, food sources, and health claims of several popular herbs are presented in Just the Facts: Some Common Herbs Sold as Nutritional Supplements on page 192.

If you decide to take an herb, here are some tips:

- Check with your physician before taking herbs, especially for serious conditions. Inform your physician of herbs you are taking, as you would for prescribed medicines. There are many potential interactions with other supplements and medicines.
- Avoid using herbs if you are pregnant or nursing.
- Check the label for the abbreviation *USP*. This means that the manufacturer has met the stringent guidelines of the U.S. Pharmacopoeia, ensuring the quality, strength, purity, and consistency of the product. The letters *NF,* which stand for *National Formulary,* also ensure that the product meets minimum standards. Presently, only a handful of herbs have been subjected to review using USP standards.
- Do your homework. Read about the herb; ask your pharmacist for information. There are several Web sites that provide helpful information:
  - U.S. Pharmacopoeia: **www.usp.org**
  - American Botanical Council: **www.herbal-gram.org**
  - The Herb Research Foundation: **www.herbs.org**
- Monitor your body's response. Start with lower than the recommended dose. Stop taking an herb if you have an adverse reaction.
- Don't expect miracles. Herbs take longer to work than prescribed and over-the-counter medicines.

**TABLE 6-6** Health Benefits of Selected Phytochemicals, Phytonutrients

| Phytochemical/ Phytonutrient | Food Source | Possible Benefit |
|---|---|---|
| Allyl sulfide | Garlic, onions, leeks, chives | Decreases reproduction of tumor cells; facilitates excretion of carcinogens; blocks nitrite formation in stomach |
| Caffeic acid | Fruits | Facilitates excretions of carcinogens |
| Capsaicin | Hot peppers | Acts as an antioxidant; inhibits carcinogenesis |
| Coumarin | Citrus fruit, tomatoes | Prevents blood clotting; stimulates anticancer enzymes |
| Dithiolthione | Cruciferous vegetables | Stimulates anticancer enzymes |
| Phytoestrogen (isoflavones) | Soybeans, dried beans | Helps prevent breast cancer by stopping the estrogen produced by the body from entering cells |
| Flavonoids | Fruits, vegetables, red wine, grape juice, green tea | Act as an antioxidant |
| Phenolic acids (ellagic acid, ferulic acid) | Fruits, grains, nuts | Prevent DNA damage in cells; bind to iron, which may inhibit the mineral from creating free radicals; bind to nitrites in the stomach, preventing them from being converted into nitrosamines |
| Indoles, isothiocynates, sulforaphane | Cruciferous vegetables | Stimulate anticancer enzymes |
| Limonene | Citrus fruits | Stimulates anticancer enzymes |
| Phytic acid | Grains | Binds to iron, which may inhibit the mineral from creating cancer-causing free radicals |
| Terpenes (lycopene, lutein, carotenoids) | Tomatoes, watermelon, sweet potatoes, carrots, spinach, cantaloupe | Neutralize free radicals and help repair DNA |

- Take specific herbs for specific needs. Avoid taking herbs continuously.

## Fiber

One advantage of a complex carbohydrate diet is that it will likely be high in fiber unless the foods are refined or highly processed.

*Fiber* (formerly called *roughage*) is a general term that refers to the substances in food that resist digestion. The amount of fiber in a food is determined by its plant source and the amount of processing it undergoes. In general, the more a food is processed, the more the fiber is broken down or removed and the lower its fiber content. Fiber comes only from plant foods. Meat, dairy products, and fats do not provide any natural fiber.[120]

There are two kinds of fiber: soluble fiber and insoluble fiber. **Soluble fiber** dissolves or swells in water and has a gel-like consistency. One of its health benefits is its ability to bind with cholesterol and subsequently excrete it. Because soluble fiber slows down the rate the stomach empties, it has an added advantage of contributing to a feeling of fullness. Fruits, legumes, barley, and oats are good sources of soluble fiber. **Insoluble fiber** does not dissolve in water. One of its health benefits is its ability to move food through the digestive system. Vegetables, whole-grain foods, and nuts are good exam-

ples of insoluble fiber[121] (see Just the Facts: Sample Ingredient List for a Whole-Grain Food). From a practical, dietary perspective, it is unnecessary to distinguish between the two types of fiber. Every plant food usually contains a mixture of fiber types, and there is significant overlap in the health benefits of soluble and insoluble fiber-rich foods[122–125] (see Table 6-7 on page 193).

Fiber may also be available as an additive or supplement. Fiber that is extracted from food because of its health benefits and then added to a food is referred to as **functional fiber**.[126] Dietary supplements, fortified foods and beverages, and bulk laxatives are some examples of food that include functional fiber.[127]

Food package labels use the term *dietary fiber* to indicate fiber content per serving. **Dietary fiber** is an umbrella term that refers to the amount of fiber found naturally in food. The amount of soluble fiber is usually listed on food labels as a subtype of dietary fiber. Food labels indicate the amount of soluble fiber and total dietary fiber in a food but do not yet distinguish between insoluble fiber and functional fiber.

### Health Benefits of Fiber

Dietary fiber is an important part of a healthy diet. To quote a leading nutrition expert, "It's hard to eat a high-fiber diet that isn't healthy."[128] Health benefits include a reduced risk for heart disease, improvement in blood

# [ JUST THE FACTS ]

## Some Common Herbs Sold as Nutritional Supplements

The following are possible benefits and problems[134,135] of various herbs:

- Black cohosh

  *Possible benefits:* reduce, relieve symptoms of menopause

  *Potential problem:* mild gastrointestinal distress, nausea, fall in blood pressure

- Cranberry

  *Possible benefits:* prevention or treatment of urinary tract infections

  *Potential problem:* concentrated cranberry tablets may increase the risk for kidney stones

- Echinacea

  *Possible benefits:* immune booster for colds, flus, and respiratory infections

  *Potential problem:* some allergic reactions reported in people with autoimmune disorders, such as lupus or multiple sclerosis

- Feverfew

  *Possible benefits:* prevention and treatment of migraines and associated nausea

  *Potential problem:* a potential allergen for people sensitive to ragweed

- Garlic

  *Possible benefits:* may promote antibacterial, antifungal, and antiviral activity, including those associated with the common cold; may have cardiovascular benefits

  *Potential problem:* in excess, possible interactions with other herbs and/or medicines

- Ginger

  *Possible benefits:* treatment of motion sickness, nausea, indigestion

  *Potential problem:* may aggravate gallstones, heartburn; acts as a blood thinner

- *Ginkgo biloba*

  *Possible benefits:* may improve memory and mental functioning; acts as an antioxidant; aids blood flow to the brain and to the legs

  *Potential problem:* acts as a blood thinner; may cause gastrointestinal upset, headaches, allergic skin reactions

- Ginseng

  *Possible benefits:* may enhance immunity

  *Potential problem:* may increase blood pressure; may cause headaches and skin problems

- Glucosamine and chondroitin

  *Possible benefits:* may stimulate cartilage growth and relieve pain associated with arthritis and stiff joints

  *Potential problem:* reduced insulin secretions

- Saw palmetto

  *Possible benefits:* may improve urinary flow in men with enlarged prostate

  *Potential problem:* may cause inaccurate readings on PSA tests

- Soy isoflavones

  *Possible benefits:* reduce postmenopausal symptoms, prevent breast or prostate cancer, promote cartilage formation, decrease joint inflammation, prevent bone loss, and act as a mildantidepressant

  *Possible problem:* mild headaches

- St. John's wort

  *Possible benefits:* may alleviate mild to moderate depression

  *Potential problem:* not useful for severe depression; may cause complications with prescription antidepressants

- Valerian

  *Possible benefits:* treatment for insomnia, mild anxiety, restlessness

  *Potential problem:* may cause complications withsedatives or antidepressants

---

sugar control, prevention and relief of constipation, and reduced risks of developing precancerous polyps in the intestines.[129] High-fiber diets may also be a key strategy for weight management because fiber delays stomach emptying, which, in turn, promotes a feeling of *satiety,* or fullness, and diminishes the appetite.

If you are not accustomed to eating fiber-rich foods, gradually add them to your diet over time, following these suggestions:[130–133]

- Eat whole-wheat bread rather than white bread. Look for bread that provides at least 3 grams of fiber per slice.
- Look for whole grains, such as whole wheat, on food labels. Foods "made with whole-wheat flour" are mostly refined. The American Heart Association recommends that at least half of grain intake come from whole grains.[136] If the food label doesn't list whole wheat first, its fiber content has

## [ JUST THE **FACTS** ]

### Sample Ingredient List for a Whole-Grain Food[137]

- Ingredients: whole-wheat flour, water, high fructose corn syrup, wheat gluten, soybean and/or canola oil, yeast, salt, honey
- Note: "Wheat flour," "enriched flour," and "degerminated corn meal" are not whole grains.

likely been compromised. Wheat flour and unbleached wheat flour are not whole grain. Color is not an indication of whole grain. Bread can be brown because of molasses or other ingredients.

- Substitute brown rice, millet, and bulgur wheat for white rice and potatoes.
- Snack on popcorn instead of potato chips (popcorn is a whole grain).
- Eat whole fruit instead of drinking juice.
- Use raspberries as a topping for ice cream and yogurt.
- Snack on an unpeeled fruit.
- Top your salads and casseroles with a whole-grain cereal, such as Shredded Wheat.
- Choose a cereal that has at least 3 grams of fiber and less than 3 grams of fat, 9 grams of sugars, and 200 calories.[138]
- Drink plenty of fluids.
- Eat the skin on your potato.
- Include beans in soups and vegetable salads.
- Eat more legumes.

### How Much Fiber?

The daily recommendation is 25 grams of fiber for women and 38 grams for men. This is based on 14 grams of fiber per 1,000 calories. After age 50, recommended fiber intake falls to 21 and 30 grams per day for women and men, respectively. The Daily Value of fiber listed on food labels is 25 grams for a 2,000-caloric diet. Most Americans consume half the recommended levels. Women average about 13 grams a day compared to men's 17 grams.[139] Most Americans have trouble meeting this recommendation because of their heavy intake of meat products.

Meat provides little or no fiber; consequently, only vegetarians are likely to get enough fiber. Eating naturally high-fiber foods, such as whole grains, fruits, vegetables, and beans, is a good way to increase fiber intake. Whole grains may include barley, buckwheat, bulgur, corn, millet, rice, rye, oats, sorghum, wheat, and wild rice. "Enriched" wheat flour is not whole grain; foods labeled as "stone-ground," "100% wheat," "bran," "multigrain," "7-grain," or "made from whole grain" usually aren't 100% whole grain.[140,141] Starting or ending the

**TABLE 6-7**  Fiber Content of Selected Foods

| Food | Fiber (g) |
| --- | --- |
| **Fruits** | |
| Apple, with peel | 4.2 |
| Banana | 3.3 |
| Blackberries (1 cup) | 9.7 |
| Dates, chopped (1 cup) | 15.5 |
| Grapes | 1.0 |
| Orange | 2.9 |
| Peach, peeled | 2.0 |
| Pear, with skin | 4.9 |
| Prunes, dried, pitted (10) | 13.5 |
| Raisins, seedless (1 cup) | 9.6 |
| **Breads** | |
| Oatmeal (1 cup) | 0.86 |
| Pumpernickel (1 slice) | 1.33 |
| Rye (1 slice) | 1.65 |
| Wheat (1 slice) | 1.40 |
| White (1 slice) | 0.68 |
| Whole-wheat (1 slice) | 3.17 |
| **Cereals** | |
| All-Bran (1/3 cup) | 10.1 |
| Bran Chex (2/3 cup) | 5 |
| Bran flakes (2/3 cup) | 5 |
| Cheerios (1 1/4 cup) | 3 |
| Corn flakes (1 cup) | 1 |
| Grape-nuts (1 1/4 cup) | 2 |
| Life (2/3 cup) | 3 |
| Raisin Bran (1/2 cup) | 4 |
| Rice Krispies (1 cup) | Trace |
| Shredded Wheat (1 biscuit) | 3 |
| **Vegetables** | |
| Baked potato, with skin | 4.4 |
| Carrot | 2.0 |
| Cauliflower (1/2 cup) | 1.3 |
| Corn, canned (1/2 cup) | 6.3 |
| Garbanzo beans (1 cup) | 8.6 |
| Green beans (1 cup) | 3.1 |
| Greens (1 cup) | 2.9 |
| Lima beans (1 cup) | 9.2 |
| Navy beans (1 cup) | 16.5 |
| Split peas (1 cup) | 16.4 |
| Tomato | 2.2 |

day with a high-fiber cereal is another convenient way to increase your consumption not only of fiber but also of many vitamins and minerals. Check food labels, which identify the amount of fiber per serving.

As with most other nutrients, fiber can be consumed in excess. Indiscriminate consumption of fiber may interfere with the body's ability to absorb other essential nutrients. A person who eats bulky foods but has only a small capacity may not be able to take in enough food energy or nutrients. A high intake of dietary fiber, such as 60 grams per day, also requires a high intake of water.[142]

## Putting Nutrition to Work

Nutrition is a complex science and involves the study of thousands of nutrients and a countless number of possible interactions, all of which take place at the cellular level. Many of the results of nutritional practices, good or bad, take years or even decades to become apparent. Fortunately, it isn't necessary to be a biochemist to understand and follow nutritional practices that promote health and prevent the early onset of many health problems. The benchmark for developing a plan for good nutrition is *Dietary Guidelines for Americans*.[143]

Which are based on the simple assumption that good health means getting nutrients from food. Food comprises thousands of natural plant chemicals that interact with vitamins and minerals in ways that promote health and prevent many chronic diseases. Dietary approaches that focus on a single nutrient or on supplements, to the exclusion of the vast array of foods in the various food groups, are the antithesis of good nutrition. While dietary supplements may be useful and even recommended in some instances, they cannot replace a healthy diet.

*Dietary Guidelines* offers 41 recommendations that are grouped in nine categories (see Just the Facts: *Dietary Guidelines for Americans*). These recommendations serve as the framework of a plan for good nutrition.

## Aim for a Healthy Weight

A healthy weight is key to a long, healthy life. To be at their best, adults need to avoid gaining weight, and many need to lose weight. Being obese increases the risk for many chronic diseases. The principle behind weight management is simple: balance calories consumed with calories expended. To lose weight, decrease intake of calories and increase physical activity. Adhering to this principle is difficult for most Americans and is influenced by complex issues. For a complete discussion of the principles of weight management and desirable body composition, refer to Chapters 7 and 8.

## Adopt a Physically Active Lifestyle

To promote health and reduce the risk of chronic disease, aim for a physically active lifestyle. Adults should engage in at least 150 minutes (2 hours and 30 minutes) a week of moderate-intensity physical activity. In addition, adults should participate in muscle-strengthening activities at least two times a week (see physical activity guidelines in Chapter 1, page xx, and Just the Facts: Light-Intensity vs. Moderate-Intensity vs. Vigorous-Intensity Physical Activity, in Chapter 1, page 14).

Choose activities that you enjoy and that you can do regularly. Some people prefer activities that fit into their daily routine, such as gardening or taking extra trips up and down stairs. Others prefer a regular exercise program, such as a physical activity program at their worksite. Some do both. All contribute to an active lifestyle. The important thing is to be physically active every day. The more exercise you get, the better. If you don't get any exercise at all, any amount of physical activity will yield health benefits. Incorporate physical activity into your lifestyle, so that it is fun and sustainable. If you are already physically active, the goal is one of maintenance and consistency.

The benefits of exercise are discussed throughout this text; specific principles and applications of exercise and physical activity are discussed in depth in Chapters 3, 4, and 5.

## Choose Nutrient-Dense Foods Within Calorie Needs

**Nutrient-dense foods** are foods that provide substantial amounts of vitamins and minerals and relatively few calories.[145] Conversely, foods that are low in nutrient density supply calories but little or no nutrients. Americans' propensity for foods that are low in nutrients and high in calories is a major contributing factor to the obesity epidemic. If nutrient-dense foods are chosen wisely and consistently, there is a small allowance for discretionary calories. **Discretionary calories** refer to the amount of energy allowed in a diet after meeting overall nutrition needs.[146] Usually, this refers to foods rich in fat and/or sugar. Stated another way, discretionary calories are the "pleasure calories." Discretionary calories provide some flexibility to consume small amounts of calories in foods and beverages such as desserts, alcohol, and snack foods, assuming, of course, that nutrient-dense foods are the hallmark of the diet. (See Just the Facts: Nutrient Density on page 198.)

The best way to ensure a nutrient-dense diet is to use one of the two diet plans recommended by *Dietary Guidelines*: USDA Food Guide and the DASH (Dietary Approaches to Stop Hypertension) Eating Plan (see Real-World Wellness: What Is the Essence of the New Recommendations in *Dietary Guidelines for Americans 2005*?). While both plans provide a balanced diet consistent with the *Dietary Guidelines*, the USDA Food Guide serves as the foundation for this chapter. Neither the DASH nor the USDA Food Guide is presented as a weight-loss plan. Instead, they are eating plans that provide nutrient-dense foods in the right amounts and in the right proportions according to a range of calorie

# [ JUST THE FACTS ]

## Dietary Guidelines for Americans 2005[144]

*Dietary Guidelines for Americans 2005* presents 41 recommendations, grouped in 9 categories, 18 of which address the needs of specific population groups.

### Weight Management (Aim for a Healthy Weight)

**Key Recommendations**
- To maintain body weight in a healthy range, balance calories from foods and beverages with calories expended.
- To prevent gradual weight gain over time, make small decreases in food and beverage calories and increase physical activity.

**Key Recommendations for Specific Population Groups**
- *Those who need to lose weight.* Aim for a slow, steady weight loss by decreasing calorie intake while maintaining an adequate nutrient intake and increasing physical activity.
- *Overweight children.* Reduce the rate of body weight gain while allowing growth and development. Consult a health care provider before placing a child on a weight-reduction diet.
- *Pregnant women.* Ensure appropriate weight gain as specified by a health care provider.
- *Breast-feeding women.* Moderate weight reduction is safe and does not compromise weight gain of the nursing infant.
- *Overweight adults and overweight children with chronic diseases and/or on medication.* Consult a health care provider about weight loss strategies prior to starting a weight-reduction program to ensure appropriate management of other health conditions.

### Physical Activity (Adopt a Physically Active Lifestyle)

**Key Recommendations**
- Engage in regular physical activity and reduce sedentary activities to promote health, psychological well-being, and a healthy body weight.
  - To reduce the risk of chronic disease in adulthood: Engage in at least 30 minutes of moderate-intensity physical activity, above usual activity, at work or home on most days of the week.
  - For most people, greater health benefits can be obtained by engaging in physical activity of more vigorous intensity or longer duration.
  - To help manage body weight and prevent gradual, unhealthy body weight gain in adulthood: Engage in approximately 60 minutes of moderate- to vigorous intensity activity on most days of the week while not exceeding caloric intake requirements.
  - To sustain weight loss in adulthood: Participate in at least 60 to 90 minutes of daily moderate-intensity physical activity while not exceeding caloric intake requirements. Some people may need to consult with a health care provider before participating in this level of activity.
- Achieve physical fitness by including cardiovascular conditioning, stretching exercises for flexibility, and resistance exercises or calisthenics for muscle strength and endurance.

**Key Recommendations for Specific Population Groups**
- *Children and adolescents.* Engage in at least 60 minutes of physical activity on most, preferably all, days of the week.
- *Pregnant women.* In the absence of medical or obstetric complications, incorporate 30 minutes or more of moderate-intensity physical activity on most, if not all, days of the week. Avoid activities with a high risk of falling or abdominal trauma.
- *Breast-feeding women.* Be aware that neither acute nor regular exercise adversely affects the mother's ability to successfully breast-feed.
- *Older adults.* Participate in regular physical activity to reduce functional declines associated with aging and to achieve the other benefits of physical activity identified for all adults.

### Adequate Nutrients Within Calorie Needs (Choose Nutrient-Dense Foods Within Calorie Needs)

**Key Recommendations**
- Consume a variety of nutrient-dense foods and beverages within and among the basic food groups while choosing foods that limit the intake of saturated and trans fats, cholesterol, added sugars, salt, and alcohol.
- Meet recommended intakes within energy needs by adopting a balanced eating pattern, such as the USDA Food Guide or the DASH Eating Plan.

**Key Recommendations for Specific Population Groups**
- *People over age 50.* Consume vitamin $B_{12}$ in its crystalline form (i.e., fortified foods or supplements).
- *Women of childbearing age who may become pregnant.* Eat foods high in heme-iron and/or consume iron-rich plant foods or iron-fortified foods with an enhancer of iron absorption, such as vitamin C–rich foods.

## [ JUST THE **FACTS** ]

### *Dietary Guidelines for Americans 2005*[144]

· *Women of childbearing age who may become pregnant and those in the first trimester of pregnancy.* Consume adequate synthetic folic acid daily (from fortified foods or supplements) in addition to food forms of folate from a varied diet.

· *Older adults, people with dark skin, and people exposed to insufficient ultraviolet band radiation (i.e., sunlight).* Consume extra vitamin D from vitamin D–fortified foods and/or supplements.

#### Carbohydrates (Choose Fiber-Rich Carbohydrates, Especially Whole Grains)

**Key Recommendations**

· Choose fiber-rich fruits, vegetables, and whole grains often.

· Choose and prepare foods and beverages with little added sugars or caloric sweeteners, such as amounts suggested by the USDA Food Guide and the DASH Eating Plan.

· Reduce the incidence of dental caries by practicing good oral hygiene and consuming sugar- and starch-containing foods and beverages less frequently.

#### Food Groups to Encourage (Choose Food Groups Wisely)

**Key Recommendations**

· Consume a sufficient amount of fruits and vegetables while staying within energy needs. Two cups of fruits and 2½ cups of vegetables per day are recommended for a reference 2,000-calorie intake, with higher or lower amounts depending on the calorie level.

· Choose a variety of fruits and vegetables each day. In particular, select from all five vegetable subgroups (dark green, orange, legumes, starchy vegetables, and other vegetables) several times a week.

· Consume three or more ounce-equivalents of whole-grain products per day, with the rest of the recommended grains coming from enriched or whole-grain products. In general, at least half the grains should come from whole grains.

· Consume three cups per day of fat-free or low-fat milk or equivalent milk products.

**Key Recommendations for Specific Population Groups**

· *Children and adolescents.* Consume whole-grain products often; at least half the grains should be whole grains. Children 2 to 8 years should consume 2 cups per day of fat-free or low-fat milk or equivalent milk products. Children 9 years of age

and older should consume 3 cups per day of fat-free or low-fat milk or equivalent milk products.

#### Food Safety (Keep Food Safe to Eat)

**Key Recommendations**

· To avoid microbial foodborne illness:
  · Clean hands, food contact surfaces, and fruits and vegetables. Meat and poultry should not be washed or rinsed.
  · Separate raw, cooked, and ready-to-eat foods while shopping, preparing, or storing foods.
  · Cook foods to a safe temperature to kill microorganisms.
  · Chill (refrigerate) perishable food promptly and defrost foods properly.
  · Avoid raw (unpasteurized) milk or any products made from unpasteurized milk, raw or partially cooked eggs or foods containing raw eggs, raw or undercooked meat and poultry, unpasteurized juices, and raw sprouts.

**Key Recommendations for Specific Population Groups**

· *Infants and young children, pregnant women, older adults, and those who are immunocompromised.* Do not eat or drink raw (unpasteurized) milk or any products made from unpasteurized milk, raw or partially cooked eggs or foods containing raw eggs, raw or undercooked meat and poultry, raw or undercooked fish or shellfish, unpasteurized juices, and raw sprouts.

· *Pregnant women, older adults, and those who are immunocompromised:* Only eat certain deli meats and frankfurters that have been reheated to steaming hot.

#### Fats (Choose the Right Fats)

**Key Recommendations**

· Consume less than 10% of calories from saturated fatty acids and less than 300 mg/day of cholesterol, and keep trans fatty acid consumption as low as possible.

· Keep total fat intake between 20 and 35% of calories, with most fats coming from sources of polyunsaturated and monounsaturated fatty acids, such as fish, nuts, and vegetable oils.

· When selecting and preparing meat, poultry, dry beans, and milk or milk products, make choices that are lean, low-fat, or fat-free.

· Limit intake of fats and oils high in saturated and/or trans fatty acids, and choose products low in such fats and oils.

**Key Recommendations for Specific Population Groups**

• *Children and adolescents.* Keep total fat intake between 30 and 35% of calories for children 2 to 3 years of age and between 25 and 35% of calories for children and adolescents 4 to 18 years of age, with most fats coming from sources of polyunsaturated and monounsaturated fatty acids, such as fish, nuts, and vegetable oils.

## Sodium and Potassium (Choose Less Sodium and More Potassium)

### Key Recommendations

• Consume less than 2,300 mg (approximately 1 tsp. of salt) of sodium per day.
• Choose and prepare foods with little salt. At the same time, consume potassium-rich foods, such as fruits and vegetables.

### Key Recommendations for Specific Population Groups

• *Individuals with hypertension, blacks, and middle-aged and older adults.* Aim to consume no more than 1,500 mg of sodium per day, and meet the potassium recommendation (4,700 mg/day) with food.

## Alcoholic Beverages (If You Drink Alcoholic Beverages, Do So in Moderation)

### Key Recommendations

• Those who choose to drink alcoholic beverages should do so sensibly and in moderation—defined as the consumption of up to one drink per day for women and up to two drinks per day for men.
• Alcoholic beverages should not be consumed by some individuals, including those who cannot restrict their alcohol intake, women of childbearing age who may become pregnant, pregnant and lactating women, children and adolescents, individuals taking medications that can interact with alcohol, and those with specific medical conditions.
• Alcoholic beverages should be avoided by individuals engaging in activities that require attention, skill, or coordination, such as driving or operating machinery.

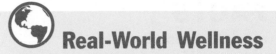

## Real-World Wellness

### What Is the Essence of the Recommendations in *Dietary Guidelines for Americans 2005*?

Dietary Guidelines *includes 41 recommendations. For the average person, that's too much to remember. Can these guidelines be reduced to a simple statement?*

While there is a risk in trying to simplify a complex subject, if the dietary guidelines were to be captured in a single statement, it would be to "eat nutrient-dense foods such as fruits, vegetables, and whole grains, switch to monounsaturated and polyunsaturated fats in place of saturated and trans fat, limit added sugar and salt, and keep calories under control." Of course, this is easier said than done. Applying some basic principles, as presented in this chapter, should move you in the right direction.

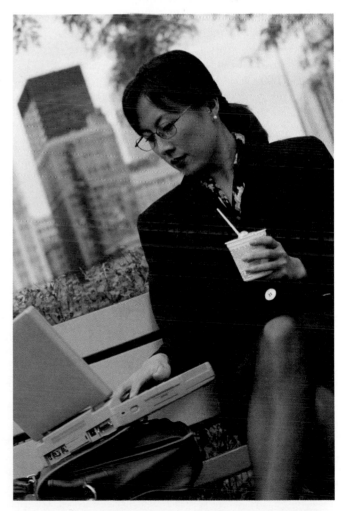

Starting your day with low-fat dairy products, such as milk and yogurt, is a good way to add calcium to your diet.

# [ JUST THE ] FACTS

### Nutrient Density

A key strategy for eating well is to select foods that offer significant amounts of nutrients but small numbers of calories. If a particular food has a high ratio of nutrients to calories, it is a nutritionally dense food. You can determine the nutrient density of food by adding the percentages of the RDA for the essential nutrients and dividing by the number of calories per serving (see the following example). The higher the score, the higher the nutrient density. The concept of nutrient density can help the health-conscious and weight-conscious person make informed choices.

Calculating the Nutrient Density of Pizza (Cheese)

| Calories | RDA % | 354 |
|---|---|---|
| Protein | 28 | |
| Vitamin A | 19 | |
| Vitamin C | 20 | |
| Thiamin | 25 | |
| Riboflavin | 29 | |
| Niacin | 19 | |
| Calcium | 33 | |
| Iron | 15 | |
| **Total** | | **188** |

**Nutrient density = 53%** (188 ÷ 354 × 100)

levels. Most dietary recommendations presented in this chapter are based on a 2,000-calorie diet. The appropriate calorie level for an individual is influenced by age, gender, activity level, health status, and whether or not weight loss is a goal. (See Wellness for a Lifetime: The Nutrient Gap on page 200.) Table 6-8 estimates the calorie level according to age, gender, and activity level.

MyPyramid embraces physically active lifestyles and eating a variety of foods in moderation.

The USDA Food Guide portrays dietary guidelines in picture form in MyPyramid: Steps to a Healthier You (see Figure 6-2 on page 199). MyPyramid is actually 12 pyramids geared to different lifestyles and nutritional needs. Consumers can determine MyPyramid's recommendations for their individual lifestyle by going to **http://mypyramid.gov** (see Just the Facts: Dietary Guidelines: Just One Click Away on page 199).

**Variety.** Variety is one of the major themes of MyPyramid (see Just the Facts: Variety: The Cornerstone of a Healthy Diet on page 202). It is symbolized by the six color bands, each representing one of the five basic

**TABLE 6-8** Estimated Calories[a] to Maintain Energy Balance (Rounded to the Nearest 200 Calories)

| Gender | Age (years) | Activity Level Sedentary[b] | Moderately Active[c] | Active[d] |
|---|---|---|---|---|
| Child (male and female) | 2–3 | 1,000 | 1,000–1,400[e] | 1,000–1,400[e] |
| Female | 4–8 | 1,200 | 1,400–1,600 | 1,400–1,800 |
| | 9–13 | 1,600 | 1,600–2,000 | 1,800–2,200 |
| | 14–18 | 1,800 | 2,000 | 2,400 |
| | 19–30 | 2,000 | 2,000–2,200 | 2,400 |
| | 31–50 | 1,800 | 2,000 | 2,200 |
| | 51+ | 1,600 | 1,800 | 2,000–2,200 |
| Male | 4–8 | 1,400 | 1,400–1,600 | 1,600–2,000 |
| | 9–13 | 1,800 | 1,800–2,200 | 2,000–2,600 |
| | 14–18 | 2,200 | 2,400–2,800 | 2,800–3,200 |
| | 19–30 | 2,400 | 2,600–2,800 | 3,000 |
| | 31–50 | 2,200 | 2,400–2,600 | 2,800–3,000 |
| | 51+ | 2,000 | 2,200–2,400 | 2,400–2,800 |

[a]Based on estimated energy requirements using the Institute of Medicine Equation.

[b]Sedentary means less than 30 minutes a day of moderate physical activity in addition to daily activities.

[c]Moderately active means at least 30 minutes a day of moderate physical activity in addition to daily activities.

[d]Active means 60 or more minutes a day of moderate physical activity in addition to daily activities.

[e]Calorie ranges accommodate needs of different ages within the group. For children and adolescents, more calories are needed at older ages. For adults, fewer calories are needed at older ages.

source: U.S. Department of Health and Human Services, U.S. Department of Agriculture. (2005). Dietary Guidelines for Americans 2005. Washington, DC: U.S. Government Printing Office.

## [ JUST THE FACTS ]

### Dietary Guidelines: Just One Click Away

*MyPyramid.gov* makes it easy to personalize dietary guidelines. Go to www.mypyramid.gov, (choose link: Get a personalized plan), enter age, gender, and physical activity level, and click on "submit." Within a few seconds your personalized Pyramid plan appears with recommended amounts and kinds of foods from each food group. Experiment with different physical activity levels to determine their effects on dietary recommendations. *MyPyramid Tracker*, one of the links on the home page of mypyramid.gov, provides additional information on the quality of your diet, physical activity status, related

nutrition messages, and links to nutrient and physical activity information. Click on other links to get a meal tracking worksheet, a list of foods contained in each food group, diet tips, and much more. Finally, click on *Inside MyPyramid* to learn about the food groups and to see how much physical activity you should be getting.

Another Pyramid is available for children and is called MyPyramid for Kids and Pre-schoolers. Developed for children, parents, and teachers, this resource is also online at www.mypyramid.gov/kids/index.html.

## Anatomy of MyPyramid

### One size doesn't fit all

USDA's new MyPyramid symbolizes a personalized approach to healthy eating and physical activity. The symbol has been designed to be simple. It has been developed to remind consumers to make healthy food choices and to be active every day. The different parts of the symbol are described below.

**Activity**
Activity is represented by the steps and the person climbing them, as a reminder of the importance of daily physical activity.

**Moderation**
Moderation is represented by the narrowing of each food group from bottom to top. The wider base stands for foods with little or no solid fats or added sugars. These should be selected more often. The narrower top area stands for foods containing more added sugars and solid fats. The more active you are, the more of these foods can fit into your diet.

**Personalization**
Personalization is shown by the person on the steps, the slogan, and the URL. Find the kinds and amounts of food to eat each day at MyPyramid.gov.

**Proportionality**
Proportionality is shown by the different widths of the food group bands. The widths suggest how much food a person should choose from each group. The widths are just a general guide, not exact proportions. Check the Web site for how much is right for you.

**Variety**
Variety is symbolized by the 6 color bands representing the 5 food groups of the Pyramid and oils. This illustrates that foods from all groups are needed each day for good health.

**Gradual Improvement**
Gradual improvement is encouraged by the slogan. It suggests that individuals can benefit from taking small steps to improve their diet and lifestyle each day.

# MyPyramid.gov
## STEPS TO A HEALTHIER YOU

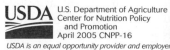

U.S. Department of Agriculture
Center for Nutrition Policy and Promotion
April 2005 CNPP-16
*USDA is an equal opportunity provider and employer.*

| GRAINS | VEGETABLES | FRUITS | OILS | MILK | MEAT & BEANS |

**FIGURE 6-2**  *My Pyramid* presents in picture form the dietary recommendations of the *USDA Food Guide*: it replaces the *Food Guide Pyramid* that was introduced to consumers in the early 1990s.

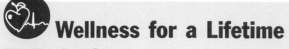

## Wellness for a Lifetime

### The Nutrient Gap

It has been estimated that as many as 25 percent of Americans 60 and older are malnourished. They do not suffer from nutritional diseases, such as scurvy or pellagra; rather, they consume insufficient amounts of key nutrients that have a direct effect on health and body function. Older adults usually expend less energy to meet the demands of their lifestyle than do their younger peers and therefore require fewer calories. This presents a dilemma because, as their need for energy decreases, their need for nutrients increases or stays the same. Unfortunately, a decrease in caloric intake is usually associated with a decrease in key nutrients. There is a gap between what older adults need and what they get from food, as shown in the table below.[154] Older adults, especially those who are 70 years old or older, should discuss with their health care provider the idea of taking supplements for the nutrients listed.[155]

| Nutrient | What They Need (Age 50+) | How They're Doing | Why Adults Age 50+ Need It |
|---|---|---|---|
| Calcium | 1,200 mg | The average intake is 400–600 mg. | The capacity to absorb calcium declines with age. |
| Folate | 400 µg | Only one-fourth of older adults get 400 µg. | Reducing homocysteine levels becomes more important as heart disease risks increase. |
| Riboflavin | 1.1 mg, women 1.3 mg, men | Only one-third get enough. | The body's need is the same throughout adulthood. |
| Vitamin $B_6$ | 1.5 mg, women 1.7 mg, men | 50–90% don't get enough. | The body's metabolism changes with age. |
| Vitamin $B_{12}$ | 2.4 µg | 20% of adults over 60 and 40% over 80 are deficient. | Increased difficulty in absorbing vitamin $B_{12}$ comes with age. |
| Vitamin D | 400 IU, ages 51–69 600 IU, 70+ | The average intake is 100–125 IU. | Decreased ability of skin to synthesize vitamin D from sunlight comes with age. |

food groups: grains, vegetables, fruits, milk, and meat and beans.[147] Oils are also depicted in MyPyramid, although they are not a food group.

- **Grain Group:** The largest area of MyPyramid is the grain group and includes foods made from wheat, rice, oats, cornmeal, and barley, such as bread, pasta, oatmeal, breakfast cereals, tortillas, and grits. In general, 1 slice of bread, 1 cup of ready-to-eat cereal, or ½ cup of cooked rice, pasta, or cooked cereal can be considered as 1-ounce equivalents from the grains group. At least half of all grains consumed should be whole grains.
- **Vegetable Group:** Includes all fresh, frozen, canned, and dried vegetables and vegetable juices. In general, 1 cup of raw or cooked vegetables or vegetable juice, or 2 cups of raw leafy greens can be considered as 1 cup from the vegetable group.
- **Fruit Group:** Includes all fresh, frozen, canned, and dried fruits and fruit juices. In general, 1 cup of fruit or 100% fruit juice, or 1/2 cup of dried fruit can be considered as 1 cup from the fruit group.
- **Milk Group:** Includes all milks, yogurts, frozen yogurts, dairy desserts, and cheeses (except cream cheese). Lactose-free and lactose-reduced products are included in this food group. Most choices should be fat-free or low-fat. A serving of milk is 1 cup of milk or yogurt, 1½ ounces of natural cheese such as cheddar cheese, or 2 ounces of processed cheese. Discretionary calories are counted for all choices, except fat-free milk.
- **Meat and Beans Group:** Includes meat, poultry, fish, dry beans and peas, eggs, nuts, and seeds. Most choices should be lean or low-fat. Dry beans and peas and soybean products are part of this group as well as the vegetable group, but should be counted in one group only. In general, 1 ounce of lean meat, poultry, or fish, 1 egg, 1 tbsp. peanut butter, ¼ cup cooked dry beans, or ½ ounce of nuts or seeds can be considered as 1-ounce equivalents.

Suggested amounts of food to consume from the basic food groups are presented according to 12 different calorie levels (see Table 6-9 on page 201). Together, fruits and vegetables make up nearly 40% of the recommended diet. For example, someone on a 2,000-calorie food plan should consume 2 cups of fruits and 2½ cups of vegetables. This is equivalent to 9 servings of fruits and vegetables. The vegetable group is further divided into subgroups with weekly recommendations for dark green vegetables, orange vegetables, legumes,

**TABLE 6-9**   USDA Food Guide

**Daily Amount of Food from Each Group**

| Calorie Level | 1,000 | 1,200 | 1,400 | 1,600 | 1,800 | 2,000 | 2,200 | 2,400 | 2,600 | 2,800 | 3,000 | 3,200 |
|---|---|---|---|---|---|---|---|---|---|---|---|---|
| Fruits | 1 cup | 1 cup | 1.5 cups | 1.5 cups | 2 cups | 2 cups | 2 cups | 2.5 cups | 2.5 cups | 2.5 cups | 2.5 cups | 2.5 cups |
| Vegetables | 1 cup | 1.5 cups | 1.5 cups | 2 cups | 2.5 cups | 2.5 cups | 3 cups | 3 cups | 3.5 cups | 3.5 cups | 4 cups | 4 cups |
| Grains | 3 oz-eq | 4 oz-eq | 5 oz-eq | 5 oz-eq | 6 oz-eq | 6 oz-eq | 7 oz-eq | 8 oz-eq | 9 oz-eq | 10 oz-eq | 10 oz-eq | 10 oz-eq |
| Meat and Beans | 2 oz-eq | 3 oz-eq | 4 oz-eq | 5 oz-eq | 5 oz-eq | 5.5 oz-eq | 6 oz-eq | 6.5 oz-eq | 6.5 oz-eq | 7 oz-eq | 7 oz-eq | 7 oz-eq |
| Milk | 2 cups | 2 cups | 2 cups | 3 cups | 3 cups | 3 cups | 3 cups | 3 cups | 3 cups | 3 cups | 3 cups | 3 cups |
| Oils | 3 tsp | 4 tsp | 4 tsp | 5 tsp | 5 tsp | 6 tsp | 6 tsp | 7 tsp | 8 tsp | 8 tsp | 10 tsp | 11 tsp |
| Discretionary calorie allowance | 165 | 171 | 171 | 132 | 195 | 267 | 290 | 362 | 410 | 426 | 512 | 648 |

**Vegetable Subgroup Amounts Are per Week**

| Calorie Level | 1,000 | 1,200 | 1,400 | 1,600 | 1,800 | 2,000 | 2,200 | 2,400 | 2,600 | 2,800 | 3,000 | 3,200 |
|---|---|---|---|---|---|---|---|---|---|---|---|---|
| Dark green veg. | 1 c/wk | 1.5 c/wk | 1.5 c/wk | 2 c/wk | 3 c/wk | 3 c/wk | 3 c/wk | 3 c/wk | 3 c/wk | 3 c/wk | 3 c/wk | 3 c/wk |
| Orange veg. | .5 c/wk | 1 c/wk | 1 c/wk | 1.5 c/wk | 2 c/wk | 2 c/wk | 2 c/wk | 2 c/wk | 2.5 c/wk | 2.5 c/wk | 2.5 c/wk | 2.5 c/wk |
| Legumes | .5 c/wk | 1 c/wk | 1 c/wk | 2.5 c/wk | 3 c/wk | 3 c/wk | 3 c/wk | 3 c/wk | 3.5 c/wk | 3.5 c/wk | 3.5 c/wk | 3.5 c/wk |
| Starchy veg. | 1.5 c/wk | 2.5 c/wk | 2.5 c/wk | 2.5 c/wk | 3 c/wk | 3 c/wk | 6 c/wk | 6 c/wk | 7 c/wk | 7 c/wk | 9 c/wk | 9 c/wk |
| Other veg. | 3.5 c/wk | 4.5 c/wk | 4.5 c/wk | 5.5 c/wk | 6.5 c/wk | 6.5 c/wk | 7 c/wk | 7 c/wk | 8.5 c/wk | 8.5 c/wk | 10 c/wk | 10 c/wk |

Source: U.S. Department of Health and Human Services. (2005). *Dietary guidelines for Americans 2005.* Washington, DC: U.S. Government Printing Office.

Many studies link a specific nutrient to good health. But the study of an isolated nutrient, when removed from its original food source, often yields misleading results and sometimes does more harm than good. For example, beta-carotene has long been reputed as a nutrient that prevents lung cancer. In a famous 1994 study, however, male smokers who took a 20-mg supplement of beta-carotene surprisingly ended up with a higher incidence of lung cancer than the placebo group. As a result, the study was stopped midstream. Researchers concluded that, if beta-carotene prevents and/or delays lung cancer, it does so in combination with other foods.

The only sure way to realize the benefits of various nutrients is to eat a variety of foods. No single nutrient or food can supply all of the essential nutrients in the right proportion needed by the body. Variety is the essence of a healthy diet and may be the only practical way of making sure you're getting the full healthful effects of various nutrients.

and starchy vegetables. The grain group makes up 25% of the recommended diet. Together, fruits, vegetables, and grains make up approximately two-thirds of the USDA Food Guide and reinforce the concept that a healthy food plan emphasizes a varied plant-based diet.

**Moderation.** Moderation is another important characteristic of the healthy diet. There is a place in the diet for almost any food if it is consumed prudently—the Food Guide doesn't label food "good" or "bad." Moderation means exercising good judgment regarding quantity and frequency. It doesn't mean avoidance. The idea that a particular food is good or bad can be destructive to anyone trying to eat more healthfully. For example, a person with rigid attitudes who thinks that cheesecake is "bad" and then indulges in eating it might think, I am bad, I have no willpower, and I am a weak person. The behavioral result might be a cheesecake binge, because the forbidden nature of the food makes it harder to resist. A more positive approach is to understand that cheesecake is not "bad" and that eating a slice does not make the eater a bad person.

Another reason for moderation is that even nutritionally dense foods can be consumed in excess. The interaction of the various substances in food can cause one nutrient to overpower or nullify the effects and benefits of another. The body's processes may be compromised or the nutrients in foods may interfere with the desired effects of medicines. Following are several examples of the negative effects of excessive consumption of various nutrients:

- Too much protein from animal sources may cause the body to lose extra calcium.[148]
- Botanicals such as garlic, ginger, and ginseng, when combined with vitamin E, fish oils, or blood-thinning medicines (e.g., aspirin, Coumadin), may inhibit the blood-clotting mechanism of the body and cause internal bleeding.[149]
- Megadoses of vitamin A can cause birth defects.
- Megadoses of vitamin C can cause diarrhea and stomach inflammation.[150]
- Excessive intake of vitamin D may cause overabsorption of calcium and lead to calcium deposits in the kidneys and other organs. Calcium deposits in organs may lead to cell death.[151]
- High intake of folate may mask the symptoms of pernicious anemia, a condition associated with a vitamin $B_{12}$ deficiency.[152]
- Excess niacin may aggravate glucose intolerance associated with noninsulin-dependent diabetes.
- Foods high in vitamin K, such as broccoli, spinach, and turnip greens, may neutralize the effectiveness of blood-thinning medicines.

These examples are not meant to discourage your consumption of a particular food. Each food offers a unique contribution to health. Vitamin D, for instance, is required for calcium metabolism; however, too much of it may result in a depletion of calcium. Moderation is an important concept that applies to essential nutrients, just as it applies to nutrients with bad reputations. Choosing foods from the Food Guide, with an emphasis on variety and moderation, not only satisfies the body's need for essential nutrients but also helps prevent problems associated with dietary excess.

## Choose Fiber-Rich Carbohydrates, Especially Whole Grains

Grain products (bread, cereal, rice, and oats) help form the foundation of a nutritious diet. They are rich in vitamins, minerals, complex carbohydrates, dietary fiber, and other substances essential for good health. The Food Guide recommends at least six ounces per day for a 2,000-calorie diet.[153] Unrefined, whole-grain foods such as whole-grain bread, pasta, and cereals should be emphasized over refined grain products— white bread, white rice, white flour, and pasta. Refined grains are not good sources of fiber. Remember, it's hard to eat a high-fiber diet that isn't healthy.

Meeting this dietary guideline is a formidable challenge to most Americans. For example, in planning meals, Americans often think first of the entrée, which is typically a meat dish. This is usually true whether we're eating at home or dining out. The Food Guide challenges us to reverse this approach by thinking of plant products first.

**TABLE 6-10**   Types of Vegetarians

| Type | What Is Excluded from Diet | What Is Included in Diet |
|---|---|---|
| Vegans | All animal products | Fruits, vegetables, grains, legumes, nuts, and seeds |
| Lactovegetarians | Eggs, fish, poultry, and meat | Milk products and fruits, vegetables, grains, legumes, nuts, and seeds |
| Ovolactovegetarians | Fish, poultry, and meat | Eggs (*ova*), milk products (*lacto*), fruits, vegetables, grains, legumes, nuts, and seeds |
| Pescovegetarians | Poultry and meat | Fish (*pesco*), eggs, milk products, fruits, vegetables, grains, legumes, nuts, and seeds |
| Pollovegetarians | Red meat | Poultry (*pollo*), fish, eggs, milk products, fruits, vegetables, grains, legumes, nuts, and seeds |
| Semi- or demi-vegetarians | Same as vegan, except meat may be eaten occasionally | Same as vegan |

## The Vegetarian Alternative

The importance of a plant-based approach to eating is evidenced by the fact that a properly planned vegetarian diet is now viewed as a healthful and acceptable way of meeting all nutritional needs. Some vegetarians avoid all animal products, including dairy products, poultry, eggs, and fish. Others include eggs and milk products but exclude fish, poultry, and red meat. There are many variations of vegetarian diet. The more common types are presented in Table 6-10.

With the exception of vegans, most types of vegetarians have little trouble getting all of the essential nutrients, including protein. Milk products, eggs, fish, and poultry are sources of complete, high-quality protein. *Vegans,* who eat all-plant diets, need to be discriminating in their food selections because most plants are sources of incomplete protein. One notable exception, as mentioned earlier, is soy protein. Vegans who don't consume soy products need to combine complementary foods, such as grains and legumes, to obtain all of the essential amino acids.

The nutritional problem most likely to occur in a strict vegetarian diet is a deficiency in vitamin $B_{12}$, which occurs naturally only in animal products. Vegans can get vitamin $B_{12}$ by taking a supplement or consuming food fortified with $B_{12}$. Vitamin D is another potential problem to the vegan if he or she has limited exposure to the sun. Milk products, fortified with vitamin D, are about the only dietary source of vitamin D. However, the body can produce adequate amounts of this vitamin if the skin receives sufficient exposure to sunlight. During periods of limited sunlight exposure, vegans may need to take vitamin D supplements. Other essential nutrients richly supplied by animal products and thus of concern to vegans, such as riboflavin, iron, zinc, and calcium, can be easily derived from a variety of plant sources.

Following are some practical tips for adding fruits, vegetables, and grains to the diet that should be helpful for people opting for a meatless meal, choosing to eat vegetarian for a day, or favoring vegetarianism as a lifestyle:

- Start off the day with fruit juice.
- Add fruit to a salad.
- Serve fruit for dessert.
- Have a smoothie (blend fruit juice, ice, and a banana).
- Add fruit to cereal.
- Eat cereal as a snack.
- Eat vegetable snacks.
- Aim for a colorful plate, with dark green, yellow, and red vegetables.
- Increase the number of vegetables in a salad by adding tomatoes, carrots, cucumbers, peppers, spinach, or broccoli.
- Eat a vegetable pizza.
- Make a soup with leftover vegetables.
- Eat an all-vegetable meal.
- Mix legumes with a salad.
- Try a new fruit or vegetable.
- Top fat-free frozen yogurt with low-fat granola and berries.
- Top salad with whole-wheat cereal.

A properly selected vegetarian diet has many health benefits. Recent reports from the medical community indicate a higher mortality risk for people who consume red meat and a lower incidence of some chronic diseases among vegetarians.[156–159] People who have health conditions associated with diets high in fat and saturated fat and low in folate, carotenoids, phytochemicals, and antioxidants stand to benefit from a plant-based diet.

## Added Sugars

Sugars are carbohydrates and a source of energy (calories). Dietary carbohydrates also include the complex carbohydrates (starch) and dietary fiber. During digestion, all carbohydrates except fiber break down into sugars.[160] Americans eat sugars in many forms, and most people enjoy the taste of sugars. Some sugars are used as natural preservatives, thickeners, and baking aids in foods. Most of the simple sugar eaten by Americans has been added to foods and beverages during processing and manufacturing. A food is likely to be high in sugars if one of the following is listed first or second in the ingredients list on a food label: brown sugar, corn sweetener, corn syrup, fructose, fruit juice concentrate, glucose (dextrose), high-fructose corn syrup, honey, invert sugar, lactose, maltose, molasses, raw sugar, sucrose (table sugar), or syrup. Many foods contain a combination of sugars.

The World Health Organization recommends that added sugars comprise no more than 10% of total calories. The Food and Nutrition Board sets an upper limit of 25%. The American Heart Association offers even more stringent recommendations. It recommends that sugars added in processing, cooking, or at the table should not total more than 100 calories a day for women and 150 calories a day for men. This is roughly the amount of sugar in a 12-ounce can of sweetened cola.[161] Americans get 16% of their calories from added sugars.[162] This translates to about 66 pounds of added sugar annually per person.

An excess intake of added sugars compromises a healthy diet and is linked to obesity-related diseases.[163] The presence of added sugar in the diet is accompanied by an increase in the number of Americans who are overweight or obese. When people consume food or beverages high in added sugars, they tend to consume more calories and fewer nutrients. In the Food Guide, added sugars comprise a portion of discretionary. A person on a 2,000-calorie diet is limited to 267 discretionary calories, assuming that calories from other food groups stay within recommended levels. Given the ubiquity of super-size meals and especially beverages, keeping discretionary calories in the form of added sugar under control is a major challenge for many Americans. This is a problem as noted by a prominent nutrition newsletter that labeled sugared soft drinks "liquid candy" and the quintessential junk food—just sugar calories and no nutrients.[164] Americans consume far more calories than their peers of 40 years ago, and soft drinks and fruit drinks account for 70% of this increase.[165]

The intake of added sugars is associated with dental caries (cavities).[166] The main offenders are sweet and gummy foods. They stick to the teeth and supply bacteria with a steady source of carbohydrate from which to make acids that can dissolve tooth enamel. Foods that promote caries are termed *cariogenic*.

Contrary to popular belief, there is little or no evidence that high sugar intake causes hyperactivity in children, heart disease, diabetes, or obesity.[167,168] If that were the case, most Americans would have all of these

conditions. The major nutritional problem of a high-sugar diet occurs when sugar is substituted for more nutritionally dense foods. When this happens, the result may be insufficient vitamin and mineral intake.

## Sugar Intake, Glycemic Index, Glycemic Load

Some health experts are exploring the relationship between blood sugar and chronic diseases from a different angle. It has been observed that sugar and starch cause a surge of glucose into the bloodstream. The glucose, in turn, stimulates the pancreas to make insulin, the hormone that converts glucose to energy. Chronically high insulin levels are linked to high blood triglycerides, increased fat deposition, increased tendency for blood to clot, and a more rapid return of hunger after a meal. Eventually, the body may develop a resistance to its own insulin and lead to Type 2 diabetes in some people.[169] The **Glycemic Index (GI)** reflects how much sugar and starches are in food. More specifically, it is a measure of how much blood sugar rises 2 hours after eating 50 grams of that food.[170] Foods with a high GI typically are high in sugars and starches and cause a rapid surge in blood sugar compared to foods with a lower GI.[171] A 50-gram serving of glucose or white bread has a GI of 100.[172] Most foods have a GI between 10 and 92.[173] A major limitation of GIs is that they don't provide comparisons of foods in terms of the way they are consumed. **Glycemic Load (GL)** is based on the same concept but takes into account how much food is usually eaten. For that reason, GL is regarded as a more realistic measure of a food's effect on blood sugar surges. GLs usually range between 1 and 35.[174] Like GIs, the lower the GL, the less likely the food will prompt a quick surge in blood sugar. From a health perspective, our diets should favor foods with a low GI and/or low GL. As a general rule, the more processed the food, the higher the GI or GL[175,176] (see Just the Facts: Strategies for Lowering Glycemic Index or Glycemic Load). However, as a way to lose weight, the jury is still out on low-GL diets despite all the claims in the popular literature.[177] GI and GL values are not included on food labels because there are many complicating factors involved in carbohydrate metabolism. But the Glycemic Load does give a more complete picture of a food's effect on blood sugar levels and eventually may turn out to be a more useful concept than is the chemical classification of carbohydrate as simple or complex, or as sugars or starches.

## Choose Food Groups Wisely

Fruits and vegetables are key parts of a nutritious diet. To promote health, at least 2 cups of fruits and 2½ cups of vegetables should be consumed daily for a person on a 2,000-calorie food plan. In general, 1 cup of fruits or vegetables is equivalent to two servings. The recommendation for fruit and vegetable consumption is nearly double those of previous food plans issued by the USDA. Why the increase? Fruits and vegetables provide essential vitamins and minerals, fiber, phytochemicals, antioxidants, and other substances good for health. They are naturally low in fat and calories and are filling. Some are high in fiber, and many are quick to prepare and easy to eat.

In choosing fruits and vegetables, aim for variety. Try many colors and kinds. The Food Guide recommends that over the course of a week, a minimum of 3 cups of dark green vegetables, 2 cups of orange vegetables, 3 cups of legumes (dried beans), and 3 cups of starchy vegetables should be consumed. That leaves 61/2 of "other" vegetables per week. Choose fresh, frozen, canned, or dried fruits and vegetables. All forms provide vitamins and minerals, and all provide fiber except for most juices.

Most Americans will be challenged to consume recommended amounts of fruits and vegetables. Less than 20% of adults consume 2 to 4 servings of fruit per day,

and less than 30% consume 3 to 5 servings of vegetables per day.[178] It will take a conscious effort to achieve dietary recommendations of this food group—an extra apple as a mid-morning snack, an extra cup of mixed vegetables in your stew, a handful of fruit in your salad. One way to get started is to add fruits and vegetables to the grocery cart so that they are always available at home, work, or school. Even if a combined daily total of 5½ cups of fruits and vegetables seems too ambitious, strive to increase your consumption of these food groups, regardless of amount.

Whole grains represent another important food group and are discussed in a previous section of this chapter. It is sufficient to state that the grain food group is the largest band in MyPyramid.gov and the consumption of whole grains is fundamental to a healthy diet.

Another major source of nutrients is milk and milk products. The Food Guide recommends 3 cups of milk daily for food plans of 1,600 calories or more. Concern about the calories in milk products and possible weight gain should not discourage milk consumption because there are many fat-free and low-fat choices. Lactose-free milk and yogurt are options within the milk food groups for people who are lactose intolerant. The nutrients in milk are important to bone health and contribute to bone mineral content or bone mineral density. Food plans that include milk consumption are associated with overall diet quality and better nutrition.[179]

One way to cultivate a taste for a variety of vegetables and fruits (and grain products) is to acquire a taste for ethnic food. The typical diets of many other countries favor grains, fruits, and vegetables and place less emphasis on animal fats. This may explain why people from Asia have lower rates of most cancers and people from the Mediterranean area have less heart disease.[180] However, watch out for the Americanization of ethnic foods. For example, the traditional Italian pasta dish comes with a tomato-based sauce containing small amounts of meat or meatballs on the side, served with crusty Italian bread or pizza with an extra-thick crust and a mere sprinkle of tomato sauce, herbs, and cheese. Americanized, the same pasta dish comes with less pasta, more creamy sauces, and more meat and is served with buttery garlic toast or pizza with a thin crust, pepperoni, sausage, olives, and extra cheese. For additional comparisons, see Just the Facts: Do You Eat Real Ethnic Food?

## Keep Food Safe to Eat

Americans face a paradox: We are urged to eat more fruits, vegetables, fish, and poultry, but we are warned about contamination and foodborne illness. **Foodborne**

## [ JUST THE FACTS ]

### Do You Eat Real Ethnic Food?

The typical diets of many other countries tend to contain more high-carbohydrate foods and fewer foods high in animal fats than does the common American diet. However, when ethnic foods are prepared in the United States, especially in restaurants, they are often Americanized by the inclusion of larger portions of meat and cheese and the addition of sauces. What follows are descriptions of some traditional, high-carbohydrate ethnic foods and their higher-fat, Americanized versions. Which versions of these ethnic foods do you tend to eat?

*Chinese*

- Traditional: large bowl of steamed rice with small amounts of stir-fried vegetables, meats, and sauces as condiments
- Americanized: several stir-fried or batter-fried entrées in sauces, with a small bowl of fried rice on the side

*German*

- Traditional: large portions of potatoes, rye and whole-grain breads, stew with dumplings, and sauerkraut
- Americanized: fewer potatoes, less bread, more sausage and cheese

*Japanese*

- Traditional: large bowl of steamed rice with broth-based soups containing rice noodles, vegetables, and small amounts of meat

- Americanized: tempura (batter-fried vegetables and shrimp), teriyaki chicken, oriental chicken salad with oil-based dressing

*Italian*

- Traditional: large mound of pasta with tomato-based sauce containing small amounts of meat or meatballs on the side, served with crusty Italian bread or pizza with an extra-thick crust and mere sprinkle of tomato sauce, herbs, and cheese
- Americanized: less pasta, more creamy sauces, and more meat, served with buttery garlic toast or pizza with a thin crust, pepperoni, sausage, olives, and extra cheese

*Mexican*

- Traditional: mostly rice, beans, and warmed tortillas and lots of hot salsa and chiles
- Americanized: crispy fried tortillas, extra ground beef, added cheese, sour cream, and guacamole (avocado dip)

*Middle Eastern*

- Traditional: pita bread (round bread), pilaf (rice dish), hummus (chickpea dip), shaved slices of seasoned meat, diced vegetables, and yogurt-based sauces, all seasoned with garlic
- Americanized: meat kebabs, salads drenched in olive oil, less bread and pilaf

**illness** is a condition caused by eating food that contains harmful bacteria, toxins, parasites, viruses, or chemical contamination (see Just the Facts: Foodborne Illness: Food Sources and Symptoms). Each year, salmonella and campylobacter, the leading bacterial causes of foodborne disease, infect 3.4 million Americans, send 25,500 to hospitals, and cause 500 deaths.[181] In a 2010 analysis of chicken purchased at stores nationwide, only 34% of the tested samples were free of both of these pathogens.[182] Contrary to popular belief, foodborne illnesses are not confined to protein-rich foods such as chicken, beef, pork, seafood, and eggs. Recent outbreaks involving spinach, strawberries, tomatoes, peanut butter, onions, and cantaloupe, some of which were grown organically, confirm the pervasiveness of pathogens even in fresh fruit and produce. Foodborne illnesses are difficult to prevent because they involve different kinds of organisms infecting food of all types grown in many parts of the world and delivered to consumers through national distribution centers.

With the exception of hepatitis A, the organisms that cause foodborne illness are bacterial. For most

of them, treatment consists of hydration and the administration of antibiotics. Other types of organisms are involved in foodborne illnesses. Parasites, such as *Trichinella spiralis* (found in pork and wild game) and tapeworms (found in beef, pork, and fish), also infect many people. The same is true of fungi, which produce mold spores that yield toxins such as aflatoxin.

Most foodborne illnesses can be prevented by observing some basic rules for storing, handling, and preparing food:

- Avoid cross-contamination: Do not prepare foods in an unclean sink and do not allow utensils that have come into contact with an unclean surface to touch food.
- Wash hands when first starting to handle food and after handling garbage or dirty dishes.
- Use separate cloths, sponges, and towels for washing dishes, wiping counters and tabletops, wiping hands, and drying clean dishes.

# [ JUST THE FACTS ]

## Foodborne Illness: Food Sources and Symptoms

Following is a short list of organisms that are common culprits of foodborne illness, along with their food sources and symptoms.

*Staphylococcus* toxins are usually present in meats, poultry, egg products, tuna, potato and macaroni salads, and cream-filled pastries. Symptoms occur 2 to 6 hours after exposure and include diarrhea, vomiting, nausea, and abdominal cramps. Recovery normally takes place in 24 to 36 hours.

*Salmonella* infections are associated with eggs, poultry, meat, dairy products, seafood, and fresh produce. Symptoms usually occur within 6 to 48 hours and include nausea, vomiting, abdominal cramps, diarrhea, fever, headache, and sometimes a rash. *Salmonella* infections may be serious, even fatal, in infants, the elderly, and the sick.

*Clostridium botulinum,* usually referred to as *botulism,* occurs in an anaerobic environment, such as in canned goods, and affects low-acid foods, such as green beans, mushrooms, spinach, olives, and beef. Symptoms occur 12 to 36 hours after exposure and affect the central nervous system. Paralysis and death may follow. Infected food usually has an odor. Avoid canned goods that show any signs of damage.

*Campylobacter jejuni* contamination is linked to raw and undercooked poultry, unpasteurized milk, and untreated water. Symptoms usually occur in 2 to 5 days and include diarrhea, fever, abdominal pain, nausea, headache, and muscle pain. Infections may last 7 to 10 days.

*E. coli* O157:H7 is typically present in undercooked and raw ground beef, raw milk, lettuce, untreated water, and unpasteurized fruit juices. Symptoms include severe abdominal pain and cramping and diarrhea (first watery, then bloody).

*Listeria monocytogenes* is associated with soft cheeses, poultry, fish, and raw meats and vegetables. The illness causes flu-like symptoms, including fever, and may progress to fatal infections of the blood and central nervous system.

*Hepatitis A virus* comes from contaminated fecal material from people who harvest, process, or handle food, including workers on farms, in food-processing plants, and in restaurants. Symptoms, which may not occur for several weeks, include fever, nausea, abdominal discomfort, and sometimes jaundice. The infection is usually mild, though symptoms can be severe.

- Measure the temperature of cooked or held foods to make sure they're hot enough to destroy bacteria (see Figure 6-3 on page 208).
- Do not consume foods whose "use by" dates have expired.
- Transfer leftovers from deep pots and casseroles to shallow pans before refrigeration to speed cooling (and thereby slow bacterial growth).
- Quickly freeze or refrigerate all ground meat and other perishable foods after shopping.
- Wash hands, utensils, and work areas with hot, soapy water after contact with raw meat to keep bacteria from spreading. Also wash your hands after using the bathroom; diapering a child; using the telephone; handling garbage; or touching your face, your hair, or other people.
- Keep the refrigerator temperature below 40° (37 °F is optimal). Keep the freezer at or below 0 °F.
- Wash whole produce. This includes melons and citrus fruits before cutting them open, to prevent the transfer of bacteria from the fruit's skin to the edible part.
- Wash or sanitize cutting boards between each use.
- Store meat products in containers separate from fruits and vegetables.

- Flip steaks with tongs or a spatula rather than with a fork during cooking. Unlike ground beef, in which bacteria are mixed throughout the meat during the grinding process, steak harbors bacteria only on the surface. Sticking a fork into meat before it is cooked injects the interior with bacteria from the outside.
- Cook fish until it flakes with a fork.
- Put your sponge or scouring pad in the dishwasher every time you run it. Or microwave your sponge on high for 30 to 60 seconds.
- Don't store raw foods on the refrigerator shelf above ready-to-eat foods.
- Don't thaw frozen food on the kitchen counter or at room temperature. Thaw frozen food in the refrigerator or microwave.
- Don't eat hamburgers or any other form of ground beef until the juices run yellow, with no trace of pink left. A single hamburger may contain meat from hundreds of animals, creating an increased risk for contamination.[183] (The color of the meat isn't a reliable indicator of doneness. Check the juice.)
- Don't let juice from raw meat, poultry, or fish drip on your hands or any fresh foods in your grocery cart.

- Don't consume unpasteurized milk and juice or foods made with raw eggs.
- Don't use tasting utensils that have touched food under preparation.
- Don't serve or transport cooked food on the plate used for raw meat.
- Don't trust your sense of smell to determine if food is bad. Food that doesn't smell bad can make you sick, and food that smells bad may not necessarily make you sick.[184]
- Don't leave leftovers or perishable food out of the refrigerator for more than 2 hours, even if it doesn't include meat. Bacteria that might be present on foods grow fastest at temperatures between 40 °F and 140 °F and can double in number every 20 minutes. Use cooked, refrigerated leftovers within four days.[185]
- Don't store raw fish in your refrigerator for more than 24 hours. Raw poultry or ground beef will keep for 1 to 2 days and raw red meat for 3 to 5.
- Reheat leftovers thoroughly to at least 165 °F.[186] Avoid coughing or sneezing over foods, even when you're healthy. Cover cuts on hands with a sterile bandage.[187]
- When eating out, do your homework regarding the health inspections of restaurants. Most states require restaurants to post in a visible place their most recent health inspection score. Remember, almost half of foodborne illnessses are linked to restaurant food.[188]

## Choose the Right Fats

Some dietary fat is needed for good health. Fats and oils supply energy and essential fatty acids and promote absorption of the fat-soluble vitamins. Whether from plant or animal sources, fat contains more than twice the number of calories as its carbohydrate and protein equivalents. Fats, the smallest band in MyPyramid, are generically referred to as oils. No more than 6 teaspoons of fats and oils are recommended for a person on a daily food plan of 2,000 calories. Very few Americans have trouble satisfying the body's needs for essential fatty acids. Perhaps one of the greatest shortcomings of the American diet is the abundance of fat, especially saturated fat. Nearly two-thirds of adults are not able to keep their saturated fat consumption under the recommended maximum of 10% of total calories.[189] Compounding this problem is that fat is usually consumed at the expense of fruits, vegetables, and grains.

What are the right fats to choose? Think polyunsaturated and monounsaturated fats. Trans fat consumption should be kept to a minimum. Food labels now make it possible to identify trans fat in packaged foods. For many people, reducing both the amount and the type of dietary fat eaten is a formidable challenge. Table 6-4 on

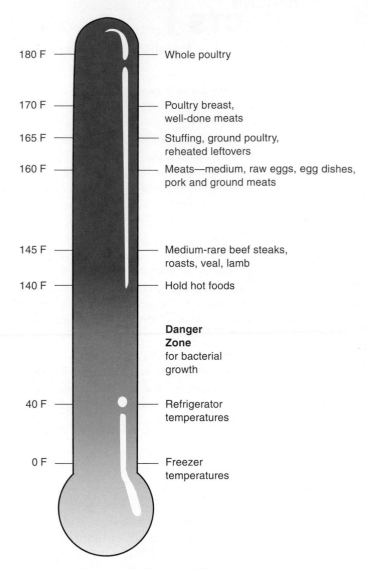

**FIGURE 6-3** How Hot Is Hot Enough?

These recommended safe cooking and storage temperatures are not intended for processing, institutional, or food service preparation.

SOURCE: U.S. Department of Health and Human Services. 2000. *Nutrition and health: Dietary guidelines for Americans.* Washington, DC: U.S. Government Printing Office.

p. 182 presented a quick reference of maximum fat intake for selected caloric intakes. You can estimate your personal maximum fat intake by completing Assessment Activity 6-2. You can learn how fatty your eating habits are by completing Assessment Activity 6-4.

### Tips for Reducing Dietary Fat

The following are some suggestions for reducing total dietary fat consumption, lowering saturated fat intake, and replacing saturated fats with unsaturated fats:

- Assess your fat intake. Complete the assessments at the end of this chapter, along with those in the nutrition software that accompanies this text, to determine your fat intake. Compare your fat intake with the recommendations in Table 6-4.
- Read labels and become familiar with the fat content of food. Try to identify foods that should be consumed in limited amounts; also identify foods that are low in fat (see Table 6-3 on p. 180).
- Become familiar with sources of saturated, monounsaturated, and polyunsaturated fats (see Figure 6-1 on p. 182).
- Check for the presence of trans fatty acids by reading food labels. Look for the word *hydrogenated* or *partially hydrogenated* to identify foods that should be consumed in limited amounts.
- Limit meat, seafood, and poultry to no more than 5 to 7 ounces per day.
- Eat chicken or turkey (without the skin) or fish instead of red meat in most meals.
- Substitute one or two meals of fish per week for red meats. Choose fish high in omega-3 fatty acids and low in saturated fat, such as Atlantic cod, haddock, salmon, shrimp, scallops, sardines, tuna, red snapper, and trout.
- Choose lean cuts of meat, trim all the visible fat, and throw away the fat that cooks out of the meat.
- Substitute meatless or low-meat main dishes for regular entrées.
- Substitute legumes for meat one or two times per week.
- Eat a vegetarian diet at least one day a week.
- Use no more than 6 teaspoons of fats and oils per day for cooking, baking, and preparing salads.
- Choose foods that contain fewer than 3 grams of fat per 100-calorie serving.
- Choose foods that contain less than 1 gram of saturated fat per 100-calorie serving.
- Use low-fat dairy products (whole milk has more than eight times the fat calories of skim milk).
- Substitute pureed fruit, such as applesauce, when cooking from a recipe that calls for cooking oil (equal substitution).
- Use soft margarine in place of hard margarine.
- Use liquid or spray margarine when possible.
- Serve dressings and condiments (for salads, potatoes, etc.) on the side. Try to cut these servings in half.
- Avoid fried foods. Substitute another cooking method (baking, grilling, broiling, or roasting) for frying.
- Eat more vegetables and fruits.
- Eat low-fat foods that have a high satiety value, such as whole grains and high-fiber foods.
- Substitute olive oil or canola oil for margarine, butter, or lard.

- Try to add diversity to your diet. Cultivate a taste for low-fat ethnic foods.
- Avoid a "forbidden fruit" approach to food selection. Any food can be enjoyed in moderation. If you consume an unusually high-fat food or meal, try to compensate with more prudent choices during the week.

## Choose Less Sodium and More Potassium

Salt, also called sodium chloride, contains about 40% sodium by weight and 60% chloride. Sodium and potassium work together in regulating muscle contraction, nerve impulses, and the body's fluid level. Sodium and potassium are electrolytes, meaning they are compounds that are able to conduct an electrical current. As sodium and potassium pass through cells, they create an electrical potential charge that allows muscles to contract and nerve impulses to be conducted.[190] Sodium and potassium also help regulate the body's fluid level, a key factor in blood pressure. For many people, high sodium intake is associated with high blood pressure or hypertension (see Chapter 2); conversely, high potassium intake helps offset the rise in blood pressure caused by sodium intake.[191] This explains why potassium is sometimes referred to as the sodium antidote.[192]

Sodium and potassium are essential nutrients. Most Americans consume too much sodium and too little potassium. Average daily consumption of sodium is 3,500 mg, substantially higher than the recommended intake of 2,300 mg, about 1 teaspoon of salt.[193] The American Heart Association recommends no more than 2,000 mg of sodium per day for people with heart disease. The Centers for Disease Control (CDC) recommends a much more stringent sodium intake, primarily because it estimates that 70% of American adults are at special risk of sodium sensitivity. CDC recommends at-risk adults to consume no more than 1,500 mg of sodium each day.[194]

The majority of sodium consumed is in the form of hidden salt added during the processing of food. Just how much sodium is in a processed food can be determined by reading the package label.

Taste buds cannot always judge salt content. Some foods that taste salty may be lower in salt content than foods that do not. For example, peanuts taste salty because the salt is on the surface where the taste buds immediately detect it. However, cheese contains more salt than peanuts or potato chips, and chocolate pudding contains even more salt. To cut down on salt consumption, you should do the following:

- Avoid adding salt before tasting food.
- Add little or no salt to food at the table.

- Season food with sodium-free spices, such as pepper, allspice, onion powder, garlic, mustard powder, sage, thyme, and paprika.
- Avoid smoked meats and fish.
- Cut down on canned and instant soups.
- Read labels for sodium content, especially on frozen dinners or pizza, processed meat, processed cheese, canned or dried soup, and salad dressing. When shopping for canned and processed foods, select foods with no more than 200 mg of sodium per 100 calories.

Average daily consumption of potassium is 2,000 to 3,000 mg per day, far short of the recommended 4,700 mg.[195] Potassium should come from food sources. Good food sources of potassium include fruits, vegetables, yogurt, beans, and seafood (see Table 6-11).

## If You Drink Alcoholic Beverages, Do So in Moderation

*Dietary Guidelines for Americans 2005* defines *alcohol moderation* as no more than one drink per day for women and no more than two drinks per day for men.[196] This limit is based on differences between men and women in both weight and metabolism. (A drink is defined as 12 ounces of beer, 5 ounces of wine, or 1.5 ounces of 80-proof spirits.) The allowance for women is smaller because women, on average, are smaller than men; they have less muscle and, therefore, less water than men (so alcohol does not get diluted as well in their bodies); and they have less of an enzyme that breaks down alcohol before it reaches the bloodstream. A maximal level of alcohol consumption has not been set for women during pregnancy, so pregnant women and women who have a high chance of becoming pregnant should not use alcohol.

From a health perspective, alcohol has both advantages and serious risks. On the one hand, it is associated with drunken-driving injuries and deaths, cirrhosis of the liver, cancer, and a host of social ills caused by alcoholism.[197–200] On the other hand, when consumed in moderate amounts as recommended by *Dietary Guidelines*, it offers protection from heart disease and stroke, improvement in bone density, higher levels of heart-healthy omega-3 fatty acids, and high-density lipoproteins.[201,202] Studies that compare moderate drinking to nondrinking show that men who consume one-half to two alcoholic drinks a day were 40 to 60% less likely to suffer a heart attack than nondrinkers.[203]

Several theories have been advanced to explain alcohol's benefit: It may improve blood levels of high-density lipoproteins, and it may serve as a blood thinner by inhibiting the blood-clotting mechanism often associated with atherosclerosis.

**TABLE 6-11** Food Sources of Potassium[210]

| Food, Standard Amount | Potassium (mg) | Calories |
|---|---|---|
| Baked sweet potato, 1 potato (146 g) | 694 | 131 |
| Tomato paste, ¼ cup | 664 | 54 |
| Baked potato, flesh, 1 potato (156 g) | 610 | 145 |
| White beans, canned, ½ cup | 595 | 153 |
| Yogurt, plain, nonfat, 8 oz | 531 | 143 |
| Prune juice, ¾ cup | 530 | 136 |
| Yellowfin tuna, cooked, 3 oz | 484 | 118 |
| Lima beans, cooked, ½ cup | 484 | 104 |
| Winter squash, cooked, ½ cup | 448 | 40 |
| Banana, 1 medium | 422 | 105 |
| Spinach, cooked, ½ cup | 419 | 21 |
| Peaches, dried, uncooked, ¼ cup | 398 | 96 |
| Prunes, stewed, ½ cup | 398 | 133 |
| Pork chop, center lion, cooked, 3 oz | 371 | 190 |
| Cantaloupe, ¼ medium | 368 | 47 |
| 1%–2% milk, 1 cup | 366 | 102–122 |
| Kidney beans, cooked, ½ cup | 358 | 112 |
| Orange juice, ¾ cup | 355 | 85 |
| Split peas, cooked, ½ cup | 355 | 116 |

Regardless of alcohol's potential health benefits, experts don't recommend alcohol consumption for everyone. The American Heart Association[204] does not recommend that abstainers begin drinking alcohol to reduce their risks of heart disease and strokes. Instead, they should follow the suggestions in Chapters 2 and 3 of this text to reduce their risk. Some people have medical, religious, and personal reasons for abstaining. People with uncontrolled hypertension, liver disease, pancreatitis, or strong family histories of addiction should avoid alcohol. The same is true for women during pregnancy and lactation. Also, some medicines may have a potentiating effect when taken with alcohol. For women there is also some concern about the link between moderate consumption of alcohol and breast cancer.[205] Remember that the health benefits associated with alcohol come from a moderate level of consumption. Alcohol consumption in excess of that recommended in *Dietary Guidelines* can cause a variety of health problems that outweigh the potential benefits. As is the case with many health issues, moderation serves as the guiding principle for alcohol consumption.

**TABLE 6-12**   Weight-Gain Guidelines During Pregnancy

The 2009 weight-gain recommendations established by the National Institutes of Medicine are listed below and are based on a woman's pre-pregnancy body mass index (BMI).

| Weight Status and Pre-Pregnancy BMI | Recommended Weight Gain (in lbs)* |
|---|---|
| Underweight (BMI: < 18.5) | 28–40 |
| Normal weight (BMI: 18.5–24.9) | 25–35 |
| Overweight (BMI: 25.0–29.9) | 15–25 |
| Obese (BMI: > 30.0) | 5–9 |

*Recommended weight gain assumes 1.1–4.4 lbs weight gain in the first trimester. Most of the weight gain occurs in the second and third trimesters.

Source: Rasmussen, K., & A. L. Yaktine. (Ed.) (2009). *Weight gain during pregnancy: Reexamining the guidelines.* Washington, DC: National Academies Press.

# Other Nutrition Issues of Concern

## Nutrition and Pregnancy

Good nutrition is crucial to a successful pregnancy, and a healthy pregnancy starts before conception. Alcohol consumption, smoking, an inadequate diet, dietary excesses of some nutrients, drug abuse, and the interactions of a host of medicines are some of the factors that may threaten a pregnancy even before conception is known or confirmed. Poor health habits throughout pregnancy, especially during the first 3 months, can harm the mother and developing baby. Although genetic and environmental influences introduce some risk factors beyond the mother's control, there is a considerable amount of medical advice about weight gain and the nutritional needs unique to pregnant women.

## Weight Gain

Adequate weight gain for a mother is one of the best predictors of pregnancy outcome. The National Institutes of Medicine recently revised its weight-gain guidelines for women during pregnancy. These guidelines are based on differences in body type as measured by pre-pregnancy body mass index (see Chapter 7 for discussion and calculation of body mass index). Women in the normal-weight category should gain 25 to 35 pounds to ensure optimal health for both mother and fetus.[206] In comparison to normal-weight women, underweight women need to gain 3-5 pounds more; overweight women need to gain 10 pounds less; and women who are obese need to gain 20 to 26 pounds less (see Table 6-12: Weight-Gain Guidelines During Pregnancy). Most of the weight gain occurs during the second and third trimesters. Additional calories may be required to accommodate the extra demands for energy during pregnancy, especially in the second and third trimesters. Caloric needs don't change much in the first trimester. During the second and third trimesters, it may be necessary for the expectant mother to increase her caloric intake approximately 350 to 450 calories per day, depending on her status in meeting the recommended weight-gain goal.[207] Inadequate weight gain can lead to many problems. It is important to monitor weight throughout the pregnancy. Large fluctuations in the recommended weight-gain pattern should be brought to the attention of the health care provider.

## Nutrient Needs

The RDAs for many nutrients increase during pregnancy:[208]

- The protein RDA increases by 25 grams daily.
- Because of its role in DNA synthesis, folate is a crucial nutrient during pregnancy. The RDA for folate during pregnancy increases to 600 mg per day. Folate deficiencies have been linked to some neural tube birth defects, such as spina bifida. The increased need for folate can be achieved through the diet or a prenatal vitamin and mineral supplement.
- Iron intake should double during the final 6 months of pregnancy to achieve the RDA of 27 milligrams per day. The extra iron is needed to synthesize the additional hemoglobin required during pregnancy and to provide iron for the developing fetus. Women often need an iron supplement if their typical iron intake is marginal. Iron deficiencies during pregnancy may threaten the health of both the baby and the mother.
- Calcium is needed during pregnancy for skeletal and tooth development of the fetus, especially during the last 3 months, when growth of these tissues is most prolific. The DRI for calcium is 1,000 to 1,300 mg, depending on age. A prenatal supplement usually contains 200 mg of calcium and may be recommended for women who are calcium deficient.[209]
- The zinc RDA increases 35% (to 11–12 mg) during pregnancy to satisfy the requirements for growth and development of the fetus. Foods rich in protein also supply zinc. Zinc deficiencies increase the chance of a low-birth-weight baby.

- Prenatal supplements may contribute to a successful pregnancy for some women and, with the possible exception of vitamin A, provide benefits that outweigh potential risks. Because of its role in cell differentiation, megadoses of vitamin A from both supplements and dietary sources are associated with birth defects, particularly when the vitamin A is consumed during the first 3 months of pregnancy. It is recommended that women set their limit of vitamin A according to the RDAs.

Recommended servings in the Food Guide should satisfy women's unique nutritional needs during pregnancy. During the second and third trimesters when more energy is required, the Food Guide (see Table 6-9) can be used to identify the food groups that should be increased to correspond with the higher calorie level. For example, a woman on a 2,000-calorie food plan during the first trimester should consume 2½ cups of vegetables. If her intake increases to 2,400 calories per day during the second and third trimesters, she should consume 3 cups of vegetables. Women who practice either ovolactovegetarianism or lactovegetarianism generally do not have difficulty meeting their nutritional needs during pregnancy. Vegans, on the other hand, must plan their diets carefully to ensure adequate amounts of protein, vitamin D, vitamin $B_6$, iron, calcium, zinc, and vitamin $B_{12}$. Vegans need to increase their intake of grains, beans, nuts, and seeds to supply the required amounts of nutrients. In addition, supplements of vitamin $B_{12}$, iron, and calcium along with a multipurpose prenatal supplement will probably also be necessary.[210]

## Nutrition and Physical Activity

The relationship between physical activity and nutrition is obvious. The ability to engage in physical activity, whether it is low-intensity and recreational or high-intensity and competitive, is influenced by dietary intake. Conversely, nutritional needs change, depending on the type, intensity, and duration of activity. Nutrition and athletic performance are complex subjects involving not only the science of nutrition but also the sciences of biochemistry and physiology. While a presentation of the intricacies of sports nutrition is beyond the scope of this text, the following information should help you plan to meet your nutrient needs when you participate in regular physical activities.

### Type of Activity and Energy Source

The body's use of carbohydrates, fats, and protein for energy depends on the type of activity and the level of physical fitness. For high-intensity, anaerobic activities lasting for only a minute or less, such as a 100-yard sprint, carbohydrates are the major fuel source. For aerobic activities lasting from several minutes to 4 or 5 hours, a combination of carbohydrates, fats, and protein provides fuel for work. If the activity is intense, such as that of a runner trying to achieve a personal best in a 1-mile run, carbohydrates will be in greater demand. If the activity is moderately intense, such as jogging or brisk walking, fats and carbohydrates are used evenly. If the activity lasts more than a few minutes and is less intense, such as easy walking, fat becomes a major source of energy.[211] Energy from protein is minimal during most activities because protein functions as a fuel source primarily after carbohydrate fuel is depleted, such as might occur in activities of long duration (such as long-distance running), and then its contribution accounts for only about 3 to 10% of the energy. In general, carbohydrates are the main fuel source for both anaerobic and high-intensity aerobic activities; fat is the main fuel source for prolonged, low-intensity exercise; and protein is a minor fuel source, primarily for endurance activities.[212]

### Recommended Sources of Energy

The diet of a physically active person should favor carbohydrates. The body is capable of converting carbohydrates to a usable form of energy more quickly and more efficiently than it can fats or protein. As a general rule, dietary intake of carbohydrates should account for 60% of the energy.[213] Tables 6-13 and 6-14 present some high-carbohydrate meal options that are appropriate as preactivity meals. An increase in carbohydrate intake should be accompanied by a decrease in fat intake.

Carbohydrate loading provides some advantages for athletes participating in intense aerobic events lasting more than 60 minutes or in shorter events repeated over a 24-hour period. **Carbohydrate loading** (also called **glycogen loading**) is the practice of increasing carbohydrate intake for 6 days before an event while decreasing exercise duration.[214] The purpose of carbohydrate loading is to increase the availability of glycogen stores in the muscles. A typical regimen[215] consists of a carbohydrate intake of 45 to 50% of calories during the first 3 days, followed by a carbohydrate intake of 70 to 80% of calories during the next 3 days. At the same time, the duration of workouts is gradually decreased. For example, a 60-minute workout on the sixth day before an athletic event is decreased to 40, 40, 20, and 20 minutes, respectively, on the following days. The sixth day is a day of rest.

Carbohydrate loading is recommended for endurance activities such as cycling, running, swimming, and similar activities.[216] However, it doesn't improve actual performance for everyone. Athletes should first experiment with carbohydrate loading during training to determine if it improves actual performance. A new trend that involves increasing carbohydrate intake dur-

**TABLE 6-13**    Two High-Carbohydrate Preactivity Meals

| | Calories | Protein (grams) | Fat (grams) | Carbohydrate (grams) |
|---|---|---|---|---|
| **Menu 1** | | | | |
| White bread, 2 slices | 123 | 4 | 2 | 22 |
| Peanut butter, 1 tbsp. | 95 | 4 | 8 | 3 |
| Grape jelly, 1 tbsp. | 56 | 0 | 0 | 14 |
| 2% milk, 1 cup | 125 | 8 | 5 | 12 |
| Orange, 1 medium | 60 | 1 | 0 | 15 |
| **Meal total** | 459 | 17 | 15 | 66 |
| **Menu 2** | | | | |
| Vegetable lo mein (soft noodles with stir-fried vegetables), 2 cups | 352 | 11 | 15 | 47 |
| Fresh papaya, 1 cup | 54 | 1 | 0 | 14 |
| Herbal iced tea, sweetened with honey, 12 oz. | 56 | 0 | 0 | 13 |
| **Meal total** | 462 | 12 | 15 | 74 |

The timing of the preactivity meal depends on the amount of calories consumed. Allow 4 hours for a big meal (about 1,200 calories), 3 hours for a moderate meal (about 800 to 900 calories), and an hour or less for a snack (about 300 calories).

**TABLE 6-14**    Convenient Preactivity Meals

| | Energy Content |
|---|---|
| **Breakfast (McDonald's)** | |
| Hot cakes with syrup and margarine | 900 cal |
| Orange juice, 2 servings | 67% from carbohydrates |
| English muffin (whole) with 2 tsp. margarine and 2 tsp. jam | (150 g) |
| ••• | |
| Cheerios, 3/4 cup | 450 cal |
| Low-fat milk, 1 cup | 82% from carbohydrates |
| Blueberry muffin | (92 g) |
| Orange juice, 1 serving | |
| **Lunch or Dinner (Wendy's)** | |
| Chili, 8-oz. portion | 900 cal |
| Baked potato with sour cream and chives | 65% from carbohydrates |
| Chocolate Frosty, 10 oz. | (150 g) |
| ••• | |
| Grilled chicken sandwich | 425 cal |
| Cola, 12 oz. | 65% from carbohydrates |
| | (70 g) |

ing activities may provide the same advantage as carbohydrate loading prior to activities.[217]

## Protein Supplement

Many physically active people, especially athletes, have the mistaken notion that intense physical activities impose a greater than usual demand for protein. This idea stems partly from the perception that if a modest amount of a nutrient is good for you, large amounts must be even better, and partly because protein is needed for the synthesis of new tissue. Both of these ideas can lead to mistaken conclusions. What athletes and others engaged in intense activities need is not extra protein but extra carbohydrates. The body's need for protein is biologically driven, and any excess in this amount is inefficiently converted to energy or stored as fat.

Two exceptions to this protein guideline occur for athletes engaged in endurance sports and athletes starting weight training programs. The recommendations for protein range from 1.0 to 1.6 grams of protein per kilogram of body weight for the athlete. For athletes beginning a weight training program, 1.7 grams of protein per kilogram of body weight is recommended.[218] This represents a substantial increase of the RDA for protein. Experts disagree about the importance of excessive protein intake for weight training.

## Vitamins and Minerals

Vitamin and mineral needs of the physically active person are about the same as those of the sedentary person. People who exercise usually eat more than sedentary people do and therefore get more vitamins and minerals. Contrary to popular belief, especially among athletes, there is no need to take vitamin and mineral supplements if adequate servings of food from the Food Guide are consumed. Two exceptions are athletes on low-calorie diets (fewer than 1,200 calories/day) and vegetarian athletes. In these cases, taking vitamin and mineral supplements and consuming fortified food, such as breakfast cereals, are recommended.[219]

If a mineral deficiency occurs, it is most likely to involve iron and calcium, especially for women athletes. A deficiency of either of these minerals not only impairs athletic performance but also may lead to serious medical conditions. Dietary intake of these two minerals should be monitored regularly.

### Fatty Acids and Activity

Most of the body's energy reserve is in its fat stores. When fat stores are broken down, fatty acids move through the bloodstream and enter muscle cells, where they are converted to energy. Well-trained muscles have a greater capacity to execute this conversion process and the ability to burn more fat. Thus, improved physical fitness causes more fat to be used for energy.[220-222] Also, the body's use of fat stores is affected by the duration of the activity. Prolonged activities (lasting more than 20 minutes) cause fat storage to be tapped for energy, particularly when the activity remains at a low intensity level. Unlike carbohydrate stores, which are limited, an unlimited amount of fatty acids are available to sustain the energy needs of low-intensity activities. Weight-conscious people interested in physical activity as a strategy for using fat, therefore, are better served by low-intensity to moderate-intensity activities that can be endured for a long period.

### Fluid Intake and Activity

Consuming the right amount of fluids before, during, and after physical activity, which is addressed in Chapter 3, is crucial for the regulation of body temperature and the dissipation of heat.

## Food Labels

The FDA oversees the labeling of food products other than meat and poultry. Virtually all processed and packaged foods are required to have uniform labels. These foods include processed meat and poultry, regulated by the USDA. Foods with little nutritional value, such as coffee, don't have labels, but do have "sell by" dates.[223] Guidelines for voluntary labeling of raw vegetables and fruits and fish are also available and will likely be displayed in most supermarkets.

Food labels must indicate the manufacturer and the packer or distributor; declare the quantity of contents, either by net weight or by volume; and list the common name of each ingredient in descending order of prominence. Information about those nutrients most closely associated with chronic disease risk factors—the amount of total fat, saturated fat, trans fat, cholesterol, sodium, sugar, dietary fiber, total carbohydrate, and protein—must also be included.

Labels are divided into two parts (Figure 6-4) and present information according to generic standards called **Daily Values** (DVs). Daily Values are benchmarks for evaluating the nutrient content of foods. They express this content as a percentage of a 2,000-calorie diet (Recommended Dietary Allowances are not used as the standards because they are age- and gender-specific). Information in the top part of a label will vary according to the contribution one serving of that food makes to the Daily Values listed in the bottom part of the label.

The DV standards located on the bottom panel are the same on all food labels and are based on two calorie levels: 2,000 and 2,500 (Table 6-15). This means that total fat intake should be fewer than 65 grams for a 2,000-calorie diet and fewer than 80 grams for a 2,500-calorie diet. Dividing the nutrient content listed in the top panel by the DVs listed in the bottom panel yields the percent Daily Value for one serving. For example, a serving of mac 'n cheese contains 15 grams of fat, or 23% of the Daily Value of 65 g for a person on a 2,000-calorie diet. With the application of simple arithmetic, you can calculate the Daily Value percents for any food with a breakdown of nutrient content.

Standard food labels are useful if daily caloric intake is approximately 2,000 or 2,500 calories and if the goal is to conform to minimum dietary recommendations. If your diet calls for significantly more or less of a nutrient, your DVs will differ. If that is the case, keep track of the total amount of a nutrient. For example, if you are on a 1,500-calorie diet and are trying to limit fat intake to 20%, keep a running total of fat grams to determine when 33 grams have been reached.

In the past, manufacturers often used labeling ploys to deceive consumers. Currently, the FDA has approved health claims that link the following foods and diseases.[224]

- Calcium-rich foods and reduced risk for osteoporosis
- Low-sodium and high-potassium foods and reduced risk for high blood pressure and stroke
- Low-fat diet and reduced risk for cancer

**TABLE 6-15    Standardized Daily Values on Food Labels***

| | Calorie Levels | |
| --- | --- | --- |
| | 2,000 | 2,500 |
| Total fat | < 65 g | < 80 g |
| Saturated fat | < 20 g | < 25 g |
| Cholesterol | < 300 mg | < 300 mg |
| Sodium | < 2,400 mg | < 2,400 mg |
| Total carbohydrates | 300 g | 375 g |
| Fiber | 25 g | 30 g |

*The Daily Values on food package labels have not yet been updated to reflect the current state of knowledge (see Table 6-1).

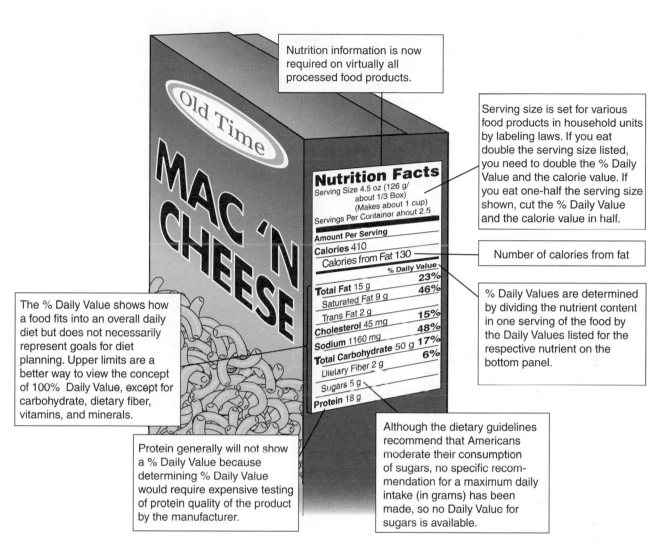

Nutrition information is now required on virtually all processed food products.

Serving size is set for various food products in household units by labeling laws. If you eat double the serving size listed, you need to double the % Daily Value and the calorie value. If you eat one-half the serving size shown, cut the % Daily Value and the calorie value in half.

**Nutrition Facts**
Serving Size 4.5 oz (126 g/ about 1/3 Box) (Makes about 1 cup)
Servings Per Container about 2.5

Amount Per Serving

Calories 410
Calories from Fat 130

% Daily Value

Total Fat 15 g — 23%
Saturated Fat 9 g — 46%
Trans Fat 2 g
Cholesterol 45 mg — 15%
Sodium 1160 mg — 48%
Total Carbohydrate 50 g — 17%
Dietary Fiber 2 g — 6%
Sugars 5 g
Protein 18 g

Number of calories from fat

% Daily Values are determined by dividing the nutrient content in one serving of the food by the Daily Values listed for the respective nutrient on the bottom panel.

The % Daily Value shows how a food fits into an overall daily diet but does not necessarily represent goals for diet planning. Upper limits are a better way to view the concept of 100% Daily Value, except for carbohydrate, dietary fiber, vitamins, and minerals.

Protein generally will not show a % Daily Value because determining % Daily Value would require expensive testing of protein quality of the product by the manufacturer.

Although the dietary guidelines recommend that Americans moderate their consumption of sugars, no specific recommendation for a maximum daily intake (in grams) has been made, so no Daily Value for sugars is available.

**FIGURE 6-4**   Food Label Showing Daily Values

Food labels provide information about those nutrients most associated with chronic disease risk factors.

- Diet low in saturated fat and cholesterol and reduced risk for heart disease
- High-fiber foods and reduced risk for some cancers
- Soluble fiber in fruits, vegetables, and grains and reduced risk for heart disease
- Soluble fiber in oats and psyllium seed husk and reduced risk for heart disease
- Fruit- and vegetable-rich diet and reduced risk for cancer
- Folate-rich foods and reduced risk for neural tube defects
- Less sugar and reduced risk for dental caries
- Low-saturated-fat and low-cholesterol diet that includes 25 grams of soy protein and reduced risk for cardiovascular disease
- Omega-3 fatty acids from oils present in fish and a reduced risk for cardiovascular disease
- Margarines containing plant stanols and sterols and a reduced risk for cardiovascular disease

The FDA has defined commonly used words describing calories, sodium, sugar, fiber, fat, and cholesterol in food. For example, when the word *free* is highlighted on a package in reference to calories, it means that the product yields fewer than 5 calories per serving; in reference to sodium, it means the product contains fewer than 5 milligrams; and in reference to fat, it means the product contains less than 0.5 gram. When *light* or *lite* is used on a package label, it means that the product has one-third fewer calories or 50% less fat than a similar product. *Low-calorie* foods can have no more than 40 calories per serving; *low-fat* foods can have no more than 3 grams of fat per serving. *Healthy* means that a food meets the criteria for low fat and low saturated fat, does not exceed maximum levels for sodium and cholesterol, and contains at least 10% Daily Value for at least one of the following: vitamins A and C, calcium, iron, protein, or fiber. The word *organic* can be used when no more than 5% of a food product's ingredients have been exposed to pesticides, chemical fertilizers, genetic engineering, sewage sludge, antibiotics, or irradiation in their production. In other words, 95% of the ingredients in a food product must be free of these exposures. If a food product meets the U.S. Department of Agriculture's (USDA) certified organic criteria, it can include the USDA organic seal on the package label (see Figure 6-5). If only 70% of the ingredients meet USDA's criteria, it can show "made with organic ingredients" on the label.[225]

Freshness dates are often stamped on a product's package, especially for refrigerated food and perishable foods with a short shelf life, such as meat, milk, and bread. A "sell by" date indicates how long the product is available for purchase. The product should be purchased before the date expires. Well-managed stores will usually pull the product from the shelf on or shortly after the sell date. A "best if used by (or before)" date tells when the product has its best flavor. It is not a purchase or safety date; it is more of a high-quality date. If a sell-by or best-if-used-by date expires during home storage, it should still be safe if it is handled properly and kept at 40 °F or below. A "use by" date indicates the last day recommended for the product while at peak quality. If a product has a use-by date, follow that date for consumption.[226]

Even with the improvements in label laws, the unwitting consumer can still be misled. A frozen dinner package displays in large, bold red letters that it has "0 percent trans fat," even though the nutritional details on the back of the package shows 40% of its calories come from saturated fat. The makers of a brand of brownie mix claim that it is low-fat. But the fine print says that the low-fat designation pertains only to each serving of the mix alone. Once an edible brownie is created by adding vegetable oil, its fat-gram content more than triples. Some foods promise fruit or other ingredients but deliver only flavor. One brand of strawberry frozen yogurt has no real strawberries, despite pictures on the label of real strawberries; a brand of blueberry pancakes has no berries. A bag of chips brags on its front that it is "made with all **Natural** oil" because it contains no trans fat, but its label shows that it has the same amount of fat, saturated fat, sodium, and calories as a competing brand of chips sitting next to it but without the "natural" claim. (There is no standard definition for the term *natural*.)[227] Clearly, although labels have improved dramatically during the past several years, they still fall short in several areas. To quote the editor of a leading consumer magazine: "I think it's unfair that manufacturers are obligated to tell the truth only in small print of the nutrition label and ingredients list but are free to deceive us in large letters."[228] Deception in old labels was more obvious; today's labels challenge consumers to apply a higher level of discrimination to sort between fact and fantasy.

# Changes in American Eating Patterns

Changes in the American family are mirrored in the trend toward convenience-food eating. For many families, time is a precious commodity that has a dramatic influence on how, where, when, and what people eat. Family meals at home are being replaced by a quick-stop, eat-on-the-go trend. Dining out has become a part of the quintessential American lifestyle. On average, Americans dine out six times a week, or nearly one of every three meals.[229] In terms of good health, this is a questionable trend because eating at home is associated with better nutrition. When people eat at home, they tend to consume less fat and calories, and more fruits, vegetables, whole grains, and calcium, compared to eating out.[230] One explanation for the negative effects of eating out is that it invites a splurge mentality because many people still view it as a special occasion.[231] Weight-conscious consumers are challenged to apply a higher level of discrimination when eating out, especially considering that restaurant food is often served in large portions and loaded with fat, sodium, and sugar and accompanied by high-calorie beverages.

Not only do many people eat away from home, but they also skip meals. This is a questionable practice. The idea that skipping meals, for example, facilitates weight loss is dabatable. Often, it has the opposite effect by encouraging binge eating, increased snacking, or overcompensatory eating. Skipping breakfast is troublesome in that the body is denied a source of energy to replace carbohydrate stores used during the night's sleep. It should be of little surprise, therefore, that mid-morning sluggishness is a common experience of students and workers. Evidence from the research community consistently indicates that eating breakfast, including consumption of high-fiber, ready-to-eat cereals and milk, is associated with improved overall nutrition and weight maintenance.[232]

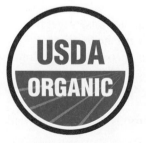

**FIGURE 6-5**    The U.S. Department of Agriculture's Organic Seal When this seal appears on a food package, it means the product is certified "organic."

## Snacking

*Snacking* refers to consuming food between the three main meals of the day. Most Americans have at least one snack per day, and snack foods contribute 21 to 25% of total daily caloric intake.[233] From a nutrition point of view, snacking is neither good nor bad. The three meals a day standard is based more on social custom than on physiology. The issue is not the time or frequency of eating but what is eaten. Nutritionally dense foods eaten as snacks are as good for health as they are when consumed as meals. The converse is also true; foods low in nutrient density eaten at mealtime are as worthless as when they are eaten as snacks. With the exception of foods restricted for medical reasons, all foods can contribute to a healthful diet. Problems occur when a person's diet is dominated by foods low in nutrient density. Rather than rule out snacking, consume snack foods that enhance wellness. The most direct way to improve snacking behavior is the most obvious one: Purchase and make nutritionally dense foods available (see Real-World Wellness: Snack Ideas).

From a nutritional viewpoint, the criticisms of fast-food eating are the same as those of the rest of the American diet: too much fat, too many calories, too much sodium, and not enough complex carbohydrates and fiber. The average meal of a cheeseburger, milkshake, and fries supplies about 1,500 calories, 43% of which come from fat. Chicken and fish are as fatty as other protein sources offered by fast-food restaurants because they are breaded and fried. Frying has the same effect on potatoes. Milkshakes get most of their calories from sugars. Food composition search engines such as USDA's National Agricultural Library (**www.nal.usda. gov**) (select links: *Food and Nutrition > Look up Calories or Nutrients in a Food*) provide detailed information that can be used to compare many fast food menu items.

Eating at fast-food restaurants does not have to be a nutritionally worthless activity. Many restaurants are aware that Americans are more knowledgeable about the nutrient content of food and are demanding wholesome, safe, and nutritious foods. Consequently, there has been a trend toward more nutritious menus, including salad, pasta, and potato bars. Guided by good judgment in the choice of foods, an occasional meal at a fast-food chain does not have to compromise a well-balanced diet.

## Planning a Nutrition Strategy for Wellness

It is not necessary to be a nutritionist to form a nutrition strategy that works for you. A nutrition plan will work only if it is personalized. Several strategies should be helpful in personalizing your nutrition plan.

### Assess Your Nutrition

You should take an honest look at your eating choices and analyze your nutrition profile through Assessment

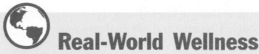

## Real-World Wellness
### Snack Ideas

*After completing a thorough 3-day dietary analysis, I was surprised to learn that the key to improving my overall nutritional profile is to make changes in my snack food choices. My meals are fairly well balanced, but my snacks are typically high in fat, high in sodium, high in sugar, and low in nutrient density. What are some examples of nutritionally dense snacks?*

The following snacks are surprisingly flavorful and satisfying and will help you improve your overall nutrition:

- Fresh raw vegetables served with a cottage cheese dip
- Fresh fruit, prewashed and cut into bite-size pieces
- Fruit dipped in yogurt
- Bagels topped with reduced-fat cream cheese
- Breadsticks
- Air-popped popcorn seasoned with herbs
- Frozen fruit-juice bars
- Low-fat frozen yogurt
- Pita chips with salsa
- Pretzels
- Rye crisps or rice cakes spread with a little peanut butter or low-fat cheese
- Broth-based soup
- Cereal (low-sugar, low-fat)
- Shelled sunflower seeds
- Gelatin with added fruit
- English muffins
- Flour tortillas with canned chili and grated low-fat cheese
- Pita bread topped with spaghetti sauce and grated low-fat cheese
- Fruit juice with added club soda
- Hot cocoa (low-sugar, low-fat)
- Milkshake made with low-fat milk and frozen fruit

Activities 6-3, 6-5, and 6-6 to determine whether you are doing the following:

- Eating a variety of foods every day from MyPyramid or the USDA Food Guide
- Avoiding high-fat foods (more than the equivalent of 3 grams of fat per 100 calories)

- Including sufficient fiber in the form of whole grains, dried beans, and fresh fruits and vegetables
- Consuming 11 and 15 cups of water (8 ounces each) daily (women and men, respectively)
- Consuming no more than three or four high-sugar desserts or sweets each week
- Restricting your intake of high-salt foods, such as processed meats
- Consuming no more than one or two alcoholic drinks a day and not letting drinking interfere with your appetite

## Make Small Adjustments

The principle of changing health behavior is that the smaller the change, the longer it lasts (see Chapter 1). For example, rather than vowing to abstain from eating ice cream, reduce the amount or number of servings at first and substitute a low-fat brand. If your diet is heavy in salt, you can gradually substitute sodium-free seasonings. If you have a sweet tooth, you can try low-sugar snacks. If you eat for fullness, you can prepare less food or leave food on your plate. You should plan an approach that builds on the cumulative effect of many small successes.

Think of balancing your diet over a long period rather than in a day or a meal. Try to meet the dietary guidelines over several days or a week. For example,

not every meal needs to contain less than 30% fat. Keep portions of favorite high-fat foods small and limit other sources of fat. Check labels to get an idea of what nutrients you are consuming, but don't keep a calculator by your plate. If you eat foods from the Food Guide, you will get all the vitamins, minerals, and protein you need.

## Choose Foods for Wellness

Choosing foods for wellness means following the *Dietary Guidelines for Americans 2005*. Your diet should

- Emphasize fiber-rich fruits, vegetables, and whole grains
- Be low in sodium and added sugars
- Provide iron, calcium, and potassium
- Limit alcohol consumption to one to two drinks a day
- Be low in saturated fats
- Avoid trans fats
- Provide plenty of water (11 and 15 cups for women and men, respectively)
- Stress nutrient-dense foods chosen within calorie needs
- Observe guidelines for the safe preparation and storage of food

Finally, make sure when choosing foods for wellness to enjoy what you eat (see Nurturing Your Spirituality: Enjoy Your Food—the Missing Dietary Guideline).

## Nurturing Your Spirituality

### Enjoy Your Food—the Missing Dietary Guideline

The fast-paced, eat-on-the-run trend among Americans comes with a high price: Fewer and fewer people spend time preparing good, home-cooked meals, and even fewer use mealtime as a time for relaxation and social bonding. Other cultures recognize that mealtime is a key social time of the day and reflect this value in the dietary recommendations health experts offer their citizens:[234]

- In Japan, immediately following the guideline to avoid too much sodium comes the advice "Happy eating makes for a happy family life; sit down and eat together and talk; treasure family taste and home cooking."
- In Great Britain, the first guideline is "Enjoy your food."
- Korea tells its citizens to "Enjoy meals and keep harmony between diet and daily life."

- In Norway, people are told, "Food and joy equal health."
- In Vietnam, the advice is to "Serve a healthy family meal that is delicious and served with affection."

The greatest nutrition challenge for Americans may not be to reduce fat intake or cut back on sodium. It may be to construct a positive view of food and of mealtime. Two highly respected nutrition publications remind us, "Healthful eating is about more than eating the right mix of nutrients. It's also about sustaining well-being in a way that can't be measured on a blood test but that is just as important to overall health as vitamins and minerals."[235] "Taking pleasure in food is part of the formula for living a healthy, happy life."[236]

# Summary

- The six classes of nutrients are carbohydrates, fat, protein, vitamins, minerals, and water. The nutrients that provide energy in the form of calories are carbohydrates, fat, and protein.
- The recommended diet for Americans in *Dietary Guidelines for Americans 2005* emphasizes complex carbohydrates as the major source of energy. A diet high in complex carbohydrates is likely to be lower in fat, lower in calories, and higher in fiber. A low-carbohydrate diet is not necessarily low in calories.
- A complete protein is one that provides all of the amino acids in amounts proportional to the body's need for them. Protein sources from animals are complete proteins. Plant sources of complete protein, such as soy protein, come from the legume family.
- One of the greatest shortcomings of the American diet is its excessive intake of fat, especially saturated fat, and trans fat.
- The amount of saturated, monounsaturated, and polyunsaturated fat in foods varies considerably. Most food contains a mixture of these fats.
- The process of hydrogenation increases the saturated fat content of polyunsaturated and monounsaturated fats and yields small amounts of fat not found in nature called trans fatty acids. No more than 10% of calories should come from saturated fats. Less than 1% should come from trans fats.
- Dietary fat intake should favor foods high in omega-6 and omega-3 fatty acids.
- The consumption of antioxidant vitamins, especially in fruits and vegetables, is associated with health benefits.
- Adequate folate consumption is thought to lower the concentration of homocysteine, an amino acid associated with an increased risk for heart disease.
- Vitamin D is an essential nutrient associated with helping the immune system combat infections, preventing and slowing down some forms of cancer and osteoarthritis, and helping the body absorb calcium. Vitamin D

- deficiency is sometimes referred to as the hidden epidemic because deficiencies easily go unnoticed.
- Two minerals of special concern are calcium and iron. Most women fall short of the RDA for calcium. People at risk for low iron levels include young children, early teens, menstruating women, and people with health conditions that cause internal bleeding.
- Daily Recommended water intake is 15 cups for men, 11 cups for women and includes water in food and beverages.
- Phytochemicals, or phytonutrients, are plant chemicals found naturally in foods. They play an important role in preventing many diseases.
- Enhanced foods are foods that have been modified and/or supplemented to achieve a health benefit.
- Many botanicals are thought to have health benefits. Because they are considered nutritional supplements and are not regulated with the same rigor as drugs, there is debate about their effectiveness and safety. Twenty to 30 botanicals are backed by well-conducted research.
- Soluble fiber forms a gel-like consistency in the body and is associated with helping the body excrete cholesterol. Insoluble fiber resists digestion and helps the body move food through the digestive tract. Plant foods contain a mixture of soluble and insoluble fiber, and their health benefits overlap.
- A good nutrition plan is one that consists of a variety of foods from the USDA Food Guide or MyPyramid.
- A food is nutrient dense when it has a high ratio of nutrients to calories.
- Variety and moderation are principles that should most influence eating habits. There is room in the diet for any food as long as it is consumed in moderation in quantity and frequency.
- *Dietary Guidelines for Americans 2005* recognizes a vegetarian diet as a healthful and acceptable way of meeting all of our nutritional needs.
- The health benefits of a vegetarian diet include a lower cholesterol level; lower levels of LDLs; reduced

- incidence of hypertension and lung, colorectal, and breast cancer; and fewer complications from non-insulin-dependent diabetes mellitus.
- Americans consume sugar and sodium in excessive amounts. The major health issue associated with high sugar intake is dental caries; for sodium, it's hypertension.
- Glycemic index is a scale that reflects how much blood sugar rises after consuming 50 grams of a food. Foods with a high glycemic index are high in sugars and starches and cause a rapid surge in blood sugar, compared to foods with a low glycemic index. In terms of health, our diets should favor foods with a low glycemic index.
- Moderate consumption of alcohol may be beneficial for some people at risk for cardiovascular disease and stroke.
- Pregnancy imposes a greater demand for some nutrients, including protein, vitamin D, folate, iron, calcium, and zinc. Recommended weight gain during pregnancy varies according to the expectant mother's prepregnancy body mass index (BMI). Women with a BMI of 18.5 to 24.9 should gain 25–35 pounds during pregnancy, primarily in the second and third trimesters. Underweight expectant mothers should gain more; women who are overweight or obese should gain less during pregnancy.
- Carbohydrates are the main source of energy for both anaerobic and high-intensity aerobic activities; fat is the main energy source for prolonged, low-intensity exercise; and protein is a minor fuel source, primarily for endurance activities.
- The risk for foodborne illness can be reduced by preventing cross-contamination of food; by washing hands, fruits, produce, and meats; and by exercising caution in the way food is prepared and stored.
- Food labels provide helpful information about nutrients associated with the common chronic health problems of Americans as well as about essential nutrients. Deceptive and misleading words, slogans, and claims are

still common on food package labels and are often subtle in their message.
• The criticisms of snacking and fast-food eating are the same as those of the rest of the American diet: too much fat, sodium, and sugar; too many calories; and not enough complex carbohydrates and fiber.

• Americans are challenged not only to eat more healthfully but also to construct a positive attitude about food and mealtimes.

# Review Questions

1. What is meant by "nutritional diseases of the past have been replaced by diseases of dietary excess and imbalance"?
2. Explain the meanings of the following nutrition acronyms: DRI, RDA, AI, UL, and DV.
3. Identify three nutrients that most Americans do not consume in sufficient amounts.
4. How many calories are supplied by carbohydrates, fat, and protein? What percentage of total calories should come from each of these sources? How does Americans' intake of energy nutrients compare with dietary recommendations?
5. Why are carbohydrates the preferred source of energy?
6. What is the difference between simple carbohydrates and complex carbohydrates? Which type should be favored in our diet? Why?
7. What is the difference between a high-quality, complete protein and a low-quality, incomplete protein?
8. What plant sources of protein are unique in that they are considered complete proteins?
9. What are the differences among saturated, monounsaturated, and polyunsaturated fats? What are some food sources of each? What percentage of fat calories should come from each type?
10. What are trans fatty acids? Why should they be avoided?
11. List five dietary practices that will help lower consumption of fat, especially saturated fat.
12. What are the similarities and differences between water-soluble and fat-soluble vitamins?
13. Which vitamins are classified as antioxidants? What is the relationship between antioxidants and health?
14. What role does folate play in preventing disease?
15. Identify three situations or circumstances that would justify the use of a vitamin or mineral supplement.
16. What are phytochemicals? How are they different from botanicals? How do they contribute to health?
17. What two minerals are Americans most likely to be consuming in insufficient amounts? Which segments of the population are most likely to be affected?
18. What vitamin deficiency is often referred to as the hidden epidemic? Why?
19. What are the major health benefits of a high-fiber diet?
20. What is the rationale for the assertion that variety and moderation are the most important principles for a healthy diet?
21. Distinguish among the different types of vegetarianism. Which types are most likely to require some form of vitamin or mineral supplementation? What are the health benefits of a vegetarian diet?
22. Identify four nutrients that pregnant women require in larger amounts than those in the RDAs.
23. How do the intensity and duration of physical activities affect the way the body uses carbohydrates, fat, and protein for energy? What type of physical activity is most conducive to burning fat calories?
24. List six things a person can do to help prevent unnecessary exposure to foodborne illness.
25. To what does the Glycemic Index (GI) of food refer? Glycemic Load (GL)? What are the health implications of GI and GL?
26. What are the main criticisms of snacking and fast-food eating?

# References

1. U.S. Department of Health and Human Services, U.S. Department of Agriculture. (2005). *Dietary guidelines for Americans 2005.* Washington, DC: U.S. Government Printing Office.
2. U.S. Department of Health and Human Services. (2000). *Healthy people 2010* (2nd ed.). With *Understanding and improving health and objectives for improving health* (2 vols.). Washington, DC: U.S. Government Printing Office.
3. U.S. DHHS (2005).
4. Ibid.
5. Harvard Health Publications. (2008). *Vitamins and minerals: What you need to know, a Harvard Medical School special health report.* Boston: Harvard Health Publications.
6. Liebman, B. (2008). Fiber free-for-all: Not all fibers are equal. *Nutrition Action Health Letter, 35(6)*, 1,3–8.
7. Wright, J. D., R. Hirsch, & C. Wang. (2009). One-third of U.S. adults embraced most heart healthy behaviors in 1999–2002. *NCHS Data Brief No 17.* Hyattsville, MD: National Center for Health Statistics.
8. Ibid.
9. Neville, K. (2008). Vitamin C seesaw: Why more is better, but not a cure-all. *Environmental Nutrition, 31(5)*, 1,6.
10. Byrd-Bredbenner, G. Moe, D. Beshgetoor, & J. Berning. (2009). *Wardlaw's Perspectives in Nutrition* (8th ed.). New York: McGraw-Hill.
11. Wardlaw, G., & A. Smith. (2011). *Contemporary Nutrition* (8th ed.). New York: McGraw-Hill.
12. U.S. Department of Agriculture, Agricultural Research Service. (2008). *Nutrient intakes from food: Mean amounts consumed per individual, by race/ethnicity and age, one day, 2005–06.* Retrieved January 23, 2010, from www.ars.usda.gov/ba/bhnrc/fsrg.

13. U.S. DHHS (2005).

14. Wright et al. (2009).

15. Tufts Media. (2009). Americans failing on grain goals. *Tufts University Health and Nutrition Letter,* 27(9), 3.

16. Popkin, Barry M. (2006). Pour better or pour worse: How beverages stack up. *Nutrition Action Healthletter,* 33(5), 3–7.

17. Wardlaw & Smith (2011).

18. Ibid.

19. Wardlaw, G., & J. Hampl. (2007). *Perspectives in nutrition* (7th ed.). New York: McGraw-Hill.

20. Schardt, D. (2009). Soy what? *Nutrition Action Healthletter,* 36(11), 8–10.

21. Welland, D. (2006). Savor soy: 9 super sources for protein, phytonutrients. *Environmental Nutrition,* 29(12), 2.

22. Consumer Union. (2010). Should you eat more soy? *Consumer Reports on Health,* 22(1), 10.

23. Gorman, R. (2009). Are some foods more equal than others? *Heart Insight,* 3(4), 14–16.

24. Wardlaw & Smith (2011).

25. Wardlaw & Hampl (2007).

26. Kraus, W. (2009). Triglycerides: The forgotten lipid. *Healthnews,* 15(7), 4.

27. Hernandez, A. (2010). Omega-3s stand out in preventing and treating heart disease. *Duke Medicine Health News,* 16(2), 1–2.

28. Cheskin, L, C. Roberts, & S. Margolis. (2010). *The Johns Hopkins white papers: Nutrition and weight control for longevity.* Baltimore: Johns Hopkins Medicine.

29. Tufts Media. (2007). Studies find new omega-3 benefits. *Tufts University Health and Nutrition Letter,* 25(5), 4–5.

30. Cheskin et al. (2010).

31. Editor. (2009). Americans only vaguely aware where to find trans fats; Do you know? *Environmental Nutrition,* 32(5), 3.

32. Cheskin, et al. (2010).

33. U.S. DHHS (2005).

34. Cheskin et al. (2010).

35. Byrd-Bredbenner et al. (2009).

36. Cheskin et al. (2010).

37. Ibid.

38. Ibid.

39. Byrd-Bredbenner et al. (2009).

40. Cheskin et al. (2010).

41. Ibid.

42. Tufts Media. (2008). Recipe for maximum nutrition. *Tufts University Health and Nutrition Letter,* 26(10:Special Report), 4   5.

43. Editors. (2005). A radical notion: Maybe antioxidants can't protect us after all. *Environmental Nutrition,* 28(3), 1,6.

44. Byrd-Bredbenner et al. (2009).

45. Cheskin et al. (2010).

46. Mozaffarian, D., M. B. Katan, A. Ascherio, M. J. Stampfer, & W. C. Willett. (2006). Trans fatty acids and cardiovascular disease. *New England Journal of Medicine,* 354(15), 1601–13.

47. Cheskin et al. (2010).

48. Tufts Media. (2007). Antioxidant supplements—now what? *Tufts University Health and Nutrition Letter,* 25(4), 4–5.

49. Tufts Media. (2008). "Fountain of youth" fact and fantasy. *Tufts University Health and Nutrition Letter,* 26(3, Special Supplement), 1–4.

50. Consumer Union. (2007). Antioxidant reality check. *Consumer Reports on Health,* 19(9), 1,4.

51. Cheskin et al. (2010).

52. Nevell, K. (2008). Vitamin C seesaw: Why more is better, but not a cure-all. *Environmental Nutrition,* 31(5), 1,6.

53. Ibid.

54. Byrd-Bredbenner et al. (2009).

55. Consumer Union. (2010). Herbs and supplements: Don't expect too much. *Consumer Reports on Health,* 22(1), 9.

56. Wardlaw & Smith (2009).

57. Ibid.

58. Tufts Media. (2008). "Sunshine" vitamin's healthy glow. *Tufts University Health and Nutrition Letter,* 26(7), 1–2.

59. Mayo Clinic Health Solutions. (2008). Study suggests vitamin D may play a role in arterial disease. *Mayo Clinic Health Letter,* 26(9), 4.

60. Belvoir Media Group. (2010). Low levels of vitamin D linked to heart and stroke death. *Duke Medicine Health News,* 16(2), 5.

61. Tufts Media. (2007). Cancer study supports higher vitamin D levels. *Tufts University Health and Nutrition Letter,* 25(7), 1–2.

62. Tufts Media. (2007). Are you getting enough vitamin D? *Tufts University Health and Nutrition Letter,* 25(10), 1–2.

63. Tufts Media. (2009). Are you vitamin D-deficient? *Tufts University Health and Nutrition Letter,* 27(4:Special Report), 4   5.

64. Harvard Health Publications. (2010). Vitamin D may prevent falls. *Harvard Health Letter,* 35(3), 3.

65. Liebman, B. (2007). Confusion at the vitamin counter. *Nutrition Action Health Letter,* 34(9), 1,3–6.

66. Consumer Union. (2009). The ABCs of vitamin D. *Consumer Reports on Health,* 21(11), 1,4,5.

67. Ibid.

68. Harvard Health Publications. (2008). The sunshine D-lemma. *Harvard Health Letter,* 33(10), 6,8.

69. Tufts Media (2009). Are you vitamin D-deficient? *Tufts University Health and Nutrition Letter,* 27(4:Special Report), 4–5.

70. Ibid.

71. Harvard Health Publications. (2009). Nutrition's dynamic duos. *Harvard Health Letter,* 34(9), 6–7.

72. Liebman (2007).

73. Tufts Media. (2009). Are you vitamin D-deficient? *Tufts University Health and Nutrition Letter,* 27(4:Special Report), 4–5.

74. Consumer Union. (2009). The ABCs of vitamin D. *Consumer Reports on Health,* 21(11), 1,4,5.

75. Ibid.

76. Harvard Health Publications. (2008). Vitamin E: Separate and unequal? *Harvard Health Letter,* 33(3), 6.

77. Harvard Health Publications. (2008). *Vitamins and minerals: What you need to know.* Boston: Harvard Health Publications.

78. Byrd-Bredbenner et al. (2009).

79. Harvard Health Publications. (2009). Nutrition's dynamic duos. *Harvard Health Letter,* 34(9), 6–7.

80. Mayo Clinic Health Solutions. (2009). The B vitamins: Simplifying the complex. *Mayo Clinic Health Letter,* 27(4), 4–5.

81. Consumer Union. (2008). Folic acid concern. *Consumer Reports on Health,* 20(2), 10.

82. McDowell, M., D. Lacher, C. Pfeiffer, et al. (2008). Blood folate levels: The latest NHANES results. *NCHS Data Brief No. 6.* Hyatts-

ville, MD: National Center for Health Statistics.

83. Harvard Health Publications. (2008). *Vitamins and minerals: What you need to know.* Boston: Harvard Health Publications.

84. Cheskin et al. (2010).

85. Byrd-Bredbenner et al. (2009).

86. Palmer, S. (2009). Key to good health: Why whole foods have the edge over supplements. *Environmental Nutrition, 32*(5) 1,4.

87. Ibid.

88. Consumer Union. (2010). One a day—or none a day? *Consumer Reports on Health, 22*(2), 1,4–5.

89. Tufts Media. (2009). Multivitamins fall short in biggest study of its kind. *Tufts University Health and Nutrition Letter, 27*(3), 1–2.

90. Palmer (2009).

91. Harvard Health Publications. (2009). Vitamins: Benefit of the doubt vs. doubts about benefit. *Harvard Health Letter, 34*(6), 6–7.

92. Consumer Union. (2010). One a day—or none a day? *Consumer Reports on Health, 22*(2), 1,4–5.

93. Harvard Health Publications. (2008). *Vitamins and minerals: What you need to know.* Boston: Harvard Health Publications.

94. Cheskin et al. (2010).

95. Wardlaw & Smith (2011).

96. Ibid.

97. Ibid.

98. Ibid.

99. Ibid

100. Ibid.

101. Ibid.

102. Ibid.

103. Ibid.

104. Ward. E. (2007). Selenium protects joints, prostate: Could it do more? *Environmental Nutrition, 30*(3), 1,6.

105. Ibid.

106. Tufts Media. (2008). Water, water everywhere; But how much should you drink? *Tufts University Health and Nutrition Letter, 26*(5:Special Report), 4–5.

107. Byrd-Bredbenner et al. (2009).

108. Ibid.

109. Tufts Media. (2008). Water, water everywhere; But how much should you drink?

110. Byrd-Bredbenner et al. (2009).

111. Cheskin et al. (2010).

112. Tufts Media. (2008). Water, water everywhere; But how much should you drink?

113. Byrd-Bredbenner et al. (2009).

114. Ibid.

115. Schardt, D. (2000). Water, water, everywhere.... *Nutrition Action Healthletter, 27*(5), 1–7.

116. Byrd-Bredbenner et al. (2009).

117. Cheskin et al. (2010).

118. Palmer, S. (2010). The top functional foods of 2010. *Environmental Nutrition, 33*(2), 1,4.

119. Synder, D. (2010). Functional foods: What it means, what they do, what they are. *Duke Medicine Health News, 16*(2), 4–5.

120. Tufts Media. (2009). The facts on fiber. *Tufts University Health and Nutrition Letter, 26*(12:Special Report), 4–5.

121. Ibid.

122. Cheskin et al. (2010).

123. Byrd-Bredbenner et al. (2009).

124. Wardlaw & Smith (2011).

125. Consumers Union. (2003). Are you getting enough fiber? *Consumer Reports on Health, 15*(11), 7.

126. Wardlaw & Smith (2011).

127. Byrd-Bredbenner et al. (2009).

128. Tufts Media. (2004). Tufts nutrition: Translating the research for use at your table. *Tufts University Health & Nutrition Letter, 21*(12:Special Supplement), 1–4.

129. Tufts Media. (2009). The facts on fiber.

130. U.S. DHHS (2005).

131. Wardlaw & Smith (2011).

132. Cheskin et al. (2010).

133. American Heart Association Nutrition Committee of the Council on Nutrition, Physical Activity and Metabolism, Council on Cardiovascular Disease in the Young, Council on Arteriosclerosis, Thrombosis and Vascular Biology, Council on Cardiovascular Nursing, Council on Epidemiology and Prevention, and Council for High Blood Pressure Research: Gidding, S. S., et al. (2009). AHA Scientific Statement: Implementing American Heart Association Pediatric and Adult Nutrition Guidelines. *Circulation, 119,* 1161–75. Retrieved January 31, 2010, from http://circ.ahajournals.org/cgi/content/full/119/8/1161.

134. Byrd-Bredbenner et al. (2009).

135. Mayo Clinic Health Solutions. (2009). Herbal supplements. *Mayo Clinic Health Letter, 27*(8), 4–5.

136. Lichtenstein, A. H., et. al. (2006). AHA scientific statement: Diet and lifestyle recommendations revision 2006. *Circulation, 114,* 82–96.

137. Broihier, K. (2006). Breads that give you a true whole-grain advantage. *Environmental Nutrition, 29*(4), 5.

138. Consumer Union. (2006). Cereals and cereal bars: Better granolas, cheaper flakes. *Consumer Reports, 71*(9), 16–19.

139. Liebman, B. (2008). Fiber free-for-all. *Nutrition Action Healthletter, 35*(6), 1,3–7.

140. Broihier (2006).

141. Consumer Union. (2006). The whole truth about whole grains. *Consumer Reports on Health, 18*(1), 9.

142. Wardlaw & Hampl (2007).

143. U.S. DHHS (2005).

144. Ibid.

145. Ibid.

146. Wardlaw & Smith (2011).

147. U.S. DHHS (2005).

148. Wardlaw & Smith (2011).

149. Center for Science in the Public Interest. (2003). Are your supplements safe? *Nutrition Action Healthletter, 30*(9), 3–7.

150. Wardlaw & Smith (2011).

151. Ibid.

152. Ibid.

153. U.S. DHHS (2005).

154. Tufts Media. (2003). Growing older presents new nutrition challenges. *Tufts University Health and Nutrition Letter, 21*(8), 1,8.

155. Tufts Media. (2008). Pyramid modified for older adults. *Tufts University Health and Nutrition Letter, 26*(1), 1–2.

156. Belvoir Media Group. (2010). Vegetarian diets may prevent and treat some chronic diseases. *Duke Medicine Health News, 16*(1), 1–2.

157. Tufts Media. (2009). Some cancers less likely to strike vegetarians. *Tufts University Health and Nutrition Letter, 27*(8), 7.

158. Tufts Media. (2009). Meat lovers' mortality risk is higher. *Tufts University Health and Nutrition Letter, 27*(4), 1–2.

159. Belvoir Media Group. (2010). Hold the beef, live longer. *Duke Medicine Health News, 15*(8), 3.

160. Wardlaw & Smith (2011).
161. Tufts Media. (2009). Heart experts: Cut way back on sugar to fight obesity. *Tufts University Health and Nutrition Letter*, 27(9), 3.
162. Wardlaw & Smith (2011).
163. Center for Science in the Public Interest. (2010). Sugar overload: Curbing America's sweet tooth. *Nutrition Action Healthletter* 37(1):3–8.
164. Center for Science in the Public Interest. 2005. Liquid candy. *Nutrition Action Healthletter*, 32(6), 2.
165. American Heart Association Nutrition Committee of the Council on Nutrition, Physical Activity and Metabolism (2009).
166. Wardlaw & Smith (2011).
167. Ibid.
168. Consumer Union. (2008). Shaking salt and sugar from your diet. *Consumer Reports on Health*, 20(1), 8–10.
169. Byrd-Bredbenner et al. (2009).
170. Wardlaw & Smith (2011).
171. Ibid.
172. Tufts Media. (2009). Does glycemic index really make a difference? *Tufts University Health and Nutrition Letter*, 27(1:Special Report), 4–5.
173. Environmental Nutrition. (2002). Glycemic index: Gateway to good health or grand waste of time. *Environmental Health*, 25(11), 1,6.
174. Webb, D. (2006). Better blood sugar for better health. *Environmental Nutrition*, 29(12), 1,4.
175. Ibid.
176. Ibid.
177. Mayo Clinic Health Solutions. (2008). Health tips: Low glycemic index diet. *Mayo Clinic Health Letter*, 26(6), 3.
178. Tufts Media. (2009). Does glycemic index really make a difference?
179. Wright et al. (2009).
180. U.S. DHHS (2005).
181. Consumer Union. (2006). Good eating, global style. *Consumer Reports on Health*, 18(9), 1–5.
182. Consumer Union. (2010). How safe is that chicken? *Consumer Reports*, 75(1), 19–23.
183. Ibid.
184. Belvoir Media Group. (2004). Food irradiation: A recipe for safer food? *Duke Medicine Health News*, 10(6), 4–5.
185. Consumer Union. (2006). Is that safe to eat? A guide to the funky

foods in your kitchen. *Consumer Reports*, 71(12), 6.
186. Ibid.
187. Wardlaw & Smith (2011).
188. Ibid.
189. Jacobsen, M. (2008). You say serrano, I say salmonella. *Nutrition Action Healthletter*, 35(7), 2.
190. Wright et al. (2009).
191. Byrd-Bredbenner et al. (2009).
192. Harvard Health Publications. (2007). Reaching for the anti-salt. *Harvard Health Letter*, 32(5), 3.
193. Liebman, Bonnie. (2005). Pressure cooker: The scoop on salt. *Nutrition Action Healthletter*, 32(6), 1,3–7.
194. Tufts Media. (2009). New reasons to be wary of hidden salt. *Tufts University Health and Nutrition Letter*, 27(3:Special Report), 4–5.
195. Ibid.
196. Wardlaw & Smith (2011).
197. Ibid.
198. Mayo Clinic Health Solutions. (2009). Any alcohol consumption increases women's cancer risk. *Mayo Clinic Health Letter*, 27(6), 4.
199. Editors. (2009). Raise your glass to wine's health benefits. *Environmental Nutrition*, 32(12), 1.
200. Tufts Media. (2009). Moderate drinking linked to better bone density. *Tufts University Health and Nutrition Letter*, 27(4), 1–2.
201. Editors. (2009). Balancing alcohol's unique mix of health benefits and health risks. *Environmental Nutrition*, 32(5), 3.
202. Tufts Media. (2009). Wine could help maximize healthy omega-3s. *Tufts University Health and Nutrition Letter*, 27(2), 1–2.
203. Tufts Media. (2009). Moderate drinking linked to better bone density.
204. Tufts Media. (2007). Up to two drinks a day help even healthy men avoid heart attacks. *Tufts University Health and Nutrition Letter*, 24(9), 6.
205. Wilder, L. B., L. J Cheskin, & S. Margolis. (2006). *The Johns Hopkins white papers: Nutrition and weight control for longevity*. Baltimore: Johns Hopkins Medicine.
206. Cheskin et al. (2010).
207. Rasmussen, K., & A. L. Yaktine (eds.). (2009). *Weight gain during pregnancy: Reexamining the guidelines*. Washington, DC: National Academies Press.

208. Wardlaw & Smith (2011).
209. Ibid.
210. Wardlaw & Hampl (2007).
211. Wardlaw & Smith (2011).
212. Ibid.
213. Byrd-Bredbenner et al. (2009).
214. Wardlaw & Smith (2011).
215. Wardlaw & Hampl (2007).
216. Nieman, D. (2007). *Exercise testing and prescription: A health-related approach* (6th ed.). New York: McGraw-Hill.
217. Wardlaw & Smith (2011).
218. Ibid.
219. Ibid.
220. Ibid.
221. Byrd-Bredbenner et al. (2009).
222. Nieman (2007).
223. Tufts Media. (2006). Smarter—and healthier—supermarket shopping made simple. *Tufts University Health and Nutrition Letter*, 24(7), 4–5.
224. Wardlaw & Smith (2011).
225. Ibid.
226. U.S. Department of Agriculture. (2007). *Fact sheets: Food labeling; Food product dating*. Washington, DC: Food Safety and Inspection Service. Retrieved February 4, 2010, from www.fsis.usda.gov/Factsheets/Food_Product_Dating/index.asp.
227. Tufts Media. (2008). Why "natural" labels don't necessarily mean healthy. *Tufts University Health and Nutrition Letter*, 26(6:Special Report), 4–5.
228. Sandroff, Ronni. (2006). Read the fine print. *Consumer Reports on Health*, 18(9), 2.
229. Welland, D. (2008). Menus magic: 7 strategies for dining out healthfully. *Environmental Nutrition*, 31(5), 2.
230. Consumer Union. (2007). Home cooking is healthier. *Consumer Reports on Health*, 19(6), 7.
231. Ibid.
232. American Heart Association Nutrition Committee of the Council on Nutrition, Physical Activity and Metabolism (2009).
233. Ibid.
234. Tufts Media. (1998). The missing dietary guideline; enjoy your food. *Tufts University Health and Nutrition Letter*, 16(5), 3.
235. Ibid.
236. Eberle, S. (2009). Learning to enjoy food, for health and pleasure. *Environmental Nutrition*, 32(9), 1,6.

# Suggested Readings

Cheskin, L., L. Roberts, & S. Margolis. (2010). *The Johns Hopkins white papers: Nutrition and weight control for longevity.* Baltimore, MD: Johns Hopkins Medical School.

This 85-page monograph is a concise, no-nonsense presentation on basic nutrition and weight control facts and guidelines. Written by medical doctors at the highly respected Johns Hopkins Medical School, this book presents guidelines that are backed by recent scientific studies in the medical world. The latest information on fat, carbohydrates, vitamins, minerals, antioxidants, phytochemicals, enhanced foods, organic foods, and food safety are discussed.

Editors. (2008). *Disease-fighting foods: Smart eating choices.* Rochester, MN: Mayo Clinic Health Solutions.

Long recognized as a leader in medicine and health education, Mayo Clinic gives nutrition advice based on its own food pyramid, called the Mayo Clinic Healthy Weight Pryamid. Included among its topics are food supplements, antioxidants, legumes, fortified foods, omega-3 and omega-6 fatty acids, food and drug interactions, and common diseases associated with the typical American diet (such as hypertension, cancer, and diabetes).

This 31-page booklet serves as a quick reference on principles of nutrition and presents them in understandable language.

Wardlaw, G., & A. Smith. (2011). *Contemporary nutrition* (8th ed.). New York: McGraw-Hill.

This book provides in-depth, comprehensive information on all aspects of nutrition. It is a "must have" book for students and laypeople alike who have more than a casual interest in the science and health applications of nutrition. It is also a good introductory book for anyone preparing for advanced study in nutrition or possibly considering a career in dietetics.

Warshaw, H. 2008. *Eat out, eat right: The guide to healthier restaurant eating* (3rd ed.). Chicago: Surrey Books.

An author and registered dietician, Warshaw offers tips and strategies to guide the reader through dining options ranging from fast-food restaurants to fine dining. Mexican, Italian, Chinese, Thai, Japanese, Indian, and Middle Eastern cuisine is included. Special sections on beverages, soup 'n sandwich style, and pizza style are also presented.

U.S. Department of Health and Human Services, U.S. Department of Agriculture. (2005). *Dietary guidelines for Americans 2005.* Washington, DC: U.S. Government Printing Office.

Every 5 years, the U.S. Department of Health and Human Services teams up with the U.S. Department of Agriculture to update dietary guidelines for Americans. The 2005 edition was a major revision to previous editions and serves as a major reference for health professionals, students, and laypeople. This book includes a separate chapter on each of the nine major topics discussed in Chapter 6 of *Wellness: Concepts and Applications.* In addition to the USDA Food Guide, *Dietary Guidelines for Americans 2005* presents the DASH Eating Plan and numerous charts and tables that identify good food sources of essential nutrients.

Willett, W., & M. Katzen. (2006). *Eat, drink, and weigh less: A flexible and delicious way to shrink your waist without going hungry.* New York: Hyperion.

Walter Willett, Harvard professor and nationally known nutrition researcher, teams up with a famous cookbook author to offer diets that are recommended for anyone, regardless of weight. The diets, like those in the USDA Food Guide, are heavy on vegetables, fruit, whole grains, cooking oils, nuts, and beans.

# Assessment Activity 6-1

## Assessing Your Carbohydrate and Protein Recommended Intake

### Assessing Your Carbohydrate Intake Goal

**Directions:** Complete the following steps to determine your goal for carbohydrate intake in grams to meet the recommended intake of 45 to 65% of total calories from carbohydrate (including sugar and complex carbohydrates).

1. *Total caloric intake:* There are two options to estimate your caloric intake:
a. Go to **www://mypyramid.gov**, (Link: Get a Personal Plan), enter your age, gender, and physical activity level, and click Submit. The recommended caloric intake will be displayed under "My Pyramid Plan."
b. Go to Table 6-8 on page 198. Identify the recommended caloric intake range for your age, gender, and activity level. The ranges vary for the "moderately active" and "active" levels. Choose the midpoint of the range unless you believe the lower or upper end of the range is more representative of your activity level.
c. Recommended caloric intake = _____ calories

2. *Carbohydrate calories:* Multiply your total caloric intake times 0.45 and 0.65 to determine the range of carbohydrate calories.

   _____ calories × 0.45 = _____ carbohydrate calories
   (minimum)

   _____ calories × 0.65 = _____ carbohydrate calories
   (maximum)

3. *Carbohydrate (grams):* Your recommended carbohydrate calories divided by 4 equals recommended carbohydrate intake in grams.

   Minimum carbohydrate calories ÷ 4 = _____ grams
   Maximum carbohydrate calories ÷ 4 = _____ grams

**EXAMPLE:** For a 19-year-old male who participates in 30 minutes a day of moderate physical activity in addition to daily activities,

Calorie requirement =   2,700 calories (see Table 6-8; range is 2,600 to 2,800 calories, midpoint is 2,700 calories)

Recommended carbohydrate calories

   2,700 × 0.45 = 1,215 calories
   2,700 × 0.65 = 1,755 calories

Recommended carbohydrate grams (rounded to nearest whole number)

   1,215 ÷ 4 = 304 grams
   1,755 ÷ 4 = 439 grams

This amounts to approximately 11 to 16 ounces of carbohydrate (304 and 439 divided by 28, respectively = 11 to 16 ounces) (28 grams = 1 ounce).

### Assessing Your Protein RDA

**Directions:** Adults require 0.36 gram of protein per pound of body weight. For example, a 20-year-old person who weighs 150 pounds needs 54 grams of protein (150 × 0.36 = 54).

Complete the following steps to determine your RDA for protein.

   Your weight      _____ pounds
                    × 0.36
   Protein RDA = _____ grams

Name _____ Date _____ Section _____

# Assessment Activity 6-2

## Assessing Your Maximum Fat and Saturated Fat Intakes

### Assessing Your Maximum Fat Intake

**Directions:**   Complete the following steps to determine your estimated maximum fat intake in grams to stay within the dietary guidelines of 35% of total calories from fat.

1. **Caloric Intake** = _____ calories
   (see Assessment 6-1)

2. **Maximum Fat Calories**

   Your caloric intake multiplied by 35% equals maximum fat calories:

   _____ calories × 0.35 = _____ calories

3. **Maximum Fat (Grams)**

   Your maximum fat calories divided by 9 equals maximum fat in grams.

   _____ calories ÷ 9 = _____ grams

**EXAMPLE:** For a moderately active male, 19 years old,

| | |
|---|---|
| 1. Caloric intake: | 2,700 calories |
| | × 0.35 |
| 2. Maximum fat calories: | 945 calories |
| | ÷ 9 |
| 3. Maximum fat: | 105 grams |

This amounts to approximately 4 ounces of fat (105 ÷ 28 = 3.75 ounces).

### Assessing Your Maximum Saturated Fat and Trans Fatty Acid Intake

**Directions:**   Complete the following steps to determine your estimated maximum saturated fat intake in grams to stay within the dietary guidelines of 10% of total calories from fat.

1. **Caloric Intake** = _____ calories
   (see Assessment 6-1)

2. **Maximum Saturated Fat Calories**

   Your caloric intake multiplied by 10 percent equals maximum saturated fat calories:

   _____ calories × 0.10 = _____ calories

3. **Maximum Saturated Fat (Grams)**

   Your maximum saturated fat calories divided by 9 equals maximum saturated fat in grams.

   _____ calories ÷ 9 – _____ grams

**EXAMPLE:** For a moderately active male, 19 years old,

| | |
|---|---|
| 1. Caloric intake: | 2,700 calories |
| | × 0.10 |
| 2. Maximum saturated fat calories: | 270 calories |
| | ÷ 9 |
| 3. Maximum saturated fat: | 30 g |

This amounts to about 1 ounce of saturated fat (30 ÷ 28 = 1.1 ounces).

# Assessment Activity 6-3

## Nutrient Intake Assessment

One way to determine if you are getting sufficient quantities of the proper nutrients is to keep a record of your diet. Ideally, this record will cover a time span of at least 1 week. However, in this exercise you are asked to assess your dietary selections for only 1 day. Therefore, choose a day representative of your overall nutritional practices. (Your instructor may ask you to conduct a 2- or 3-day assessment.)

**Directions:** To complete this assessment you will use the *NutritionCalc Plus* Web site that accompanies this textbook. Record all of the foods and beverages that you consume during one day with the exception of vitamin or mineral supplements. Be specific regarding the amount eaten, how it is cooked, and so on. List condiments and seasonings, such as mustard, ketchup, and butter, and dressings and trimmings, such as lettuce, onions, marshmallows, and sugar. The more detailed your record, the more accurate it will be and the more you will learn from it. Remember, the quality of the results is dependent on the quality of the information entered. A carefully and thoroughly prepared dietary recall will yield an accurate nutritional profile.

**Instructions for Computer Analysis Using NutritionCalc Plus:** Once foods have been listed, you are ready to use the *NutritionCalc* Plus Web site to generate your personal nutrition assessment report. The address is **http://nutritioncalc.mhhe.com/**. Click on *First Time User* and enter the registration code that accompanies your textbook. Enter a user name and password. Be sure to make note of your user name and password. These will be needed to log in each time you return to the program. Next, click on *Intakes* and begin entering your data. When you have completed data entry, print and arrange the results in the following order:

1. **User Profile:** Click on *profiles*. Print profile information, recommended intake of calories, protein, carbohydrates, fiber, total fats, saturated fat, mono fat, poly fat, cholesterol, water, vitamins and minerals, BMI.

2. **Reports:** Click on *reports*. Print the following reports:
a. **Bar Graph Report:** Bar graph that displays comparison of macronutrients, vitamins, minerals with dietary recommendations. *Vitamins* and minerals bars that extend to the 100% mark meet dietary

recommendations. Click on a particular nutrient to identify the contributions of foods in your 1-day food plan.
b. **Nutrient Spreadsheet Report:** Spreadsheet displays the nutrient breakdown of every food item listed in your 1-day food plan.
c. **Pyramid Report:** The pyramid report displays a comparison of the number of servings in your 1-day food plan with those recommended in the food pyramid. Note: The comparison may refer to the 2000 Food Pyramid rather than the 2005 MyPyramid. If this is the case, compare the number of servings in your food plan with those in Table 6-9 on p. 201 of this textbook. Your instructor may ask you to enter your 1-day food plan at **www.mypyramid.gov** to display the contributions of your diet to *Dietary Guidelines for Americans 2005*.
d. **Calories and Fat Report:** This table presents percentage of recommended water intake, breakdown of calorie source, and breakdown of fat.
e. **Nutrition Facts Report:** This table transfers the information on your one-day food plan to a food label graphic. Print this graphic so that it includes all meals (see pull-down menu).

3. **Food Prescription for Nutrient Deficiencies:** Refer to **Bar Graph Report (2a)** to identify vitamins and minerals that do not meet dietary recommendations (bar graph falls short of the 100% mark). Also, include fiber and protein in this analysis. For each nutrient, identify five good food sources. Go to the following Web site: **http://www.nal.usda.gov/fnic/foodcomp/search/**. Click on the *Nutrient Lists* link, identify the nutrient(s), click on *sorted by nutrient content*. This search will produce a rank-order list of foods according to nutrient content. From this list, identify five foods that you would consider adding to your diet.

4. **Follow-Up Questions:**
a. How many calories are recommended daily for your current age and activity level, assuming you are not in a weight-gain or weight-loss program?
b. What is your BMI and physical activity level?
c. What vitamins fall below recommended amounts?
d. What minerals fall below recommended amounts?

e. How does your protein intake compare to recommendation?

f. How does your fiber intake compare to recommendation?

g. What food groups in your one-day food plan meet dietary recommendations in MyPyramid or the USDA Food Guide?

h. How does your breakdown of calories compare with dietary recommendations?

i. How does your breakdown of fat calories compare with dietary recommendations?

j. Identify five foods you would consider adding to your diet to satisfy most of your nutritional deficiencies.

k. Complete the following open-ended sentences: After completing this one-day diet analysis:

i. I learned that I need to eat more _____

_____

ii. I learned that I need to eat less _____

_____.

iii. I was surprised to learn that _____

_____.

iv. I was disappointed that _____

_____.

v. I learned that some examples of foods I should cultivate a taste for to improve my diet include _____

_____.

**Name** _____   **Date** _____   **Section** _____

# Assessment Activity 6-4

## Do You Have Fatty Habits?

Fat has earned a bad reputation because of the health problems it contributes to in high-fat diets. The following questionnaire will help you think about the amounts and types of fat that you generally eat. For each general type of food or food habit, circle the category that is more typical for your diet. If you never or almost never eat any items of a particular food type, skip it.

| Food Type/Habit | High-Fat | Medium-Fat | Low-Fat |
|---|---|---|---|
| Chicken | Fried with the skin | Baked, broiled, or barbecued with the skin | Baked, broiled, or barbecued without the skin |
| Fat present on meats | Usually | Sometimes | Never |
| Fat used in cooking | Butter, lard, bacon grease, chicken fat | Margarine, oil | Nonstick cooking spray or no fat used |
| Additions to rice, bread, potatoes, vegetables, etc. | Butter, lard, bacon grease, chicken fat, coconut oil | Margarine, oil, peanut butter | Butter-flavored granules or no fat used |
| Pizza toppings | Sausage, pepperoni, extra cheese, combination | Canadian bacon | Vegetables (e.g., peppers, onions, mushrooms) |
| Sandwich spreads | Mayonnaise or mayonnaise-type dressing | Light mayonnaise, oil and vinegar | Mustard, fat-free mayonnaise |
| Milk and milk products (e.g., yogurt) | Whole milk and whole-milk products | Low-fat dairy products | Skim milk and milk products |
| Sandwich side orders | Chips, potato salad, macaroni salad with creamy dressing | Coleslaw, pasta salad with clear dressing | Vegetable sticks, pretzels, pickle |
| Salad dressings | Blue cheese, Ranch, Thousand Island, other creamy type | Oil and vinegar, clear-base dressing | Oil free dressing, lemon juice, flavored vinegar |
| Typical meat portion | 6–8 oz. or more | 4–5 oz. | 2–3 oz. |
| Sandwich fillings | Beef or pork hot dogs, salami, bologna, pepperoni, cheese, tuna or chicken salad | Turkey hot dogs, 85% fat-free lunch meats, corned beef, peanut butter, hummus (chick-pea paste) | 95% fat-free lunch meats, roast turkey, roast beef, lean ham |
| Ground meats | Regular ground beef, sausage meat, ground meat, ground pork (about 30% fat) | Lean ground beef, ground chuck, turkey sausage meat (20–25% fat) | Ground turkey, extra-lean ground beef, ground round (about 15% fat) |
| Deep-fried foods (e.g., french fries, onion rings, fish or chicken patties, egg rolls, tempura) | Eat every day. | Eat once a week. | Eat once a month or never. |
| Bread for sandwiches | Croissant | Biscuit | Whole-wheat, French, tortilla, pita or pocket bread, bagel, sourdough, English muffin |
| Cheeses | Hard cheeses (e.g., cheddar, Swiss, provolone, Jack, American, processed) | Part-skim mozzarella, part-skim ricotta, low-fat cheeses | Nonfat cheese, nonfat cottage cheese, no cheese |
| Frozen desserts | Premium or regular ice cream | Ice milk or low-fat frozen yogurt | Sherbet, Italian water ice, nonfat frozen yogurt, frozen fruit whip |

| Food Type/Habit | High-Fat | Medium-Fat | Low-Fat |
|---|---|---|---|
| Coffee lighteners | Cream, liquid or powdered creamer | Whole milk | Low-fat or skim milk |
| Snacks | Chips, pies, cheese and crackers, nuts, doughnuts, chocolate, granola bars | Muffins, toaster pastries, unbuttered commercial popcorn | Pretzels, vegetable sticks, fresh or dried fruit, air-popped popcorn, bread sticks, jelly beans, hard candy |
| Cookies | Chocolate-coated, chocolate chip, peanut butter, filled sandwich type | Oatmeal | Ginger snaps, vanilla wafers, graham crackers, animal crackers, fruit bars |
| **Scoring** | (_____ × 2)          + | (_____ × 1)          + | (_____ × 0)          = |

Total score: _____

Once you have completed the questionnaire, count the number of circles in each column and calculate your score as follows: Multiply the number of choices in the left-hand (High-Fat) column by 2 and multiply the number of choices in the middle (Medium-Fat) column by 1; then add these two values together. Based on your total score, rate yourself as follows:

| Less than 10 | = Excellent fat habits |
|---|---|
| 10 to 19 | = Good fat habits |
| 20 to 30 | = Fat habits needing improvement |
| Over 30 | = Very high-fat diet |

If your score is 20 or higher, try to substitute more foods from the middle (Medium-Fat) column or, better still, the right (Low-Fat) column for foods in the left-hand (High-Fat) column.

**Name** _____ **Date** _____ **Section** _____

# Assessment Activity 6-5

## Eating Behaviors to Consider

**Directions:**   Answer the following questions to reveal information about your eating habits, how you developed certain tastes, and your attitude about various foods.

1. When was the last time you tried a new food? What was the food? What were the circumstances? _____

   _____

2. What new foods have you learned to eat during the past year? _____

   _____

3. Name the foods that have been on your "will not try" list (that is, foods that you will not eat under any circumstances). _____

   _____

4. What special events do you celebrate in some way with food? _____

   _____

5. Where is your favorite place to eat? _____

6. If you were to go on an eating binge, what foods would you be most likely to eat? _____

   _____

7. Describe in detail your favorite meal. _____

   _____

8. Do you consider yourself a slow eater, moderately fast eater, or gulper? What do you think is responsible for your eating pattern? _____

   _____

9. To what extent, if any, are your eating habits related to stress? Emotions? _____

   _____

10. What do you consider to be your good eating habits? Poor eating habits? _____

   _____

**Name** _____    **Date** _____    **Section** _____

# Assessment Activity 6-6

## Estimating Calorie Source

**Directions:**   The purpose of this assessment is to determine what percentage of a food's calories come from carbohydrates, protein, and fats. Complete columns 6, 7, and 8 by calculating the percentage of calories that comes from protein, carbohydrates, and fat. Theoretically, columns 6, 7, and 8 should total 100% but may not because of rounding errors. Your instructor may identify additional foods for this assessment.

Example of calculation for plain baked potato:

| | | |
|---|---|---|
| 4 grams of protein × 4 calories/gram | = 16 protein calories | ÷ 188 = 8% protein |
| 43.5 grams of carbohydrate × 4 calories/gram | = 174 carbohydrate calories | ÷ 188 = 92% carbohydrate |
| 0.2 gram of fat × 9 calories/gram | = 1.8 fat calories | ÷ 188 = < 1% fat |

| | (1) Food (1 Serving) | (2) Calories | (3) Protein g | (4) Carbohydrate g | (5) Fat g | (6) % Protein | (7) % Carbohydrate | (8) % Fat |
|---|---|---|---|---|---|---|---|---|
| | **Baked potato with skin** | **188** | **4** | **43.5** | **0.2** | **8%** | **92%** | **< 1%** |
| 1 | Ice cream, vanilla, rich | 357 | 5.2 | 33.2 | 24 | | | |
| 2 | Nuts, cashew, dry-roasted | 262 | 7 | 14.9 | 21.2 | | | |
| 3 | Arby's Jamocha Shake | 500 | 13 | 81 | 13 | | | |
| 4 | Burger King Whopper | 800 | 35 | 53 | 49 | | | |
| 5 | KFC Sub Extra Crispy Chicken Breast | 460 | 34 | 19 | 28 | | | |
| 6 | Taco Bell Sub Mexican Pizza | 550 | 21 | 47 | 31 | | | |
| 7 | Taco Bell Fiesta Taco Salad | 870 | 31 | 80 | 47 | | | |
| 8 | Bread, whole-wheat | 69 | 2.7 | 12.9 | 1.2 | | | |
| 9 | Beans, lima, cooked | 108 | 7.3 | 19.6 | 0.4 | | | |
| 10 | Bagel, plain | 245 | 9.3 | 47.5 | 1.4 | | | |
| | **To be assigned:** | | | | | | | |
| 11 | | | | | | | | |
| 12 | | | | | | | | |
| 13 | | | | | | | | |
| 14 | | | | | | | | |
| 15 | | | | | | | | |

# Understanding Body Composition

## ONLINE LEARNING CENTER

Log on to our Online Learning Center (OLC) for access to these additional resources:

- Chapter key term flashcards
- Learning objectives
- Additional goals for behavior change
- Concentration game
- Self-scoring chapter quizzes
- Additional lab activities

The OLC also offers Web links for study and exploration of wellness topics. Access these links through **www.mhhe.com/anspaugh8e**.

## GOALS FOR BEHAVIOR CHANGE

- Use Table 7-5 to calculate your body mass index and interpret your results.
- Make a commitment to either maintain your existing weight or select a healthier weight.
- Formulate a long-range plan to achieve or maintain an ideal body weight and improve your body composition.

## Objectives

After completing this chapter, you will be able to do the following:

✔ Define *body composition*.
✔ Define *essential fat* and *storage fat*.
✔ Define and differentiate between *obesity* and *overweight*.
✔ Discuss the health implications of regionally distributed fat.
✔ Discuss the limitations of height/ weight tables for weight management.
✔ Calculate body mass index and interpret the results.
✔ Describe hydrostatic weighing, bioelectrical impedance, and skinfold measurements as methods for determining body composition.

### [ Key Terms ]

| | |
|---|---|
| adipose cells | obesity |
| amenorrheic | overfat |
| body composition | overweight |
| body mass index (BMI) | sarcopenia |
| essential fat | |

**B**ody tissues are characterized by a four-compartment model: water, fat, protein, and minerals. But from the perspective of health and fitness, the composition of the body may be categorized as a two-compartment model: fat and fat-free mass. **Body composition** is defined as the ratio of fat to fat-free mass. Considerable attention is also directed to the way fat is distributed throughout the body.[1] Excessive fat stored in the intra-abdominal or visceral region of the body (also called android or male pattern fat) is most dangerous because it significantly increases the risk for such chronic diseases as Type 2 diabetes, hypertension, hyperlipidemia (elevated cholesterol and/or triglycerides), coronary artery disease, metabolic syndrome, and some forms of cancer.

The Centers for Disease Control and Prevention estimated that 400,000 obesity-related deaths occurred during the year 2004. The surgeon general stated that obesity was "going to overtake tobacco as the number one cause of preventable death."[2] However, later studies indicated that flawed research methodology resulted in a substantial overestimation of obesity-related deaths. Today that figure ranges from 110,000 to 149,000. Conversely, being underweight as measured by a body mass index of less than 18.5 kg/m$^2$ was responsible for approximately 33,746 premature deaths during the same year.[3] However, leanness per se was not the direct cause of death. Instead, excessively low body weight and body fat were associated with and probably caused by chronic illness and/or cigarette smoking, both of which are responsible for **sarcopenia** or body wasting.[4]

Fat-free weight includes all tissues—muscle, bone, blood, organs, fluids—exclusive of fat. Fat is found in the organs (such as the brain, heart, liver, and lungs) and adipose cells.[5] **Adipose cells** are fat cells located subcutaneously (beneath the skin) and surrounding various body organs. They are an insulator against heat loss and a protection for the internal organs against trauma. The majority of body fat is found in adipose cells, where it acts as a vast storage depot for energy.

A certain amount of fat is required for normal biological functions. This is referred to as **essential fat.** Essential fat is located in the bone marrow, organs, muscles, and intestines; it is a component of cell-membrane structure as well as of brain and heart tissue.[6] The amount of essential fat in the male and female bodies differs. Essential fat constitutes 3 to 5% of the total weight of men and 8 to 12% of the total weight of women.[7] Total body fat includes adipose fat plus essential fat.

The higher female requirement for essential fat is directly related to fertility and childbearing. Women whose body fat drops below essential requirements, such as gymnasts, ballerinas, long-distance runners, and anorexics, often become **amenorrheic;** that is, they stop having a menstrual cycle. The period of infertility continues until they gain weight and their essential fat is restored. In both genders, essential fat represents a minimal threshold, or lower limit, for the maintenance of health.

## Obesity

Obesity, or overfatness, is gender-specific. For men, **obesity** is defined as body fat equal to or greater than 25% of total body weight, and for women, it is equal to or greater than 32% of total body weight.[8] These values are arbitrary because the point at which fat storage increases health risks has not been determined. Contributing further to the confusion is the fact that methods of assessing the amount of body fat are indirect, and each contains a degree of measurement error. Another complicating factor is that all obesity is not the same. The distribution of body fat in the abdominal area is highly correlated with illness and premature death.[9] A discussion of this topic occurs later in the chapter.

Acceptable body fat percentages have been derived from young adult subjects, and these standards have been applied to all age groups—age-specific standards have yet to be determined, and it is possible that such standards will vary somewhat with age. Optimal body fat for males ranges from 5 to 15%, and optimal body fat for females is between 12 and 23%.[10] But, the optimal level of body fat for physical fitness or athletic performance is considerably less—12 to 22% for female athletes and 5 to 13% for male athletes.[11] The ranges are based on the type of activity. For example, long-distance running requires extreme leanness whereas golf does not. On the other hand, there are at least two types of athletes who benefit from having a higher percentage of body fat: sumo wrestlers and long-distance swimmers, who perform in cold water for extended periods of time.

Recent body fat health standards based on age and gender allow for an increase in percent body fat with age. This allowance amounts to a trade-off in risks for chronic diseases, especially for women. Low body fat among middle-aged women is associated with losses of bone mineral content, which can lead to osteoporosis and bone fractures.[12] However, leanness, or low body fat, helps protect these women against heart disease. It is best for women to be lean enough to prevent heart disease yet not so lean as to risk the development of osteoporosis. This is particularly problematic for small-framed women, whose bone mineral content is already low. See Tables 7-1 and 7-2 for recommended body fat percentages for women and men of different ages.[13] These are only recommendations designed to recognize

**TABLE 7-1**   Recommended Body Fat Percentages for Adult Women

| Age | Essential Fat % | Minimal Fat % | Recommended Fat % | Obese Fat % |
|---|---|---|---|---|
| 34 or younger | 8–12 | 10–12 | 20–35 | 38 or higher |
| 35 to 55 | 8–12 | 10–12 | 23–38 | 40 or higher |
| 56 and over | 8–12 | 10–12 | 25–38 | 41 or higher |
| Athletic | 8–12 | 10–12 | 12–22 | 38 or higher |

Source: Adapted from Ratamess, N. (2010). Body composition status and assessment. In ACSM's resource manual (6th ed.), edited by J. K. Ehrman. Philadelphia: Wolters Kluwer/Lippincott Williams and Wilkins.

**TABLE 7-2**   Recommended Body Fat Percentages for Adult Men

| Age | Essential Fat % | Minimal Fat % | Recommended Fat % | Obese Fat % |
|---|---|---|---|---|
| 34 or younger | 3–5 | 5 | 8–22 | 25 or higher |
| 35 to 55 | 3–5 | 5 | 10–25 | 28 or higher |
| 56 and over | 3–5 | 5 | 10–25 | 28 or higher |
| Athletic | 3–5 | 5 | 5–13 | 25 or higher |

Source: Adapted from Ratamess, N. (2010). Body composition status and assessment. In ACSM's resource manual (6th ed.), edited by J. K. Ehrman. Philadelphia: Wolters Kluwer/Lippincott Williams and Wilkins.

differences between males and females, and increasing age is taken into account. Whether these recommendations are accepted or rejected by the scientific community will become evident in the near future. See also Nurturing Your Spirituality: Setting Realistic Fitness and Weight-Loss Goals on page 240.

## Overweight

**Overweight** refers to excessive weight for height without consideration of body composition. Because the term *overweight* makes no allowances for body composition, it is a poor criterion for determining the desirability of weight loss. For example, a well-muscled person may be overweight but lean in regard to body fat. By American social standards, such body mass is healthy, aesthetically pleasing, and desirable. It is also possible for a person to be well within the norms for total body weight but **overfat;** that is, such a person carries a large proportion of body weight in the form of fat rather than lean tissue. Overfat is unhealthy and, according to American social standards, unattractive.

See Real-World Wellness: Practical Ways to Estimate Overweight and Obesity on page 241.

## Regional Fat Distribution

Deposition of fat varies among people. The amount of fat and the storage sites are influenced by heredity and gender (Figure 7-1). After puberty, women generally deposit fat in the buttocks, hips, breasts, and thighs. These preferential sites are largely dictated by the female hormone estrogen.[17] This tendency is known as the *gynoid,* or feminine, pattern of fat deposition. It is also referred to as "pear shaped." Gynoid fat is not confined exclusively to women; a few men deposit fat in this configuration as well.

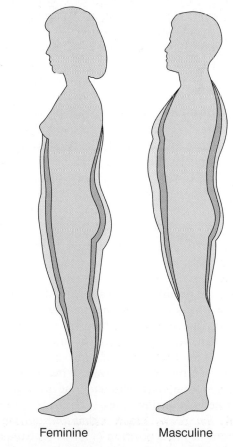

Feminine          Masculine

**FIGURE 7-1**   Feminine Versus Masculine Deposition of Fat

## Nurturing Your Spirituality

### Setting Realistic Fitness and Weight-Loss Goals

Success in any endeavor requires the establishment of long-term goals. Goals that are challenging and worthwhile but not impossible to accomplish are the keys to success. For instance, it would be unrealistic to expect to run a marathon after a few months of sporadic training or to lose 30 pounds in 1 month and keep it off.

A more feasible approach is to set realistic short-term goals that can be accomplished relatively easily and quickly. The accomplishment of these will provide the feedback you need to stay on track and the reinforcement to continue the program.

Attainable, realistic goals for exercise should be consistent with the American College of Sports Medicine guidelines for exercise, and realistic weight loss should not exceed 1.5 to 2 pounds per week. People often throw themselves into exercise with a vengeance, as if to wipe out years of inactivity with a frenzied few weeks of activity. The same degree of impatience surfaces with weight-loss attempts.

The following guidelines increase the likelihood of succeeding with exercise and weight loss:

1. Genetics is responsible for 40 to 50% of the factors that determine how aerobically fit we may become.[14,15] We can achieve our aerobic potential with regular exercise, but world-class endurance performances are beyond the reach of most of us. Exercise and enjoy it, be as good as you can, and be satisfied with a significant accomplishment. You should be encouraged to know that you are in the select 15% of the adult population who exercise regularly and vigorously.
2. Studies suggest that 25 to 40% of obesity can be explained by genetics.[16] The reason for this wide divergence relates to the fact that obesity is a complex, multifactorial disease that has defied the best efforts of scientists to accurately pin down the ratio of risks. Most scientists do agree that genetics probably explains about 25% of obesity. Most scientists also agree that the genes involved in weight gain do not cause obesity directly, because it appears that only the tendency for becoming obese is inherited. Therefore, people who inherit the tendency and who are exposed to an environment that is characterized by limited physical activity and an abundance of food may very well become obese. Conversely, these same people may potentially avoid obesity, and possibly any weight gain, through healthy eating (a diet relatively low in calories and high in nutrient density) and participating in a moderately intense physical fitness program for 60 minutes per day on most, preferably all, days of the week.

3. For weight loss or physical fitness, participate in moderate physical activity (preferably low impact if you are a beginner) that builds exercise into your daily life, such as mowing the lawn, washing the car by hand, and climbing stairs instead of taking elevators; plus participate in a structured exercise program (walking, walking/jogging, cycling, swimming, aerobics, etc.). Sixty minutes or more of exercise per day, preferably 5 days per week, plus eating nutritious meals based on the Food Guide, will improve physical fitness and produce sensible weight loss that can be maintained for life.
4. Avoid the inflexible pursuit of artificial aesthetic ideals and aim for reasonable goals. Don't pressure yourself to achieve your goals too rapidly. Remember, healthy eating and sensible, regular exercise are for a lifetime, not just a few weeks or months. Let the body changes that result from this lifestyle occur slowly, and you will be able to enjoy them for a lifetime.

Taking care of your body does not result in instant health. To make real changes in your lifestyle, you must change the way you think. You must do more than nurture your body; you must nurture your mind as well.

---

Because they produce little estrogen, and much testosterone, men usually deposit minimal amounts of fat in the female pattern. Instead, they store fat primarily in the abdomen, lower back, chest, and nape of the neck.[18] This is referred to as "apple shaped." Some women store fat this way as well. After menopause, estrogen production decreases and the prevalence of *android* fat deposition increases.

Although the general claim is that *android,* or masculine, pattern of fat deposition (sometimes called *central fat*) is harmful, newer evidence indicates that not all android fat is equal.[19–21] Intra-abdominal fat, stored deep within the abdominal cavity, carries a much higher risk than does subcutaneous abdominal fat, stored directly beneath the skin. Intra-abdominal fat, also known as visceral fat, surrounds the internal organs and forms adipose deposits that may lead to endothelial dysfunction, insulin resistance, glucose intolerance, diplipidemia, hypertension, and coronary artery disease.[22] Physical activity and calorie reduction tend to reduce intra-abdominal fat as well as subcutaneous fat. Moderately intense physical activities, such

## Real-World Wellness

### Practical Ways to Estimate Overweight and Obesity

*What are some practical techniques I can use to determine whether I'm overweight or obese that don't require much time, a technician, or sophisticated measuring equipment?*

Practical sources for measuring overweight and overfatness rely on subjective observations and other sensory information. These estimates do not quantify, in a real sense, the extent of the problem, should one exist.

Our mirrors supply us with visual feedback. Stand naked in front of a full-length mirror and, as objectively as possible, observe the shape of your body, determine where fat has accumulated, and estimate the amount of muscle you have. Use a tape measure to measure the circumference of your waist and hips. Your hips should be larger than your waist. While you have the tape measure in your hands, measure the circumference of your ankle according to the directions in Table 7-3. This will estimate your skeletal size, or frame size. People with large frame sizes can carry more weight than can people of the same height with small frame sizes. Knowing your frame size may help you more accurately interpret the results from the bathroom scale in conjunction with height/weight charts.

A few years ago the slogan "pinch an inch" became popular. If you can pinch an inch at various sites on the body, you are probably somewhat overweight.

The fit of your clothes will provide other clues. If your pants or dress size is increasing steadily, you are gaining weight. Conversely, if the sizes are getting smaller, you are successfully losing weight, changing your body composition, or both. If you are not consciously trying to lose weight and don't need to lose but are doing so, anyway,

this could be a sign of emerging disease and should be evaluated by a physician.

There is always the feedback you receive from other people. They may tell you that you appear to have either gained or lost some weight. Their perceptions may or may not be correct, but your size has led them to their conclusions.

After all is said and done, remember this: About 40% of men are dissatisfied with their appearance and two-thirds of young women between 13 and 19 years think they weigh too much. Millions of normal-weight Americans, particularly young women, are also attempting to lose weight.

We are preoccupied with thinness in the United States. Beauty is in the eye of the beholder, but the vision has been distorted by Madison Avenue's preoccupation with excessive leanness. We need to be realistic and understand that excessive leanness is not within the grasp of most people, nor should it be. Thinness does not always go hand in hand with robust health.

**TABLE 7-3**   Measurement of Ankles to Determine Body Frame Size

Measure the ankle at the smallest point above the two bones that protrude on each side of the ankle. The tape measure should be pulled very tightly. Read the tape measure in inches and see the table for an interpretation.

| Gender | Small Frame | Medium Frame | Large Frame |
|--------|-------------|--------------|-------------|
| Male | < 8 inches | 8–9¼ inches | > 9¼ inches |
| Female | < 7½ inches | 7½–8¾ inches | > 8¾ inches |

as gardening and casual walking, may not improve one's cardiorespiratory endurance, but when coupled with modest caloric restriction, they can decrease abdominal fat. Since there is a dose-response relationship between exercise and visceral fat, more vigorous exercise of longer duration will more effectively contribute to a reduction of abdominal fat and overall fat.

The waist-to-hip ratio (WHR) is a simple method for determining the distribution of body fat. It requires an accurate measurement of the circumference of the waist at the narrowest point between the rib cage and the navel and of the hips at the largest circumference of the hip/buttocks region. The waist measurement is then divided by the hip measurement. The resulting value may be interpreted by comparing the WHR with the following standard:[23]

*MALES*

a. Ages 20–70 (WHR of 0.89 to 0.99 or higher is a high risk for disease)

b. Younger adults (WHR greater than 0.95 is a very high risk)

c. Ages 60–69 (WHR of 1.03 or higher is a very high risk)

*FEMALES*

a. Ages 20–70 (WHR of 0.78 to 0.84 or higher is a high risk for disease)

b. Younger adults (WHR of 0.86 or higher is a very high risk)

c. Ages 60–69 (WHR of 0.90 or higher is a very high risk)

The WHR has been criticized for failing to recognize factors other than abdominal fat, such as skeletal size and muscle mass in the buttocks. An expert panel convened by the National Heart, Lung, and Blood Institute in 1998 concluded that a circumference measure of only the waist is more highly predictive of disease risk than is the WHR.[24] For males, a high waist circumference is greater than 40 inches, and for females it is greater than 35 inches. The power of waist circumference to predict heart disease is unaffected by height, and its predictive power is increased if combined with a body mass index greater than 25 kg/m². **Body mass index (BMI)** is the ratio of body weight to height calculated in kilograms per meter squared (kg/m²) (BMI 5 wt [kg]/ht[m²]).

Evidence has emerged from the large international INTERHEART Study, which indicated that the waist-to-hip ratio was a better predictor of future heart attacks than body mass index.[25,26] The authors of this 52-country study recommended a redefinition of obesity based on waist-to-hip ratio instead of BMI because it estimated myocardial infarction (heart attack) was attributed to obesity more accurately in most ethnic groups. The scientific community will weigh this evidence and determine whether a change in the manner in which obesity is measured and expressed is warranted.

The android pattern of deep fat deposition is related to an increase in the risk for heart disease, stroke, Type 2 diabetes, and some forms of cancer.[27] There are several reasons for this increased risk. First, enzymes in abdominal adipose cells are active, so fat moves in and out easily. In sedentary people, abdominal fat enters the bloodstream and is routed directly to the liver, where it becomes the raw material for the manufacture of very low-density lipoprotein (VLDL) triglycerides.[28] Later these are converted to low-density lipoprotein cholesterol (LDL-C), and this increases the risk for cardiovascular disease. Conversely, active people direct abdominal fat to the muscles, where it is used as fuel for physical work.

Second, abdominal fat cells are larger than other fat cells. Large fat cells are associated with blood glucose (sugar) intolerance and excessive amounts of insulin in the blood. Such an environment is conducive to the development of Type 2 diabetes because the cells' receptor sites become resistant to insulin. Higher than normal amounts of insulin must be secreted to transport sugar from the blood to the cells, but excessive insulin remains in the blood. The body's cells continue to resist insulin, so blood sugar also remains high. This sequence of events is characteristic of glucose intolerance, or poor regulation of sugar. Over the years these factors can lead to Type 2 diabetes. A person does not have to be excessively overweight to be at risk for Type 2 diabetes; it is enough that fat be concentrated in the deep abdominal region. Additionally, deep abdominal fat may spawn a cascade of inflammatory events resulting in dangerous metabolic modifications, plaque deposition, and ultimately cardiovascular disease.[29] Extra fat that accumulates in the hips (gynoid pattern) also increases the risk for metabolic diseases, but not quite as much as the android pattern of fat deposition.

Third, excessive insulin in the blood interferes with the removal of sodium by the kidneys, possibly leading to hypertension. Concurrently, the high circulating level of insulin stimulates the overproduction of epinephrine and norepinephrine, both of which raise the blood pressure. This cluster of disorders—high blood pressure, high blood sugar (glucose intolerance), abnormal blood lipids (cholesterol and triglycerides), and abdominal obesity—has deadly consequences. Researchers refer to this combination as *metabolic syndrome*.[30] Too much visceral fat migrates throughout the splanchnic beds promoting cellular resistance to insulin and putting undue strain on the heart, which consequently might result in elevating the blood pressure. Deep abdominal fat is dangerous for a number of reasons. First and foremost, it is more metabolically active than subcutaneous abdominal fat.[31] Deep fat settles in the abdominal region adjacent to the liver, kidneys, and intestines. This type of fat in excess can intrude upon and crowd out the internal organs. Additionally, the deep abdominal fat cells release chemicals that stimulate the liver to ramp up its production of cholesterol and triglycerides.

The good news about android fat is that it is more easily removed from the body than is fat stored in the gynoid pattern. Fat stored in the feminine pattern is highly resistant to removal from its storage depots. Losing gynoid fat usually requires calorie restriction and exercise. Even the best effort may not result in the removal of enough fat from the lower half of the body to satisfy the dieter. Lower-extremity fat is stubborn and much more difficult to lose than is upper-body fat.[32]

# Methods for Measuring Body-Weight Status

## Height/Weight Tables

Optimal body weight is not necessarily reflective of optimal body composition. This was illustrated by a comparison of young and middle-aged men within 5% of their ideal weight as determined by height, weight, and frame-size charts. Although both groups were within the ideal range, the middle-aged subjects had twice the amount of fat as the young subjects.[33]

Height/weight tables do not measure body composition. They act as a standard for total body weight based on height and gender without regard to the composition of weight. Some of the height/weight tables also require users to know their body frame sizes. One method for determining body frame size is found in Table 7-3 on page 241.

## Body Mass Index

Another method for measuring body-weight status is to calculate body mass index. As previously mentioned, body mass index is the ratio of body weight in kilograms to height in meters squared. There are several body mass index protocols, all of which originate from height/weight measurements. These protocols represent an attempt to adjust body weight to derive a height-free measure of obesity. Although BMI does not measure percent body fat and although BMI uses height/weight data, it is more useful than the height/weight tables[34] and it can be used to compare population groups. It also correlates fairly well ($r = 0.70$) with percentage of fat derived from underwater weighing.[35] The $r$ is a coefficient of correlation between two variables; in this particular case, it is between BMI and underwater weighing.

In June 1998, the American Heart Association added *obesity* to its list of major controllable risk factors for heart disease.[36] Obesity is now viewed as a chronic disease that represents a "dangerous epidemic" in this country. Later the same month, The National Heart, Lung, and Blood Institute (NHLBI) issued its initial clinical recommendations on obesity (see Table 7-4).[37] A panel of 24 experts commissioned by the NHLBI conducted an extensive review of the research literature on obesity and concluded that people with BMIs of 25.0 to 29.9 kg/m$^2$ should be classified as overweight. The panel recommended that people whose BMIs fall in this category should attempt to lose weight if they have two or more weight-related risk factors for illness. These include high blood pressure, diabetes, impaired glucose tolerance, and a waist circumference of greater than 40 inches for men and greater than 35 inches for women.

People whose BMIs are 30 kg/m$^2$ and higher are considered to be obese, and the panel advises these people to make serious attempts to lose weight.[38] According to the new BMI guidelines, approximately 65% of Americans are currently overweight.[39] This figure was recently reported by the Centers for Disease Control and Prevention. This value reflects the increasing number of Americans who have become overweight, up 10%, compared with the recent past.

There are two major limitations to using BMI measurements: (1) The technique is misleading for people

**TABLE 7-4** Disease Risk Based on Body Mass Index (BMI) and Waist Circumference

| Class | BMI (kg/m$^2$) | Men ≤ 40 in.** Women ≤ 35 in. | Men > 40 in.** Women > 35 in. |
|---|---|---|---|
| | | **Disease Risk Based on Waist Circumference*** | |
| Underweight | < 18.5** | | |
| Normal | 18.5–24.9 | | |
| Overweight | 25.0–29.9 | Increased | High |
| **Stages of Obesity** | | | |
| I | 30.0–34.9 | High | Very high |
| II | 35.0–39.9 | Very high | Very high |
| III | > 40 | Extremely high | Extremely high |

*Disease risk is for cardiovascular disease, hypertension, and Type 2 diabetes.

**Increased waist circumference may be a marker for an elevated risk even for people of normal weight.

Source: Adapted from National Heart, Lung, and Blood Institute. (1998). *Obesity education initiative expert panel clinical guidelines on the identification, evaluation, and treatment of overweight and obesity in adults.* Washington, DC: National Heart, Lung, and Blood Institute.

with greater than average muscle mass because it measures overweight rather than overfat; and (2) the results are difficult for the general public to interpret, and the average person does not know how to apply BMI values to weight loss. The first limitation is easily surmounted. People with large amounts of muscle tissue should be directed to use a technique such as skinfold measurements or underwater weighing to measure their body composition.

The second limitation is more challenging. Follow these guidelines to establish and interpret BMI measurement. Calculate BMI, taking care to accurately measure weight and height. Weigh yourself in the morning after voiding and prior to breakfast. Wear light clothing and no shoes. For the height measurement, take off your shoes and stand with your back against a flat wall with your heels, buttocks, shoulders, and head against it. Have another person establish your height by using an object that has a right angle, such as a carpenter's square, a textbook, a clipboard on edge, or any other rigid item that is rectangular and has a 90° angle. The person doing the measuring should place the right angle against the wall and slide it down to the top of your head, mark the wall at the bottom of the right angle, and use a tape measure to measure from the mark to the floor.

The simplest way to calculate BMI is to bypass the formula and use Table 7-5 (page 244). Find your height in the left column and move across to your weight in

**TABLE 7-5** Calculating Body Mass Index (BMI)

Each entry gives the body weight in pounds for a person of a given height and BMI. Pounds have been rounded off. To use the table, find the appropriate height in the far-left column. Move across the row to a given weight. The number at the top of the column is the BMI for that height and weight.

| Height (Inches) | BMI (kg/m²) | | | | | | | | | | | | | |
|---|---|---|---|---|---|---|---|---|---|---|---|---|---|---|
| | 19 | 20 | 21 | 22 | 23 | 24 | 25 | 26 | 27 | 28 | 29 | 30 | 35 | 40 |
| | Body Weight (Pounds) | | | | | | | | | | | | | |
| 58 | 91 | 96 | 100 | 105 | 110 | 115 | 119 | 124 | 129 | 134 | 138 | 143 | 167 | 191 |
| 59 | 94 | 99 | 104 | 109 | 114 | 119 | 124 | 128 | 133 | 138 | 143 | 148 | 173 | 198 |
| 60 | 97 | 102 | 107 | 112 | 118 | 123 | 128 | 133 | 138 | 143 | 148 | 153 | 179 | 204 |
| 61 | 100 | 106 | 111 | 116 | 122 | 127 | 132 | 137 | 143 | 148 | 153 | 158 | 185 | 211 |
| 62 | 104 | 109 | 115 | 120 | 126 | 131 | 136 | 142 | 147 | 153 | 158 | 164 | 191 | 218 |
| 63 | 107 | 113 | 118 | 124 | 130 | 135 | 141 | 146 | 152 | 158 | 163 | 169 | 197 | 225 |
| 64 | 110 | 116 | 122 | 128 | 134 | 140 | 145 | 151 | 157 | 163 | 169 | 174 | 204 | 232 |
| 65 | 114 | 120 | 126 | 132 | 138 | 144 | 150 | 156 | 162 | 168 | 174 | 180 | 210 | 240 |
| 66 | 118 | 124 | 130 | 136 | 142 | 148 | 155 | 161 | 167 | 173 | 179 | 186 | 216 | 247 |
| 67 | 121 | 127 | 134 | 140 | 146 | 153 | 159 | 166 | 172 | 178 | 185 | 191 | 223 | 255 |
| 68 | 125 | 131 | 138 | 144 | 151 | 158 | 164 | 171 | 177 | 184 | 190 | 197 | 230 | 262 |
| 69 | 128 | 135 | 142 | 149 | 155 | 162 | 169 | 176 | 182 | 189 | 196 | 203 | 236 | 270 |
| 70 | 132 | 139 | 146 | 153 | 160 | 167 | 174 | 181 | 188 | 195 | 202 | 207 | 243 | 278 |
| 71 | 136 | 143 | 150 | 157 | 165 | 172 | 179 | 186 | 193 | 200 | 208 | 215 | 230 | 286 |
| 72 | 140 | 147 | 154 | 162 | 169 | 177 | 184 | 191 | 199 | 206 | 213 | 221 | 258 | 294 |
| 73 | 144 | 151 | 159 | 166 | 174 | 182 | 189 | 197 | 204 | 212 | 219 | 227 | 265 | 302 |
| 74 | 148 | 155 | 163 | 171 | 179 | 186 | 194 | 202 | 210 | 218 | 225 | 233 | 272 | 311 |
| 75 | 152 | 160 | 168 | 176 | 184 | 192 | 200 | 208 | 216 | 224 | 232 | 240 | 279 | 319 |
| 76 | 156 | 164 | 172 | 180 | 189 | 197 | 205 | 213 | 221 | 230 | 238 | 246 | 287 | 328 |

the same row. The number at the top of this column is your BMI. For example, a man who is 71 inches tall and weighs 200 pounds has a BMI of 28 kg/m². This man is in the "overweight" category. How much weight would he need to lose if he wanted to achieve a BMI of 24 kg/m²? He can easily calculate this from the table. Find the column with the desired BMI of 24 kg/m² and drop down in the table to the row with his height (71 inches). He should weigh 172 pounds to achieve a BMI of 24 kg/m². Then subtract his desired weight (172 pounds) from his current weight (200 pounds). He needs to lose 28 pounds to reach his goal. Turn to Assessment Activity 7-1 to calculate your BMI and your desired body weight.

## Measurement of Body Fat

The only direct means to measure the fat content of the human body is to perform chemical analysis on cadavers. The information obtained from cadaver studies has been used to develop indirect methods for estimating fat content. Because these estimates are indirect, they contain some degree of measurement error and should be interpreted accordingly. These indirect methods are commonly used in exercise physiology laboratories and fitness and wellness centers. See Wellness for a Lifetime: Body Composition of Children and Adolescents.

## Selected Methods for Measuring Body Composition

### Underwater Weighing

*Underwater weighing,* one of the most accurate of the measurement techniques, involves weighing subjects both on land and while completely submerged in water (Figure 7-2).

Whole-body density is calculated from body volume according to Archimedes' principle of displacement. Several thousand years ago, Archimedes discovered that a body immersed in water loses an amount of weight equal to the weight of the displaced water. The loss of weight in water is directly proportional to the volume of the water displaced or the volume of the body that displaces that water. The density of bone and muscle is higher than that of water and tends to sink. The density of fat is lighter than water and tends to float. Therefore, people with more muscle mass weigh more in water than do those who have less. Formulas have been developed that use weight on land and weight in water to determine the percentage of the total weight that consists of fat.

Underwater weighing has an inherent error of measurement that can be minimized when the residual vol-

## Wellness for a Lifetime
### Body Composition of Children and Adolescents

The body composition of children changes during the growth process. It has been well established that obese children and adolescents have a higher probability of becoming obese adults than do normal-weight children and that dramatic changes in body fat and body composition can occur during the peripubertal years (the time before, during, and after puberty). The proportion of body fat in young children ranges from 10 to 15%, with boys toward the lower end and girls toward the upper.[40]

Body fat generally increases in adolescent boys and girls and continues to do so into young adulthood, so that the percentage of fat in males increases to 15 to 20%, whereas that of females increases to 20 to 25%. As we age, the percentage of fat continues to increase while muscle mass decreases. By middle age, fat accumulation exceeds 25% of the total weight of many men and 30 percent of the total weight of many women. The reason is a growing disparity between energy intake (food consumption) and energy expenditure (level of physical activity). We become less active with age. Television, computers, automobiles, elevators, escalators, remote controls, golf carts, riding mowers, and a lack of quality physical education programs in the public schools have diminished the energy expended by American children and adults.

Skinfold measurements made on children and adolescents in the 1960s and 1970s have been compared with those made on similar subjects in the 1980s. A trend surfaced in this comparison, indicating that a systematic increase in body fat percentage had occurred during the interim.[41] There is not a generally accepted definition of *obesity* that distinguishes it from overweight among children and adolescents.[42] Therefore, the term *overweight* is used to determine cutoff points at which health can be negatively affected. In 2000, the incidence of overweight among children (aged 6 to 11) was 15.3% and among adolescents (aged 12 to 19) was 15.5%.[43] An additional 15% of children and 14.9% of adolescents were just below the cutoff point for being overweight.[44]

One study examined the relationship between body fatness and health status among children and adolescents.[45] The risks for high blood pressure, high total and LDL cholesterol (the harmful form), and low HDL cholesterol (the protective form) were associated with body fat above 25% for men and 30% for women. These levels have subsequently been proposed as useful health standards for those between 6 and 18 years of age.

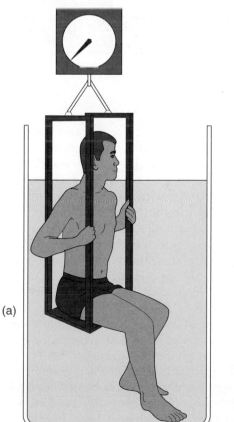

(a)

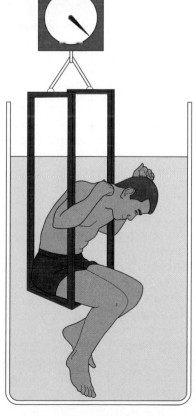

(b)

**FIGURE 7-2**  Underwater Weighing Apparatus
(a) The subject is in the ready position for underwater weighing.
(b) The subject is being weighed.

ume of air (the air left in the lungs after a maximal expiration) is accurately measured. If residual air is measured, the error is approximately 2.7%.[46] Accuracy also depends on the subject's ability to exhale maximally on each trial and to sit still while completely submerged for 6 to 10 seconds.

The equipment required for underwater weighing includes an autopsy scale with a capacity of approximately 9 kg (about 20 lbs.). The scale is suspended over a tank of water at least 4 feet deep. The subject sits suspended chin-deep, exhales completely, and bends forward from the waist until entirely submerged. This position is maintained for 6 to 10 seconds to allow the scale to stabilize. Five to 10 trials are required, and the underwater weight is attained by averaging the three heaviest readings. The subject's net underwater weight is calculated by subtracting the weight of the seat, its supporting structure, and a weight belt (if needed) from the gross underwater weight. Percentage of body fat can be calculated from body density by using appropriate formulas.

## Bioelectrical Impedance Analysis

Bioelectrical impedance analysis (BIA) is a relatively new and simple method of determining body composition. The equipment is portable and computerized but fairly expensive. It is safe, noninvasive, quick, and convenient to use (Figure 7-3). Additionally, it does not require a high degree of technical skill, it intrudes less on the subject's privacy than other methods, and it is generally more comfortable.

The most common application of BIA employs a harmless, low-level, single-frequency electric current. This current is passed through the body of the person being measured via electrodes attached to specific sites on the right hand and foot, as shown in Figure 7-3. Impedance represents resistance to the transmission of an electrical current. Impedance is least in lean body tissues because of their high water content (approximately 73% water). Water is an excellent conductor of electricity. Conversely, fat contains only 14 to 22% water and is resistant to electrical flow.[47]

A major limitation of BIA is that it does not accurately estimate fat-free mass in very lean or very fat subjects. Body fatness is generally overestimated for lean subjects and underestimated in obese subjects.[48]

Recent advances in BIA instrumentation have improved the technique. The newer instruments use multiple frequency bioelectrical impedance analysis (MFBIA), which seems to be less susceptible to the hydration status of subjects. As a result, a better estimate of lean body mass can be achieved.[49]

Conventional BIA systems employ an arm-to-leg protocol to indirectly measure body fat. Two new BIA

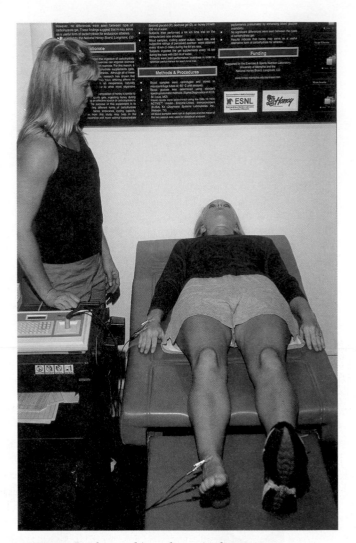

**FIGURE 7-3**  Bioelectrical Impedance Analysis

systems have been developed in recent years: one measures leg-to-leg impedance and the other measures arm-to-arm impedance. The leg-to-leg system combines a digital scale equipped with two stainless steel pressure contact footpad electrodes with a BIA system. Subjects stand barefooted on the foot pads while their body weight and impedance are measured simultaneously.

A handheld bioelectrical analyzer has been developed that measures arm-to-arm impedance. Both of the new BIA systems appear to produce valid estimates of body composition. In general, the standard error of measurement for BIA is 3.5 to 5.0%, which is a bit higher than the error of measurement for skinfold calipers.[50] The main sources of error are the hydration state of the subject and the prediction equation used. Hydration is affected by eating, drinking fluids, urination, and exercise, and it significantly influences the results. Technician error is relatively minor, provided standard procedures for electrode placement and body position of the subject are followed. To reduce error, the temperature of the testing room should be comfortable, and the following guidelines should be given to subjects the day before they are scheduled for testing:

- No eating or drinking within 4 hours of the test
- No exercise within 12 hours of the test
- No urination within 30 minutes of the test
- No alcohol consumption within 48 hours of the test
- No diuretic medicines within 7 days of the test

## Skinfold Measurements

Skinfold measurements are one of the least expensive and most economical methods of measuring body composition. The cost of skinfold calipers can be as low as $10. Computerized models, however, can run as high as $600. The most accurate calipers maintain a constant jaw pressure of 10 g/mm$^2$ of jaw surface area.

The thumb and index finger are used to pinch and lift the skin and the fat beneath it. The caliper is placed beneath the pinch (Figures 7-4 through 7-8). Tables 7-6 and 7-7 (pages 249 and 250) show how to convert the sum of millimeters of skinfold thickness to percentage of body fat. When performed by skilled technicians,

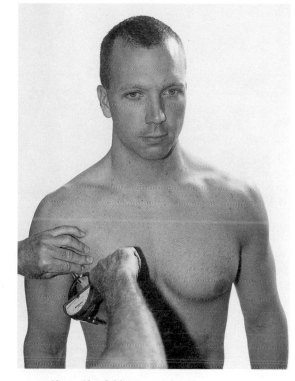

**FIGURE 7-5** Chest Skinfold Measurement
Take a diagonal fold half the distance between the anterior axillary line and the nipple.

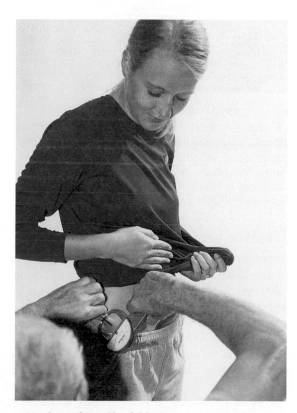

**FIGURE 7-4** Suprailium Skinfold Measurement
Take a diagonal fold above the crest of the ilium, or upper portion of the hip bone, directly below the midaxilla (armpit).

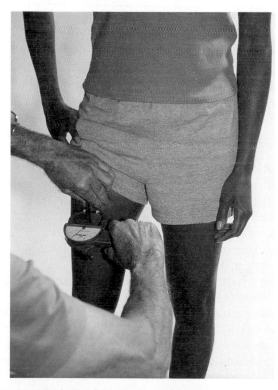

**FIGURE 7-6** Thigh Skinfold Measurement
Take a vertical fold on the front of the thigh midway between the hip and the knee joint. The midpoint should be marked while the subject is seated.

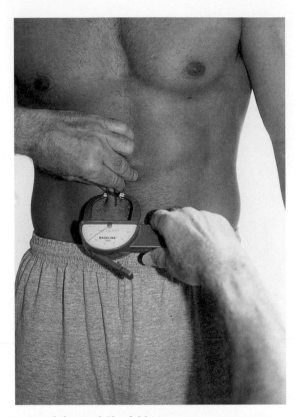

**FIGURE 7-7** Abdominal Skinfold Measurement
Take a vertical fold about 1 inch from the navel.

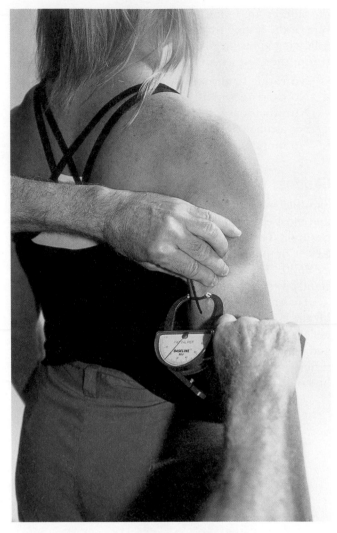

**FIGURE 7-8** Triceps Skinfold Measurement
Take a vertical fold on the midline of the upper arm over the triceps, halfway between the acromion and olecranon processes (tip of the shoulder to the tip of the elbow). The arm should be extended and relaxed when the measurement is taken. All skinfold measurements should be taken on the right side.

skinfold measurements correlate well (0.70–0.90) with body density calculated from underwater weighing.[51] It is very important that technicians receive adequate practice and training under a qualified instructor before performing skinfold measurements.

As suggested by the American College of Sports Medicine, these guidelines should be followed when taking skinfold measurements:[52]

1. All measurements should be made on the right side of the body.
2. The caliper heads should be placed about 1/4 to 1/2 inch below the thumb and index finger, perpendicular to the fold, and halfway into the length of the fold.
3. The pinch should be held continuously while reading the caliper.
4. Wait no more than 1 to 2 seconds before reading the caliper.
5. Take duplicate measures at each site, and retest if the measures are farther than 1 to 2 millimeters (mm) apart.
6. Measure each of the sites one time, and then repeat the measurements again. This will allow time for the skinfold to return to normal before the next measurement.[53]

## Air-Displacement Plethysmography

Air-displacement plethysmography is one of the more recent methods developed to measure body composition through densiometry techniques. In lieu of being submerged in water, subjects sit inside a precisely calibrated chamber, marketed commercially as the BodPod (Figure 7-9, page 251), where they displace air instead of water.[54] The volume of air displaced when the subject sits inside the chamber is equal to body volume. This value is calculated indirectly by subtracting the volume of air remaining in the chamber while the subject is inside from the volume of air in the chamber when it is empty.[55] Subjects should wear a bathing cap and a Lycra-type bathing suit to avoid air being trapped

**TABLE 7-6**   Percentage of Fat Estimated for Men (Sum of Chest, Abdomen, and Thigh Skinfolds)

| Sum of Skinfolds (mm) | Age to Last Year | | | | | | | | |
|---|---|---|---|---|---|---|---|---|---|
| | Under 23 | 23–27 | 28–32 | 33–37 | 38–42 | 43–47 | 48–52 | 53–57 | Over 57 |
| 8–10 | 1.3 | 1.8 | 2.3 | 2.9 | 3.4 | 3.9 | 4.5 | 5.0 | 5.5 |
| 11–13 | 2.2 | 2.8 | 3.3 | 3.9 | 4.4 | 4.9 | 5.5 | 6.0 | 6.5 |
| 14–16 | 3.2 | 3.8 | 4.3 | 4.8 | 5.4 | 5.9 | 6.4 | 7.0 | 7.5 |
| 17–19 | 4.2 | 4.7 | 5.3 | 5.8 | 6.3 | 6.9 | 7.4 | 8.0 | 8.5 |
| 20–22 | 5.1 | 5.7 | 6.2 | 6.8 | 7.3 | 7.9 | 8.4 | 8.9 | 9.5 |
| 23–25 | 6.1 | 6.6 | 7.2 | 7.7 | 8.3 | 8.8 | 9.4 | 9.9 | 10.5 |
| 26–28 | 7.0 | 7.6 | 8.1 | 8.7 | 9.2 | 9.8 | 10.3 | 10.9 | 11.4 |
| 29–31 | 8.0 | 8.5 | 9.1 | 9.6 | 10.2 | 10.7 | 11.3 | 11.8 | 12.4 |
| 32–34 | 8.9 | 9.4 | 10.0 | 10.5 | 11.1 | 11.6 | 12.2 | 12.8 | 13.3 |
| 35–37 | 9.8 | 10.4 | 10.9 | 11.5 | 12.0 | 12.6 | 13.1 | 13.7 | 14.3 |
| 38–40 | 10.7 | 11.3 | 11.8 | 12.4 | 12.9 | 13.5 | 14.1 | 14.6 | 15.2 |
| 41–43 | 11.6 | 12.2 | 12.7 | 13.3 | 13.8 | 14.4 | 15.0 | 15.5 | 16.1 |
| 44–46 | 12.5 | 13.1 | 13.6 | 14.2 | 14.7 | 15.3 | 15.9 | 16.4 | 17.0 |
| 47–49 | 13.4 | 13.9 | 14.5 | 15.1 | 15.6 | 16.2 | 16.8 | 17.3 | 17.9 |
| 50–52 | 14.3 | 14.8 | 15.4 | 15.9 | 16.5 | 17.1 | 17.6 | 18.2 | 18.8 |
| 53–55 | 15.1 | 15.7 | 16.2 | 16.8 | 17.4 | 17.9 | 18.5 | 19.1 | 19.7 |
| 56–58 | 16.0 | 16.5 | 17.1 | 17.7 | 18.2 | 18.8 | 19.4 | 20.0 | 20.5 |
| 59–61 | 16.9 | 17.4 | 17.9 | 18.5 | 19.1 | 19.7 | 20.2 | 20.8 | 21.4 |
| 62 64 | 17.6 | 18.2 | 18.8 | 19.4 | 19.9 | 20.5 | 21.1 | 21.7 | 22.2 |
| 65–67 | 18.5 | 19.0 | 19.6 | 20.2 | 20.8 | 21.3 | 21.9 | 22.5 | 23.1 |
| 68–70 | 19.3 | 19.9 | 20.4 | 21.0 | 21.6 | 22.2 | 22.7 | 23.3 | 23.9 |
| 71–73 | 20.1 | 20.7 | 21.2 | 21.8 | 22.4 | 23.0 | 23.6 | 24.1 | 24.7 |
| 74–76 | 20.9 | 21.5 | 22.0 | 22.6 | 23.2 | 23.8 | 24.4 | 25.0 | 25.5 |
| 77–79 | 21.7 | 22.2 | 22.8 | 23.4 | 24.0 | 24.6 | 25.2 | 25.8 | 26.3 |
| 80–82 | 22.4 | 23.0 | 23.6 | 24.2 | 24.8 | 25.4 | 25.9 | 26.5 | 27.1 |
| 83–85 | 23.2 | 23.8 | 24.4 | 25.0 | 25.5 | 26.1 | 26.7 | 27.3 | 27.9 |
| 86–88 | 24.0 | 24.5 | 25.1 | 25.7 | 26.3 | 26.9 | 27.5 | 28.1 | 28.7 |
| 89–91 | 24.7 | 25.3 | 25.9 | 26.5 | 27.1 | 27.6 | 28.2 | 28.8 | 29.4 |
| 92–94 | 25.4 | 26.0 | 26.6 | 27.2 | 27.8 | 28.4 | 29.0 | 29.6 | 30.2 |
| 95–97 | 26.1 | 26.7 | 27.3 | 27.9 | 28.5 | 29.1 | 29.7 | 30.3 | 30.9 |
| 98–100 | 26.9 | 27.4 | 28.0 | 28.6 | 29.2 | 29.8 | 30.4 | 31.0 | 31.6 |
| 101–103 | 27.5 | 28.1 | 28.7 | 29.3 | 29.9 | 30.5 | 31.1 | 31.7 | 32.3 |
| 104–106 | 28.2 | 28.8 | 29.4 | 30.0 | 30.6 | 31.2 | 31.8 | 32.4 | 33.0 |
| 107–109 | 28.9 | 29.5 | 30.1 | 30.7 | 31.3 | 31.9 | 32.5 | 33.1 | 33.7 |
| 110–112 | 29.6 | 30.2 | 30.8 | 31.4 | 32.0 | 32.6 | 33.2 | 33.8 | 34.4 |
| 113–115 | 30.2 | 30.8 | 31.4 | 32.0 | 32.6 | 33.2 | 33.8 | 34.5 | 35.1 |
| 116–118 | 30.9 | 31.5 | 32.1 | 32.7 | 33.3 | 33.9 | 34.5 | 35.1 | 35.7 |
| 119–121 | 31.5 | 32.1 | 32.7 | 33.3 | 33.9 | 34.5 | 35.1 | 35.7 | 36.4 |
| 122–124 | 32.1 | 32.7 | 33.3 | 33.9 | 34.5 | 35.1 | 35.8 | 36.4 | 37.0 |
| 125–127 | 32.7 | 33.3 | 33.9 | 34.5 | 35.1 | 35.8 | 36.4 | 37.0 | 37.6 |

within clothing and body hair. Preliminary investigations have shown that this method of assessing body composition is highly compatible with underwater displacement. The difference in body fat measured between the two methods was quite small.[56]

The BodPod has several advantages over underwater weighing: (1) The measurement takes only about 5 minutes, (2) the system is easy to operate, (3) the device is mobile, (4) minimal technical training is required due to the menu-driven software, and (5) it may more effectively accommodate special popula-tions, including, but not limited to, the disabled, the obese, children, the elderly, and nonswimmers afraid to submerge completely in a water tank. This technique seems to have a great deal of promise. The major disadvantage is its cost—approximately $34,000.

## Dual-Energy X-Ray Absorptiometry (DXA)

Dual-energy X-ray absorptiometry was originally developed to measure bone mineral density, but advances in technology have allowed for the quantification of fat and

**TABLE 7-7** Percentage of Fat Estimated for Women (Sum of Triceps, Suprailium, and Thigh Skinfolds)

| Sum of Skinfolds (mm) | Age to Last Year | | | | | | | | |
|---|---|---|---|---|---|---|---|---|---|
| | Under 23 | 23–27 | 28–32 | 33–37 | 38–42 | 43–47 | 48–52 | 53–57 | Over 57 |
| 23–25 | 9.7 | 9.9 | 10.2 | 10.4 | 10.7 | 10.9 | 11.2 | 11.4 | 11.7 |
| 26–28 | 11.0 | 11.2 | 11.5 | 11.7 | 12.0 | 12.3 | 12.5 | 12.7 | 13.0 |
| 29–31 | 12.3 | 12.5 | 12.8 | 13.0 | 13.3 | 13.5 | 13.8 | 14.0 | 14.3 |
| 32–34 | 13.6 | 13.8 | 14.0 | 14.3 | 14.5 | 14.8 | 15.0 | 15.3 | 15.5 |
| 35–37 | 14.8 | 15.0 | 15.3 | 15.5 | 15.8 | 16.0 | 16.3 | 16.5 | 16.8 |
| 38–40 | 16.0 | 16.3 | 16.5 | 16.7 | 17.0 | 17.2 | 17.5 | 17.7 | 18.0 |
| 41–43 | 17.2 | 17.4 | 17.7 | 17.9 | 18.2 | 18.4 | 18.7 | 18.9 | 19.2 |
| 44–46 | 18.3 | 18.6 | 18.8 | 19.1 | 19.3 | 19.6 | 19.8 | 20.1 | 20.3 |
| 47–49 | 19.5 | 19.7 | 20.0 | 20.2 | 20.5 | 20.7 | 21.0 | 21.2 | 21.5 |
| 50–52 | 20.6 | 20.8 | 21.1 | 21.3 | 21.6 | 21.8 | 22.1 | 22.3 | 22.6 |
| 53–55 | 21.7 | 21.9 | 22.1 | 22.4 | 22.6 | 22.9 | 23.1 | 23.4 | 23.6 |
| 56–58 | 22.7 | 23.0 | 23.2 | 23.4 | 23.7 | 23.9 | 24.2 | 24.4 | 24.7 |
| 59–61 | 23.7 | 24.0 | 24.2 | 24.5 | 24.7 | 25.0 | 25.2 | 25.5 | 25.7 |
| 62–64 | 24.7 | 25.0 | 25.2 | 25.5 | 25.7 | 26.0 | 26.7 | 26.4 | 26.7 |
| 65–67 | 25.7 | 25.9 | 26.2 | 26.4 | 26.7 | 26.9 | 27.2 | 27.4 | 27.7 |
| 68–70 | 26.6 | 26.9 | 27.1 | 27.4 | 27.6 | 27.9 | 28.1 | 28.4 | 28.6 |
| 71–73 | 27.5 | 27.8 | 28.0 | 28.3 | 28.5 | 28.8 | 29.0 | 29.3 | 29.5 |
| 74–76 | 28.4 | 28.7 | 28.9 | 29.2 | 29.4 | 29.7 | 29.9 | 30.2 | 30.4 |
| 77–79 | 29.3 | 29.5 | 29.8 | 30.0 | 30.3 | 30.5 | 30.8 | 31.0 | 31.3 |
| 80–82 | 30.1 | 30.4 | 30.6 | 30.9 | 31.1 | 31.4 | 31.6 | 31.9 | 32.1 |
| 83–85 | 30.9 | 31.2 | 31.4 | 31.7 | 31.9 | 32.2 | 32.4 | 32.7 | 32.9 |
| 86–88 | 31.7 | 32.0 | 32.2 | 32.5 | 32.7 | 32.9 | 33.2 | 33.4 | 33.7 |
| 89–91 | 32.5 | 32.7 | 33.0 | 33.2 | 33.5 | 33.7 | 33.9 | 34.2 | 34.4 |
| 92–94 | 33.2 | 33.4 | 33.7 | 33.9 | 34.2 | 34.4 | 34.7 | 34.9 | 35.2 |
| 95–97 | 33.9 | 34.1 | 34.4 | 34.6 | 34.9 | 35.1 | 35.4 | 35.6 | 35.9 |
| 98–100 | 34.6 | 34.8 | 35.1 | 35.3 | 35.5 | 35.8 | 36.0 | 36.3 | 36.5 |
| 101–103 | 35.3 | 35.4 | 35.7 | 35.9 | 36.2 | 36.4 | 36.7 | 36.9 | 37.2 |
| 104–106 | 35.8 | 36.1 | 36.3 | 36.6 | 36.8 | 37.1 | 37.3 | 37.5 | 37.8 |
| 107–109 | 36.4 | 36.7 | 36.9 | 37.1 | 37.4 | 37.6 | 37.9 | 38.1 | 38.4 |
| 110–112 | 37.0 | 37.2 | 37.5 | 37.7 | 38.0 | 38.2 | 38.5 | 38.7 | 38.9 |
| 113–115 | 37.5 | 37.8 | 38.0 | 38.2 | 38.5 | 38.7 | 39.0 | 39.2 | 39.5 |
| 116–118 | 38.0 | 38.3 | 38.5 | 38.8 | 39.0 | 39.3 | 39.5 | 39.7 | 40.0 |
| 119–121 | 38.5 | 38.7 | 39.0 | 39.2 | 39.5 | 39.7 | 40.0 | 40.2 | 40.5 |
| 122–124 | 39.0 | 39.2 | 39.4 | 39.7 | 39.9 | 40.2 | 40.4 | 40.7 | 40.9 |
| 125–127 | 39.4 | 39.6 | 39.9 | 40.1 | 40.4 | 40.6 | 40.9 | 41.1 | 41.4 |
| 128–130 | 39.8 | 40.0 | 40.3 | 40.5 | 40.8 | 41.0 | 41.3 | 41.5 | 41.8 |

lean tissue as well. DXA uses an X-ray generator and two energy levels as the source radiation. The subject lies on a table while a series of transverse scans are made 1 centimeter (cm) apart from head to toe. This system allows for the simultaneous measurement of bone mineral, fat, and nonbone lean tissue. The radiation exposure is very low, and technicians can stay in the room while the procedure is in progress (see Figure 7-10).

The advantages of DXA are the following:

1. The subject simply lies on a table while the scan is in progress.

2. The procedure takes 10 to 20 minutes.
3. The elderly, the young, and the disabled can be measured with this technique.
4. It estimates bone mineral, fat, and nonbone lean tissue at the same time.

Research indicates that DXA provides accurate and reliable estimates of body composition.[57,58] But its use is possibly limited by the price of the equipment, which runs $75,000 to $150,000. Also, some authorities suggest that the equations used to assess body composition need some refinement.

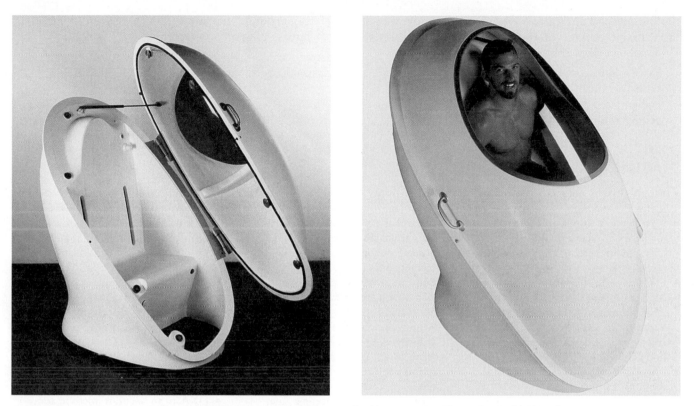

**FIGURE 7-9**   A Subject Prepared for Air-Displacement Plethysmography Measurement Using the BodPod Body Composition System

## Determining Desired Body Weight from Body Fat

Calculating desirable body weight is a simple procedure when the percentage of body fat is known. The following example is for a 148-pound woman whose body fat is equal to 30% of her total body weight, based on her skinfold measurements. She wishes to reduce her body fat to 23%.

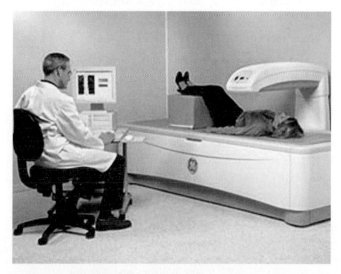

**FIGURE 7-10**   The Dual-Energy X-Ray Absorptiometry (DEXA) System

Find fat weight (FW) in pounds:

$$FW \text{ (lbs.)} = \frac{\text{Body weight (BW) (lbs.)} \times \% \text{ fat}}{100}$$

$$= \frac{148 \text{ lbs.} \times 30}{100}$$

$$= \frac{4,400 \text{ lbs}}{100}$$

$$= 44.4 \text{ lbs.}$$

Find lean weight (LW) in pounds:

$$LW \text{ (lbs.)} = BW - FW$$
$$= 148 \text{ lbs.} - 44.4 \text{ lbs.}$$
$$= 103.6 \text{ lbs.}$$

Find desirable body weight (DBW) in pounds:

$$DBW \text{ (lbs.)} = \frac{LW \text{ (lbs.)}}{1.0 - \% \text{ fat desired}}$$

$$= \frac{103.6 \text{ lbs}}{1.0 - 0.23}$$

$$= \frac{103.6 \text{ lbs}}{0.77}$$

$$= 134.5 \text{ lbs.}$$

She needs to lose 13.5 lbs to reach her DBW (148 − 134.5 = 13.5).

The method for calculating desirable body weight based on percentage of body fat is relatively effective if the subject does the following:

- Exercises to maintain muscle tissue
- Loses no more than 1.5 pounds per week
- Is evaluated for body fatness two or three times during the weight-loss period

- Understands that indirect measurements of body fatness contain some error

Complete Assessment Activity 7-2 to determine your desirable body weight.

## Summary

- Essential fat is necessary for normal biological function.
- Men carry 3 to 5% of their weight in the form of essential fat; women carry 11 to 14% of their weight as essential fat.
- *Obesity* is defined as overfatness.
- Men are obese when fat constitutes 25% or more of the body's weight, and women are obese when fat constitutes 32% or more of the body's weight.
- The majority of women store fat in the hips, buttocks, thighs, and breasts (gynoid fat).

- The majority of men store fat in the abdomen, lower back, chest, and nape of the neck (android fat).
- Height/weight tables are limited and poor instruments for weight-loss recommendations.
- Body mass index correlates fairly well with percent fat derived from hydrostatic weighing.
- A high body mass index correlates with hypertension, high total cholesterol, low HDL cholesterol, high serum triglycerides, and poor glucose tolerance.
- Bioelectrical impedance is a safe, quick, and relatively accurate method for assessing percentage of body fat.

- Skinfold measurements are one of the most economical methods of measuring body composition in terms of the cost of equipment and the time required to determine percentage of body fat.
- Underwater weighing is still considered the "gold standard" for measuring body composition.
- Air-displacement plethysmography is one of the newest techniques for measuring body composition, and it correlates highly with underwater weighing.
- DXA is an accurate method for measuring body composition.

## Review Questions

1. What is essential fat, and how is it distributed in men and women?
2. How would you define *obesity* and *overweight*?
3. At what level of fat deposition does obesity become a health hazard for men and women?
4. What are *gynoid obesity* and *android obesity*? Which is a greater health risk and why?
5. What are the limitations of height/weight tables for recommending weight loss?
6. What is body mass index, and how is it classified for men and women?
7. How are underwater weighing, bioelectrical impedance, and skinfold measurements used to determine percentage of body fat?
8. How is healthy body weight determined when the percentage of body fat is known?

## References

1. Ratamess, N. (2010). Body composition status and assessment. In *ACSM's resource manual* (6th ed.), edited by J. K. Ehrman. Philadelphia: Wolters Kluwer/Lippincott Williams and Wilkins.
2. Center for Consumer Freedom. (2005, February 17). A detailed analysis of the CDC's 'Obesity Kills' statistics. Retrieved from www.consumerfreedom.com/article detail.cfm/a/165_1_detailed analysis of the cdcs obesity kills statistics.
3. Flegal, K. M., et al. (2005, April 20). Excess deaths associated with underweight, overweight and obesity. *Journal of the American Medical Association,* 293, 1861.
4. Editors. (2005, August). Hefty is healthy? *Harvard Health Letter,* 30(10), 7.
5. ACSM. (2010). *ACSM's guidelines for exercise testing and prescription.* Philadelphia: Wolters Kluwer/Lippincott Williams and Wilkins.
6. Mac, B. (2010, March 8). Facts about fat. Retrieved from www.brainmac.co.uk/fat.htm.
7. Ibid.
8. Nieman, D. C. (2007). *Exercise testing and prescription* (6th ed.). Boston: McGraw-Hill.
9. Powers, S. K., & E.T. Howley. (2009). *Exercise physiology* (7th ed.). Boston: McGraw-Hill.
10. Nieman (2007).
11. Ratamess (2010).
12. Kaminsky, L., & G. Dwyer. (2006). Body composition. In *ACSM's resource manual* (5th ed.), edited by L. A. Kaminsky. Philadelphia: Lippincott Williams and Wilkins.
13. Ratamess (2010).
14. Powers & Howley (2009).

15. Wilmore, J. H., D. L. Costill, & W. L. Kenney. (2008). *Physiology of sport and exercise* (4th ed.). Champaign, IL: Human Kinetics.
16. Nieman (2007).
17. Byrd-Bredbenner, C., et al. (2009). *Wardlaw's perspectives in nutrition.* New York: McGraw-Hill.
18. Ibid.
19. Editors. (2009, January). Measuring how fat we are. *Harvard Health Letter, 34(3),* 1.
20. Wikipedia. (2010, March 3). Adipose tissue. Retrieved from http://enwikipedia.org/wiki/Adipose_tissue.
21. Jacquescoley, E. (2008, March 31). Subcutaneous vs. visceral fat: Which matters most when battling the bulge? Retrieved from www.scienceblog.com/cms/subeutaneous-vs-visceral-fat-which-matters-most-when-battling-bulge-15764.html.
22. Ratamess (2010).
23. Ibid.
24. National Heart, Lung and Blood Institute. (1998). Obesity education initiative expert panel clinical guideline on the identification, evaluation and treatment of overweight and obesity in adults. Washington, DC: National Heart, Lung and Blood Institute.
25. Powers & Howley (2009).
26. Nieman (2007).
27. Weil, A. (2005, June). The battle of the belly bulge. In *Dr. Andrew Weil's Self-Healing, 3.*
28. Byrd-Bredbenner (2009).
29. NBC and iVillage. (2008, February 22). Pot bellies point to heart risk. *Your Total Health. Retrieved from* http://yourtotalhealth.ivillage.com/pot_bellies_point_to_heart-risk_.html.
30. Ryan, A., & L. Joseph. (2010). Pathophysiology and treatment of metabolic disease. In *ACSM's resource manual* (6th ed.), edited by J. K. Ehrman. Philadelphia: Wolters Kluwer/Lippincott Williams and Wilkins.
31. Weil (2005).
32. Nieman (2007).
33. Ibid.
34. Blair, S. N., et al. (1995). Changes in physical fitness and all-cause mortality. *Journal of the American Medical Association, 273(14),* 1093.
35. Nieman (2007).
36. Editors. (1998). Guidelines call more Americans overweight. *Harvard Health Letter, 23(10),* 7.
37. Expert panel on the identification, evaluation, and treatment of overweight and obesity in adults. 1998 Executive Summary. *Archives of Internal Medicine, 158,* 1855.
38. Ibid.
39. American College of Sports Medicine. (2010). *ACSM's guidelines for exercise testing and prescription* (8th ed.). Philadelphia: Wolters Kluwer/Lippincott Williams and Wilkins.
40. Powers & Howley (2009).
41. Wilmore (2008).
42. Nieman (2007).
43. American Obesity Association. (2006, July 20). Obesity in youth. Retrieved from www.obesity.org/subs/fastfacts/obesity-youth.shtml.
44. Ibid.
45. Eisenmann, J. C., et al. (2005). Relationships between adolescent fitness and fatness and cardiovascular disease risk factors in adulthood: The Aerobics Center Longitudinal Study (ACLS). *American Heart Journal,* 149(1), 46.
46. Nieman (2007).
47. Ibid.
48. Ratamess (2010).
49. Ibid.
50. Ibid.
51. ACSM (2010).
52. Ibid.
53. Ratamess (2010).
54. Powers & Howley (2009).
55. Ratamess (2010).
56. Powers & Howley (2009).
57. Ibid.
58. Ratamess (2010).

## Suggested Readings

Benardot, D. (2010, March 15). Dual energy X-ray absorptiometry (DEXA). Healthline. Retrieved from www.healthline.com/hcbook/nut-dual-energy-x-ray-absorptiometry-dexa.

According to the author, DEXA is the latest, most accurate, and most expensive method for determining body composition. It is generally considered the gold standard, and is replacing underwater weighing for calculating body composition. The article discusses how DEXA works to separate and calculate bone density, lean body mass, and fat mass.

Department of Health and Human Services, National Center for Health Statistics. (2008, December). Prevalence of overweight, obesity and extreme obesity among adults: U.S. trends 1960–62 through 2005–2006.

This article shows that the prevalence of obesity in the United States has more than doubled since 1980.

However, the rate of overweight has remained stable during this time. A brief description of the survey technique is given. The cut-points for BMI are identified, and a very good chart of obesity trends is presented.

New York Obesity Research Center: St. Lukes Roosevelt Hospital Center. (2010, March 15). Anthropometry lab. Retrieved from www.nyorc.org/bcu/labs/anthropometry.html.

Anthropometric measurements include body weight, height, skinfold measurements, circumferences, and various body diameters. These types of measurements have a long history of use. When performed accurately, they provide a reasonable prediction of body composition in nonobese subjects. There is a brief description of each of these measurements.

Staff. (2010, March 15). Body composition: Skin-fold measurements.

Retrieved from www.-rohan.sdsu.edu/~ens3041?skinfold.htm.

This article provides a brief history of skinfold measurements and emphasizes the importance of training. It also provides instructions and illustrations of some of the most common sites used for skinfold measurements.

Wikipedia. (2010, March 6). *Wikimedia Foundation, Inc.* Body fat percentage. Retrieved from http://en.wikipedia.org/wiki/body_fat_percentage.

This article covers total fat and essential fat for males and females and makes recommendations for acceptable body fat for health or fitness or for athletes. It provides information on the following techniques for measuring body fat: near-infrared interactance, DEXA, body average density measurement, bioelectrical impedance analysis, skinfold methods, height and circumference methods, and body mass index.

**Name** _____   **Date** _____   **Section** _____

# Assessment Activity 7-1

## Using BMI to Estimate Body-Weight Status and Calculate Desirable Body Weight

**Directions:**  Calculate your BMI:

1.  Your body weight: _____ lbs.

2.  Your height: _____ in.

3.  Use the nomogram in Table 7-5 to calculate your BMI.

    Your BMI:  kg/m2

4.  Your desired BMI: _____ kg/m$^2$

5.  Once again, use the nomogram to calculate your desired body weight. Connect your desired BMI to your height and extend the line through the weight column.

    Your desired weight: _____ lbs.

6.  Subtract your desired body weight from your current body weight to determine how much weight you need to lose or gain.

    Current weight − desired weight = weight to gain or lose

    _____ lbs. − _____ lbs. = _____ lbs.

Name _____    Date _____    Section _____

# Assessment Activity 7-2

## Calculating Desirable Body Weight from Percentage of Body Fat

**Directions:**  To find your desirable body weight, insert your current weight, your percentage of body fat, and the desirable body fat that you wish to attain in the appropriate spaces. Then calculate fat weight, lean weight, and desirable body weight. Subtract desirable body weight from current weight. This figure tells you how much weight you must lose to achieve your desirable percentage of body fat.

Current weight = _____ lbs.

Current percentage of body fat = _____ %

Desirable body fat = _____ %

1. Fat weight

$$= \frac{\text{Body weight} \times \text{percentage of fat}}{100}$$

= _____ lbs.

2. Lean weight

= Body weight − fat weight

= _____ lbs.

3. Desirable body weight

$$= \frac{\text{Lean weight}}{1 - \text{percentage of fat desired}}$$

= _____ lbs.

4. Amount of weight to lose = _____ lbs.

# Achieving a Healthy Weight and Body Composition

 **ONLINE LEARNING CENTER**

Log on to our Online Learning Center (OLC) for access to these additional resources:

- Chapter key term flashcards
- Learning objectives
- Additional goals for behavior change
- Concentration game
- Self-scoring chapter quizzes
- Additional lab activities

The OLC also offers Web links for study and exploration of wellness topics. Access these links through **www.mhhe.com/anspaugh8e.**

**GOALS FOR BEHAVIOR CHANGE**

- Compare physical characteristics of your ideal body image with your actual body image.
- Estimate caloric expenditure for your basal metabolism and physical activity level.
- Adjust your caloric intake and physical activity as necessary to achieve a healthy weight.
- Formulate a plan for achieving a healthy weight.

## Objectives

After completing this chapter, you will be able to do the following:

- ✔ Define *obesity* and *overweight*.
- ✔ Differentiate between hypertrophic and hyperplastic development of adipose cells.
- ✔ Identify and discuss the health aspects of obesity.
- ✔ Discuss biological and behavioral causes of obesity.
- ✔ Discuss the relationship of genetics, set point, overeating, and physical activity to body shape, fat distribution, and obesity.
- ✔ Define, identify, and distinguish among various forms of eating disorders and disordered eating.
- ✔ Calculate the caloric cost of physical activities.
- ✔ Compare and contrast dieting and physical activity as strategies for weight management.
- ✔ Identify principles of weight management.

## [ Key Terms ]

anorexia nervosa
bariatric surgery
basal metabolic rate (BMR)
binge eating disorder
body dysmorphic disorder (BDD)
bulimia nervosa
caloric deficit

caloric expenditure
caloric intake
defended weight
diet resistance
disordered eating
eating disorder
fasting
female athlete triad
gastroplasty

healthy weight
hyperplasia
hypertrophy
hypokinesis
liposuction
metabolism
normal weight
obesity
obesogenic environment

obesogens
overcompensatory eating
overweight
set point
thermic effect of food (TEF)
weight maintenance

Theoretically, achieving a healthy weight and body composition is a simple issue (see Just the Facts: "Healthy Weight" vs. "Ideal Weight" vs. "Desirable Weight"). A person balances **caloric intake,** calories supplied by food, with **caloric expenditure,** calories expended by physical activity and metabolism. In practice, however, people vary considerably in their responses to caloric intake and caloric expenditure. No two people have identical experiences with dieting or physical activity regimens. Some people who chronically face body composition and body-weight problems eat no more and sometimes less than their normal-weight peers. Conversely, some normal-weight people have voracious appetites and do not expend any more calories than their overweight peers.

How can this be explained? Are the differences due to heredity, metabolism, or errors in reporting food intake and physical activity expenditures? Although on the surface body weight appears to be a function of the basic laws of nature (caloric intake vs. caloric expenditure), in truth it is a complex issue still not fully understood by medical experts. For many people, self-improvement goals involving weight management are achievable and worthwhile. For others, formulating weight-management goals means first constructing a realistic view of body image (see Nurturing Your Spirituality: Body Image Is About More Than Losing Weight). This chapter addresses some of the complexities of body composition and body-weight issues and presents basic principles for achieving a healthy weight.

## Defining the Problem

For many Americans, improving body composition and losing weight are healthy goals. Losing weight often means reducing the risk of developing common chronic health problems. However, many people who are not overweight and have good body composition try to lose weight. For them, losing weight offers no health benefits and may even be harmful.

The number of people who stand to benefit from weight loss is at an all-time high. A **healthy weight** is defined as a body mass index (BMI) equal to or more than 18.5 and no more than 24.9 (see Chapter 7, Table 7-4, page 243). Being **overweight** is defined as having a BMI between 25 and 29.9. **Obesity** is defined as having a very high amount of body fat or adipose tissue in relation to lean body mass, or a BMI of 30 or higher.[7] By these definitions, more than two-thirds of American adults are overweight or obese.[8] These figures are significantly higher than comparison figures for each of the previous decades since data have been collected. Adult obesity rates have grown from 13% in 1960 to 34% in 2008.[9] The trend toward obesity applies to Americans regardless of where they live. Some geographic regions

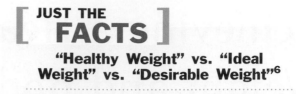

such as the Southeast United States lead the way toward obesity (see Figure 8.1, page 263).[10] Experts suggest that obesity in the United States may actually be worse than publicized because much of the data come from self-reported telephone surveys. Self-reported data show that women tend to underreport their weight and men tend to report they are taller than they are.[11] Both of these tendencies lead to lower BMI scores and lower rates of obesity than actually exist.

Adults are not the only ones overweight or obese. Among children and adolescents aged 2 through 19 years, 32% are overweight and/or obese. Seventeen percent of children and adolescents have a BMI of 30 or higher and fall in the BMI classification of "obesity."[12] These obesity trends are troublesome especially considering that childhood obesity is predictive of teen obesity, and teen obesity is predictive of adult obesity (see Just the Facts: Are U.S. Children and Adults of Today Heavier Than Their Peers of 50 Years Ago?).[13] The dramatic increase in obesity suggests that obesity is epidemic in the United States, regardless of age.

Americans are getting heavier for two reasons: too little energy going out (as exercise) and too much energy going in (as food). The majority of Americans are sedentary; at the same time they are consuming extra calories. Overall, two-thirds of adults, including young adults 18–29 years of age, do not participate in regular leisure-time light or moderate physical activity for at least 150 minutes per week.[14] (See Chapter 1, Just the Facts: Light-Intensity vs. Moderate-Intensity vs. Vigorous-Intensity Physical Activity.) How do adults and children in the United States spend their discretionary time? Rather than participating in physical activities, Americans spend much of their time using a computer and other forms of media and technology, and watching television. Passive, sedentary activities have become the norm. American society has become an obesogenic environment. **Obesogenic environment** refers to environments that promote increased food intake, nonhealthful foods, and physical inactivity.[15] Obesogenic environments are not conducive to physical activity, healthy eating habits, weight loss, or weight maintenance; instead, they are associated with a sedentary lifestyle, weight gain, and overeating. Addressing obesogenic environments has become a national health priority that has produced many school, university, worksite, and community initiatives. Several examples: Employees are petitioning office cafeterias to offer low-calorie, nutritionally dense food options;

workers are asking management to clean and paint stairways so they become more aesthetic options to the elevator; students are forming walking clubs; PTA groups are substituting fruits and healthy snacks for cake and doughnuts at school birthday parties; elementary schools are adding physical activity to the school day curriculum; universities are stocking vending machines with healthy food choices. These initiatives, along with many others, are showing signs of success. Between 2003 and 2006, the prevalence of obesity did not increase from one year to the next.[16] While obesity rates remain at an all-time high, health experts are hopeful that obesity rates are now leveling off.

## Nurturing Your Spirituality
### Body Image Is About More Than Losing Weight[1-4]

Body image involves our perception of and about our bodies. For most Americans, this perception is not positive. The majority of Americans are unhappy with their physical appearance and even more are dissatisfied with their body weight. This is particularly true for young women who are willing to subject themselves to elective surgery to improve some aspect of their appearance. Fifty percent of women don't like their weight, in many cases, even if their body mass index indicates "healthy weight."[5]

Why are so many people unhappy with their appearance or weight? Why do people tend to focus on their physical imperfections? Why does such a large discrepancy exist between the ways people see their bodies and the ways others see them? Body-image studies identify the following factors as being responsible for negative body images:

- The media's preoccupation with thinness as the trademark for beauty
- The plethora of messages in the media about the prevalence of obesity
- Disapproving messages from others
- Physical changes, such as pregnancy
- Chronic illness
- Childhood teasing
- Weight gain
- Sexual abuse
- Cultural pressures

What are the costs of an exaggerated negative body image? People who are deeply troubled about their appearance or preoccupied with selected physical "flaws" often limit their social activities; may not be assertive at work, at school, or in personal relationships; may experience difficulty in forming a positive sexuality; may engage in high-risk behaviors; and often become victims of unrealistic fad diets. Studies of adolescents indicate that body dissatisfaction is the single strongest predictor of eating disorders and excessive dieting. Extreme cases may involve a psychological disorder called **body dysmorphic disorder (BDD)**. People with this condition are so preoccupied with what they see as a disfiguring flaw that they avoid social activities, including school and work.

Although self-improvement is a worthy goal for many people, when it comes to body image it is important to separate nature from nurture, heredity from environment. The challenge for many people with negative body images is to set realistic goals about what can be changed and to accept what can't be changed. Every one of us has a natural, unique size and shape. While it is true that more and more Americans are challenged to lose weight and improve body composition, it is important to remember that our self-esteem depends on accepting the physical features unique to each of us. Improving body composition and losing weight are not likely to change physical features that set us apart from others. Changing what and how we think about our bodies can be healthier than constantly working to change our body weight and shape by diet and exercise. Having a positive body image is not just about losing weight.

**Sources:** Veale, D. (2004). Body dysmorphic disorder. *Postgraduate Medical Journal, 80*(940), 67–71.
Tiggemann, M., & D. Hargreaves. (2003). The effect of "thin ideal" television commercials on body dissatisfaction and schema activation during early adolescence. *Journal of Youth and Adolescence, 32*(5), 367–74.
MayoClinic.com. (2010). Body dysmorphic disorder. Retrieved February 16, 2010, from www.mayoclinic.com/health/body-dysmorphic-disorder/DS00559.
National Institutes of Health. (2009). How you see yourself: When your body image doesn't measure up. NIH News in Health. Retrieved February 16, 2010, from http://newsinhealth.nih.gov/2009/July/feature1.htm.

# [ JUST THE FACTS ]

## Are U.S. Children and Adults of Today Heavier Than Their Peers of 50 Years Ago?

The answer to the above question is an unequivocal yes. Health experts are troubled by the pattern of consistent weight gain among U.S. children, adolescents, and adults.

| Age Group, Gender | Percent Overweight/Obese | | |
| --- | --- | --- | --- |
| | 1960 | 2006 | Change |
| **Overweight (Includes Obesity)** | | | |
| Boys, 6–11 years old | 4% | 18% | +14% |
| Girls, 6–11 years old | 4.5% | 15.8% | +11.3% |
| Both sexes, combined | 4.2% | 17% | +12.8% |
| Adolescent boys, 12–19 years old | 4.6% | 17.6% | +13% |
| Adolescent girls, 12–19 years old | 4.7% | 16.8% | +12.1% |
| Both sexes, combined | 4.6% | 17.6% | +13% |
| Adult men, 20–74 years old | 49.5% | 72.6% | +23.1% |
| Adult women, 20–74 years old | 40.2% | 61.2% | +21% |
| Both sexes, combined | 44.8% | 66.9 | +22.1% |
| **Obese** | | | |
| Men, 20–74 years old | 10.7% | 33.1% | +22.4 |
| Women, 20–74 years old | 15.7% | 35.2% | +19.5% |
| Both sexes, combined | 13.3% | 34.1% | +20.8% |

Source: National Center for Health Statistics. (2009). *Health, United States, 2008 with special feature on the health of young adults.* Hyattsville, MD: U.S. Department of Health and Human Services.

Although BMI provides a basis for classifying levels of overweight and obesity, it is not without its limitations. It is just one predictor. Rather than relying solely on BMI, the National Heart, Lung, and Blood Institute recommends assessing waist circumference because abdominal fat is associated with increased risk of contracting obesity-related diseases[17,18] (see Chapter 7). It is also important to remember that BMIs of 25 and 30 (for overweight and obesity, respectively) are not precise points on a scale that, when exceeded, magically increase a person's risk for health problems. For example, although a BMI of 29.9 does not technically fall into the category of obesity, it is a small step away from the "magic number" of 30, the cutoff point for obesity. For all practical purposes, a BMI of 29.9 carries the same risk for obesity as a BMI of 30.

## Health Aspects of Obesity

In declaring obesity a disease, the NIH signaled a new approach toward obesity. Medical experts no longer regard being obese as a failure of willpower. Instead, obesity is considered a chronic disease. This is a radical departure from traditional thinking. Like any other chronic disease, obesity is a complex issue with multiple causes and diverse treatments. No single cause-and-effect relationship has been established that accounts for the wide variance in eating and activity patterns among the obese. What we know today about

obesity is the tip of the iceberg and represents a small portion of this evolving and growing medical field.

One aspect of obesity that has not changed is its medical consequences. Morbidity occurs more frequently and with greater severity and death occurs at an earlier age among obese people than among those of normal weight.[19] The magnitude of the risk for morbidity and premature death is dependent on the degree of obesity and the distribution and location of excess fat cells. Fortunately, losing as little as 5 to 10% of body weight can yield significant improvement in health and self-esteem.[20]

Obesity is highly correlated with coronary heart disease and stroke. LDL cholesterol, which contributes to the development of atherosclerosis, is associated with obesity. Hypertension is also related to obesity. Many lifestyle factors are related to hypertension but, overall, obesity is considered the one with the most influence. Many hypertensive people experience a decline in systolic and diastolic blood pressures during the early stages of a weight-loss program.

Obesity is also a major risk factor for some forms of cancer. Topping the list are colorectal, uterine, breast, esophageal, and kidney cancer.[21] Preventing obesity and controlling weight may be the second most important anticancer step, after smoking cessation.[22]

Type 2 diabetes, the most common type of diabetes, is highly associated with obesity and/or being overweight. In many cases, the fat cells in people with Type 2 diabetes become resistant to insulin. In the absence of insulin, the cells cannot make full use of circulating blood sugar (glucose), so the affected person develops *hyperglycemia*, or high blood sugar, as a result of glucose remaining in the bloodstream. Sustained levels of blood glucose lead to full-blown Type 2 diabetes. Type 2 diabetes linked to obesity often disappears as weight is lost. Even if diabetes persists after weight loss, the body's need for insulin often drops dramatically.[23,24]

Other conditions associated with obesity include osteoarthritis, gallbladder disease, dyslipidemia, and sleep apnea. *Dyslipidemia* occurs when various blood lipids or fats, such as LDL cholesterol or triglycerides, are elevated or, in the case of HDL cholesterol, very low[25] (see Chapter 2). *Sleep apnea* is a condition characterized by loud snoring and brief interruptions in breathing. It is thought to be caused by the accumulation of fat in the upper airway, which interferes with breathing.

Obesity, combined with high blood sugar, hypertension, and abnormal blood fat levels, is highly related to a condition referred to as *metabolic syndrome* (see Chapter 2). Approximately one-third of American adults have metabolic syndrome, which increases the risk for diabetes, heart disease, and stroke.[26]

For some people, the first symptom of strain placed on the body by excess fat is shortness of breath. As fat accumulates, it crowds the space occupied by organs. Some people cannot sit comfortably because of fat accumulation in their abdomens. In a sitting position, a person's lungs have limited space in which to expand.

Postsurgical complications occur more often in overweight people than in those who are not overweight. Wounds don't heal as well or as fast. Infections are more common.

In addition to suffering from medical hazards, some obese people suffer psychological stress, depression, social discrimination, and reduced income. They pay higher premiums for health insurance or are denied coverage. Obese children are often ridiculed by their normal-weight peers. Armed forces personnel are forced out of the military if they gain weight beyond an acceptable level.

The link between obesity and chronic disease is well established, but evidence has emerged indicating that the *distribution* of fat is equally important to the development of disease. Studies have confirmed that abdominal fat is associated with a higher rate of heart attack and stroke than is fat distributed around the hips and

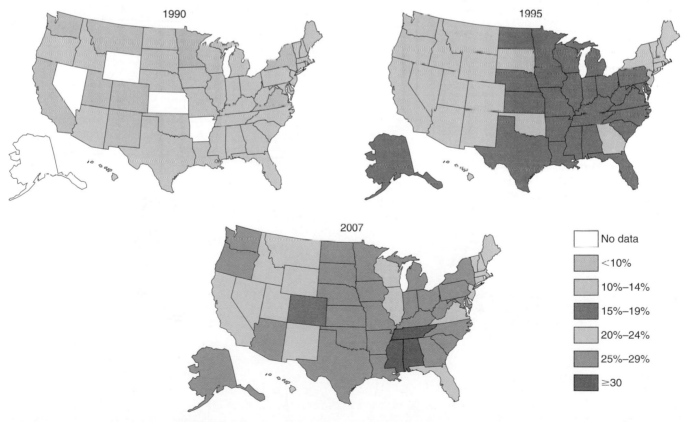

**FIGURE 8-1**   Obesity Trends* Among U.S. Adults
(Percentage of U.S. adults with BMI of ≥30 by state in 1990, 1995, and 2007)

Sources: Behavioral Risk Factor Surveillance System, CDC.

National Center for Disease Prevention and Health Promotion. (2009). Obesity: Halting the epidemic by making health easier. Atlanta: Centers for Disease Control an Prevention.

thighs (see Chapter 7). Guidelines for doctors now suggest that, in addition to calculating BMI, they should assess waist circumference. A waist measurement more than 40 inches in men and 35 inches in women is considered a predictor of health risks, especially if it is combined with a BMI of 25 or more.[27] (See Just the Facts: Waist Size Matters at **www.mhhe.com/anspaugh8e** Student Center, Chapter 8, Just the Facts.)

In summary, the medical community clearly concurs that the health risks and complications of obesity are associated with premature death. Overweight is a different matter. People who are overweight, but not obese, live as long as people of normal weight. The health implications of being overweight, but not obese, are mixed and complex and are influenced by such things as fat distribution, fitness level, diet, heredity, environment, and health conditions[28] (see Just the Facts: Overweight and Health—What Are We to Believe?).

## Weight Loss: A New Attitude Emerges

The term *weight loss* lacks specificity, and it is often used in such a way to imply that indiscriminate weight loss—of body fluids, protein, and fat—is desirable. A more appropriate weight-related goal is to measure success by the amount of fat lost, not by weight loss. The term *weight loss* should be replaced by the more specific term *fat-weight loss*.

Until recently, advice to overfat people was imprecise. For example, the suggestion to "cut back on calories" reinforces the misconception that diet alone can lead to fat-weight loss. Successful weight management is rarely the result of following a diet or counting calories for a specific period. Successful weight management usually requires a lifelong lifestyle change. The loss or gain of body weight, the development of fat cells, and the causes of obesity are complex issues related to the interaction of three factors—heredity, diet, and exercise.

## Development of Obesity

The body consists of 30 to 40 billion adipose cells (fat cells) that provide storage space for extra energy. Adipose cells can be viewed as collapsible, thin-walled containers with unlimited storage capacities (Figure 8-2). In prehistoric humans, large fat stores developed when food was available in spring and summer, and this proved biologically advantageous when winters

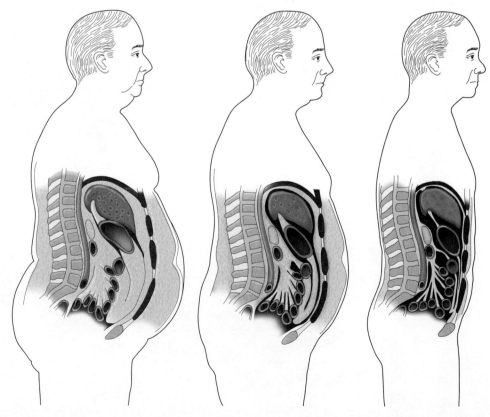

**FIGURE 8-2**   Adipose Cell Deposits

Adipose (fat) tissue can be deposited in many areas of the body. Losing fat and building lean muscle tissue boost metabolism, reduce strain on the hips and knees, and may prevent lower-back pain.

## [ JUST THE FACTS ]

### Overweight and Health—What Are We to Believe?

Until recently, experts believed that the relationship between health and overweight was dependent on fitness. Overweight people who are physically active live longer than their healthy-weight but sedentary peers. In terms of mortality, therefore, it is better to be overweight and fit than to be healthy-weight and unfit. This thinking led to the claim that you can be fat and fit. However, this claim was later refuted when scientists suggested that the more accurate conclusion is just the opposite. Being overweight or obese increases the risk of many chronic conditions and premature death even if you are physically active. Regardless of fitness level, if you are overweight, weight loss should be a primary goal. Now, studies recently reported in the scientific journal *Obesity* suggest a different conclusion. In a surprising reversal of previous findings, one large study[29] reported that overweight people had a lower mortality than those who were healthy-weight. In fact, being overweight was said to be protective against mortality. In the same study, underweight and obesity class II or higher (see Chapter 7, Table 7-4) were clearly linked to mortality. However, class I obesity was not linked to increased mortality. Another large-scale study[30] found similar findings, with a slightly different twist. As waist circumference increased, the risk of mortality increased for both the healthy-weight and obese. However, in older adults (65 years of age and older), being overweight was associated with increased longevity, compared to people who were healthy-weight or underweight.

What are we to make of these seemingly contradictory findings? First and foremost, mortality, overweight, obesity, fitness, and health status are complex phenomena and difficult to measure and predict. Some contradictions should not surprise us. Second, weight classification measurement techniques that are used in most large-scale studies are not perfect assessments of body fat. BMIs, waist, and waist-hip measurements, for example, come with their own unique advantages and disadvantages (see Chapter 7). Third, recent findings still don't change the consensus opinion among medical experts about the strong positive relationship that exists between obesity and many of the common chronic diseases in the United States. Fourth, body fat measurements may not be as good at predicting mortality and longevity as physical fitness. For example, recent studies support early claims that cardiorespiratory fitness may be a better predictor of mortality and once again suggest that it is better to be fit and fat than to be inactive and at a healthy weight.[31] And, fifth, it is possible that what experts consider to be a healthy weight (or BMI) needs to be reexamined. A healthy weight (and BMI) for senior adults may turn out to be different from a healthy weight and BMI for young adults, adolescents, and children. It is conceivable that future norms may differentiate weight and BMI recommendations according to age, gender, and other factors, such as fitness levels. Instead of referring to one chart for body fat classifications, we may have two, three, or more. Until then, while the research jury is still out, if you are overweight, as are most Americans, take comfort in the fact that from a health perspective, physically active lifestyles improve health, regardless of body weight status.

Sources: Orpana, H., J. Berthelot, M. Kaplan, D. Feeny, B. McFarland, & N. Ross. (2010). BMI and mortality: Results from a national longitudinal study of Canadian adults. Obesity, 18(1), 214–18.
Reis, J., C. Macera, M. Araneta, S. Lindsay, S. Marshall, & D. Wingard. (2009). Comparison of overall obesity and body fat distribution in predicting risk of mortality. *Obesity*, 17(6), 1232–39.
Tufts Media. (2008). What does the latest research on weight mean to you? *Tufts University Health and Nutrition Letter*, 25(11), 6.

were long and harsh and food was scarce. Energy stored in fat cells could be tapped for use later. This is not the case today. Food is available year-round for most Americans and surplus fat storage is not advantageous.

Obesity occurs when adipose cells increase excessively in size (**hypertrophy**), in number (**hyperplasia**), or both. Obesity that results from an increase in the size of fat cells is hypertrophic, obesity that results from an increase in the number of fat cells is hyperplastic, and obesity that results from an increase in both is hypertrophic/hyperplastic.

Adipose cells follow a normal pattern of growth and development. Once developed, fat cells do not disappear.

Gender differences in depositing fat become noticeable during and after puberty. Men distribute fat primarily in the upper half of the body, and women tend to deposit it in the lower half. The percentage of fat in the body reaches peak values during early adolescence for boys and then declines during the remainder of adolescent growth. Girls experience a continuous increase in the percentage of fat from the onset of puberty to age 18–20.

Excessive fat cell development during childhood is a cause for concern because childhood obesity is a predictor of obesity later in life.[32] The risk of obesity in adulthood is greater for the most obese children and adolescents and for those with obese parents and grandparents.[33]

## Causes of Obesity

The laws of thermodynamics state that energy cannot be destroyed; it is used for work or converted into another form. Accordingly, the progressive accumulation of stored fat in the body is the result of consumption of more calories (energy) than are expended. Food energy in excess of the body's need results in storage of fat in adipose cells (Figure 8-3). This relationship is demonstrated in almost all people. Excessive caloric intake and deficient energy expenditure are responsible for most obesity. What is more difficult to explain, however, is the difference among people's responses to the laws of energy conservation and expenditure. Two people may be overfed the same number of calories and yet differ in the amount of weight gained, even if their activity levels are held constant. What accounts for these differences? The answer suggests that obesity is a complex issue, involving both biological and behavioral theories.

### Biological Theories

Age, metabolism, gender, disease, heredity, and set point, the body's internal signal for the level of fatness it tries to defend, are biological factors that influence body weight and obesity. As people age, their amount of muscle tends to drop, and fat accounts for a greater percentage of their body weight. Metabolism also slows naturally with age (see Just the Facts: Metabolism Basics). The metabolism of adults typically declines at the rate of about 2% a decade.[34] Women usually have higher fat-to-muscle ratios than men because of the influence of hormones unique to fertility and the female reproductive system. Also, men typically have higher muscle-to-fat ratios than women, which increases metabolism and caloric expenditure. Diseases that affect the thyroid gland may have a dramatic impact on body weight. An overactive thyroid gland (hyperthyroidism) increases the resting metabolic rate (RMR) and may cause weight loss. Conversely, an underactive thyroid gland (hypothyroidism) lowers RMR and may lead to overweight or obesity.

Infections may also be a factor in obesity. This is not altogether unexpected, because a number of chronic conditions have been connected to viral and/or bacterial infections. Atherosclerosis and ulcers are two examples. Viral infections have been shown to cause

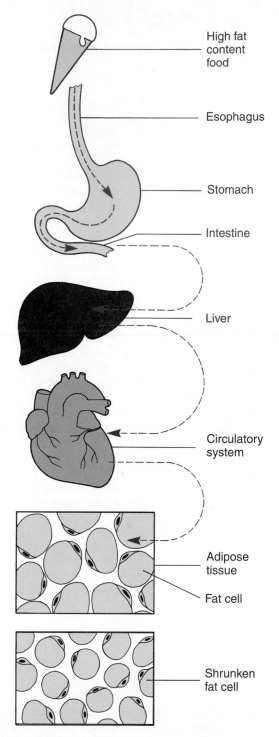

**FIGURE 8-3** Fat Storage

Fat can be manufactured in the body from any food and stored when caloric intake exceeds expenditure. Fat droplets travel to the liver from the stomach and intestines and then enter the circulatory system, where they are delivered to the cells and organs. Excess fats are stored in adipose tissue. When more energy is needed, fats are released from adipose cells. If the energy needs continue, the cells shrink.

## [ JUST THE ] FACTS
### Metabolism Basics

A common misconception is that most people become overweight and/or obese because they were born with a low metabolism. Metabolism may influence weight gain but it is not the direct cause of obesity for most people. One possible exception is someone who has *hypothyroidism* or an underactive thyroid gland. A blood test can determine if this condition exits. It is uncommon for hypothyroidism to be the cause of overweight and obesity. Most obese people don't have an underactive thyroid gland.[35]

What is metabolism, how does it influence weight gain and/or loss, and is it possible to increase metabolism through lifestyle changes?

**Metabolism** refers to the complex chemical processes in the body that provide energy necessary to sustain life.[36] These processes enable the body to use energy, so it stands to reason that anything affecting metabolism may also affect weight gain. A high metabolism causes the body to use more energy and works against weight gain; a low metabolism causes the body to use less energy and promotes weight gain.

When the body is at complete rest, such as in sleeping and fasting, a minimum level of energy is required to maintain the vital life processes of breathing, circulation, and cell generation and repair. Energy required to sustain basic life processes is called *basal metabolism*. Basal metabolism accounts for most of the energy expended by most people. Nearly three-fourths of the calories used each day are expended to support basal metabolism.[37]

The process of digesting food also requires energy and refers to the *thermic effect of food* (TEF) (see High Fat intake, page 269). This process accounts for about 10 to 15% of the calories used each day.[38]

Physical activity accounts for the remainder of energy expended. Physical activities that improve body composition exert a major influence on basal metabolism. Muscle tissue burns more calories at rest than fat tissue, so a good strategy for losing and/or maintaining weight is to increase participation in physical activities, including resistance-type exercises. While the ability to change basal metabolism is limited, participation in physical activity offers the dual advantage of burning extra calories to sustain the activity while promoting the development of lean body tissue that burns more calories at rest than does fat.[39,40]

obesity in animals. It will take years of research to determine if there is a link between viruses and weight gain in humans.

The two major biological explanations of obesity are heredity and set point. Although they are interrelated, they are discussed separately here.

### Heredity

The study of obesity lends itself to the classic question of nature versus nurture, heredity versus environment. Does obesity run in families? If so, is it caused by eating habits learned from family influence or by genetic influence?

Studies of adoptees and identical twins help reveal the influence of the genetic component of obesity. In classic longitudinal studies when researchers follow adoptees over time, they find that their body weight classification resembles that of their biological parents, rather than that of their adoptive parents, even though they learned and practiced the lifestyles of their adoptive parents.

Identical twins are excellent subjects for these studies because they have identical genetic makeups. Any physical differences that occur can be attributed to environmental and/or lifestyle factors. Classic longitudinal studies of identical twins consistently reveal a strong genetic influence.[41] When comparing height, weight, and BMI, identical twins follow similar patterns. Each member of the pair can be expected to gain the same amount of weight at approximately the same time in life. The similarity in identical twins is twice that observed in fraternal twins (twins who emanate from separate eggs that do not have identical genes).

The connection between heredity and obesity is also confirmed in studies that correlate the prevalence of childhood obesity with the prevalence of obesity in parents. Eighty percent of children born to two obese parents will become obese, compared with 14% of children born to nonobese parents.[42] Studies support the idea that obesity and fat deposition are significantly influenced by heredity.

In addition to influencing body weight, heredity influences body shape. Body shape generally falls into one of three categories: ectomorph, endomorph, and mesomorph (see Just the Facts: Body Shapes). Most people are a combination of all three, with a tendency to be more like one or two of them. If a person's body shape strongly favors a particular classification, the person cannot realistically hope to attain another body type. It would be more appropriate for such a person to seek changes in body composition that reduce fat weight regardless of body-shape tendencies. *Shape acceptance* is essential in constructing a realistic view of body weight.

Another factor that helps explain the connection between heredity and obesity surfaced with the discovery of *leptin*, a hormone made in fat cells by a gene called *OB* (for its connection with obesity), often referred to as the *fat gene*. Leptin senses when fat cells are satisfied and signals the brain to suppress appetite. If the *ob* gene doesn't work properly, leptin is either not available to suppress appetite or the body develops a

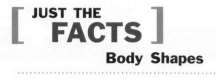

## JUST THE FACTS

### Body Shapes

According to somatotype (body-type) experts, there are three classic body shapes. Most people are a combination of all three. The body shapes/body types are as follows:

Ectomorphic    *Ectomorphs* have long, thin body frames; are slender; and have a low capacity for fat storage.

Endomorphic    *Endomorphs* have rounded physical features and large frames. Of the three classic body shapes, they have the greatest capacity for fat storage.

Mesomorphic    *Mesomorphs* have muscular, athletic body frames with an ability to store fat that falls in between ectomorphs and endomorphs.

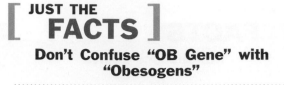

## JUST THE FACTS

### Don't Confuse "OB Gene" with "Obesogens"

They may look and sound alike, but the terms *OB gene* and *obesogens* have very different meanings. Both relate to obesity, but that's where their similarities end. *OB* genes are intrinsic to the body and produce hormones that suppress appetite. Obesogens, on the other hand, are extrinsic to the body and have little to do with genes and DNA. **Obesogens** are defined as chemicals that upset the body's hormonal systems in ways that lead to weight gain and obesity.[45] Altered hormones disrupt the metabolism of fat, which in turn facilitates the accumulation of fat. In a way, obesogens program the body to gain weight. Obesogens come from many sources commonly found in the American diet: artificial hormones fed to animals, plastic pollutants in some food packaging, chemicals added to processed foods, and pesticides sprayed on fruits and vegetables. Proponents of what is referred to as "the obesogen effect" maintain that the fewer obesity-promoting chemicals we expose our body to, the easier it is to lose weight and keep it off.[46]

Medical experts are taking note, but the obesogen effect is still not fully supported by the health community. Proving cause and effect between food, obesogens, and health is a big challenge and will require considerable time and research.

resistance to it (see Just the Facts: Don't Confuse "*OB* Gene" with "Obesogens"). The end result is the same: the brain doesn't get the signal to stop eating.[43]

Another obesity gene discovered accidently in 2007 is called *FTO*, which stands for fat mass and obesity associated. People who have two copies of this gene are more likely to be obese than people who don't have it. Most people of European descent have one or more *FTO* genes. The good news about this gene is that its ability to cause obesity is negated by physical activity, such as brisk walking, housework, and gardening.[44] While it is too early to draw any firm conclusions about the role of this gene in causing obesity, the fact that its effects may be attenuated or blocked by a physically active lifestyle should be a cause for optimism.

### Set Point Theory

The **set point** theory of weight control also reflects the role of genetics. Proponents of this theory suggest that the body works to defend a certain weight. The popular literature often refers to a person's set point as defended weight. **Defended weight** is the weight that our body strives to attain when we're not on a diet or participating in an exercise program. You might call it your "normal weight." Each body has an internal set point for the weight it defends. In any given year, it could range from plus or minus 5 pounds in one person to 20 pounds or more in another. How the body determines its set point is not known. One hypothesis is that the body is able to adjust its energy expenditure by adjusting its metabolism. Gordon Wardlaw, well-known nutrition author, provides an analogy and explanation.[47] The analogy is to view set point (i.e., defended weight) as a coiled spring: The far-

ther you stray from your usual weight, the harder the force acts to pull you back to that weight. When dieters lose weight, their metabolism slows down. When they gain weight, metabolism increases.

There is physiological evidence to support the set point explanation. If energy intake is reduced, the blood concentration of thyroid hormone falls, and the metabolic rate slows. In addition, lower body weight decreases the energy cost of activity and the total energy used by muscle tissue falls because some of these tissues are also lost. In addition, the enzyme used by fat cells and muscle cells to take up fat from the bloodstream often increases its activity. Through these changes, the body resists further weight loss.[48]

If a person overeats, in the short run the metabolic rate tends to increase because total body mass increases. This causes some resistance to further weight gain. People often recognize the body's resistance to weight loss when dieting but do not think much about the resistance to weight gain after eating a big holiday meal. However, in the long run, resistance to weight gain is much less than resistance to weight loss.[49] When a person gains weight and stays at that weight for a while, the body tends to defend the new weight.

Can a person change his or her set point? Proponents of the set point theory think that the set point does shift over time in response to behavioral factors: Eating a high-fat diet tends to raise the set point for fatness, and regular physical activity tends to lower it. This shift may be so slight and gradual as to go unnoticed for years.

Some proponents of the set point theory suggest that, because some people are genetically programmed to have unwanted pounds, efforts to eliminate fat with diet, exercise, or both are doomed. The body can shut down its calorie-losing mechanism by lowering metabolism and can stimulate appetite to the point that a person must have food (see Nurturing Your Spirituality: Nature Versus Nurture—Make Peace with Obesity or Take Action).

Other proponents of the set point theory argue that vigorous regular exercise brings about physiological changes in muscle that speed up metabolism and lower the set point, thereby lowering the level of fat the body will accept and defend. Exercise induces the body to stabilize at a lower defended weight, precisely what dieters try to do. Proponents of the set point theory argue that, while exercise cannot negate heredity, it can modify it. Obesity need not be destiny.

## Behavioral Theories

Behavioral explanations of obesity include excessive caloric intake (overeating), lack of physical activity (hypokinesis), and many other contributing factors (see Just the Facts: Obesity: Contributing Factors).

### Overeating

The basic laws of nature require that calories be consumed before energy can be stored as excess weight. The body cannot make energy on its own. For the obese and overweight, therefore, caloric intake is an important issue, especially considering that Americans are consuming more calories today than in the past. Caloric consumption averages 300 calories per day more than it did 20 years ago.[50] This is equivalent to about 3 pounds per month and 36 pounds per year of extra calories.

Does the increased caloric consumption of Americans apply to all people or just to people with obesity? This has been a controversial question, and researchers fall into two camps regarding this issue. One camp suggests that obese people eat no more and sometimes less than normal-weight people. They maintain that blaming obesity on a lack of willpower is unfair and oversimplifies the facts. The body of the obese person is more efficient at converting calories to adipose cells for reasons beyond his or her control, such as genetic

predisposition or higher set point for fatness. Stated another way, obese people may not eat more than normal-weight people; they just consume more calories than are required by their bodies.

The other camp claims that there is a tendency for people to underestimate their weight status[52] and that many obese people do not see themselves as obese.[53] They also opine that obese people underestimate their caloric intake. The farther people are from their healthy weight, the more likely they are to underreport their food consumption.[54] This helps explain the difficulty some people have losing weight despite repeated attempts. They may be consuming more calories than they realize. According to these researchers, the phenomenon referred to as **diet resistance,** the inability to lose weight by dieting, has more to do with overeating and little to do with the innate biological factors of heredity and set point.

## High Fat Intake

Although researchers are divided on the issue of overeating, they tend to agree that the abundance of food high in fat and calories is a major factor in the prevalence of obesity in the United States. In his review of the literature on obesity—a review that included more than 300 citations from the scientific literature—David C. Nieman, exercise scientist at Appalachian State University, wrote, "Of all the current theories attempting to explain the epidemic of obesity in most Western societies, the high dietary fat intake hypothesis is most widely accepted by experts."[55] Overweight people tend to eat a higher-fat diet than do people of normal weight. Ounce for ounce, fat yields more than double the number of calories than protein or carbohydrates do (9 calories versus 4). Calories from fat also appear to be more readily converted to body fat than are calories from carbohydrates and protein.

Excess carbohydrates are converted to glycogen in the liver and muscle. The body can store only a limited amount of glycogen. This is not true for fat. Fat cells are distributed throughout the body. Whereas carbohydrate storage is carefully regulated, fat storage is not, allowing a high degree of expansion. Given the sedentary lifestyles of most Americans, glycogen stores are rarely exhausted. The reality for too many people is that they burn carbohydrates and store fat.

The **thermic effect of food (TEF)** represents the amount of energy required by the body to digest, absorb, metabolize, and store nutrients. Dietary fat has less of a thermic effect than does carbohydrate or protein and can thus be easily stored as adipose tissue. The body expends 0 to 3 calories of energy to process 100 calories from fat, compared with 20 to 30 calories to process 100 calories from protein and 5 to 10 calories

## [ JUST THE FACTS ]

### Obesity: Contributing Factors

Overeating and sedentary lifestyles are emphasized in this chapter as major factors associated with the obesity epidemic in the United States. However, there are many other contributing factors, some subtle and some obvious, that influence the tendency to make poor decisions about food intake and physical activity. These factors are presented by Trust for America's Health's landmark publication titled *F as in Fat: How Obesity Policies Are Failing in America, 2006.*[51]

#### Limited Time

1. Long work hours
2. Car time and commuting

#### Family and Home Influences

1. The influence of other family members' habits on eating and exercise patterns
2. "Electronic culture" options for entertainment and free time, including TV, video games, and the Internet
3. More people work outside the home or far from home

#### Children and Schools

1. Influx of soda, juice, snack machines, and fast food
2. Reduction in the amount of physical education, recess, and recreation time

#### Workplaces Not Conducive to Health

1. Many desk jobs where activity is limited or not encouraged
2. Worksites typically not designed to foster movement

3. Limited opportunities for physical activity or recreation during the workday
4. Unhealthy options in work lunch sites

#### Communities Not Designed for Physical Activity

1. Communities are designed to foster driving rather than walking or biking
2. Lack of public transit options
3. Poor upkeep of sidewalk infrastructure
4. Walking areas often unsafe or inconvenient
5. Limited parks and recreation space, including indoor facilities
6. Lack of affordable indoor physical activity options

#### Economic Constraints

1. Health insurance coverage for obesity-preventive services is often limited or not available
2. "Value sizing" of less nutritious foods, and the higher costs of many nutritious foods
3. Lower-income neighborhoods have fewer and smaller grocery stores and less access to fruits and vegetables

#### Psychology

1. Greater advertising and marketing of less nutritious foods
2. Marketing of fad diets
3. Consumers' frustration about conflicting nutrition information and advice
4. Eating to combat stress
5. Turning to eating as a replacement for smoking or other unhealthful behaviors

---

from carbohydrates. Approximately 5 to 10% of total body energy goes to support the TEF.[56] For example, after a meal containing 1,000 calories, the body uses 100 calories to process the meal. The TEF helps explain why studies consistently show that, when adults and children overeat and consume high amounts of dietary fat, they tend to gain weight. Conversely, when the intake of dietary fat is low and the intake of protein, carbohydrate, and fiber is high from nutrient-dense foods, desirable body weight is more readily achieved.[57]

### Portion Sizes, Volume Eating, and Over Eating

Americans' obsession with fat grams and low-carbohydrate diets is misplaced because the real issue is less

about the type of food eaten and more about the quantity of food eaten. Food producers and eating establishments are cashing in on our quest to get a better value for the dollar. *Super-sized, all-you-can-eat, buffet-style eating,* and a *meal in a sandwich* are some of the catchphrases used to increase business. When it comes to calories, the phrases are not all hype (see Just the Facts: Super-Sized Calories, and also Real-World Wellness: Practical Tips for Coping with Super-Sized Foods). In response to consumers' expectations, runaway portion sizes have become the norm. For many foods, what is considered a serving size today is 63% larger than the same food of yesteryear.[58] An example is popcorn. Twenty years ago an average serving of movie theater popcorn was

## Nurturing Your Spirituality

### Nature Versus Nurture—Make Peace with Obesity or Take Action

Very few health issues fuel the debate about nature vs. nurture better than obesity. Genetic factors account for anywhere between 30 and 70% of weight differences between people, depending on which medical expert you ask. In addition, each one of us appears to have a built-in set point for fatness, which the body tries to maintain, and when we stray too far from this set point certain biological changes occur to return us to our natural weight. The genetic and set point explanations of obesity give validity to the argument that obesity is beyond individual control. Therefore, since we can't do anything about it, why fight it? Would it not be better to make peace with our body-weight status and go about the process of enjoying life, rather than constantly doing battle with obesity, inevitably losing the battle, and feeling demoralized because of it?

Arguments against genetics and the set point theory maintain that people become obese because of lifestyle choices. For some people, obesity is caused by physical inactivity or poor dietary habits; for others, obesity is explained by social, emotional, or physical environmental factors; for still others, all of these factors apply. Proponents of nurture as the cause of obesity maintain that, while nature may provide a predisposition, or set point,

for fatness, it is behavior, or what we choose to do, that determines our level of fatness.

What are we to conclude about the debate between nature and nurture, genetics and behavior, as causes of obesity, especially when all of the explanations seem plausible? It's helpful to remember several things: First, obesity is a complex disease; second, obesity is influenced by so many variables that it will likely be years before genetic and environmental factors are clearly understood; third, any attempt to oversimplify obesity is probably born out of misinformation or naïveté; and fourth, causes of obesity are theories, not proven facts.

If you are obese, or you appear to be predisposed to obesity, what's the bottom line? In the final analysis, we must assume responsibility for weight maintenance ourselves. There is little to be gained by blaming genetics or pointing a finger at biological factors for which we have little control. Rather than getting stuck in denial, blame, or rationalization and never taking action to manage our weight, we are better served by a can-do and will-do attitude, realizing that we can take steps to improve health and promote weight maintenance, even if we are obese or can't lose weight.

5 cups and provided 270 calories. Today, it is 11 cups and 630 calories. "Big buckets" hold 16 cups of popcorn and if topped off with butter provide 1,500 calories, a day's worth for some people.[59] The problem with large serving sizes is that we tend to eat what is served. For many people, it is difficult to resist the temptation of large-size portions of certain foods. Lack of self-control is not the only reason we overeat. A key factor that makes it difficult to resist food is the multisensory appeal of foods.[60,61,62] To quote David Kessler, former commissioner of the U.S. Food and Drug Administration, the sensory appeals of fat, sugar, and salt, when combined, "make food compelling and indulgent. The most palatable foods have two or three of them. They lead to a roller coaster in the mouth—the total orosensory experience. We get captured."[63] The food industry knows that sugar, fat, and salt drive consumption, and it knows exactly how to combine these foods to keep us coming back for more, even when we're not hungry.[64] People differ in their vulnerability to the multisensory appeal of food. Answer the questions in Just the Facts: Are You Vulnerable to Overeating? to see if your eating habits are influenced by the multisensory appeal of food.

Portion sizes and volume eating also apply to beverages (see Just the Facts: Solid Calories vs. Liquid Calories at **www.mhhe.com/anspaugh8e** Student Center, Chapter 8, Just the Facts). Beverages provide 22% of total calories and 50% of added sugar in the typical American diet.[65] Soft drinks make up a big part of our beverage menu, and this presents a problem because they offer little nutrition and lots of sugar calories. To exacerbate the problem, beverages come in super-size servings; and the larger the serving, the more we drink.[66] People seem to have a different attitude about beverages compared to solid food: they are unaware that liquid calories are less filling than solid food. People don't usually compensate for liquid calories by eating less solid food;[67] the end result is extra calories and added weight. Getting liquid calories under control is a good first step for people concerned about their weight. One simple solution: substitute water or low-calorie or sugar-free beverages for their sweetened versions.

Eating out also contributes to volume eating. While restaurants are serving food in larger portions than in the past, Americans are eating at restaurants more than ever before. The more people eat out, the more likely they are to consume more calories and gain weight.[68]

# [ JUST THE FACTS ]

## Super-Sized Calories

Americans are overwhelmed with super-sized servings of food, more so now than in the past and especially when eating out. Twenty years ago, coffee was typically served in 8-ounce cups with whole milk and sugar and yielded 45 calories. Today's coffee-house 16-ounce serving of mocha with steamed milk and syrup yields 350 calories. Muffins of yesteryear were typically prepared in a serving size of 1.5 ounces and yielded 210 calories compared to today's restaurant-made muffin that weighs 4 ounces and yields 500 calories. Here are more examples of supersized servings of food prepared today and 20 years ago.

| Food | 20 Years Ago | | Today | | |
| | Serving Size | Calories | Serving Size | Calories | Difference |
| --- | --- | --- | --- | --- | --- |
| Pepperoni pizza | 2 slices | 500 | 2 slices | 850 | +350 |
| Chicken Caesar salad | 1½ cups | 390 | 3½ cups | 790 | +400 |
| Popcorn | 5 cup | 270 | 11 cups | 630 | +360 |
| Chicken stir-fry | 2 cups | 435 | 41/2 cups | 865 | +430 |
| Cheesecake | 3 ounces | 260 | 7 ounces | 640 | +380 |
| Chocolate chip cookie | 1½" diameter | 55 | 3½" diameter | 275 | +220 |
| Bagel | 3" diameter | 140 | 6" diameter | 350 | +210 |
| Cheeseburger | Quantity, one | 330 | Quantity, one | 590 | +260 |
| Spaghetti with sauce | 1 cup and 3 meatballs | 500 | 2 cups and 3 large meatballs | 1,025 | +525 |
| French fries | 2.4 ounces | 210 | 6.9 ounces | 610 | +400 |
| Soda | 6.5 ounces | 85 | 20 ounces | 250 | +165 |
| Turkey sandwich | 1 sandwich | 320 | 1 sandwich | 820 | +500 |

Sources: Levi, J., C. Juliano, & L. M. Segal. (2006). *F as in fat: How obesity policies are failing in America 2006.* Washington, DC: Trust for America's Health.

Department of Health and Human Services, National Institutes of Health. (2006). *Portion distortion.* Retrieved from http://hp2010.nhlbihin.net/portion/index.htm.

What can we do to counter the volume-eating epidemic? Some states are enacting a mandatory menu-labeling law that requires restaurant chains to disclose the number of calories per menu item.[69] Additional information such as total calories, fat calories, and amounts of saturated fat, cholesterol, sodium, carbohydrates, sugar, fiber, and protein must be available in writing upon customer request. It's possible that menu-labeling laws will be enacted on a national level. Until that time, if you live in a state that does not require menu labeling at restaurants, you might refer to some of the tips for controlling portion sizes and overeating on page 289 under the heading: Principles of Weight Management: Putting It All Together.

## Hypokinesis (Physical Inactivity or Sedentary Lifestyle)

Obesity is in large part caused by the sedentary lifestyle of most Americans. Scientific improvements have led to modern conveniences and labor-saving devices that decrease the need for physical activity. Advancements in technology make it possible to bank, shop, and even complete college courses without leaving the desktop computer. Devices such as motorized golf carts have made leisure activities less strenuous. Each new invention fosters a receptive attitude toward a life of ease. Take Americans' favorite pastime: watching television. Much ado has been made in the research community about the amount of time Americans spend watching television, and how this has contributed to obesity.[70,71] People who watch television 2 hours a day have higher rates of obesity than their peers who substitute other sedentary activities such as sewing, reading, or writing[72] (see Just the Facts: Watching Too Much TV? Try a "Commercial-Break Workout"). Each new invention fosters a receptive attitude toward a life of ease. The technological way is generally the most expedient way in the time-oriented American society.

## Real-World Wellness

### Practical Tips for Coping with Super-Sized Foods

*My friends and I enjoy eating out and prefer fast-food or casual dining restaurants. The local restaurants provide some super-sized bargains that fit a college budget. My problem is that I am a volume eater—I eat what is served, usually much more than I need and certainly more than is good for my waistline. But I live on a tight budget and refuse to throw away good food. What are some strategies that will help me manage my tendency for volume eating without being wasteful?*

Following are some suggestions for volume purchasing without waste:

- Eat what you need, not necessarily what is served. Take the rest home.

- Share an entrée, an appetizer, or dessert. This saves calories and money. (Some restaurants add a surcharge for sharing meals.)

- Start each day with a plan. Think first of your main meal and work around it. If you're planning a prime rib dinner, for example, favor vegetables and fruits for breakfast and lunch. One serving of prime rib is plenty of meat for one day.

- At a buffet, serve yourself small portions and eat slowly. Give your food time to digest. Emphasize vegetables and fruits in your food selections.

- Ask for a half order of an entrée.

- Order only appetizers.

- When grocery shopping, plan ahead. Make a list of the amount or quantity of each item to buy. Stick to your list.

- If you're watching calories, learn what makes a serving. One small fistful of candy, french fries, or nuts is a serving.

- Picture what you think is a reasonable serving before food is served. If more is served, take it home.

Exercise for fitness is now separate from other parts of life. Even when people do exercise during their leisure time, their total daily energy expenditure still falls far short of what was typical several decades ago. Some experts believe that lack of physical activity is the factor that distinguishes the obese from people of normal weight.[76]

The general decline in physical activity and fitness is correlated with the rise in obesity. When physical activity levels of overweight people are compared with those of normal-weight people, normal-weight people are about twice as active as their overweight peers.[77] On the average, Americans take about 2,000 to 3,000 steps daily or roughly 1 to 1.5 miles (2,000 steps are equivalent to a mile, depending on stride).[78] This is far short of the minimum recommendation of 10,000 steps a day (5 miles) that is typical of people who are physically active.

To state that obese people are less physically active than normal-weight people is one thing; to claim that lack of physical activity causes obesity is different. Researchers are not clear which comes first: Does obesity lead to physical inactivity or does physical inactivity lead to obesity? The cause-and-effect nature of the relationship between these two factors has yet to be determined and is complicated by the fact that energy expenditure from exercise differs very little between the obese and the normal-weight. Because of their extra weight, the obese expend more energy when they participate in physical activity. In other words, even though they exercise less, they expend more energy in the course of activity. For this reason, overeating is considered by most experts to be more important than inactivity as a determinant of obesity.[79] Calorie control is needed.[80] While there is general agreement that exercise is an important complement to calorie control in weight-loss efforts, it is considered especially important for weight maintenance.[81] However, it is unclear just how much physical activity is needed, given the typical American diet, to maintain weight.[82]

## [ JUST THE FACTS ]

### Are You Vulnerable to Overeating?

Approximately 50% of obese, 30% of overweight, and 20% of healthy-weight individuals score very high on three characteristics of overeating, which are represented in the questions below. If you have a history of overeating, it is very likely that your answers are "yes," suggesting you are vulnerable to the multisensory appeal of food.

1. Is it hard to resist certain foods? Do you lose control in the face of highly palatable foods?

2. Do you feel a lack of satiation—a lack of feeling full—when you're eating?

3. Do you think about food between meals, or about what you're going to eat next while you're eating?

Sources: Kessler, D. (2009). *The end of overeating.* New York: Rodale Inc.
Liebman, B. (2009). Why we overeat. *Nutrition Action Health Letter,* 8(11), 1,3–5.
Strecker, L. (2010). The science behind overeating. *UpdatePlus,* January/February, 4,37.

## [ JUST THE FACTS ]

### Watching Too Much TV? Try a "Commercial-Break Workout"

A large-scale study[73] that tracked nearly 9,000 people for 6 years concluded that sitting still for prolonged periods of time contributes to increased obesity and mortality (see Chapter 1, page 13). Most of that time was spent watching television. Why is watching television worse for us than other sedentary activities, such as sewing, reading, or writing? The few calories used in writing, for example, is still more than watching television. Plus, when people watch TV, they tend to snack on high-calorie foods.[74] And, they sit in one position for long periods of time. Sitting for prolonged periods of time affects the body's processing of fats and other substances that contribute to obesity and mortality.[75] People can offset this risk by avoiding long periods of time sitting still. Intersperse TV watching with periods of standing, walking around the room, and anything that requires movement. Think of how much energy you can burn by starting a "commercial-break workout." Short commercials usually last 2–3 minutes; longer ones may go for 5 minutes. A 60-minute show will likely include at least 15–20 minutes of commercial time. You can get a good workout and burn lots of energy during an evening of TV viewing, even if you exercise in increments of 2 to 5 minutes. Buy a dumbbell for muscular strength and endurance exercises, do some floor exercises, or take a brisk walk in or around your home. If you have a stationary bicycle or a treadmill, you can use them during commercials and beyond. You're only limited by your imagination.

## Dieting and Exercise: Strategies for Weight Maintenance or Weight Loss

To maintain weight, caloric intake must be balanced by caloric expenditure. To lose weight, a person has to achieve a **caloric deficit,** in which the number of calories burned exceeds the number of calories consumed. This is the basic principle of weight management. It is simple and straightforward, and it includes three obvious strategies: (1) the restriction of caloric intake by dieting, (2) the increase of caloric expenditure through physical activity, and (3) a combination of dieting and physical activity. What is not so easy to explain is how two people can respond so differently to dieting and exercise weight-loss strategies. Complex forces, many of which are still not clearly understood, influence the success of weight-management/weight-loss efforts.

The loss of 1 pound of body fat requires a caloric deficit of 3,500 calories. (The loss of 1 pound of adipose tissue yields more than 1 pound of body weight because fat storage includes some lean support tissue—muscle, connective tissues, blood supply, and other body components.) A caloric deficit of 3,300 calories results in a loss of 1 pound of body weight.[83] A loss of 1 pound of body fat per week is a good goal and requires an average daily caloric deficit of 500 calories. A caloric deficit of more than 500 calories per day, unless medically supervised, borders on the extreme and is difficult to sustain over long periods. A loss of 2 pounds of body fat per week is considered a maximum goal.

A desirable long-term goal for a person trying to lose weight is 1 to 2 pounds per week. Body fat loss in excess of 2 pounds per week is not practical for most people. For example, diets that promise a fat-weight loss of 10 pounds per week require a caloric deficit of 35,000 calories per week; that is an average of 7,000 calories per day. For that kind of caloric deficit, a person would have to go to the extremes of fasting while running two marathons in one day. Weight loss in excess of a couple of pounds per week usually involves lean tissue weight, which should be retained, and fluid weight, which needs to be replaced to prevent health consequences ranging from dehydration to electrolyte imbalance.

### Dieting

Statistics show that dieting is the method of choice for most Americans trying to lose weight. Although dieting usually works only temporarily, most people who fail to maintain weight loss are willing to try again. Many people seek the miraculous diet that will transform them from fat to thin, preferably with minimal effort and in the shortest time possible.

The success rate of diet-only strategies is dismal. Only 5% of people who lose weight keep it off for at least a year, a standard definition of weight-loss success.[84] Typically, one-third of the weight lost during dieting is regained within the first year, and almost all weight lost is regained within 3 to 5 years.[85] Maintaining postdiet weight is one of the major failures of weight loss through dieting because dieters do not learn the habits and behaviors needed to remain at the new weight. The high recidivism rate of diet-only weight-loss programs confirms that for most dieters, losing weight is easier than keeping it off. When dieters are successful at keeping their weight off, it is usually because they emphasize a low-fat, high-carbohydrate diet consisting mainly of fruits, vegetables, and whole grains; they don't skip meals, especially breakfast; they weigh themselves regularly (once a day or at least once a week) so they can take action immediately when their weight increases even a little bit; they keep food jour-

# [ JUST THE FACTS ]

## Should Weight Maintenance Be Your Goal?

The average weight gain of Americans over 10 years is approximately 8 pounds, a little less than 1 pound per year.[88] Few of us would become overly concerned with a 1-pound weight gain over the course of a year. Most of us probably wouldn't even notice a gain of just 1 pound and, if we did, would prefer to view it as a temporary occurrence that would even out over time. However, we would probably notice a 16-pound weight gain 20 years later or a 24-pound weight gain 30 years later. But by that time, eating habits and activity patterns are deeply entrenched in our being and more difficult to change. For many adults, weight maintenance, or weight stability, is a preferred goal. If, after an 8-pound weight gain

over 10 years, a 30-year-old adult focuses on weight maintenance, creeping obesity can be prevented with very slight changes in lifestyle. For example, a daily drop of 100 calories in food intake is not much and can be as little as one serving of a sweetened beverage. The result is a 700-calorie deficit over the course of a week; 3,500 calories, or 1 pound, in 5 weeks; and a little more than 10 pounds in a year. A modest plan of this nature won't sell books or make headlines and it doesn't promise huge weight loss. But it is doable and will be an effective strategy for curbing the weight-gain cycle of the previous decade.

---

nals; and they complement their dieting efforts with a planned program of physical activity.[86,87]

A better goal for many people is weight maintenance, or weight stability. **Weight maintenance** is consistently maintaining weight within certain limits between any two points in time. The concept of weight maintenance is not popular, doesn't make headlines, and doesn't require weight loss. For people with creeping weight gain, however, it will curb the tendency to gain weight over time (see Just the Facts: Should Weight Maintenance Be Your Goal?)

In diet-only strategies, the caloric intake should not drop below 1,200 per day in women or 1,500 per day in men, unless the diet is medically supervised (see Table 8-1).[89,90] Gender differences in caloric intake are due to differences in physical activity patterns, metabolism (from more or less muscle tissue), and size. Because fat is more than twice as energy dense as carbohydrates, many experts recommend concentrating on limiting fat intake rather than on counting calories. If an eating plan calls for a caloric intake below 1,200 calories for women and 1,500 calories for men per day, discuss it with your health care provider. You may need to take vitamin and/or mineral supplements. One last caveat for people frustrated because they can't lose weight on a 1,200- or 1,500-calorie diet: If you can't lose weight at this caloric level, you probably don't need to lose weight. You might be better served by reexamining your reasons for losing weight.

In structuring a diet, some modification in the USDA Food Guide is recommended (see Chapter 6). Figure 8-4 presents the Mayo Clinic Healthy Weight Pyramid and recommends food selections that start first with fruits and vegetables.[91] At least 4 servings of vegetables and at least 3 servings of fruit are recommended each day, but you are allowed to eat an unlimited number of servings of both. Next in ascending

order is the carbohydrate group (grains, pasta, etc.) with 4 to 8 servings recommended. This represents a 33% reduction in the number of servings of carbohydrates in comparison with the USDA Food Guide. Whole-grain, high-fiber foods are the preferred source of carbohydrates. Protein and dairy foods are combined as one food category, with a recommendation of 3 to 7 servings.

The Mayo Clinic Healthy Weight Pyramid emphasizes foods that promote both healthy weight and good nutrition. Hunger should not be an issue with this approach. Also, in the center of the pyramid is the recommendation to engage in physical activity on a daily basis.

## Popular Diets

Many diets on the market are nutritionally sound, and many are not. Some are potentially hazardous, and many are based on faulty nutritional and physiological concepts. Some require that food be eaten in a certain order and severely restrict foods. Some require medical supervision. Others impose unrealistic caloric restrictions, and still others make promises based more on fantasy than facts. (You can explore a list of popular diets that includes descriptions, the type of weight loss expected, health drawbacks, and pros and cons for each diet on this text's Online Learning Center at **www.mhhe.com/anspaugh8e** Student Center, Chapter 8, Popular Diets.) The Food and Drug Administration (FDA) does not investigate every new fad diet, and many diet plans are published without the FDA's endorsement. If a diet is published, it is usually because a publisher sees potential profits from its sales. Publishers know that the advice to "eat fewer calories and increase physical activity" will not sell books, but fad diets with secret ingredients or magic formulas will.

**TABLE 8-1** Food Substitutions That Reduce Fat, Cholesterol, and Calories

| Instead of eating . . . | Substitute . . . | To save* |
|---|---|---|
| 1 croissant | 1 plain bagel | 35 calories, 10 g fat, 13 mg cholesterol |
| 1 cup cooked egg noodles | 1 cup cooked macaroni | 50 mg cholesterol |
| 1 whole egg | 1 egg white | 65 calories, 6 g fat, 220 mg cholesterol |
| 1 oz. cheddar cheese | 1 oz. part-skim mozzarella | 35 calories, 4 g fat, 15 mg cholesterol |
| 1 oz. cream cheese | 1 oz. cottage cheese (1% fat) | 74 calories, 9 g fat, 29 mg cholesterol |
| 1 tsp. whipping cream | 1 tbsp. evaporated skim milk, whipped | 32 calories, 5 g fat |
| 3.5 oz. skinless roast duck | 3.5 oz. skinless roast chicken | 46 calories, 7 g fat |
| 3.5 oz. beef tenderloin, choice, untrimmed, broiled | 3.5 oz. beef tenderloin, select, trimmed, broiled | 75 calories, 10 g fat |
| 3.5 oz. lamb chop, untrimmed, broiled | 3.5 oz. lean leg of lamb, trimmed, broiled | 219 calories, 28 g fat |
| 3.5 oz. pork spare ribs, cooked | 3.5 oz. lean pork loin, trimmed, broiled | 157 calories, 17 g fat |
| 1 oz. regular bacon, cooked | 1 oz. Canadian bacon, cooked | 111 calories, 12 g fat |
| 1 oz. hard salami | 1 oz. extra-lean roasted ham | 75 calories, 8 g fat |
| 1 beef frankfurter | 1 chicken frankfurter | 67 calories, 8 g fat |
| 3 oz. oil-packed tuna, light | 3 oz. water-packed tuna, light | 60 calories, 6 g fat |
| 1 regular-size serving french fries | 1 medium-size baked potato | 125 calories, 11 g fat |
| 1 oz. oil-roasted peanuts | 1 oz. roasted chestnuts | 96 calories, 13 g fat |
| 1 oz. potato chips | 1 oz. thin pretzels | 40 calories, 9 g fat |
| 1 oz. corn chips | 1 oz. plain air-popped popcorn | 125 calories, 9 g fat |
| 1 tbsp. sour cream dip | 1 tbsp. bottled salsa | 20 calories, 3 g fat |
| 1 glazed doughnut | 1 slice angel-food cake | 110 calories, 13 g fat, 21 mg cholesterol |
| 3 chocolate sandwich cookies | 3 fig bars | 4 g fat |
| 1 oz. unsweetened chocolate | 3 tbsp. cocoa powder | 73 calories, 13 g fat |
| 1 cup ice cream (premium) | 1 cup sorbet | 320 calories, 34 g fat, 100 mg cholesterol |

*The values listed are the most significant savings; smaller differences are not shown. Weights given for meats are edible portions.

Because fad diets are unlikely to disappear, identifying some of the characteristics and marketing strategies used by diet promoters to appeal to unwitting consumers is helpful.[92] Fad diets do the following:

- Promote quick results
- Stress eating one type of food to the exclusion of others
- Emphasize gimmick approaches, such as eating food in a particular order
- Cite anecdotes and testimonials, usually involving well-known people
- Claim to be a panacea for everyone
- Often promote a secret ingredient
- Often recommend expensive supplements
- Rarely emphasize permanent changes in eating habits
- Usually show little concern for accepted principles of good nutrition (see Chapter 6)
- Are usually cynical about the evidence that comes from the scientific community
- Often claim there is no need to engage in physical activities

If you're committed to losing weight, what diet plan is best for you? Should it be a low-carbohydrate diet, low-fat diet, low-sugar diet, vegetarian diet, high-fiber diet, volume diet, detox diet, a subscription diet with pre-prepared meals, or some kind of novelty diet that emphasizes a particular type of food? Studies that compare the weight loss of dieters who follow the instructions and guidelines of a particular diet regimen for a year lose weight, regardless of the eating plan. No one particular diet is necessarily any better than another.[93,94,95] Studies reveal a common theme among successful dieters: they cut calories. It's not the diet per se; it's the caloric deficit that matters, whether the deficit comes from carbohydrates, fats, sugars, or some combination. (Table 8-1 demonstrates how to reduce calories that come from fat by making appropriate substitutions.) The best diet is one that fits your personality and personal food preferences and one you can stick with until you reach your goal. You don't have to purchase a commercial weight-loss program to succeed. A survey of 32,000 dieters found that 80% of those who successfully lost weight and kept it off did so without subscribing to a copyrighted, commercial plan.[96] Successful dieters follow the simple and practical principles of reducing portion size, monitoring volume eating, modifying food intake, cutting back on high-fat and sugar-loaded foods, and increasing participation in physical activities.[97] In structuring or choosing a diet plan, there is one

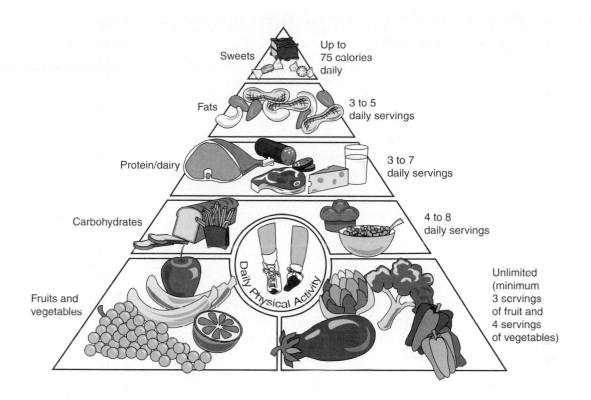

**FIGURE 8-4** Mayo Clinic Healthy Weight Pyramid

The Mayo Clinic Healthy Weight Pyramid shows you where to focus when selecting foods that help promote healthy weight. What's more, you'll never be hungry with this dining approach. When a range of servings is shown, the lower number is based on 1,200 calories and the higher number is based on 2,000 calories.

caveat: avoid very low-calorie diets, which are diets containing fewer than 800 calories a day. These are extreme diets that should be implemented under medical supervision. It's important to remember: The more extreme the diet, the less likely resultant weight loss will be permanent. Often, extreme diets lead to overcompensatory eating. **Overcompensatory eating** typically occurs when certain high-calorie foods are avoided entirely but the dieter ends up consuming more calories. This often occurs with very low-fat diets, but it can occur with any diet or any food. Overcompensatory eaters might rationalize that since they chose a low-fat version of a food in place of their preferred high-fat version, they saved calories and can therefore indulge in more of other foods. If there is a strong sense of denial associated with the low-fat version, they may end up consuming more calories than they would have with the high-fat version. Extreme diets represent the antithesis of the approach recommended in this text. The key to successful weight management is making gradual and progressive changes in eating behaviors and physical activity that can be sustained over a lifetime. These principles are summarized beginning on page 289, Principles of Weight Management: Putting It All Together.

## Diet Drugs

If recent history is a good predictor of the future, American dieters can anticipate a new arsenal of drug solutions for losing weight. Drugs that suppress appetite by stimulating the satiety center in the brain have helped many dieters lose weight temporarily. Drugs marketed under the names *fen-phen* (fenfluramine) and *redux* (dexfenfluramine) during the mid-1990s quickly sold in huge quantities. The popularity of these drugs did not last long, however, because of the plethora of side effects, including death, which eventually led to their withdrawal from the marketplace. Diet drugs typically work in one of three ways. They (1) block the absorption of some of the dietary fat in the intestine (e.g., Xenical), suppress appetite (e.g., Didrex), or promote feelings of fullness (e.g., Meridia).[98] It is important to remember that diet drugs have many potential side effects and require close medical supervision. They are not intended for people who are marginally obese. Instead, they are intended for the management of severe obesity that does not respond to dieting and exercise regimens and for people whose obesity causes serious health risks that outweigh the possible risks of the medication. Unfortunately, many people are drawn to the quick fix of a drug, and many physicians are willing to provide a prescription.

**TABLE 8-2** Classification of Herbs and Unproven but Purported Weight-Loss Mechanisms

| Classification | Common Herbs | Weight-Loss Mechanism |
| --- | --- | --- |
| Thermogenics | Conjugated linoleic acid (CLA) and products containing 5-hydroxytryptophan (5-HTP) | Burn fat and/or help draw fat from cells |
| Diuretics | Buchu, celery seed, dandelion, juniper, parsley, uva ursi | Increase urine production and water-weight loss |
| Stimulants | Ephedra, caffeine, guarana, yerba mate, yohimbine, bitter orange, hot and spicy herbs such as red pepper, mustard, and cayenne | Increase metabolism and suppress appetite |
| Laxatives | Mucilaginous herbs such as psyllium seed (used in Metamucil) | Inhibit appetite by producing feeling of fullness |

The reality is that drugs offer only a temporary solution. They do not correct the underlying cause of persistent weight gain. People who take weight-loss medications can anticipate the typical weight-cycling effect of other dieting strategies with an added problem: Diet drugs are powerful medicines that tamper with the body's delicate balance of hormones and body chemicals. Except for the severely obese, long-term exposure to diet drugs creates harmful effects that may far outweigh the health benefits of fewer pounds of body weight.

## Surgery

The most extreme treatment for obesity is surgery. Surgery to reduce weight is called **bariatric surgery**.[99] Bariatric surgery performed to limit the size of the stomach is called **gastroplasty**.[100] The popular literature often refers to gastroplasty as stomach stapling. Its popularity as an option was given a boost with the development of laparoscopic procedures that require small incisions. There are several variations of gastroplasty; for example, one variation of this surgery decreases the size of the stomach to limit the volume of food that can be processed by the body; another variation involves bypassing the stomach by rerouting the small intestines to a portion of the stomach about the size of an egg.[101] The latter method is call *gastric bypass*. There are more than a dozen variations of bariatric surgery, but gastric bypass is the most commonly used procedure (see Figure 8-5).[102] Regardless of the procedure recommended, surgery is a drastic approach to weight loss and is recommended as a last resort for people classified as morbidly obese or for people with significant complications of obesity. Specifically, it is considered a treatment option for people who either have a BMI of 40 or greater or are 100 pounds overweight (men) or 80 pounds overweight (women) and have been unable to lose weight through nonsurgical means. It may also be appropriate for people with a BMI between 35 and 40 who have serious obesity-related complications.[103] For many people, the results

of bariatric surgery are dramatic, helping people lose on average 61% of excess weight.[104] That translates to 61 pounds for someone who is 100 pounds overweight. However, there are many disadvantages, including follow-up surgery to correct stretched skin, previously filled with fat. Surgery also requires major and dramatic lifestyle changes.[105]

Another surgical procedure that is less invasive than gastric bypass surgery and promoted as an option for mildly to moderately obese people is laparoscopic adjustable banding (LAP-BAND[R] surgery). In LAP-BAND surgery an adjustable band is surgically inserted around the upper part of the stomach to form a small pouch. Unlike other gastric surgeries, LAP-BAND surgery is reversible.[106]

**Liposuction** is the surgical removal of fat tissue, but it is not to be confused with gastroplasty. Liposuction is primarily a cosmetic procedure that helps remove stubborn fat deposits. Common sites of liposuction include the abdomen, hips, buttocks, legs, and upper arms. Although the extracted fat cells will not return, weight can still be gained at other sites in the body.[107] Fat removal by liposuction has no proven health benefits.[108] Liposuction is typically performed by plastic surgeons.

## Diet Supplements and Herbal Remedies

Numerous supplements and herbal versions of prescription drugs used for losing weight are available in health food stores, many drugstores, and online. Some are promoted as thermogenics or "fat burners," while others act as diuretics, stimulants, and/or laxatives. Table 8-2 presents the classification of some common herbs that are promoted as weight-loss products.

The view that herbs are safe because they come from nature is misleading. When packaged in large, concentrated doses and taken as pills or supplements, they should be viewed as drugs with potential side effects. From a medicinal point of view, a major shortcoming of herbs is that they are classified as supplements and, therefore, are not subjected to the same scientific testing

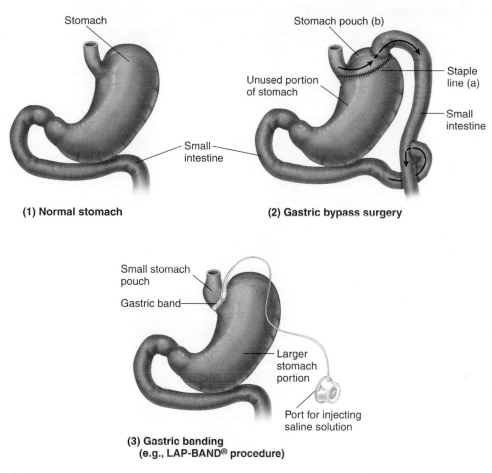

Stomach

Small
intestine

**(1) Normal stomach**

Stomach pouch (b)

Unused portion
of stomach

Staple
line (a)

Small
intestine

**(2) Gastric bypass surgery**

Small stomach
pouch

Gastric band

Larger
stomach
portion

Port for injecting
saline solution

**(3) Gastric banding
(e.g., LAP-BAND® procedure)**

**FIGURE 8-5**  Gastroplasty

In gastric bypass surgery (2) the surgeon staples (a) off a large section of the stomach, leaving a tiny pouch (b). In gastric LAP-BAND surgery (3) an adjustable band is placed around the upper portion of the stomach, creating a small pouch. A salt solution can be injected into the band through a port to adjust the size of the pouch over time.

SOURCE: Wardlaw, G., and Hampl, J. 2007. *Perspectives in Nutrition* (7th ed.), New York: McGraw-Hill.

as are FDA-approved drugs. Consumers cannot be sure what they are getting. In 2009, the FDA warned consumers that at least 70 nonprescription weight loss products contained potentially harmful ingredients not listed on the package label.[109] The Federal Trade Commission (FTC) conducted a study on the claims of weight-loss ads, including the use of supplements and herbs, and found that 40% of them were definitely false and 55% of them were likely to be false.[110] Medical groups usually recommend that herbal weight-loss products be avoided.

## Fasting

**Fasting,** or complete starvation, has been practiced throughout history. Traditionally, people fasted for religious reasons. Although fasting is still used to achieve spiritual enlightenment by some people, a growing number of people fast for dubious physical reasons: to lose weight, to detoxify their bodies of impurities, and to cure everything from allergies to chronic diseases.

The physical benefits of fasting have not been demonstrated in carefully planned studies. Most people who are in good health can tolerate a 24-hour fast without a problem as long as they drink plenty of water. If you decide to try a short fast, first consult with your physician, especially if you are taking medicines. However, prolonged fasting can be harmful and even fatal.

## Physical Activity

The optimal approach to weight loss combines mild caloric restriction with regular physical activity. A weight loss of 1 pound per week requires a caloric deficit of 3,500 calories, or 500 calories per day. This can be accomplished by the following:

- Reducing caloric intake by 500 calories per day
- Reducing daily caloric intake by 250 calories and increasing daily energy expenditure 250 calories or any combination that equates to 500 calories per day

**TABLE 8-3**  Caloric Expenditure of Common Physical Activities

| Activity | Calories/ Min/Lb. | Calories/ Hr./Lb.* | Approx. Calories for 150-Lb. Person** |
|---|---|---|---|
| Aerobics (heavy) | 0.060 | 3.60 | 540 |
| Aerobics (light) | 0.023 | 1.38 | 207 |
| Aerobics (medium) | 0.038 | 2.28 | 342 |
| Basketball (vigorous) | 0.048 | 2.88 | 432 |
| Bed making (and stripping) | 0.031 | 1.86 | 279 |
| Bicycling (< 10 mph) | 0.031 | 1.86 | 279 |
| Bicycling (> 10 mph) | 0.064 | 3.84 | 576 |
| Bowling | 0.029 | 1.74 | 261 |
| Cooking | 0.021 | 1.26 | 189 |
| Dancing | 0.036 | 2.16 | 324 |
| Driving | 0.013 | 0.78 | 117 |
| Golf (walking, carrying clubs) | 0.036 | 2.16 | 324 |
| Hiking | 0.040 | 2.40 | 360 |
| Light gardening | 0.036 | 2.16 | 324 |
| Mopping floors | 0.024 | 1.44 | 216 |
| Piano playing | 0.018 | 1.08 | 162 |
| Raking leaves, grass | 0.034 | 2.04 | 306 |
| Running/jogging | 0.064 | 3.84 | 576 |
| Sleeping | 0.009 | 0.54 | 81 |
| Stretching | 0.019 | 1.14 | 171 |
| Swimming (slow freestyle) | 0.055 | 3.30 | 495 |
| Walking (3.5 mph) | 0.030 | 1.80 | 270 |
| Walking (4.5 mph) | 0.050 | 3.00 | 450 |
| Weight lifting (light workout) | 0.024 | 1.44 | 216 |
| Weight lifting (vigorous workout) | 0.048 | 2.88 | 432 |
| Window cleaning | 0.027 | 1.62 | 243 |
| Writing while seated | 0.013 | 0.78 | 117 |
| Yard work (light) | 0.036 | 2.16 | 324 |
| Yard work, heavy (chopping wood) | 0.048 | 2.88 | 432 |

**Sources:** U.S. Department of Health and Human Services, U.S. Department of Agriculture. (2005). *Dietary guidelines for Americans 2005.* Washington, DC: U.S. Government Printing Office.

Wardlaw, G., & A. Smith. (2011). *Contemporary nutrition* (8th ed.). New York: McGraw-Hill.

*Multiply calories/minute/pound times 60 to determine calories burned per pound in an hour.

**Multiply calories burned per hour per pound times body weight. (this example is for a 150-pound person.)

- Increasing caloric expenditure via physical activity by 500 calories per day

Any of the above options will produce a caloric deficit necessary to lose weight. For most people, a combination approach that includes both caloric restriction and physical activity works best. This is especially true for people who are severely overweight or obese and unable to sustain physical activity sufficient to burn 500 calories per day.

## Use of Calories

One of the obvious benefits of physical activity is that it burns calories. Calories are consumed according to body weight, so heavier people burn more calories per minute than do lighter people for the same activity. Table 8-3 presents the calorie consumption of some physical fitness activities and a few common physical activities. To use it, multiply your body weight by the coefficient in the calories/min./lb. column and then multiply this value by the number of minutes spent participating in the activity. For example, to determine the calories expended by a 150-pound person who walks at 4.5 mph for 30 minutes, do the following:

1. Multiply body weight by calories/min./lb.:

   150 lbs. × 0.050 = 7.5 calories/minute

2. Multiply calories/minute by the exercise time in minutes:

   7.5 calories/minute × 30 minutes = 225 calories

If this person walks daily, 1 pound will be lost in approximately 16 days, or 23 pounds will be lost in 1 year, provided caloric intake is unchanged. The annual weight loss is calculated as follows:

1.  3,500 calories/lb. ÷ 225 calories/day = 15.6 days/lb.
2.  365 days/year ÷ 15.6 days/lb. = 23.4 lbs./year

The landmark document, *2008 Physical Activity Guidelines for Americans*,[111] emphasizes the importance of physical activity in weight control. However, just how much physical activity is needed to maintain weight or lose weight is unclear. The recommendation that adults do at least 150 minutes a week of moderate-intensity or 75 minutes a week of vigorous-intensity physical activity may offer health benefits, but it may not be sufficient for weight control in some people (see Chapter 1, page 13, for physical activity recommendations, and Just the Facts: Light-Intensity vs. Moderate-Intensity vs. Vigorous-Intensity Physical Activity on page 14). There is wide variation from one person to the next in how much physical activity is required to prevent weight gain, to lose weight, and to maintain their body weight after it is lost. Some people can meet their weight-control goals by doing between 150 to 300 minutes of moderate-intensity physical activity each week. Other people may require much more. And for people trying to lose a substantial amount of weight, defined as 5% of body weight, a greater time investment, more than 300 minutes each week, in moderate-intensity physical activity may be required. An example of a 5% weight loss goal is a 200-pound person who is trying to lose more than 10 pounds. People who strive for weight maintenance after reaching their weight loss goal also may require more than 300 minutes of moderate-intensity physical activity each week. The best way to determine what works best for you is to monitor the time spent in physical activity along with changes in your body weight. You can determine how many calories you burn when doing 300 minutes of various physical activities by completing Assessment Activity 8-2.

The American College of Sports Medicine (ACSM) also offers recommendations for weight control through physical activity. Its recommendations are similar to those above but more specific. ACSM states that doing 150–250 minutes per week of moderate-intensity physical activity is associated with weight maintenance. At this level, physical activity is associated with prevention of weight gain. However, it may not be sufficient for losing weight and, if it is, weight loss will likely be modest. To effectively lose weight, more than 250 minutes of physical activity per week is recommended. At this level, weight loss may be substantial in some people. For weight maintenance after a weight-loss goal has been reached, more than 250 minutes per week of moderate-intensity physical activity is recommended.[112]

To the sedentary person who is long removed from any type of physical activity, these guidelines may seem overwhelming. To accumulate the upper level of 250–300 minutes of physical activity each week may require major adjustments in your school, work, and family schedules. It may also have a major impact on your personal lifestyle. The solution: start slow and progress gradually according to the principles of exercise intensity, frequency, and duration discussed in Chapters 3 and 4 in this text. Exercising 60 minutes a day, 5 days a week may be too much at first. An initial goal of 30 minutes a day in increments of 10 minutes spread throughout the day will provide a good foundation for progressively increasing time and distance until a 60-minute-a-day workout can be sustained.

There is an unlimited number of ways to meet physical activity guidelines for weight control. Yard work, gardening, housework, shopping, swimming, hiking, and dancing all count. One of the easiest and most popular activities is walking. Many walkers use a *pedometer,* a device that counts steps (see Figure 8-6), to monitor their physical activity. Pedometers are inexpensive, convenient, accurate, and unobtrusive. Attached to a belt or waistband or carried in the pocket, or clipped to clothing, they monitor steps taken throughout the day, whether you are at work, school, store, play, or just performing routine tasks. Some pedometers have extra features that also monitor the amount of time spent walking and calories burned. Pedometers are good motivators and often encourage people to look for opportunities to add steps. Studies show that people who use pedometers increase their physical activity by more than 2,000 steps a day.[113] Adding just 2,000 steps a day offers health benefits.[114]

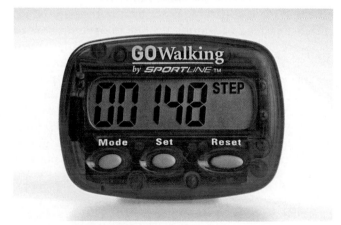

**FIGURE 8-6**  A Typical Pedometer

A pedometer is used to count the number of steps taken daily. It consists of a display, a reset button, and a clip that fastens the pedometer to clothing, usually the belt or waistband. Some are worn on the wrist like a watch. Fancy models come with built-in GPS.

## Wellness for a Lifetime
### Age and Weight Gain Do Not Have to Go Together

Weight gain is one experience people ages 25 to 65 have in common. From the time people embark on their professional careers until the time they start thinking about retirement, they often experience creeping weight gain, sometimes obesity. Often they blame the aging process. But is creeping obesity a function of biological factors that are part of the aging process, or are other factors involved? Rather than aging, a higher standard of living may be responsible for such weight gain. A higher standard of living usually results in an easier, less active life. Improvements in standard of living go hand in hand with labor-saving devices that add convenience and save energy. Many experts believe that weight gain associated with increased age is a function of the subtle changes in metabolism caused by less muscle tissue, which is caused by less physical activity.

Metabolism is an important issue for the weight-conscious person, because 70% of our energy is expended to support basic life processes. Muscle tissue burns more energy at rest than does fat tissue, so changes in body composition that favor muscle tissue over fat tissue provide a calorie-burning advantage throughout the day. Conversely, changes in body composition that favor fat over muscle lower the body's metabolism and promote weight gain. Metabolism declines with age, primarily because of the physical inactivity and muscle loss that often accompany aging. The annual decrease in BMR beginning at 25 years of age, though imperceptible, has serious ramifications for weight management and accounts for a significant amount of the weight gained with age. The loss of muscle tissue is equal to 3 to 5% every decade after age 25. The subsequent decline in BMR produces changes in body composition. Exercise and physical activities are the keys to weight management because they increase or sustain muscle tissue, thus accelerating metabolism and using calories.

---

For most people, this is equivalent to 1 mile. Most walking programs recommend building to 10,000 steps a day (about 5 miles) for good health. This can be done in increments of 200 to 300 steps a week until the goal of 10,000 steps is reached. To lose weight, a goal of 15,000 steps a day (about 7.5 miles) is recommended. And, once the weight-loss goal is reached, 20,000 steps a day (about 10 miles) is recommended to compensate for the weight gain that often occurs when the body adapts to the new weight. All steps taken during the day count. Choosing the stairs rather than the elevator, grabbing the first parking space next to the parking lot entrance instead of waiting for one to open up next to the store entrance, and walking to class rather them driving all contribute to the daily total, as does time set aside specifically for walking. For most people, walking 10,000, 15,000, and 20,000 steps a day for health, weight loss, and weight maintenance, respectively, exceed the recommendations in *2008 Physical Activity Guidelines for Americans* and ACSM's guidelines. (See Assessment Activity 8-3 to assess the number of steps you take each day.)

### Exercise Stimulates Metabolism

**Basal metabolic rate (BMR)** is the energy required to sustain life when the body is in a rested and fasted state. BMR is measured in calories and represents the energy needed to keep the heart, lungs, liver, kidneys, and all other organs functioning. More calories are used to maintain BMR than to perform any other function.

Metabolism is affected by age, gender, nervous system activity, secretions from endocrine glands, nutritional status, sleep, fever, climate, body surface area, and amount of muscle tissue. Because men have more muscle tissue than do women, their BMRs average 5 to 10% higher. See Assessment Activity 8-4 to learn how to estimate your BMR.

Muscle tissue stimulates metabolism. Therefore, physical activity is a key strategy for weight management. This is especially true for people as they get older (see Wellness for a Lifetime: Age and Weight Gain Do Not Have to Go Together). The best way to boost metabolism is to increase participation in aerobic and resistance exercise.[116]

### The Key to Weight Control

Although scientifically controlled studies have not yet proven that physical activity is instrumental in losing weight, they provide compelling evidence of its importance in weight control and weight-loss maintenance. Most people who lose weight and keep it off exercise daily. Regular physical activity is one of the best predictors for those who are able to maintain weight loss over the long term.[117] Ninety percent of people who lose weight and keep it off do so because they use physical activity as part of their weight-control program.[118] Thus, although physical activity as a singular strategy has modest effects on weight loss, it is the key strategy for lifelong weight control. Stated more directly, weight maintenance gets easier when people

## Walking for Weight Loss, Weight Maintenance: Think "More Time"[115]

Researchers at the University of Pittsburgh, Brown University, and Wake Forrest University studied the effects of exercise intensity in losing weight. They asked 184 obese women with an average weight of 190 pounds to limit their diet to 1,200 to 1,500 calories daily and to exercise 5 days a week by walking briskly.

Women who walked less than 30 minutes a day lost 5% of their body weight; those who walked between 30 and 40 minutes a day lost 10% of their body weight. In other words, for an extra 10 minutes a day spent walking, the weight-loss benefit doubled.

These results are consistent with those reported by the National Weight Control Registry, which keeps statistics on people who have lost 30 pounds and kept off the weight for at least 1 year. They walk almost every day. And the more they walk, the more they lose—and keep off.

Source: Tufts Media. (2003). Note to women: Thinner, healthier, and longer life within easy reach. *Tufts University Health and Nutrition Letter*, 21(9), 4.

exercise. More importantly, moderate exercise improves health and reduces the risk factors associated with morbidity and mortality for the obese just as it does for normal-weight people.

### Exercise Intensity and Fat Loss

In Chapter 6, a distinction is made between the intensity and duration of exercise and the accompanying use by the body of energy nutrients. In general, carbohydrates are the main source of energy for high-intensity exercise, and fat is the main source of energy for low-intensity exercise sustained for a prolonged time. (The body instinctively spares its protein reserve except when needed for activities of exceptional duration.) The fat-burning benefit of low-intensity exercise should be a source of encouragement for people trying to shed extra fat, making exercise a viable option for most people. When it comes to walking for weight loss, think "more time."[119] (See Just the Facts: Walking for Weight Loss, Weight Maintenance: Think "More Time"). When it comes to fat-weight loss, think "long and slow."[120] Walking a mile in 30 minutes may take longer than walking a mile in 20 minutes, but it burns more fat calories. If a pace of 30 minutes per mile seems too slow, walk at your normal pace. You're still burning calories. Gardening, yardwork, housework, and numer-

ous household chores also burn fat calories. To improve cardiovascular fitness, the "long-slow" pace should be supplemented with more vigorous activities.

## Regular Exercise Is the Key to Weight Management: Make It Fun

Whatever kind of exercise you do on a regular basis, it is the best strategy for weight management. If your motivation for exercise is based solely on external factors, such as losing weight or preventing disease, it is unlikely that exercise will become a permanent fixture in your lifestyle. Many experts believe that physical activity is more likely to become a lifestyle pattern if it is motivated by intrinsic factors, such as having fun, feeling pleasure, and feeling good. Losing weight is a good reason to start exercising, but you probably won't sustain exercise unless you learn to enjoy it and to value the way it makes you feel. People who are consistently physically active shift their focus from the outcome (weight loss) to the process of exercise. Regular exercisers want to work out because they like it and it makes them feel better.[121] (For tips on making exercise fun, see Nurturing Your Spirituality: Fun Is the Key to Regular Exercise for Weight Maintenance on page 284.) With this approach to exercise, even if weight loss is modest, overall health is improved.

### Combining Dietary Modification and Exercise

Because caloric consumption and expenditure are involved in weight management, both should be manipulated to be effective. Combining sensible exercise and sensible changes in eating habits that can be maintained for life is the most effective approach to permanent weight management. Dieting alone can promote significant weight loss, but a substantial component of the weight loss may be lean tissue. Physical activity alone results in modest fat loss and an increase in lean body mass. Combination strategies involving altering behavior, increasing participation in physical activity, and modifying the diet to cut caloric intake meet the goals of weight management most effectively.[123] (See Just the Facts: Six Keys to Losing Weight and Keeping It Off.) This three-pronged approach to weight loss improves the chances of both short-term and long-term success.

### Behavioral Effects

Some evidence suggests that obese people are more likely than normal-weight people to eat in response to external cues. A clock that says it is suppertime; media messages

## Nurturing Your Spirituality

### Fun Is the Key to Regular Exercise for Weight Maintenance

Experts have shifted the paradigm of weight management from counting calories burned in exercise to promoting movement that is social, playful, and pleasurable. If exercise is fun, if it makes you feel good about yourself, and if it provides that mini-vacation each day (a time and place where nothing else interferes), it is more likely to be incorporated permanently into daily living. As noted by one expert, "Inner joy is the key to dutiful exercise. The body fails to persist if the soul is in rebellion."[122]

Do you want to move from an occasional, dreaded workout to one that you look forward to on a regular basis? Following are some tips passed on by others who once were couch potatoes:

• First, examine your likes and dislikes. Think in terms of activities that are fun for you. These may be taking a stroll in a park, working in a flower garden, skating to class, or joining a fitness club.

• Build relationships with people who share your interests and goals. Workout partners often provide incentive and encouragement for working out.

• Tell people if you notice improvements in their energy level and appearance after exercising. Not only will they feel better but so will you, and the compliment will likely be returned at some point.

• Join a fitness club or participate in a structured fitness program that will increase your repertoire of skills and activities.

• Find a comfortable workout environment with a supportive staff.

• Vary your activities. Variety is the antidote for boredom; cross-training is the key for many longtime exercisers.

---

advertising food and beverages; and the sight, sound, and aroma of food are more apt to elicit eating behavior in the obese. This tendency is the basis of the "externality" hypothesis: If people can learn to eat in response to external cues, they can also learn to recognize cues that stimulate eating behavior, substitute other behaviors for eating, and use techniques that decrease the amount of food eaten. As a result of this training, the response to external cues should be reduced and replaced by attention to internal hunger signals. Many techniques have been developed to assist people in resisting the tendency to eat indiscriminately or to overeat. Generally, these techniques use one or more of the following approaches:

1. *Self-Monitoring and Assessment.* A journal or daily log records food consumption, physical activities, and circumstances related to eating. A written record provides important clues regarding eating patterns, volume eating, portion management, social factors related to eating, and events and circumstances that lead to eating and overeating. For many people, just writing down what they eat causes them to eat less. A thorough assessment not only provides valuable information to act on but also serves as an indicator of your commitment to losing weight and keeping it off. In addition, it provides a basis for evaluating your successes. The principles of lifestyle change that are presented in Chapter 1 of this text, especially the preparation and action stages starting on page xx, provides helpful advice for self-monitoring and assessment.

2. *Control and Modify Eating.* Strategies are used to control, change, or modify problem eating patterns revealed in self-monitoring and assessment. (See Real-World Wellness: Behavioral Strategies for Reshaping Your Eating Habits.) In restructuring eating habits, make gradual changes and build on successes over time. Making extreme changes is a recipe for failure. Avoid labeling foods as "off limits." Doing so creates an internal conflict that feeds an obsession for the food and may promote overcompensatory eating. Managing food choices with the principle of moderation is best.[124] Rather than depriving yourself of a favorite food, try eating it in smaller portions or less frequently. If this doesn't work, place it off limits temporarily. Avoid skipping meals.

3. *Positive Reinforcement.* Positive reinforcement includes rewards that are tied to the achievement of weight loss and physical activity goals.

4. *Support from Family and Friends.* People who elicit the support of others are more successful in changing their eating behaviors.[125] At home, you might ask for support in planning menus that are conducive to your weight-loss plan. At school, you might share your weight-loss plan with your roommate as a way to instill a degree of accountability. You might seek long-term counseling or online support, both of which are shown to boost chances of success in maintaining weight loss.[126]

## [ JUST THE FACTS ]

### Six Keys to Losing Weight and Keeping It Off

Since 1994, the National Weight Control Registry has been following thousands of people who have successfully lost 30 pounds or more and kept it off for at least a year. Two of the questions asked of people in the registry are how did you lose weight, and how did you keep it off? While no single strategy was used all of the time, about half of the participants received help from a nutritionist, doctor, or weight-loss program. The other half lost weight on their own. Some common strategies emerged whether or not participants worked alone or received help. The six keys to their success are as follows:

1. **They ate fewer calories.** Nearly all participants reduced their caloric intake. Very few used extreme diets. Instead, they emphasized low-fat foods, counted calories, counted fat grams, monitored portion sizes, limited their intake of certain foods, followed the menus of a weight-loss program, or some combination of all of these approaches. The bottom line: They consumed fewer calories.

2. **They included physical activity in their daily regimen.** Over 90% of participants burned calories by participating in physical activities equivalent to a 1-hour brisk walk every day. Many participants also engaged in resistance exercises and aerobic activities such as jogging or bicycling.

3. **They ate breakfast.** Eighty percent of participants ate breakfast every day, with an emphasis on cereal and fruit.

4. **They weighed themselves regularly.** Seventy percent of participants weighed themselves at least once a week. More than half of this group weighed themselves every day.

5. **They maintained a consistent diet on weekends, holidays, and weekdays.** Participants who were able to maintain consistency in their caloric intake day in and day out, regardless of the occasion, were least likely to regain the weight they lost.

6. **They were on guard for "slips."** Participants who took quick action to get back on track following a small weight gain improved their chances of stopping or reversing rebound weight gain.

Source: Mayo Foundation for Medical Education and Research. (2007). Losing weight, keeping if off. *Mayo Clinic Health Letter*, 25(1), 6.

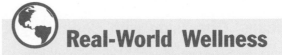

## Real-World Wellness

### Behavioral Strategies for Reshaping Your Eating Habits

*In Chapter 1, I learned about intervention strategies for changing behavior. In this chapter, I've learned about the importance of gaining control over the tendency to overeat. How can I apply behavioral principles from Chapter 1 to my goal of curbing overeating?*

Try the following strategies:

- Eat in a certain place—not in every room of your home.
- Eliminate from your immediate environment all food that can be eaten without careful preparation.
- Always eat at a carefully set place at the table, and eat only one helping of planned foods.
- Prepare only enough food for one meal.
- Eat slowly.
- Chew each bite 25 to 50 times.
- Set down your utensils after every mouthful.
- Partway through the meal, stop and relax without eating for 2 to 3 minutes.
- Leave some food on your plate at each meal.
- Plan to eat some meals alone. (There is a tendency to overeat in social situations.)
- Eat a carefully balanced diet, so that you are not deprived of a particular food element.
- Eat a nutritious breakfast every day, such as whole-grain cereals and fresh fruits.
- Eat three meals a day and nutritious snacks spread throughout the day. Eat in response to hunger cues, which are driven by internal factors, as opposed to appetite cues, which are driven by external factors such as time of day, mood, and social customs.[127] Avoid eating most of your calories in one meal.
- Serve food on a small plate or in a small bowl.
- Rinse with mouthwash or brush your teeth after a meal to break the taste sensation.
- Substitute water for sugared beverages. Add lemon for taste.
- Avoid family-style, buffet menus. If you can't resist the occasional buffet, cut back on calories the day before and/or after.
- Taste your food (and beverage) before adding butter, dressings, sauces, or sugar.

## Americans' Obsession with Body Weight

Americans are preoccupied with their body weight. At any given time, a large percentage of women and men are on a diet, often several a year. Even children are getting the message that dieting is fashionable.

The evidence for this obsession can be found in advertisements and the news. Numerous television celebrities have engaged in special diet or weight-loss programs. Both the print and video media show countless numbers of advertisements that associate supersvelte body images with almost every imaginable product. Consumers demand low-calorie versions of every consumable food, and much of this demand is motivated more by the desire to achieve an unobtainable physique than by health reasons. Consumers have been observed counting the number of calories even in a dose of laxatives. The term *calorie anxiety* applies to many Americans. Even health magazines and professional journals reinforce this preoccupation by featuring headlines of diet articles or diet studies on their covers. If some new diet finding is released by the scientific community, it will surely be headlined on national and local news shows and will quickly be followed by numerous feature stories, many of which produce misleading claims.

For some people, the obsession with weight is so intense that it causes serious body-image problems; distorts their self-esteem; and eventually leads to eating disorders, conditions almost unheard of 30–40 years ago. Extreme cases may involve body dysmorphic disorder (BDD).[128] If a slight flaw in appearance is present, the person's concern is markedly excessive. This preoccupation leads to compulsive checking and questioning; inappropriate surgeries; and occasionally, self-inflicted injury. These symptoms, in turn, may lead to social isolation. This preoccupation is not to be confused with the "normal" dislikes many people associate with one of their physical features. People often complain about the shape of their nose, the size of their ears, or skin blemishes. However, these dislikes do not seriously limit anyone's life. BDD goes far beyond mere dislike into the realm of distress and serious perceptual distortion.

The effects of weight obsession may be more subtle. Some people develop aversive attitudes toward food, eating, and mealtime. Rather than serving as a source of pleasure and enjoyment, the eating experience becomes a constant test of willpower, which rarely yields positive results. For too many people, attitudes about appearance, body weight, and food combined with the ubiquitous messages and body images promulgated by the media form a vicious cycle of guilt, denial, and unhappiness. For example, the average beauty pageant contestant has a body mass index below 18.5; this places them in the "underweight category[129] and is so low that it doesn't show up on standard BMI charts for adults. In contrast, the average BMI of an American woman ranges from 24 to 27 ("high normal weight" to "overweight" category.[130] A very small percentage of the population genetically fits the typical model's BMI zone. The rest of the population is left with unobtainable and unrealistic body images. The challenge for many people is to construct a realistic view of their body while maintaining positive attitudes toward food and formulating reasonable strategies to address the weight problem.

## Eating Disorders and Disordered Eating

Anorexia nervosa (anorexia) and bulimia nervosa (bulimia) are eating disorders familiar to most Americans. More recently, binge eating disorder and female athlete triad have emerged as health issues that require professional intervention. Full-blown anorexia and bulimia are eating disorders; binge eating disorder and female athlete triad usually involve disordered eating patterns. The major difference between the two types of conditions is that eating disorders meet certain criteria as outlined by the American Psychiatric Association. **Eating disorders** are defined as severe alterations in eating patterns linked to physiological changes. The alterations are associated with food restrictions, binge eating, purging, and fluctuations in weight.[131] **Disordered eating**, on the other hand, entails mild and short-term changes in eating patterns that occur in relation to a stressful event, an illness, or even a desire to modify the diet for a variety of health and personal appearance reasons.[132] While these conditions share some characteristics, each has some distinctive qualities.

### Anorexia Nervosa

The chief characteristic of **anorexia nervosa** is a refusal to maintain a minimally normal weight for age and height. Refusal to eat is the hallmark of the disease, regardless of whether other practices, such as binge-purge cycles, occur. Although specific causes of anorexia have not been identified, a combination of biological, social, and psychological factors contributes to the disorder. Support for an organic influence has centered on the hypothalamus (the portion of the brain reputed to house the appetite center) and the pituitary gland (the master gland of the body). Sociocultural theories focus on the compulsion of adolescent girls to become and remain lean. This exaggerated goal manifests at a time when girls are naturally depositing fat.

Anorexia is characterized by extreme weight loss, amenorrhea (absence of a menstrual period), and a variety of psychological disorders culminating in an obsessive preoccupation with the attainment of thinness.

Fortunately, most anorectics recover fully after one experience with the disease. However, the longer a person practices anorexic behaviors, the less the chance for recovery. Just the Facts: Criteria for Diagnosing Anorexia Nervosa lists the criteria that have been developed by the American Psychiatric Association for diagnosing anorexia.[134]

When confronted, anorectics typically deny the existence of a problem and the weight-loss behaviors that have resulted in their emaciated physical appearance. They also avoid medical treatment, refuse the well-intended advice of family and friends regarding professional assistance, and submit to treatment only under protest. Anorexia is a subtle disease, and anorectics become secretive in their behaviors. They are evasive, and many hide their disease in deep denial even while undergoing treatment, making the diagnosis especially difficult.

The course of treatment for anorexia is complex, involving a coordinated effort by several health care specialists. Hospitalization is often required because anorectics may have to be fed intravenously or by some other method if they cannot or will not eat. Medications that stimulate the appetite and medications that calm the patient are usually necessary. Nutritional counseling and psychological counseling—individual, group, and family—are integral components of treatment (see Real-World Wellness: Helping a Friend Overcome an Eating Disorder). Finally, behavior modification techniques are used to help change the perceptions and lifestyle of the anorectic. At this point, no single treatment has proved to be unusually successful in the treatment of anorexic patients.

## Bulimia Nervosa

**Bulimia nervosa** is characterized by alternate cycles of binge eating and restrictive eating. Binge eating is distinguished from ordinary overeating in that it involves the consumption of a large amount of food in a relatively brief time (that is, within a 1- to 2-hour period) and is accompanied by lack of control. Bingeing is nearly always done in private; in public, the bulimic tends to eat normal or even less than normal amounts. Unlike the occasional splurge almost everyone has, the bulimic becomes compulsive and habitual and often resorts to secretive eating. Binges are usually followed by purging, primarily by self-induced vomiting supplemented with laxatives and diuretics. Some people with this disorder may purge excess energy by *hypergymnasia,* or excessive exercise. The physical ramifications of bulimia include esophageal inflammation, erosion of tooth enamel caused by repeated vomiting, and the possibility of electrolyte imbalances. Psychological ramifications include guilt, shame, self-disgust, anxiety, and depression.

[ **JUST THE**
**FACTS** ]
## Criteria for Diagnosing Anorexia Nervosa

The American Psychiatric Association[133] has identified the following criteria for a diagnosis of anorexia nervosa:

- Weight change
  - Unwillingness to maintain minimal normal body weight for the person's age and height
  - Weight loss that leads to the maintenance of a body weight that is 15% below normal
  - Failure to gain the amount of weight expected during a period of growth, resulting in a body weight that is 15% below normal
- Inordinate fear of gaining weight or becoming fat despite being significantly underweight
- Disturbed and unrealistic perceptions of body weight, size, or shape; feeling of being "fat" although emaciated; possible perception of one specific part of the body as "too fat"
- Absence of at least three menstrual cycles for women when they would normally be expected to occur (amenorrheic women have a normal menstrual cycle only during administration of hormone therapy)
- Rigid dieting; maintenance of rigid control in lifestyle; security found in control and order
- Rituals involving food and excessive exercise

The diagnostic criteria for bulimia are given in Just the Facts: Criteria for Diagnosing Bulimia.[136] These criteria specify that, to be diagnosed a bulimic, a person must vomit at least twice a week for 3 months. Binge-purge cycles may occur daily, weekly, or in other intervals. Bulimic behaviors range from binge eating frequently or from time to time, binge eating with a feeling of being unable to control food intake, severe restriction of the diet between binge periods, and binge eating followed by purging. Purging in the form of laxatives, vomiting, diuretics, fasting, and excessive exercise follows in the hope that weight gain will be blunted. Because many people with bulimia engage in binge-purge practices in isolation and because bulimics are often not excessively thin, they cannot be diagnosed easily or by their appearance.

Bulimics are treated similarly to anorectics, except that hospitalization is usually not required. In addition to nutritional and psychological counseling, treatment often includes antidepressive medication because bulimia is associated with clinical depression. Treatment focuses on correcting typical bulimic behaviors, such as "all-or-none" thinking: "If I'm not perfect, I'm a failure, so one slipup—one cookie—justifies a binge." Generally, psychotherapy aims primarily to help a person with self-acceptance and to be less concerned with body weight.[137]

## Binge Eating Disorder

**Binge eating disorder** is similar to bulimia in two ways: (1) It involves eating large amounts of food in a short time, and (2) it is accompanied by a sense of lack of control regarding eating. It is different from bulimia in that it is not associated with compensatory behaviors, such as purging, fasting, and excessive exercise. When binge eating occurs on average at least 2 days a week for 6 months, it becomes an eating disorder. The American Psychiatric Association has identified additional criteria for this disorder.[138] (See Just the Facts: Criteria for Diagnosing Binge Eating Disorder.)

## Female Athlete Triad

**Female athlete triad** is a condition marked by three characteristics: disordered eating, *amenorrhea* (lack of menstrual periods), and osteoporosis (low age-adjusted bone density).[139] It most often affects women athletes engaged in appearance-based, weight-based, and endurance sports. The components of the triad are interrelated. Typically the triad begins with disordered eating. Poor nutrition combined with intense training results in an energy deficit. In time, the energy deficit can cause the body to shut down the production of estrogen, which in turn can trigger amenorrhea. The lack of estrogen combined with nutritional deficiencies, particularly in calcium and vitamin D, may lead to fragile bones. Some young women diagnosed with female athlete triad have bones equivalent to those of 50- to 60-year-olds, making them overly susceptible to fractures during both sports and general activities. Much of the bone loss is irreversible.[141] Women with this condition should seek professional help to reduce their preoccupation with food, weight, and body fat; to regain body weight; to establish regular menstrual cycles; and to increase their consumption of food.

## Underweight

Underweight is defined as a body mass index under 18.5.[142] A small number of people who are not anorexic or bulimic are naturally thin, and some of them are dissatisfied with their appearance. Being underweight presents as much of a cosmetic problem for affected people as obesity does for the obese person. For many underweight people, it is more difficult to gain a pound than it is for obese people to lose one.

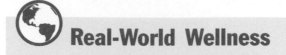

## Real-World Wellness

### Helping a Friend Overcome an Eating Disorder

*I suspect a friend of mine is struggling with an eating disorder. How can I help without making matters worse? Are there some Internet resources available?*

Try doing the following:
- Talk to the person alone.
- Tell the person why you are concerned.
- Be nonjudgmental; ask clarifying questions; listen carefully.
- Offer to go with the person to talk to someone.
- Encourage him or her to verbalize feelings.
- Show how much you care by asking frequently how the person is doing.
- Show an interest in the person's life outside of eating.
- Enlist the help of a counselor if you think the disorder is severe; however, eating disorders are usually not emergency situations.
- Anticipate and accept that denial and anger are part of the illness.

Avoid doing the following:
- Threaten or challenge the person.
- Give advice about weight loss.
- Get into an argument.
- Try to keep track of the person's food consumption.
- Try to force the person to eat.
- Be patronizing by being overly caring.
- Try to be a hero or rescuer; the person may resent such efforts.

Following are some Internet sites that serve as good resources:
- Eating Disorders Awareness and Prevention, Inc., at www.edap.org
- National Eating Disorders Information Centre at www.nedic.ca
- American Dietetics Association at www.eatright.org
- The Center for Eating Disorders at www.eatingdisorder.org

In their attempts to gain weight, many lean people consume large quantities of food, particularly those rich in calories. Unfortunately, these foods are also high in fat and sugar. This eating pattern is unhealthy for anyone, regardless of body weight. The preferred

[ **JUST THE**
**FACTS** ]
### Criteria for Diagnosing Bulimia

The American Psychiatric Association[135] has identified the following criteria for a diagnosis of bulimia:

- Episodic secretive binge eating characterized by rapid consumption of large quantities of food in a short time; never overeating in front of others

- At least two eating binges per week for at least 3 months

- Loss of control over eating behavior while eating binges are in progress

- Frequent purging after eating; using techniques such as self-induced vomiting, laxatives, or diuretics; engaging in fasting or strict dieting; or engaging in vigorous exercise

- Constant and continual concern with body shape, size, and weight

- Erosion of teeth; swollen glands

- Purchase of syrup of ipecac

[ **JUST THE**
**FACTS** ]
### Criteria for Diagnosing Binge Eating Disorder

The American Psychiatric Association[140] has identified the following criteria for a diagnosis of binge eating disorder:

- Recurrent episodes of eating an amount of food clearly larger than most people would eat in a similar circumstance

- Binge eating that occurs, on average, at least 2 days a week for 6 months

- A sense of lack of control over eating

- Binge eating associated with any three of the following:

  - Eating large amounts of food when not feeling hungry

  - Eating alone because of embarrassment over the amount of food eaten

  - Eating much more rapidly than normal

  - Eating far beyond comfort level

  - Feeling guilty or depressed after eating

approach is to combine muscle-building exercises with three well-balanced, nutritious meals supplemented by two nutritious snacks. Increasing caloric intake by 500 calories a day should yield a weight gain of about a pound a week. In doing so, emphasize calorie-rich foods from the Food Guide. Whole-grain cereals with nuts and raisins and dried fruits are examples. Also emphasize foods that are good sources of monounsaturated fats. Examples include olive oil and canola oil. Finally, plan an exercise program that includes resistance training. Instead of gaining fat as calories are increased, muscle weight will be added.

The amount and type of weight gain should be closely monitored. Fat stores should not be increased unless the person is extremely thin and on the verge of dipping into stores of essential fat.

## Principles of Weight Management: Putting It All Together

The best approach to weight management is the most obvious: maintaining a moderate lifestyle, so that excess weight is not gained. In summary, the basic principles of weight maintenance and weight loss are the following:

1. Avoid the obsession with body weight. Remember that body weight per se is not the most important issue; rather, body composition is. Modest weight gain distributed in the wrong places increases health risks. Conversely, significant weight gain in the form of muscle tissue

enhances health and well-being. You should consider losing weight if it becomes excessive or if you have a family history of disease that may be worsened by excess weight.

2. If you are satisfied with your current weight but concerned about gradual weight gain over time, think physical activity. Participating in physical activity on a consistent basis is the best way to prevent creeping weight gain. It is also the best way to maintain weight over time.

   Participation in physical activity is also a key strategy if you are trying to lose weight, especially if combined with calorie restriction. Almost all people who lose weight and keep it off exercise daily. Exercise is the best way to overpower the body's set point for fatness.

   A good weight-loss goal is 1 pound per week. This means imposing a weekly caloric deficit of 3,500 calories or a daily caloric deficit of 500 calories. This can be achieved by reducing caloric intake by 250 calories and increasing physical activity to burn an extra 250 calories. Dietary restriction of 250 calories should not impose a serious hardship to most people. Substituting one or two diet beverages may satisfy this goal for a heavy soda drinker. A 250-calorie workout may be a bit more challenging. It is equivalent to a

2.5-mile walk for most people. Remember, energy expenditure through exercise does not have to occur at one time. The effects of physical activity are cumulative and reinforce the value of activity spread throughout the day, even in 10- to 15-minute increments. The key issue in exercising is consistency and moderation. Plan an activity program that can be sustained 1 year and 5 years from now.

The American College of Sports Medicine expresses physical activity guidelines for weight control in terms of minutes. Doing 150–250 minutes per week of moderate-intensity physical activity promotes weight maintenance. More than 250 minutes per week may be required to lose weight and also to keep it off once the weight loss goal has been reached. To accumulate a weekly total of 150–250 minutes of exercise requires a time investment of 30 to 50 minutes 5 days a week.

If you enjoy walking, purchase a pedometer to monitor the number of steps you take each day. Shoot for a goal of 10,000 steps a day for weight maintenance, 15,000 steps a day to lose weight, and 20,000 steps a day after reaching your weight-loss goal to prevent weight regain. Steps taken throughout the day, at home, work, school, and play, all count. Most people walk only about 2,000 steps a day in their normal routine, so it is important to look for opportunities to accumulate more steps and to build in some walking times in your daily agenda. If long walks aren't practical, take short walks throughout the day, preferably in 10-minute increments or longer.

3. Follow the Mayo Clinic Healthy Weight Pyramid by eating nutrient-dense foods and stressing consumption of fruits and vegetables. Calories from fat convert easily to fat, with only 3% being lost in the digestive process. By comparison, 25% of carbohydrate calories are lost in the process.

Emphasize fiber in your diet. Because of fiber's high satiety value, people who eat a great deal of it usually consume fewer total calories at mealtime.

4. Avoid volume eating. Calories count, regardless of their source. The penchant to practice compensatory eating behavior may be especially common among people who choose low-fat and/or low-calorie products. People are eating food in larger quantities. Avoid buffet-style, all-you-can-eat restaurants. People eat more when they are served more.[143] Practice behavioral strategies that make volume eating more difficult. For example, split restaurant entrées with a friend or avoid the practice of cleaning your plate by taking leftovers home. When eating low-fat, low-carb, or low-calorie foods, be aware of the tendency to overcompensate by eating more food. Remember, two servings of a low-fat food that contains 5 grams of fat yields 90 total fat calories and may exceed the number of fat calories in one serving of the regular, high-fat version. The tendency to overcompensate by consuming more calories also applies to beverages. Liquid calories don't have the satiety value of solid food and often result in extra calories. Drink plenty of water and substitute calorie-free beverages or limit calorie-containing beverages.

5. Watch for "hidden sugar" in foods with a high glycemic index (see Chapter 6, page 204). Foods with a high glycemic index, such as white, refined bread, cause a quick surge in blood sugar, which in turn causes a surge in insulin (see Figure 8-7). The sugar-insulin surge stimulates appetite, which is counterproductive to anyone trying to lose weight. Choose foods with a low glycemic index, such as whole-wheat bread. Sugared beverages are common sources of hidden sugar. Remember, liquid calories don't have the satiety value of solid food and often result in extra calories. Drink plenty of water, and substitute calorie-free beverages or limit consumption of sugared beverages.

6. Set realistic goals. Don't be misled by messages and advertisements that promise huge weight loss in a short time. Weight loss per week usually should not exceed 1 to 2 pounds. The ideal approach is to lose pounds at the same rate at which they were gained. In trying to set goals, ask yourself these questions: What is the least I have weighed as an adult, for at least a year? Based on past experiences, what is the most weight I can expect to lose? A weight goal set below your lowest weight or one that was achieved for only a brief period of time following a strenuous diet is not realistic. Adjust your goals upward from your minimum weight. A realistic goal is to lose 10% of your body weight.[144] For a 200-pound person, a good weight loss goal is 20 to 30 pounds. Losing these first pounds produces the biggest health gains in lower blood pressure, lower blood cholesterol, and lower blood sugar. This is especially true for people with abdominal fat.

7. Make a gradual lifestyle change. Such change represents a calm, deliberate approach, rather than a frenetic "lose it now" attitude. A 200-pound person should exercise, reduce calories, and eat like a 180-pound person to become a

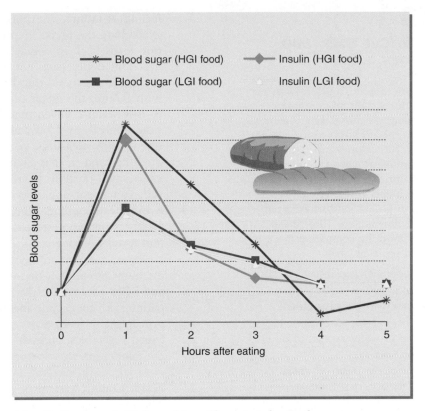

**FIGURE 8-7**  Blood Sugar and Insulin Response to High- and Low-Glycemic-Index Foods

Foods with a high Glycemic Index (HGI food)—such as white, refined bread—cause a quick surge of blood sugar and insulin to enter the bloodstream. After 3 to 4 hours, blood sugar drops below fasting level (0); circulating insulin leads to a hunger reflex and increased appetite. Foods with a low Glycemic Index (LGI food)—such as whole-wheat bread—are digested more slowly and cause less of a surge in blood sugar and insulin; blood sugar keeps pace with circulating insulin, does not drop below the fasting level, and doesn't cause increased appetite.

Source: Consumers Union. (2003). Carbohydrates without fear. Consumer Reports on Health, 15(10), 1, 4.

180-pound person. Once the weight is lost, the person must resist reverting to the habits of a 200-pound person. A diet is successful only if the weight does not return.

8. Anticipate a plateau. During the first week of a diet, weight loss comes primarily from loss of protein, glycogen, and water but little fat. As the body adjusts to a diet, fat loss increases. This adjustment takes about a week on a moderate diet and still longer when the diet is severe. Many dieters experience a plateau after about 3 to 4 weeks, not because they are suddenly cheating but because they have gained water weight while still losing body fat. If physically active, dieters may gain lean body mass and lose fat while maintaining weight. If weight loss is drastic during the early stages, it induces an adaptive response in the body that slows down metabolism. The body resists drastic change of any sort. Once its internal signals recognize a substantial reduction in caloric intake, it slows down to conserve fuel. After losing 20 to 30 pounds, expect to reach a stable plateau.

9. Avoid diet pills, special formula diets, all-you-can-eat diets, fat-burning concoctions, skin creams, and other fad diets. Some of these fads impose health risks, and others simply don't work; if they do, their results are temporary. The more extreme the diet, the less likely the weight loss will be permanent.

10. Avoid very-low-calorie diets. Diets that cut calories to under 1,200 (if you're a woman) or 1,400 (if you're a man) do not allow enough food to be satisfying over the long haul and are unlikely to meet the body's needs for nutrients. Remember, if you can't lose weight at the 1,200- or 1,400-calorie level, you probably don't need to.

11. Develop an eating plan that includes easily obtained foods.

12. Develop a less rigid lifestyle, one that reduces the need to consciously control what is eaten. Maintaining weight loss is the antithesis of counting every calorie.

13. Avoid fasting and restrictive dieting. These practices often lead to a preoccupation with

# [ JUST THE FACTS ]

## Ten Ways to Cut Back 100 Calories a Day

The recommended caloric deficit of 500 calories per day is standard advice for weight-loss programs. What about people trying to achieve weight maintenance or people who are in no hurry to lose weight? A caloric deficit of just 100 calories can result in weight loss, although it takes longer. On the positive side, a deficit of 100 calories is hardly noticeable and is sustainable. The highly respected newsletter *Environmental Nutrition* provides 20 ways to cut 100 calories a day.[146] Following are 10 of them. You can identify many more by comparing the caloric content on food package labels.

1. Substitute 2 tablespoons of jam instead of butter or margarine (100 vs. 200 calories).
2. Order an egg sandwich without the cheese (105 calories per slice).
3. Choose tuna packed in water instead of oil (175 vs. 275 calories per 6 ounces).
4. Substitute fat-free mayo in place of regular mayo (100 vs. 200 calories per 2 tablespoons).
5. Order a 12-ounce (small) beverage in place of a 21-ounce (medium) beverage (110 vs. 210 calories) or choose a sugar-free beverage (0 vs. 210 calories).
6. Choose a medium-sized baked potato over a large one (160 vs. 278 calories).
7. Enjoy two Haagen Dazs chocolate bars in place of 1/2 cup of gourmet ice cream (160 vs. 230 calories).
8. Order a McDonald's regular cheeseburger instead of a Quarter Pounder (330 vs. 430 calories).
9. Snack on a small handful of cashews instead of a large handful (163 calories for 18 nuts vs. 273 for 30 nuts).
10. Make an omelet without the egg yolks (33 vs. 149 calories for two large eggs).

food, weight, and/or dieting. Dieting should allow people to attend parties, eat at restaurants, and participate in normal activities. People erroneously assume that, if they have eaten just a little bit of a forbidden food, they have crossed the line. Foods are neither good nor bad. Labeling them as such often promotes a denial-guilt-preoccupation cycle, in which one slight deviation from a diet or food choice is interpreted as a failure: A forbidden food is eaten (denial), a sense of relief from restraint leads to a binge, the binge leads to guilt and a feeling of failure, and both denial and guilt exacerbate the preoccupation. The preoccupation leads back to denial and the cycle continues. This cycle exerts considerable pressure on the dieter. To avoid the dissonance that comes with failure, the dieter often abandons attempts to lose weight. Given moderation and discretion, almost any food can be enjoyed. Food is one of life's pleasures, so you need not avoid any one food. If it is high in fat and calories, eat a small portion. If you do not deny yourself, you might not feel compelled to cheat.

14. Avoid meal skipping. One strategy that surprises people is the advice to eat three meals a day, plus snacks. Eating small meals plus a morning, afternoon, and before-bedtime snack discourages the habit of eating a one-time, extra-heavy meal and helps prevent the usual denial-guilt-preoccupation with food cycle mentioned above (see principle 13). Keep portions small and emphasize fruits, vegetables, and whole-grain foods Resist the temptation to skip breakfast. Remember, most successful dieters eat breakfast every day

15. Form a buddy system or join a support group. The support and encouragement of a friend or relative are often the difference between success and failure.

16. If you stop smoking, don't be discouraged by subsequent weight gain. If you are a heavy smoker, you can expect on average an increase in weight of 10 pounds. That's not enough to make most smokers obese. From a health perspective, the benefits of not smoking will far outweigh the risks of gaining 10 pounds.

17. Don't indulge yourself in self-blame for past failures. View past dieting attempts objectively, as a psychologist would. Focus more on what you learned from past experiences. Most people who are successful at maintaining weight loss are not successful in their first attempt. In studies that track dieters listed in the Weight Control Registry, 90% of them are repeaters. In some studies, nearly 60% of dieters were found to have made five attempts before achieving success.[145] Rather than blaming yourself, reflect on what you learned about yourself and what worked and didn't work.

18. Weight maintenance may be a more appropriate goal than weight loss. Most people gain weight slowly and progressively over time. The first step (and the only step) for many people creeping into obesity is to stop the pattern of weight gain by stabilizing at the present weight. Weight maintenance, or weight stability, can usually be achieved with slight changes in lifestyle (see Just

the Facts: Ten Ways to Cut Back 100 Calories a Day). Even if weight loss becomes necessary, a history of weight maintenance provides a benchmark for future efforts.

19. Consult with a nutritionist, doctor, or weight-loss program provider to develop a plan for losing weight. Doing so may be the key to success, especially if you are a repeat dieter. If you want to develop your own plan, be comforted in knowing that nearly one-half of people who lose weight and keep it off are able to customize their own plan, one that fits their personal needs and preferences. In doing so, it's important to set realistic goals, cut calories, add physical activity, maintain a consistent diet, including holidays, weekends, and special occasions, watch for brief relapses and take quick action to get back on track, weigh yourself regularly, preferably daily, and keep a written record of your progress.

20. Finally, accept yourself. Before trying to lose weight, determine how great a risk your weight poses to your health. People at risk for chronic conditions, such as hypertension and Type 2 diabetes, for example, often improve dramatically with a modest weight loss. Some people, however, are overweight despite their best efforts to reduce. For such people, striving to attain a certain weight may be futile and even damaging to health. If a person was overweight throughout childhood, chances are that person will never be thin. Be realistic and aim for a healthy weight for you, not for an actor or actress. Not everyone can be skinny. Everyone can try to be healthy.

# Summary

- Americans' obsession with body weight is evidenced by the large number of women, men, and even children who are unhappy with their physical appearance and willing to subject themselves to elective surgery to improve some aspect of their body.

- A healthy weight is defined as a BMI of 18.5 to 24.9. Overweight occurs with a BMI of 25 or over. Obesity occurs with a BMI of 30 or over. By these standards, nearly two-thirds of Americans are overweight or obese. The obesity epidemic also includes children. Thirty-two percent of children and adolescents are overweight or obese; 17% are obese.

- Obesity is a risk factor for coronary heart disease, stroke, hypertension, LDL cholesterol, some forms of cancer, impaired glucose tolerance, osteoarthritis, gallbladder disease, and sleep apnea.

- *Obesogenic* is a term that refers to environments that promote increased food intake, nonhealthful foods, and physical inactivity.

- Obesity occurs when fat cells increase excessively, either in size (hypertrophy) or in number (hyperplasia).

- Waist measurements are predictive of health risks associated with overweight and/or obesity. For men, the risks increase with a waist measurement of 40 inches, for women, 35 inches.

- There is considerable controversy regarding the relationship between overweight, fitness, and mortality. Recent large-scale studies indicate that being overweight is not associated with premature mortality, and for older adults over 65 years of age it is associated with increased longevity. These findings run counter to mainstream medical opinion. Proving cause and effect between fitness, weight status, and mortality is a big challenge that will require much more research. Until then, the consensus opinion is that physically active lifestyles improve health and longevity, regardless of body-weight status.

- Heredity and set point are the major biological factors associated with obesity.

- *OB* genes, or fat genes, are intrinsic to the body and produce a hormone called leptin that suppresses appetite. In the absence of the *OB* gene, the brain doesn't get the signal to stop eating. Some people don't get enough leptin or develop a resistance to it. Obesogens are extrinsic chemicals commonly found in the diet that disrupt the metabolism of fat and facilitate the accumulation of fat. Both *OB* genes and obesogens may lead to obesity.

- Defended weight is synonymous with set point and represents the weight our body strives to attain when we're not on a diet or participating in an exercise program.

- Childhood obesity is a predictor of obesity later in life.

- The development and distribution of body fat are under substantial genetic control.

- The classic types of body shapes are ectomorph, endomorph, and mesomorph. Ectomorphs have a low capacity for fat storage; endomorphs have a larger capacity for fat storage; and mesomorphs fall somewhere in between ectomorphs and endomorphs.

- Physical activity is the best way to alter the body's set point for fatness.

- Overeating and lack of physical activities are the major behavioral explanations of obesity.

- Americans consume 300 calories per day more than their peers of 20 years ago. This is equivalent to 3 pounds per month, 36 pounds per year.

- Restaurants serve food in larger portions than ever before, and Americans are eating more than ever before. People eat more when they are served more food. Portion sizes and volume eating contribute significantly to the high caloric intake of Americans.

- The abundance of food high in fat and calories is a major factor in the prevalence of obesity in the United States.

- The multisensory appeal of salt, fat, and sugar, especially when combined, makes food difficult to resist and contributes to overeating.
- Dietary fat has less of a thermic effect than do carbohydrate and protein and therefore is more efficiently and easily stored as fat tissue.
- Soft drinks account for 22% of total calories and 50% of added sugar in the typical American diet. There is a direct relationship between the consumption of sweetened soft drinks and overweight.
- Americans are overwhelmed with supersized portions of food, more so now than in the past and especially when eating out.
- The general decline in physical activity is highly correlated with the rise in obesity.
- Sitting still for prolonged periods of time, such as in watching TV, affects the body's processing of fats and other substances in ways that contribute to obesity and mortality.
- Americans take about 2,000 to 3,000 steps a day, roughly about 1 to 1½ miles. This is far short of the minimum recommendation of 10,000 steps a day (5 miles).
- Engaging in a physically active lifestyle is the best way to prevent weight gain.
- Approximately 70% of the energy liberated from food is expended to support BMR.
- Physical activity improves body composition, increases BMR, improves insulin sensitivity, and increases oxygen capacity and glycogen storage in muscles.
- Weight loss requires a caloric deficit in which food intake and exercise are manipulated, so that caloric expenditure exceeds caloric intake.
- For many people, weight maintenance, or weight stability, is a better goal than weight loss. Because

weight-maintenance approaches usually involve only modest changes in lifestyle, they are sustainable and help curb the tendency toward creeping obesity.
- Complex forces influence the success of weight-loss efforts and help explain why people respond so differently to similar dieting strategies.
- Low-fat diets often result in overcompensatory eating behaviors, as a result of which the dieter ends up consuming more total calories.
- A good weight-loss goal is 0.5 to 1 pound per week. A weekly weight-loss goal of 1 pound requires a caloric deficit of 3,500 calories per week and can be achieved by cutting calories consumed, using more calories in physical activity, or, preferably, doing both.
- Diet-only strategies should provide at least 1,200 calories per day for women and 1,500 for men.
- Foods with a low Glycemic Index (e.g., whole-wheat bread) have an advantage over foods with a high Glycemic Index (e.g., white, refined bread) because they are digested more slowly, cause less of a surge in blood sugar and insulin, and don't cause an increase in appetite.
- The optimal approach to weight loss combines mild caloric restriction with regular physical activity. Together these two strategies should provide a caloric deficit of 500 calories per day.
- In structuring a diet to lose weight, follow the recommendations in the Mayo Clinic Healthy Weight Pyramid. Emphasize fruits and vegetables. Observe recommended servings for carbohydrates, protein sources, and fats.
- People who are successful at losing weight, and keeping it off, typically eat a low-fat, high-carbohydrate diet consisting primarily of fruits, vegetables, and whole grains; they don't

skip meals, especially breakfast; they weigh themselves regularly, usually daily; and they keep a food journal.
- Diet drugs include fat inhibitors, appetite suppressants, and antidepressants. New drugs that influence cravings are currently being studied. Diet drugs are not intended for people who are overweight or only marginally obese. The harmful effects of long-term use of diet drugs may outweigh the health benefits of losing weight.
- The American College of Sports Medicine recommends 150 to 250 minutes of moderate-intensity physical activity each week for weight maintenance. More than 250 minutes per week of physical activity may be required to lose weight and keep it off. Physical activity, combined with dietary restriction of calories, offers the best strategy for losing weight and for preventing weight regain.
- Low-intensity exercises, such as a slow walk, are effective in burning fat calories. To promote weight loss through physical activity, think: long-slow-distance rather than short, fast, and intense. However, regardless of intensity level, exercising on a consistent basis is the best strategy for managing weight.
- Surgery to reduce weight is called bariatric surgery. When the purpose of surgery is to reduce the size of the stomach, it is called gastroplasty. Surgery is recommended as a last resort for people classified as morbidly obese and for people with significant complications of obesity.
- Liposuction is a cosmetic procedure used to remove fat deposits. It yields no proven health benefits.
- Anorexia, bulimia, binge eating, and female athlete triad are four potentially destructive eating disorders and/or disordered eating patterns with complex causes.

# Review Questions

1. What evidence exists to support the idea that Americans are obsessed with weight control?
2. In terms of BMIs, what are the definitions of *healthy weight, overweight,* and *obesity*?

3. What evidence exists to support the claim that obesity in U.S. children, adolescents, and adults is epidemic?
4. What health problems and chronic conditions are associated with obesity?

5. What is the relationship between obesity and morbidity and mortality?
6. What are the major biological and behavioral factors that help explain obesity?

7. What evidence can you use to support the existence of an influential role of heredity in the development of obesity?
8. Distinguish between the terms *OB gene*, *obesogens*, and *obesogenic environment*. How do these terms relate to obesity?
9. What do the terms *set point*, *defended weight*, and *normal weight* mean in reference to body shape and body weight? What strategy is best for altering a person's set point for fatness?
10. Discuss the relationship between physical fitness, overweight, and premature mortality. How does mainstream medical opinion about the relationship between fitness, overweight, and mortality compare with the findings in recent studies?
11. What dieting strategies need to be emphasized in weight-loss programs?
12. Why are more Americans overweight today than in the past?
13. What are the major differences between the dietary recommendations in the USDA Food Guide and those in the Mayo Clinic Healthy Weight Pyramid?

14. Compare and contrast dieting and exercise as strategies for (a) losing weight and (b) maintaining weight or preventing weight gain.
15. Why is the thermic effect of food an important issue in weight management?
16. Explain the relationship between metabolism and weight gain and/or weight loss.
17. Explain the relationship among blood sugar, insulin response, low- and high-Glycemic-Index foods, and appetite.
18. Compare the physical activity recommendations for weight control presented in *2008 Physical Activity Guidelines for Americans* and by the American College of Sports Medicine. Identify similarities and differences between these two sets of recommendations.
19. In what ways do physical activity recommendations differ for the three goals of weight maintenance (i.e., preventing weight gain), losing weight, and preventing weight regain after a weight-loss goal has been achieved?

20. What is the relationship among BMR, physical activity, and body composition?
21. Explain why the walking prescription to maintain weight, once it is lost, is 20,000 steps per day while the walking prescription to lose weight is 15,000 steps per day.
22. What are the differences and similarities among anorexia, bulimia, binge eating, and female athlete triad?
23. What guiding principles should be observed in planning a reasonable approach to weight loss/weight management?
24. According to the National Weight Control Registry, there are six common themes observed in the actions of people who are successful at losing weight and keeping it off. Identify and discuss each of these themes.
25. Identify eight behavioral strategies that can be used to discourage the practice of overeating.
26. What does overcompensatory eating mean? What diet practices promote overcompensatory eating? Why?

# References

1. Veale, D. (2004). Body dysmorphic disorder. *Postgraduate Medical Journal*, 80(940), 67–72.
2. Tiggemann, M., & D. Hargreaves. (2003). The effect of "thin ideal" television commercials on body dissatisfaction and schema activation during early adolescence. *Journal of Youth and Adolescence*, 32(5), 367–74.
3. MayoClinic.com. (2010). Body dysmorphic disorder. Retrieved February 16, 2010, from www.mayoclinic.com/health/body-dysmorphic-disorder/DS00559.
4. National Institutes of Health. (2009). How you see yourself: When your body image doesn't measure up. *NIH News in Health*. Retrieved February 16, 2010, from http://newsinhealth.nih.gov/2009/July/feature1.htm.
5. Neergaard, L. (2009). Weight worries skewer priorities. *The Commercial Appeal*, May 12, 2009, p. A5.

6. Wardlaw, G., & A. Smith. (2011). *Contemporary nutrition* (8th ed.). New York: McGraw-Hill.
7. Division of Nutrition, Physical Activity and Obesity, National Center for Chronic Disease Prevention and Health Promotion. (2009). *Defining overweight and obesity*. Retrieved February 17, 2010, from www.cdc.gov/obesity/defining.html.
8. Flegal, K., M. Carroll, C. Ogden, & L. Curtin. (2010). Prevalence and trends in obesity among US adults, 1999–2008. *JAMA*, 303(3), 235–41.
9. National Center for Health Statistics. (2009). *Health, United States, 2008 with special feature on the health of young adults*. Hyattsville, MD: U.S. Department of Health and Human Services.
10. National Center for Disease Prevention and Health Promotion. (2009). *Obesity: Halting the epidemic by making health easier*. Atlanta: Centers for Disease Control and Prevention.

11. Levi, J., C. Juliano, & L. M. Segal. (2006). *F as in fat: How obesity policies are failing in America 2006*. Washington, DC: Trust for America's Health.
12. Ogden, C., M. Carroll, L. Curtin, M. Lamb, & K. Flegal. (2010). Prevalence of high body mass index in US children and adolescents, 2007–2008. *JAMA*, 303(3), 242–49.
13. Levi et al. (2006).
14. National Center for Health Statistics (2009).
15. National Center for Disease Prevention and Health Promotion (2009).
16. Ibid.
17. Harvard Health Publications. (2009). Measuring how fat we are. *Harvard Health Letter*, 34(1), 1–23.
18. Editors. (2009). Waist circumference predictive of heart failure. *Environmental Nutrition*, 32(6), 1.
19. U.S. Department of Health and Human Services, U.S. Department of Agriculture. (2005). *Dietary guidelines for Americans 2005*.

Washington, DC: U.S. Government Printing Office.

20. Cheskin, L, C. Roberts, & S. Margolis. (2010). *The Johns Hopkins white papers: Nutrition and weight control for longevity*. Baltimore: Johns Hopkins Medicine.

21. Mayo Foundation for Medical Education and Research. (2008). Cancer and weight. *Mayo Clinic Health Letter*, 26(6), 4–5.

22. Consumers Union. (2006). The new do's and don'ts for preventing cancer. *Consumer Reports on Health* 18(2), 1, 4–5.

23. Byrd-Bredbenner, G. Moe, D. Beshgetoor, & J. Berning. (2009). *Wardlaw's perspectives in nutrition* (8th ed.). New York: McGraw-Hill.

24. Wardlaw, G., & A. Smith. (2011). *Contemporary nutrition* (8th ed.). New York: McGraw-Hill.

25. National Institutes of Health. (2010). *Guidelines on overweight and obesity: Electronic textbook—dyslipidemia*. Retrieved February 19, 2010, from www.nhlbi.nih.gov/guidelines/obesity/e–txtbk/ratnl/2212.htm.

26. Ervin, R. (2009). Prevalence of metabolic syndrome among adults 20 years of age and over, by sex, age, race and ethnicity, and body mass index: United States, 2003–2006. *National Health Statistics Reports*, no. 13. Hyattsville, MD: National Center for Health Statistics.

27. Wardlaw & Smith (2011).

28. National Center for Health Statistics (2009).

29. Orpana, H., J. Berthelot, M. Kaplan, D. Feeny, B. McFarland, & N. Ross. (2010). BMI and mortality: Results from a national longitudinal study of Canadian adults. *Obesity*, 18(1), 214–18.

30. Reis, J., C. Macera, M. Araneta, S. Lindsay, S. Marshall, & D. Wingard. (2009). Comparison of overall obesity and body fat distribution in predicting risk of mortality. *Obesity*, 17(6), 1232–39.

31. Tufts Media. (2008). What does the latest research on weight mean to you? *Tufts University Health and Nutrition Letter*, 25(11), 6.

32. Levi et al. (2006).

33. Nieman, D. (2007). *Exercise testing and prescription: A health-related approach* (6th ed.). New York: McGraw-Hill.

34. Mayo Foundation for Medical Education and Research. (2005). Metabolism: How you burn calories. *Mayo Clinic Health Letter*, 23(7), 4–5.

35. Ibid.

36. Wardlaw & Smith (2011).

37. Cheskin et al. (2010).

38. Ibid.

39. Mayo Foundation for Medical Education and Research. (2005). *Mayo Clinic healthy weight for everybody*. Rochester, MN: Mayo Clinic Health Information.

40. Cheskin et al. (2010).

41. Levi et al. (2006).

42. Cheskin et al. (2010).

43. Ibid.

44. Surwit, R. (2008). Obesity gene can be blocked by high levels of physical activity. *Duke Medicine Health News*, 14(12), 6.

45. Perrine, S., & H. Hurlock. (2010). *The new American diet*. New York: Rodale Inc.

46. Ibid.

47. Wardlaw, G. M. (2003). *Contemporary nutrition: Issues and insights* (5th ed.). New York: McGraw-Hill.

48. Wardlaw & Smith (2011).

49. Ibid.

50. Levi et al. (2006).

51. Ibid.

52. Binkley, S., M. Fry, & T. Brown. (2009). The relationship of college students' perceptions of their BMI and weight status to their physical self-concept. *American Journal of Health Education*, 40(3), 139–45.

53. Ibid.

54. Tufts Media. (2003). You underestimate calorie intake, but by how much? *Tufts University Health and Nutrition Letter*, 21(9), 2.

55. Nieman (2007).

56. Wardlaw & Smith (2011).

57. Nieman (2007).

58. Consumers Union. (2010). Sizing up food portions. *Consumer Reports on Health*, 22(3), 7.

59. Broiher, K. (2009). Test your portion I.Q.: Tips to control how much you eat. *Environmental Nutrition*, 32(1), 2.

60. Kessler, D. (2009). *The end of overeating*. New York: Rodale Inc.

61. Liebman, B. (2009). Why we overeat. *Nutrition Action Health Letter*, 8(11), 1,3–5.

62. Strecker, L. (2010). The science behind overeating. *UpdatePlus*, January/February, 4,37.

63. Liebman (2009).

64. Ibid.

65. Tufts Media. (2007). Beverages total 22% of U.S. calories—but who's counting? *Tufts University Health and Nutrition Letter*, 25(1), 1–2.

66. Ibid.

67. Helm, J. (2008). Think before you drink: Watch out for covert calories. *Environmental Nutrition*, 31(4), 1,6.

68. Consumers Union (2004).

69. Palmer, S.( 2009). Calorie counts at restaurants may be sweeping the nation. *Environmental Nutrition*, 32(10), 2.

70. Dunstan, D. W., E. L. M. Barr, G. N. Healy, et al. (2010). Television viewing time and mortality: The Australian diabetes, obesity and lifestyle study. *Circulation*, 121(2), 384–91.

71. Mayo Foundation for Medical Education and Research. (2010). Is watching television really all that bad for you? *Mayo Clinic Health Letter*, 28(3), 8.

72. Ibid.

73. Dunstan et al. (2010).

74. Mayo Foundation for Medical Education and Research (2010).

75. Winslow, R. (2010, January 12). Watching TV linked to higher risk of death. *The Wall Street Journal—Business*. Retrieved February 23, 2010, from http://online.wsj.com/article/SB1000142405274870405510457465234070817 2608.html?KEYWORDS=Watching+TV+Linked+to+Higher+Risk+of+Death.

76. Nieman (2007).

77. Ibid.

78. Upton, Julie. (2005). Walk yourself well: EN's step-by-step guide to good health. *Environmental Nutrition*, 28(9), 1,6.

79. Nieman (2007).

80. Harvard Health Publications. (2008). Let's talk to an expert. *Harvard Health Letter*, 33(1), 8.

81. Wardlaw & Smith (2011).

82. Harvard Health Publications (2008).

83. Wardlaw & Smith (2011).

84. Byrd-Bredbenner et al. (2009).

85. Ibid.

86. Ibid.

87. Schardt, D. (2008). Secrets of successful losers. *Nutrition Action Healthletter*, 35(1), 8.

88. Wardlaw, G., Hampl, J., & R. DiSilvestro. (2004). *Perspectives in nutrition* (6th ed.). New York: McGraw-Hill.
89. Wardlaw & Smith (2011).
90. Cheskin et al. (2010).
91. Mayo Foundation for Medical Education and Research. (2008). Achieving a healthy weight. *Mayo Clinic Health Letter*, 26(6: Supplement), 1–8.
92. Wardlaw & Smith (2011).
93. Consumers Union. (2009). Calories, calories, calories. *Consumer Reports on Health*, 21(6), 3.
94. Editor. (2009). Bucking the trends: Calories still count. *Duke Medicine Health News*, 15(6), 5.
95. Tufts Media. (2009). For weight loss, calories count—diet plans don't. *Tufts University Health and Nutrition Letter*, 27(4), 8.
96. Consumers Union. (2007). A truce in the diet wars. *Consumer Reports on Health*, 19(5), 8–9.
97. Palmer, S. (2010). The new science behind diet and weight loss—It's all about diversity. *Environmental Nutrition*, 33(1), 1,4.
98. Cheskin et al. (2010).
99. Ibid.
100. Ibid.
101. Wardlaw & Smith (2011).
102. Consumers Union. (2006). Surgically slim: A cure for obesity and why it's risky. *Consumer Reports*, 71(2), 24–28.
103. Cheskin et al. (2010).
104. Ibid.
105. Wardlaw & Smith (2011).
106. Cheskin et al. (2010).
107. Ibid.
108. Ibid.
109. Ibid.

110. Welland, D. (2003). Researchers at international summit cite new links between diet and cancer. *Environmental Nutrition*, 26(9), 1,4.
111. Department of Health and Human Services. (2008). *2008 Physical activity guidelines for Americans*. Hyattsville, MD: U.S. Department of Health and Human Services.
112. American College of Sports Medicine. (2009). *ACSM position stand on physical activity and weight loss now available*. Retrieved February 26, 2010, from www.acsm.org/AM/Template.cfm?Section=ACSM–News–Releasts&CONTENTID=12153&TEMPLATE=/CM/ContentDisplay.cfm.
113. Tufts Media. (2008). Pedometer users walk more, lose pounds and BP. *Tufts University Health and Nutrition Letter*, 25(11)f, 1–2.
114. Editor. (2008). Pedometers lead to increased activity, better health. *Duke Medicine Health News*, 14(3), 5.
115. Consumers Union. (2003). Lose the remote control. *Consumer Reports on Health*, 15(6), 2
116. Forman, A. (2006). Boosting metabolism to lose weight: What works, what doesn't. *Environmental Nutrition*, 29(1), 1,4.
117. Nieman (2007).
118. Mayo Foundation for Medical Education and Research. (2007). Losing weight, keeping it off. *Mayo Clinic Health Letter*, 25(1), 6.
119. Upton (2005).
120. Ibid.
121. White, D. (1999). Inner joy is key to dutiful exercise. *The Commercial Appeal*, January 4, pp. C1–3.
122. Ibid.

123. Cheskin et al. (2010).
124. Wardlaw & Smith (2011).
125. Cheskin et al. (2010).
126. Ibid.
127. Wardlaw & Smith (2011).
128. Veale (2004).
129. Wardlaw & Smith (2011).
130. Ibid.
131. Ibid.
132. Ibid.
133. American Psychiatric Association. 2000. *Diagnostic and statistical manual of mental disorders* (4th ed.). Washington, DC: American Psychiatric Association.
134. Ibid.
135. Ibid.
136. Ibid.
137. Wardlaw & Smith (2011).
138. American Psychiatric Association (2000).
139. Wardlaw & Smith (2011).
140. American Psychiatric Association (2000).
141. Wardlaw, G., & J. Hampl. (2007). *Perspectives in nutrition* (7th ed.). New York: McGraw-Hill.
142. Wardlaw & Smith (2011.
143. Consumers Union. (2003). Quit the clean-plate club. *Consumer Reports on Health*, 15(9), 20.
144. Cheskin et al. (2010).
145. Tufts Media.(1998). What it takes to take off weight [and keep it off]. *Tufts University Health and Nutrition Letter*, 15(11), 4–5.
146. Environmental Nutrition. (2003). More leisurely weight loss: 20 ways to cut 100 calories a day. *Environmental Nutrition*, 26(1), 8.

# Suggested Readings

Byrd-Bredbenner, G. Moe, D. Beshgetoor, & J. Berning. (2009). *Wardlaw's perspectives in nutrition* (8th ed.). New York: McGraw-Hill.

Major reference text on nutrition with separate chapters on dieting, weight control, and eating disorders. Designed for nutrition and health science majors, this text provides an in-depth look at nearly every aspect of nutrition, including obesity, overweight, weight maintenance, and the pros and cons of many popular diet regimens. Scientific explanations of obesity and weight control include concepts related to physiology and chemistry.

Cheskin, L., C. Roberts, & S. Margolis. (2010). The Johns Hopkins white papers: Nutrition and weight Control for longevity. Baltimore: Johns Hopkins Medicine.

Designed for the lay public, this monograph presents an overview of issues related to nutrition and weight loss, compares popular weight-loss methods, describes medical conditions that may cause obesity, and outlines lifestyle treatments for weight loss. This monograph is updated annually.

Department of Health and Human Services. (2008). *2008 Physical activity guidelines for Americans*. Hyattsville,

MD: U.S. Department of Health and Human Services.

This landmark document presents the federal government's first comprehensive guidelines on physical activity and serves as a major reference for policy makers, educators, and the general public on the amount, types, and intensity of physical activity needed to achieve health benefits for Americans of all ages. The role of physical activity in weight maintenance, losing weight, and preventing weight regain is highlighted throughout the book.

Mayo Foundation for Medical Education and Research. (2010). The Mayo Clinic Diet: Eat well. enjoy life. lose weight. Rochester, MN: Mayo Clinic Health Information.

This book is designed for the lay public and provides practical and commonsense ideas on how to achieve a healthy weight. It starts out with a 2-week period of adding 5 habits, breaking 5 habits, and adopting 5 habits and then taps into areas that will likely motivate you to succeed in your efforts. This book comes with the endorsement of the famous Mayo Clinic.

Nieman, D. C. (2007). Exercise testing and prescription: A health-related approach (7th ed.). New York: McGraw-Hill Higher Education.

In this text a separate chapter is devoted to the relationship of physical activity and obesity. The author provides a comprehensive review of the literature on physical activity and obesity, citing more than 300 studies. Concepts, issues, and misconceptions are thoroughly discussed and documented.

Perrine, S., & H. Hurlock. (2010). *The new American diet*. New York: Rodale Inc.

This book discusses the obesogen effect and how it disrupts metabolism in a way that leads to obesity. It suggests that losing weight is not simply a matter of eating less and exercising more. Rather, it is about gaining control over obesity-causing chemicals commonly found in the American diet. These may be chemicals found in soy products, hormones given to our animals, plastic pollutants in food packaging, and pesticides sprayed on vegetables and fruits. A 6-week plan is offered to help rid your body of these chemicals and so break free of the obesogen effect.

Roberts, S., & B. Sargent. (2010). The "I" diet. New York: Workman Publishing.

Originally published as *The Instinct Diet*, this book shows you how to identify your five instincts that compel you to overeat and then provides an 8-week program for healthy, hunger-free, and long-term weight loss. This program is based on 20 years of research on the science of nutrition and weight loss at Tufts University. The book discusses our need to feel full, calorie density, cravings, variety, and availability. It also includes numerous healthy eating recipes.

Wardlaw, G., & A. Smith. (2011). Contemporary nutrition (8th ed.). New York: McGraw-Hill.

Comprehensive introductory reference text on nutrition that includes separate chapters on dieting, weight control, and eating disorders. This book is designed for readers with a limited background in chemistry and physiology.

# Assessment Activity 8-1

## Calculating Caloric Expenditure Through Exercise

**Directions:** This exercise illustrates the calculations used for determining weight loss through exercise. In the example in Part 1, a subject weighing 195 pounds wishes to lose 12 pounds by exercising 40 minutes per day five times per week. The form of exercise will be riding a bike at >10 mph, which burns 0.064 calories per minute per pound of body weight (see Table 8-3). Study this example and then apply it to the problem presented in Part 2 to answer the following questions:

- How many calories are expended per exercise session?

- How many pounds may be lost per week at this energy expenditure?

- How long will it take to lose 12 pounds?

**Part 1**

1. Multiply body weight by the appropriate activity coefficient:

   195 lbs. × 0.064 = 12.48 calories/min.
   12.48 calories/min. × 40 min. = 499 calories

2. Multiply the number of calories expended per workout by the number of workouts per week:

   499 calories × 5 workouts/week = 2,495 calories/week

   $$\frac{2,495 \text{ calories/week}}{3,500 \text{ calories/lb.}} = 0.71 \text{ lb. lost/week}$$

3. Divide the total pounds you want to lose (12 lbs.) by the number of pounds lost per week:

   $$\frac{12 \text{ lbs.}}{7.71 \text{ lbs. lost/week}} = 16.9 \text{ weeks (rounded to 17)}$$

This subject would lose 12 pounds in 17 weeks by riding a bike at >10 mph for 40 minutes per day five times per week. Your weight-loss goals can be determined in the same way.

**Part 2**   Now apply your knowledge of energy expenditure through exercise by solving the following problem. Jim weighs 220 pounds and wishes to lose 25 pounds by running or jogging at 5 mph for 30 minutes per exercise session 5 days per week. Do the calculations to solve Jim's problem by following these steps:

1. Multiply body weight by the appropriate calories burned per minute per lb. from Table 8-3 for running or jogging 5 mph.

   220 lbs. × _____ coefficient = _____ calories/min.

   _____ calories/min. × 30 min. = _____ calories

2. Multiply the number of calories expended per workout by the number of workouts per week:

   _____ calories × 5 workouts/week = _____

   _____ calories/week ÷ 3,500 calories/lb. = _____ lbs. lost/week

3. Divide the total pounds to be lost by the number of pounds lost per week.

   25 lbs. ÷ _____ lbs. lost/week = _____ weeks

4. 

   a. How many calories will Jim expend per exercise session? _____

   b. How many pounds will he lose per week at this energy expenditure? _____

   c. How many weeks will it take Jim to lose 25 pounds? _____

**Name** _____   **Date** _____   **Section** _____

# Assessment Activity 8-2

## Assessing Calorie Costs of 300 Minutes of Physical Activity

*2008 Physical Activity Guidelines for Americans* recommends 150–300 minutes of physical activity each week. At the 300-minute-per-week level, weight loss may be substantial for some people, especially if combined with dieting. The purpose of this assessment is to determine the number of calories expended in 300 minutes of 10 physical activities.

**Directions:** Following are listed the caloric costs for three activities (see Table 8-3). Add seven activities of your choice from Table 8-3, indicate your weight in the fourth column, and complete the information required in each column to determine the number of calories you burn in 300 minutes. An example is provided for a person weighing 180 pounds who walks at a rate of 3.5 mph (17-minute mile) for a weekly total of 300 minutes.

| Activity | Caloric Cost/ Min/Lb. | × | Weight | = | Calories/ Minute | × | 300 (minutes) | = | Total Calories |
|---|---|---|---|---|---|---|---|---|---|
| Example: (180-lb person) 1. Walking (3.5 mph) | 0.030 | × | 180 | = | 5.4 | × | 300 | = | 1,620 |
| **Personal Assessment:** 1. Walking (3.5 mph) | 0.030 | × | | = | | × | 300 | = | |
| 2. Aerobics (light) | 0.023 | × | | = | | × | 300 | = | |
| 3. Raking | 0.034 | × | | = | | × | 300 | = | |
| 4. | | × | | = | | × | 300 | = | |
| 5. | | × | | = | | × | 300 | = | |
| 6. | | × | | = | | × | 300 | = | |
| 7. | | × | | = | | × | 300 | = | |
| 8. | | × | | = | | × | 300 | = | |
| 9. | | × | | = | | × | 300 | = | |
| 10. | | × | | = | | × | 300 | = | |

**Name** _____   **Date** _____   **Section** _____

# Assessment Activity 8-3

## Walking Assessment

One way to monitor physical activity is to count the number of steps you take daily. This includes steps taken at home, work, play, or when performing chores, household tasks, yardwork, and so on. Experts recommend 10,000 steps a day to achieve health benefits associated with walking, 15,000 steps a day to lose weight, and 20,000 steps a day to maintain weight after a weight-loss goal has been reached. The purposes of this activity are to determine your "walking baseline," that is, the number of steps you take in your daily routine, excluding structured time set aside for exercise and sport activities, and start a walking program to achieve 10,000 steps per day. To complete this assessment, you will need to use or purchase a pedometer. Ask your instructor for his or her recommendation of a pedometer, or Google "pedometer" on the Internet, or shop for one at a sports retail store. Inexpensive, accurate, and reliable digital pedometers can be purchased for less than $20. Follow the instructions for attaching the pedometer and put it on when you start the day. At the end of the day, record the number of steps in Part 1 of the log. Reset the pedometer the next morning. Repeat this for 5 days. Calculate a 5-day average to determine your walking baseline. Enter this number in the "baseline" column of Part 2. If you average 10,000 steps or more and you're not trying to lose weight, continue with your present routine. If you're short of the recommended 10,000 steps, add 300 steps a day during the first week and continue in 300-step increments each subsequent week until you build up to 10,000 steps per day. Chart your walking program in Part 2. Print or make extra copies of the log to cover at least a 6-week period.

### Part 1. Walking Baseline Log

| Day | Number of Steps |
|---|---|
| 1 | |
| 2 | |
| 3 | |
| 4 | |
| 5 | |
| Total | |
| 5-Day Average (Walking Baseline) | |

### Part 2. Walking Log (10,000 Steps a Day)*

| Week/Day | Baseline (from Part 1) | Add 300 | Daily Goal (Baseline + 300) | Actual** Steps |
|---|---|---|---|---|
| **Week #1** | | | | |
| Sunday | | +300 | | |
| Monday | | +300 | | |
| Tuesday | | +300 | | |
| Wednesday | | +300 | | |
| Thursday | | +300 | | |
| Friday | | +300 | | |
| Saturday | | +300 | | |
| **Weekly Average** | | | | |

*Make extra copies of this chart as needed to monitor steps for 6 weeks (or more).
**Count and record all steps, including those taken in structured workouts, sport activities, etc.

Name _____   Date _____   Section _____

# Assessment Activity 8-4

## Estimating Your Basal Metabolic Rate

**Directions:** Study the example in Part 1 and then calculate your personal total energy expenditure in Part 2.

**Part 1** The calculations for estimating BMR use different constants for men and women. The constant for men is 1 calorie per kilogram (2.2 lbs.) per hour; for women it is 0.9 calorie per kilogram per hour. These constants are referred to as the *BMR factor.* An example for a 125-pound woman follows:

1. Convert body weight in pounds to kilograms:
   125 lbs. ÷ 2.2 lbs. = 56.8 kg
2. Multiply weight in kilograms by the BMR factor:
   56.8 kg × 0.9 calorie/kg/hr. = 51.1 calories/hr.
3. Multiply calories per hour by 24 hours:
   51.1 calories/hr. × 24 hrs./day = 1,226.4 calories/day
4. The BMR is 1,226.4 calories per day.

To determine the total daily calories expended, you need to estimate the number of calories used in muscular movement during a typical day. This is a rough approximation at best, but you should be within your range if you follow these guidelines and select the category that fits you best.

1. Sedentary—student, desk job, sitting during most of your work and leisure time: Add 40 to 50% of the BMR.

2. Light activity—teacher, assembly-line worker, walk 2 miles regularly: Add 55 to 65% of the BMR.

3. Moderate activity—food server, aerobic exercise at about 75% of maximum heart rate: Add 65 to 70% of the BMR.

4. Heavy activity—construction worker, aerobic exercise above 75% of maximum heart rate: Add 75 to 100% of BMR.

   If our subject determines that her level of activity is in the light category, she will calculate the range of her daily total caloric expenditure as follows:

1. Multiply BMR by the level of activity:
   1,226.4 calories/day × 0.55 = 674.5 calories/day
   1,226.4 calories/day × 0.65 = 797.2 calories/day

2. Add BMR calories to level of activity calories to get total calories:
   a. 1,226.4 + 674.5 = 1,900.9 calories/day
   b. 1,226.4 + 797.2 = 2,023.6 calories/day

This subject's total calorie expenditure in a day falls between 1,900.9 and 2,023.6 calories.

**Part 2** Calculate your BMR by doing the following:

1. Convert body weight (BW) in pounds to kilograms:

   _____ lbs. ÷ 2.2 = _____ kg

2. Multiply weight in kilograms by the BMR factor for your sex (male factor 1.0, female factor 0.9):

   _____ × _____ kg = _____ calories/hr.

3. Multiply calories per hour by 24 hours per day to get the number of calories burned per day:

   _____ calories/hr. × 24 = _____ calories/day

4. BMR: _____ calories/day

**Determine your level of physical activity:**

1. Multiply BMR by the level of activity factor:

   _____ × _____ – _____ calories/day

   _____ × _____ = _____ calories/day

2. Add the number of BMR calories to the level of activity calories to get the range of total calories expended in a day:

   _____ calories + _____ calories = _____ calories/day

   _____ calories + _____ calories = _____ calories/day

3. Total calories expended range from _____ to _____.

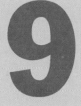
# Coping with and Managing Stress

## ONLINE LEARNING CENTER

Log on to our Online Learning Center (OLC) for access to these additional resources:

- Chapter key term flashcards
- Learning objectives
- Additional goals for behavior change
- Concentration game
- Self-scoring chapter quizzes
- Additional lab activities

The OLC also offers Web links for study and exploration of wellness topics. Access these links through **www.mhhe.com/anspaugh8e.**

## GOALS FOR BEHAVIOR CHANGE

- Identify your personal sources of stress.
- View stress as holding potential for personal growth.
- Develop a time management plan.
- Select strategies for managing stress.
- Put into action a stress management plan.

## Objectives

After completing this chapter, you will be able to do the following:

- ✔ Define *stress*.
- ✔ Identify potential stressors.
- ✔ Describe the various types of stress.
- ✔ Describe the stages of the general adaptation syndrome (GAS).
- ✔ Explain the body's physiological response to stress.
- ✔ List the short- and long-term health effects of stress.
- ✔ Identify strategies that effectively deal with stress.

### [ Key Terms ]

| | |
|---|---|
| coping | psychoneuroimmunology (PNI) |
| distress | |
| eustress | relaxation techniques |
| general adaptation syndrome (GAS) | stress |
| | stressor |

**S**tress profoundly affects people's lives. Everyone—students, businesspeople, parents, athletes—lives with stress. Stress is frequently viewed as an enemy. This is a misconception. Stress is often neither positive nor negative. How people deal with or react to what they perceive as stress is what determines its effect on their lives. As has been stated, "It is often said that stress is one of the most destructive elements in people's daily lives, but that is only a half truth. The way we react to stress appears to be more important than the stress itself."[1] The effects of stress can be either positive or negative. Positively used, stress can be a motivator for an improved quality of life. Viewed negatively, it can be destructive.

## What Is Stress?

Dr. Hans Selye was the first to define the term *stress* as the "nonspecific response of the body to any demands made upon it." It can be characterized by diverse reactions, such as muscle tension, acute anxiety, increased heart rate, hypertension, shallow breathing, giddiness, and even joy. From a positive perspective, stress is a force that generates and initiates action. Using Selye's definition, stress can accompany pleasant or unpleasant events. Selye referred to stress judged as "good" as **eustress.** This form of stress is the force that initiates emotional and psychological growth. Eustress provides the experience of pleasure, adds meaning to life, and fosters an attitude that tries to find positive solutions to complex problems. Eustress can accompany a birth, graduation, the purchase of a new car, the development of a new friendship, the accomplishment of a difficult task, and success in an area that previously produced anxiety. **Distress,** on the other hand, is stress that

results in negative responses. Unchecked, negative stress can interfere with the physiological and psychological functioning of the body and may ultimately result in a disease or disability.[2,3]

Stress also provides humans with the ability to respond to challenges or dangers. It is vital to self-protection and serves as a motivator that enhances human ability.

A **stressor** is any physical, psychological, or environmental event or condition that initiates the stress response (Figure 9-1). See Assessment Activity 9-2 to evaluate your own stress level in the different categories listed in Figure 9-1.

What is considered a stressor for one person may not be a stressor for another. Speaking in front of a group may be stimulating for one person but terrifying for another. Some people experience extreme test anxiety and others feel confident about written assessments. Fortunately, the stress response is not a genetic trait, and because it is a response to external conditions, it is subject to personal control. A person may not avoid taking a test, but he or she can apply techniques and take precautions that lessen the effects of the stress. For example, knowing the material thoroughly and engaging in deep breathing several minutes before a test help dissipate anxiety. To maximize quality of life, people can find positive ways of dealing with stress.

A stress response can enhance and increase the level of either mental or physical performance. This response is referred to as the *inverted-U theory.*[4] Not enough stress (hypostress) may result in a poorer effort, but too much stress can inhibit effort. There appears to be an optimal level of stress that results in peak performance (Figure 9-2). Achievement of an appropriate level of stress depends on the person and the type of

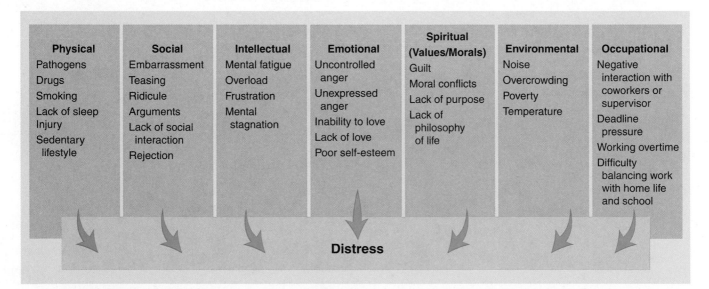

**FIGURE 9-1** Stressors That Can Create Distress

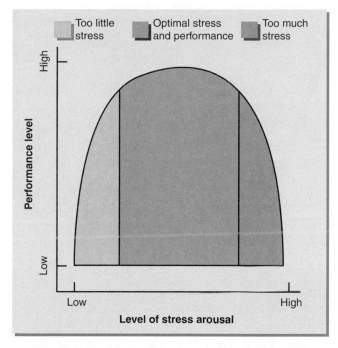

**FIGURE 9-2** The Inverted-U Theory

task. Table 9-1 lists some of the potentially positive outcomes associated with stress. Your body is constantly attempting to maintain a physiological balance. This balance is referred to as *homeostasis*. Any event or circumstance that causes a disruption (a stressor) in your body's homeostasis requires some type of adaptive behavior. Physiologically, whether a stressor is perceived as positive or negative, the body responds with the same three-stage process. This series of changes is known as the **general adaptation syndrome (GAS)**.[5] The three phases are alarm, resistance, and exhaustion (Figure 9-3, page 310).

The *alarm* phase occurs when homeostasis is initially disrupted. The brain perceives a stressor and prepares the body to deal with it, a response sometimes referred to as the *fight-or-flight response*. The subconscious appraisal of the stressor results in an emotional reaction. The emotional response stimulates a physical reaction associated with stress, such as the muscles becoming tense, the stomach tightening, the heart rate increasing, the mouth becoming dry, and the palms of the hands sweating.

The second stage is *resistance*. In this phase, the body meets the perceived challenge through increased strength, endurance, sensory capacities, and sensory acuity. Hormonal secretions regulate the body's response to a stressor. Only after meeting and satisfying the demands of a stressful situation can the internal activities of the body return to normal. Other researchers[6] argue that people have different levels of energy to deal with stressors. For short-term stressors, only a superficial level of energy is required, allowing deeper energy levels to be protected. Superficial levels of energy are readily accessible and easily renewable. Unfortunately, not all stress can be resolved with superficial energy levels. When long-term or deep levels of stress are experienced, the amount of energy available is limited. If sufficient stress is experienced for an extended period, loss of adaptation can result. Although some scientists believe that energy stores may be genetically programmed, all people can replenish their energy stores through exercise, good nutrition, adequate sleep, and other positive behaviors.

When stressors become chronic or pervasive, the third phase, *exhaustion*, is reached. In exhaustion, energy stores have been depleted and rest must occur. Although weeks to years may pass before the effects of long-term stressors occur, if a person does not learn how to deal adequately with stress, exhaustion will result. At this point, stress may affect the stomach, heart, blood pressure, muscles, and joints. Fortunately, the effects of stressors can be completely or partially reversed when adequate management techniques are initiated. The earlier these management techniques are learned and used, the fewer problems result.

## Sources of Stress and Warning Signs

Most stressful situations fall into one of three categories: (1) harm and loss, (2) threat, and (3) challenge.[7] Examples of *harm-and-loss situations* are the death of a loved one, the loss of personal property, physical assault, physical injury, and the severe loss of self-esteem. *Threat situations* may be real or perceived and can range from being caught in traffic to being unable to perceive an event. Threatening events tax a person's ability to deal with everyday life. Threat stressors are any stressors that result in anger, hostility, frustration,

**TABLE 9-1**  Positive Outcomes of Stress

| Mental | Emotional | Physical |
|---|---|---|
| Enhanced creativity | Sense of control | High energy level |
| Enhanced thinking ability | Responsiveness to environment | Increased stamina |
| Greater goal orientation | Improved interpersonal relationships | Flexibility of muscles and joints |
| Enhanced motivation | Improved morale | Freedom from stress-related disease |

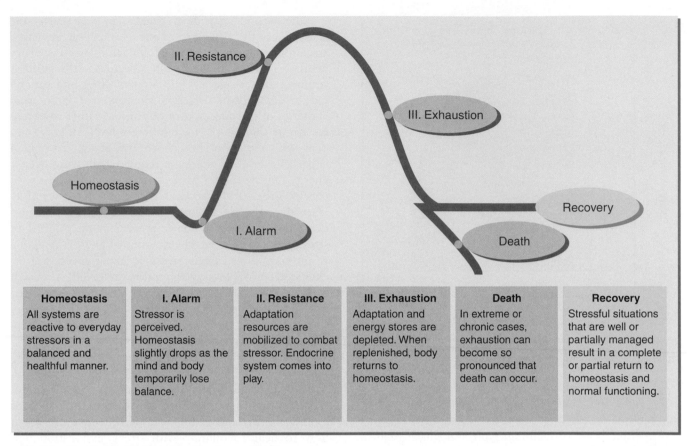

| Homeostasis | I. Alarm | II. Resistance | III. Exhaustion | Death | Recovery |
|---|---|---|---|---|---|
| All systems are reactive to everyday stressors in a balanced and healthful manner. | Stressor is perceived. Homeostasis slightly drops as the mind and body temporarily lose balance. | Adaptation resources are mobilized to combat stressor. Endocrine system comes into play. | Adaptation and energy stores are depleted. When replenished, body returns to homeostasis. | In extreme or chronic cases, exhaustion can become so pronounced that death can occur. | Stressful situations that are well or partially managed result in a complete or partial return to homeostasis and normal functioning. |

**FIGURE 9-3**  The General Adaptation Syndrome (GAS)

or depression. *Challenge situations* are catalysts for either growth or pain. These stressors often involve major life changes and include such events as taking a new job, leaving home, graduating from college, and getting married. Challenge events are usually perceived as being good but involve stress because they disrupt homeostasis and require considerable psychological and physical adjustment.

Being aware of the mental and physical signals associated with stress is the beginning step in learning how to manage it. Assessment Activity 9-1 will aid you in identifying some of the major stressors. By using self-assessments to monitor for signs of stress, you can avoid excessive stress. The negative results of distress are shown in Table 9-2. Indicators of excessive distress include the following:

- Chronic fatigue, migraine headaches, sweating, lower-back pain, sleep disturbances, weakness, dizziness, diarrhea, and constipation
- Harder and/or longer work or study while accomplishing less, an inability to concentrate, general disorientation
- Denial that there is a problem or troubling event
- Increased incidence of illness, such as colds and flu, or constant worry about illness or becoming

ill; overuse of over-the-counter drugs for the purpose of self-medication
- Depression, irritability, anxiety, apathy, an overwhelming urge to cry or run and hide, and feelings of unreality
- Excessive behavioral patterns, such as spending too much money, drinking, breaking the law, and developing addictions
- Accident proneness
- Signs of reclusiveness and avoidance of other people
- Emotional tension, "keyed up" feeling, easy startling, nervous laughter, anxiety, hyperkinesias, and nervous tics

## Factors Generating a Stress Response

As mentioned earlier, the criteria for a stressful event and the response to that event for any person are unique to the individual. Figure 9-4 provides an overview of the complexity of the stress experience and some of the many moderating effects. For instance, a dysfunctional home life (characterized by an alcoholic parent, a difficult divorce, or extreme poverty) may contribute to a personality that is more susceptible to

**TABLE 9-2**  Negative Results of Distress

| Mental | Physical | Emotional |
|---|---|---|
| **Short-Term Effects** | | |
| Poor memory | Flushed face | Irritability |
| Inability to concentrate | Cold hands | Disorganization |
| Low creativity | Gas | Conflicts |
| Poor self-control | Rapid breathing | Mood swings |
| Low self-esteem | Shortness of breath | Chronic sleep problems |
| | Dry mouth | Acid stomach |
| | | Overindulgence in alcohol or other drugs, food |
| **Long-Term Effects** | | |
| Bouts of depression | Hypertension | Overweight/underweight |
| Mild paranoia | Coronary disease | Drug abuse |
| Low tolerance for ambiguity | Ulcers | Excessive smoking |
| Forgetfulness | Migraine/tension headaches | Ineffective use of work/leisure time |
| Inability to make decisions/quickness to make decisions | Strokes | Overreaction to mild work pressure |
| | Allergies | |

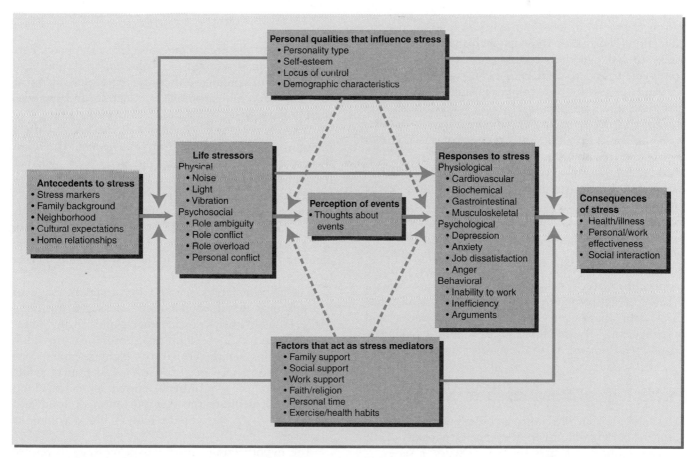

**FIGURE 9-4**  Theoretical Framework of the Stress Experience

difficult events, such as poor grades or a failed relationship. This combination of inadequate preparation for life along with an event perceived as personal failure is likely to lead to depression, anxiety, or anger. Conversely, a person whose background has fostered a deep sense of self-worth and meaningfulness will be able to handle a difficult event better and will not perceive the event as a personal failure. Poor grades may be the result of poor study habits, an undiagnosed learning behavior, or inadequate sleep, and a failed relationship may be the result of a poor match, bad timing, or immaturity.

## Sources of Stress for College Students

During the college years stress can become a major factor in the life of a student. The most obvious source of stress is the pressure to be successful in the academic arena. In fact, 33% of college students reported that stress negatively affected their academic performance and resulted in a lower grade, dropped classes, or an incomplete.[8] Pressures from parents, peers, and professors can all cause stress in the student. Other stressors can be the strain of having to work to help finance the educational costs. For students in this position there is stress to balance the expectations of their place of employment and to deal with being successful in the academic classes they are taking. Leaving home for the first time, the adjustments of living with another person for the first time, and developing a new social network are most stressful, yet necessary if success is to be obtained in college. Tied with this process of networking are the social pressures students face in terms of alcohol, other drugs, joining social groups, or the pressures and issues of dealing with their sexuality. Finally there may be family stressors such as divorce of parents, health problems of loved ones, or the death of a loved friend or family member.[9] Some common stressors of college life include academic competition, money problems, loneliness, choice of major, lack of privacy, social alienation, sexual pressures, drug pressures, and relationship decisions such as dating and marriage (see Figure 9-5 and Real-World Wellness: Stress-Free Preparation for Tests on page 313).

## Physiological Responses to Stress

Stress abounds in life and can be experienced as the result of happy and unhappy events. Regardless of the stressor, each time a stressful event occurs, a series of neurological and hormonal messages are sent throughout the body.

The nervous system serves as a reciprocal network that sends messages between the awareness centers of

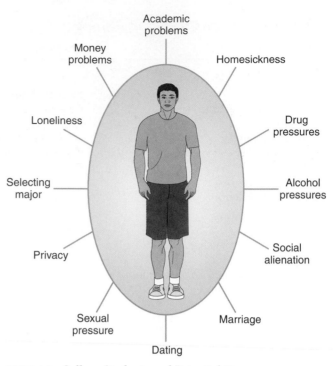

**FIGURE 9-5**  College Students and Potential Stressors

the brain and the organs and muscles of the body. Part of this system is referred to as the *limbic system*. The limbic system contains centers for emotions, memory, learning relay, and hormone production and includes the pituitary gland, thalamus, and hypothalamus.

When a stressor is encountered, the body sends a message to the brain via the nervous system. The brain then synthesizes the message and determines whether it is valid. If a message is not verified by the brain as being threatening, the limbic system overrides the initial response and the body continues to function normally. If the initial response is translated as accurate and a stressor is detected, the body responds with some emotion (fear, joy, terror), and the hypothalamus begins to act.

The hypothalamus sends a hormonal message to the pituitary gland, which then releases a hormone (ACTH), which helps signal other glands in the endocrine system to secrete additional hormones, providing fuel to respond with the fight or flight response. Systolic blood pressure may rise 15 to 20 mmHg while fluid is retained. The adrenal cortex increases blood pressure to facilitate the transportation of food and oxygen to active parts of the body.[10] Blood volume is increased.

The hypothalamus also sends a message to release the hormones epinephrine and norepinephrine, which initiate a variety of physiological changes. These changes include increased heart rate, increased metabolic rate, increased oxygen consumption, and the

## Real-World Wellness

### Stress-Free Preparation for Tests

One stressor that seems to be a constant for college students is preparing and taking tests. Here are some suggestions for making test preparation less stressful:

- Study notes every day so memorization occurs over a longer period of time and is not crammed into a brief period of time. Devote 2 hours of study outside class for every hour spent in class.

- Plan assignments and projects over the course of the semester so you won't need to work on them at the time of midterm or final tests.

- Effectively manage time. Make a schedule and create priorities of what needs to be done and in what order or time frame tasks need to be accomplished.

- Get adequate sleep (7–9 hours each night).

- Plan for an exercise time each day.

- Eat healthy meals, don't skip meals, and eliminate "junk" food.

- Stay positive.

Activities or practices to be refrained from:

- Refrain from overconsumption of caffeine drinks. Especially avoid those energy drinks that are extremely high in caffeine content; they can leave you feeling drained as the effect of the high amounts of caffeine begins to wear off.

- Don't have study parties. If you want to study with other people, do so with only one or two others. Fewer people help to maintain the focus of the study session. Dorm rooms, fast-food restaurants, or other heavy traffic areas are not recommended, since they can interfere with focus and create interruptions by others.

- Don't wait until the last minute.

release of hormones called *endorphins*, which decrease sensations of pain.

The autonomic nervous system is responsible for a second major set of physiological responses. It is referred to as autonomic because this system can function without conscious thought or voluntary control. However, it is now recognized that the autonomic system can be influenced by conscious thought[11] and works closely with the central nervous system to maintain homeostasis.

There are two components of the autonomic nervous system, the parasympathetic and sympathetic divisions.

The sympathetic division is involved in the fight-or-flight response. It accomplishes this through the release of catecholamines, specifically epinephrine (adrenaline) and norepinephrine (noradrenaline). The parasympathetic division helps constantly maintain homeostasis and returns the body to a normal state. Thus, you cannot be aroused and relaxed at the same time.

In reaction to a threat, the autonomic nervous system increases heart rate, strength of the skeletal muscles, mental activity, and basal metabolic rate; dilates the coronary arteries, pupils, bronchial tubes, and arterioles; and constricts the abdominal arteries. This system also returns the body to a normal, relaxed state.

## Stress and the Immune System

The mind and body act on each other in remarkable ways. Our immune system is a part of the body's defense against illness and disease originating from factors and conditions both outside and inside our bodies. The immune system consists of a variety of mechanical and chemical defenses that protect against such outside invaders as microorganisms, allergens, and other substances as well as such inside factors as mutating cells or improperly functioning tissue. The immune system is a functional system rather than an organ system and, as a result, seems to be prone to the effects of stress when fighting off the situations and conditions previously mentioned.[12]

The biological link between emotions and disease and even death is strong. Mortality is three times higher in people with few close relationships than in those with numerous such relationships, and people with strong support groups have additional protection against life stressors. Death rates are higher for cancer patients with pessimistic attitudes. Illness is more common among people who feel locked into strife-ridden marriages. AIDS patients with healthy psyches seem better able to withstand disease.[13]

In a study involving cancer patients with malignant melanoma, health education, enhanced problem-solving skills, and stress management techniques provided significant increases in natural killer cells and increased activity of these cells in patients receiving these behavioral interventions. A 6-year follow-up showed a trend toward greater recurrence and a statistically significant higher mortality rate in the control group as opposed to those receiving behavioral interventions.[14,15]

Another study demonstrated a system of nerve fibers that transmits messages between the brain and lymphocytes that fight infection and cancer in the body. This research found that neurotransmitters, such as epinephrine and norepinephrine, can attack immune cells and influence their ability to replicate and destroy invading pathogenic agents.[16]

The immune system becomes dysfunctional and can lead to stress-related illnesses in three ways: (1) underactivity (cancer), (2) hyperactivity (asthma), and (3) misguided activity (lupus). The immune function seems to be affected by the relationship between the brain and nervous system. This relationship among brain, nervous system, and immune response has been the outgrowth from the field of study called **psychoneuroimmunology (PNI).** This relatively new medical discipline seeks to explain the connection among the brain, the nervous system, and the body's response to infections and deviated cell division. Several studies have shown that chronic stress suppresses the body's ability to initiate an effective immune response. This suppression is attributed to an increase in corticosteroids, produced during chronic stress. This increase in corticosteroid levels delays and weakens the immune response.[17] Research has found that chronic stress suppresses the immune system, particularly when the stress is associated with social disruption (such as leaving home for the first time), psychological depression (such as feeling "down" for prolonged periods), or some negative personality attribute (lack of self-confidence).[18] It has also been found that immunosuppression is associated with loneliness and feelings of hopelessness.[19] Stress has also been demonstrated to be associated with infertility.[20,21,22] No known specific reason exists for this correlation. Whether the stress is the result of infertility problems or another source, stress-reduction intervention results in significant improvement in conception rates.

Because stress affects the immune system, the body becomes more susceptible to a multitude of ailments, from colds to cancer. Respiratory conditions, such as asthma, may become worse. The cardiovascular system reacts by constricting the blood vessels while increasing blood volume. The result is a rise in blood pressure throughout a stress-ridden day. Multiple increases in blood pressure can eventually contribute to chronic high blood pressure. More forceful contraction of the heart elevates levels of free fatty acids, enhancing the development of clogged arteries leading to and including the heart. In extreme cases, sudden death can occur, especially for a person who has been experiencing high levels of uncontrolled stress for an extended period.

Headaches, including migraines, have long been associated with stress. Tension headaches are caused by involuntary contractions of the scalp, head, and neck muscles. Typical muscular reaction to stress is contracting or tensing. When chronic stress occurs, the body reacts by being constantly ready to respond, and the muscles become braced, always in a state of tension. More stress magnifies the tension the muscles are already undergoing. Increased muscular tension manifests in headaches, backaches, neckaches, and other

### TABLE 9-3 Stress, Nutritional Status, and Immunity: An Interactive Effect

Although the mechanism is not completely understood, stress significantly affects nutritional status and therefore immunity. Several nutritional factors have implications for how your body responds to stress.

**Energy**

Stress can increase the body's basic caloric needs by as much as 200%. The stress hormones increase body heat production. When this heat is released, it is not available for cell metabolism. The caloric inefficiency induced by stress accounts for the increased need for energy intake.

**Protein**

Stress may increase the body's need for protein from 60% to as much as 500%. The integrity of the body's tissues, such as the skin and the tissue lining the mouth, lungs, and nose (called *mucosal tissue*), depends on adequate protein repair and maintenance of secretions of biochemicals that serve as protective agents. The formation of antibodies also requires protein.

**Fats**

Dietary fatty acids influence the synthesis of a group of fatty acid derivatives called *prostaglandins*. Prostaglandins stimulate or depress other cellular and immune functions in relation to stress.

**Vitamins**

Vitamin A maintains healthy skin and mucous membranes. Vitamin A–deficient individuals have fewer mucus-secreting cells and those they do have produce less mucus; thus, the protection provided by the mucous lining is diminished. Vitamin C has been shown to enhance the engulfing, or "eating," actions of the immune cells called *macrophages*. If vitamin C is deficient, macrophages are less mobile and less able to consume disease-causing organisms. Deficiencies of vitamin A, vitamin $B_{12}$, and folate can impair production of the cells that enable antibody responses. Large doses of vitamin E have been associated with suppression of B cells, vital to the immune response. Finally, metabolic requirements for thiamin, riboflavin, and niacin are increased in response to a stressful situation.

**Minerals**

Deficiencies of zinc impair immune cell reproduction and responsiveness.

pains. The smooth muscles that control internal organs also experience pains. More intense contractions can lead to stomachache, diarrhea, hypertension, heartburn, gastritis, bloating, inflammation of the pancreas, and blockage of the bile ducts.

Stress decreases saliva in the mouth, often making speaking awkward. Swallowing may become difficult, and the increase in stomach acids contributes to ulcer pain. People tend to perspire more, and electrical currents are transmitted more quickly across the skin. Skin conditions such as acne, psoriasis, herpes, hives, and eczema are exacerbated.

Stress also seems to affect the body's nutritional status. Individual nutritional patterns can also influence stress management efforts. For example, eating too much or too little, eating the wrong kinds of food, and overusing products such as caffeine or alcohol upset homeostasis. Diets high in fat, sugar, and processed foods place a heavy burden on various body systems. Ingesting too few calories can lead to the breakdown of lean tissue. To meet the demands of stress, you should maintain adequate nutrition through a balanced and varied diet. (Chapter 6 provides guidelines for developing a beneficial nutrition plan.) Table 9-3 provides some insight into the interactive natures of stress, nutritional status, and immunity.

Ultimately, no body system escapes the effects of stress. The long-term presence of certain stress-associated hormones in the brain damages receptors and cells found in the hippocampus. (The hippocampus sends messages when stress is occurring.) Because brain cells do not regenerate, these cells are lost forever. The effects of this loss are unknown, but indications are that eventually affected people become less able to respond to stress appropriately.[23] Assessment Activity 9-3 provides guidelines for identifying stress style and suggests relaxation activities.

## Self-Esteem and Stress

How people feel about themselves and others, and their perceptions of the stressors in their lives, are parts of the psychology of stress. Ability to deal with stress often hinges on impressions of how detrimental a stressor is and how adequately resources can deal with the situation. How much stress people feel themselves experiencing is closely associated with their sense of self-esteem. Self-esteem includes beliefs and attitudes about changes, personal talent, skills, and one's ability to deal with the changes and challenges that inevitably occur in life. It is also the basis of self-efficacy and the locus of control (see Chapter 1). The most influential factor in determining response to stress may be people's perceptions of themselves.

## Attitude and Stress

The question many researchers have asked is why one person is more susceptible to stress than another. The answer is not altogether clear, but evidence is mounting that one's perception, or attitude, is a key factor in the stress equation. The realization that our attitude has such a significant impact on our health has led to a new movement in psychology termed "positive psy-

chology." Dr. Martin Seligman of the University of Pennsylvania is the founder of positive psychology. He believes that optimism is a key in maintaining not only our mental health, but our physical health as well. Other writers have examined the differences between optimism and pessimism and the impact that these attitudes have on health. What researchers have found is that the fundamental difference between a pessimist and an optimist is the degree of control individuals feel over their life.[24] What is suggested is that we learn feelings of helplessness, and this becomes a major factor in depression and stress. Not surprisingly, both depression and stress are highly correlated with pessimism. Researchers report that optimists are much better at coping with the anxiety and distress associated with everything from infertility to higher grade point averages in law students. A study by Mayo Clinic researchers compared the health of 839 men and women to scores on a personality test they had taken 30 years previously. It was found that those who had an optimistic attitude in their younger years were 19% more likely to still be alive than were their pessimistic counterparts.

To help develop more positive optimistic attitudes, consider these ideas:

1. *Teach yourself a lesson.* Find something positive in a sad or stressful situation by thinking about what you have learned from the experience. Don't ignore the negatives but do learn from them without dwelling on them.

2. *Interrupt negative thoughts.* Get out of the pessimistic frame of mind. Force yourself to think positive thoughts. Think of pleasant memories. Don't allow the negative to set you off on a "pity party" or self-flagellation.

3. *Set realistic goals.* Set achievable, realistic goals. Positive thinkers have developed the art of meeting goals (see Assessment Activity 9-6).

4. *Be good to yourself.* Treat yourself to the things you love—it is essential to building confidence and creating a sense of control over your life. Keep in mind that the purpose is to take control; don't do something because it is a habit—do it because you want to.

5. *Go digging for silver.* Seek the bright side of things. Make sure you find at least one positive thing that happens each day. Take an appreciation appraisal each day. When irritating or disappointing events occur, ask yourself, "What did I learn from this that will make me a better person?"

6. *Be glad it's not worse.* When you are low, think of someone less fortunate than you. Write down or say, "I'm glad that . . . " or "I'm lucky to . . ." People who can find positives to reflect on

report more satisfaction with their lives than those who are always pointing to the negative.

7. *Reframe your perception.* What can cause stress in many of us is allowing ourselves to view the situation or event from a pessimistic perspective. Fostering a positive attitude can be a stress reliever if we practice "reframing" our thoughts and how we view the stressor. Reframing involves changing the way we perceive a situation or person. Concentrate on how to deal with the stressor to help ease the situation. Avoid allowing words such as *always*, *never*, *ought to*, or *it should have been* to be the focus of your thoughts. View yourself as being successful in dealing with the stressor, and give yourself positive self-talks. Eliminate pessimistic thinking in planning how to perceive and deal with a stressful situation—remind yourself to remain positive.

8. *Fake it.* When all else fails, keep on smiling. Project the mood you want to get back. Find something that makes you laugh. It is hard to be down if you are smiling and laughing.

## Personality and Stress

Two physicians, Friedman and Roseman,[25] have written extensively about personality, cardiovascular disease, and stress. These researchers have described two stress-related personality types—type A and type B.

Most people are neither type exclusively but fall somewhere between the two.

The type A personality is characterized by an urgent sense of time, impatience, competitiveness, aggressiveness, insecurity over status, and inability to relax. People with type A behavior characteristics are likely to be highly stressed. Type B people have a more unhurried approach to their lives. The type B personality does not become as upset at losing or not attaining a goal. Type B people also tend to set more realistic goals.[26] Researchers disagree on whether there is a possible relationship between the stress-prone type A personality and cardiovascular disease.[27]

In general, researchers believe that being a type A personality is not a problem if there is no underlying hostility. However, regardless of whether type A people are more susceptible to heart disease, they do experience more negative effects, such as tiredness and frustration, from short-term stress.[28]

There is another type of personality that some researchers refer to as the "distressed" personality or type D personality. Type D persons are socially inhibited, and their personality is pervasive with negative thoughts and emotions. Individuals who are type D demonstrate excessive dependence on others, worry excessively, fear common situations or circumstances, and have little social support. This type of person tends to view life situations much more negatively than do others. Researchers have found that the individuals

 ## Wellness for a Lifetime
### The Time of Our Lives

Although middle age is often dreaded, the changes that inevitably occur as we grow older are not necessarily bad. In fact, more and more elderly adults report that the best time in their lives was not their youth but, rather, their midlife years.

One recent study of this question involved more than 3,000 people, each of whom answered more than 1,100 questions. Researchers found that more than 70% of the respondents viewed themselves as being in excellent health and felt their lives had purpose and meaning. In fact, 9 of 10 study participants said they had never experienced the proverbial midlife crisis. Most middle-aged people reported that they had been able to make the adjustment necessary for life to remain rewarding. Most said that they did not have arthritis, backaches, skin problems, indigestion, constipation, depression, gum disease, high blood pressure, or migraines. And contrary to popular belief, most middle-aged women reported that menopause was a fairly benign experience.

One negative finding of the study is that middle-aged adults are not working hard to maintain a high quality of life. In addition, respondents reported not having enough money and sex—probably two things lacking at any age, not just middle age. However, while sexual satisfaction was low, middle-aged adults seemed to be content overall with their marriages and relationships. Seventy-two percent said that their relationships were very good or excellent, and 90% felt that their relationships were unlikely to break up.

Finally, the survey found that by the time adults reached age 65, men felt an average of 12.6 years younger than their actual age and women felt 14.7 years younger than their actual age. As we grow older, our lives can become even more fulfilling, particularly if we can maintain a sense of control over our well-being by practicing healthful lifestyle habits. How can you ensure optimal health as you age?

Source: Adapted from Johns Hopkins InteliHealth Online (www.intelihealth.com/IH?ihtIH?d5dm).

demonstrating these types of characteristics are at greater risk for heart attacks and depression.[29]

The good news concerning type A or D personalities is that they can change. Type A people can learn to let go of their hostility and to slow down, and the type D personalities can learn to modify their negativity and to find stronger social support. "Stress survivors"—people who handle stress successfully—have several common characteristics. Psychologist Suzanna Kobasa[30] has isolated these attributes and characterized the type of person who exhibits them. A hardy personality tends to remain healthy even under extreme stress. Characteristics of a hardy personality or hardiness are challenge, commitment, and control (see Assessment Activity 9-5).

*Challenge* is the ability to see change for what it is—that is, not only inevitable but an opportunity for the growth and development of unique abilities. *Commitment* is delineated by a strong sense of inner purpose. It is necessary to want to succeed to achieve success. Commitment is the ability to become involved while maintaining the discernment to know when dedication and desire are harmful. *Control* is the recognition that one has power over one's life and attitudes. People who have a sense of control act in situations rather than react to them (see Wellness for a Lifetime: The Time of Our Lives).

## Dealing with Stress

All events in life precipitate a reaction. How people react or respond to situations differs. Coping is the attempt to manage or deal with stress. Coping is independent of outcome—it does not necessarily result in success.

Dealing successfully with stress may require using a variety of techniques (see Real-World Wellness: Guidelines for Dealing with Stress). Because stress-related responses are based primarily on mental perceptions, coping strategies that achieve desirable results may need to originate in a change in attitude or outlook. If specific situations or people are perceived as disruptive, one solution is to avoid them.

Although there are no easy answers, there is always some type of answer or solution. When dealing with a stressor reaches a point where it seems there are no solutions, the tension from the situation becomes increasingly detrimental. It may then become necessary to consider changing attitudes, goals, and values.

Seeking the help of a professional counselor is frequently beneficial when attempting to resolve particularly stressful situations. Assessment Activity 9-4 identifies ways to recognize some of the positive and negative behaviors that can be used to deal with stress.

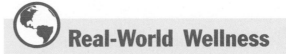

## Real-World Wellness

### Guidelines for Dealing with Stress

*Being in school can be so overwhelming. I have many classes, extracurricular activities, and a pile of homework each night. How can I balance it all?*

Following are guidelines for effectively dealing with potential harmful stress:

- *Schedule time effectively.* Practice good time management techniques by using time wisely. This means taking time out for yourself every day and scheduling work when you are usually at your peak ability (see Assessment Activity 9-7).

- *Set priorities.* Know what is important to you. Do not attempt to work on four or five projects simultaneously. Keep your efforts focused on one or two major items.

- *Establish realistic goals.* Goals must be achievable. Do not establish impossible expectations and then become frustrated when they are not accomplished as quickly as you would like. Write down long-range goals and then establish checks for keeping yourself on track and monitoring progress. Short-term goals help you see how you are moving toward your goal and provide rewards as you advance toward success.

- *See yourself as achieving the goals.* Visualize yourself as being successful. Go over in your mind what it will look and feel like to accomplish a goal.

- *Give yourself a break.* Take time every day to exercise and relax.

Engaging in positive self-talk and relabeling negative experiences (viewing difficulties as challenges rather than as problems, for example) are positive steps in reducing stress-related disorders. Eating well, taking time to enjoy life, laughing, exercising, and living in the present reduce stress. People can handle stress effectively when they work on developing all of their abilities to the fullest, when they develop lifestyles compatible with personal values, and when they develop realistic expectations for themselves. Working toward these goals is the way to establish a wellness lifestyle (see Real-World Wellness: Dealing with Technostress on page 318).

Successful coping includes being aware of incidents and situations that you might perceive as being stressful. Recognition of stressors means being aware of how

## Real-World Wellness

### Dealing with Technostress

College students have grown up with computers and are surrounded by constantly changing technology such as PDAs, e-mailing, facebooking, and twittering. This ever-changing technology can be stress producing because people are forever learning something new or having to adapt to another innovation. Today, we don't even need a hard copy of a book since we can read thousands of titles with our own personal readers. Even our recreational pursuits, such as the music we listen to and the video games we play, can be purchased online. In addition, the programs and devices we are using today will change within a matter of months. For some, all this constant change and available technology can cause a type of stress referred to as technostress. Here are some suggestions for not allowing our technology to overwhelm us.

- *Don't allow texting, or twittering to consume your day.* You might even want to make certain times of day off limits for engaging in such activities.
- *Have a set amount of time to send and answer your e-mails.* Limit the amount of time you look at your e-mail; when the time expires, end your e-mail session. It may help to prioritize your e-mails so that you address the most important ones first.
- *Limit your time on the Internet.* When using the Internet, know what your needs are. Investigate or search only for what you need. Don't allow yourself to be distracted or begin surfing for additional topics that draw your attention from tasks that need your attention now.
- *Buy the technology you need and can use effectively.* To avoid being frustrated because your technology purchases cannot be effectively used, buy only the technology needed. If all else fails, take a class; or find a "techie" to help you effectively utilize your equipment or device.
- *When using computers, back up whatever you do.* Whenever possible, leave your computer at home during semester breaks or vacations. When on vacation, don't keep your cell phone on 24-7. Turn it off and check your voicemails only at certain times each day.
- *Take a break from technology.* Turn off the cell phone, leave the computer off, and find a peaceful place to relax and get away from all your technology. Even 15 minutes will help reduce your stress.
- *Finally, exercise.* Go for a walk or play a recreational game. By walking or playing an activity-oriented game, you can escape the technology of exercise machines.

your body responds to stress. Recognition requires continuous monitoring of your body and mind for evidence of excessive stress (see Real-World Wellness: Sleep and Stress Reduction on page 319).

Successful coping takes effort. One suggestion is to focus on the signals your body is sending when experiencing stress and then to think back to the event or situation that might have triggered those feelings. Another suggestion is to re-create a recent event that has been stressful. After visualizing the episode, write down six ways that the outcome could have been different—three ways it could have been worse and three ways it could have been better. Doing so will increase awareness of how to handle similar situations better in the future. A last suggestion is to try something new. The idea is for you be challenged and to meet that challenge successfully. Trying something new and meeting the challenge reinforce your sense of being able to deal with life successfully.[31]

## Relaxation Techniques

The ultimate goal in stress coping and management is to reduce the negative effects of stress. Various **relaxation techniques** have proved successful. Brief descriptions of various techniques follow. If you are interested in pursuing the use of these techniques, you can find more information about them in books or on tapes. These books and tapes can be purchased at bookstores or may be found at your library.

### Deep Breathing

Deep breathing is the most basic technique used in relaxation and is often the foundation for other methods. The primary benefit of this technique is that it can be done anywhere and anytime. It is beneficial to practice deep breathing several times a day. The methodology consists of completely filling the lungs when breathing, so that the abdomen expands outward. Begin by

## Real-World Wellness

### Sleep and Stress Reduction

Sleep is one of those factors that we all seem to be aware of, yet we seem to do little to correct lifestyle habits that create sleep deprivation. Recently *U.S. News and World Report* featured a full-length article and an editorial on the results of sleep deprivation. Research has shown that sleep is essential not only to brain function but also to the function of every organ in the body. Additionally, researchers have found that sleep deprivation can result in heart attack, prediabetic state, slowed reaction time, and mania episodes in bipolar patients.[32]

The National Sleep Foundation (NSF) reports that 47 million adults aren't getting sufficient sleep. Sleepiness is especially acute among 18- to 29-year-olds. Forty-four percent of this age group reported experiencing tiredness a few days a month. This compares with 38% of 36- to 64-year-olds, and 23% of subjects age 65 and over. The NSF survey found that those who got fewer than 6 hours of sleep were more likely to report feeling tired than those getting 8 hours of sleep (32% vs. 15%). The group that got less than 6 hours per night more often reported feeling stressed (32% vs. 16%), sad (14% vs. 7%), and angry (11% vs. 4%). People who reported often being sleepy during the day were compared with those reporting not feeling sleepy. Those who reported feeling sleepy were more likely to describe themselves as dissatisfied with life (21% vs. 7% of nonsleepy individuals) and angry (12% vs. 4% of nonsleepy individuals).[33]

Although it is generally recommended that adults average 7 to 9 hours of sleep each night, adolescents need an additional hour of sleep—10 hours per night. Even as we age we still need 7 to 9 hours of sleep. Sleep patterns may change, but the need for sleep doesn't. The choice is either to get enough sleep or suffer the consequences.[34]

taking a deep breath and then exhaling slowly through the mouth. A hand can be placed on the stomach to ensure that it is fully expanded. If the stomach does not rise, the breath is not deep enough or the abdomen is being held too tightly. Repeat this cycle several times and then rest quietly for 3 to 5 minutes.

### Progressive Muscle Relaxation

Progressive muscle relaxation creates awareness of the difference between muscular tension and a relaxed state. This is a three-step process, which begins with tensing of a muscle group and noticing how the tension feels. Next, make a conscious effort to relax the tension and notice that feeling. The third phase consists of concentrating on the differences between the two sensations. Beginning at either the head working down or at the feet working up, tense and relax all major muscle groups (see Real-World Wellness: Progressive Muscle Relaxation on page 320).

### Autogenics

Autogenics is the use of self-suggestion to produce a relaxation response. Autogenics begins with a deep breath and a conscious effort to relax. This technique may follow a progression from head to feet or feet to head. Repeat the phrase "My arm feels heavy and warm" several times before moving on to the next muscle group. You can repeat other phrases that carry a calming message, such as "I am completely calm and relaxed." End the session by thinking, "I am refreshed and alert." Autogenics takes practice, time, and commitment and should be practiced twice a day for about 10 minutes. Commercial tapes may help guide people wanting to learn autogenics.

### Meditation

Meditation can be approached from a variety of perspectives. As a stress-reduction technique, its purpose is to help the practitioner temporarily tune out the world and to invoke relaxation. During a meditation session, the person meditating focuses his or her attention on a *mantra*, a particular word or sound, while attempting to eliminate all outside distractions.

Begin by taking a comfortable position on a couch or in a chair. Take several deep breaths, slowly inhaling and exhaling. Shut your eyes or softly focus them on an object so that the details are blurred. Concentrate all your thoughts on a word or phrase that you have selected to use, such as *peace* or *relax*, while continuing to breathe slowly and deeply.[35] The relaxation response can also be initiated by counting breaths backward from 100 or by imagining a white light that slowly travels throughout your body, letting in light and energy while expelling tension and fear. Many commercial meditation tapes are available.

### Visualization

Visualization (imagery) is a form of relaxation that uses the imagination. Begin by finding a comfortable position; then shut your eyes and take several deep breaths. Several variations of visualization can then be used. You can imagine a tranquil scene, such as a beach on a sunny day or a valley with a stream or forest, and then place yourself in the scene. Imagine all of the scene's sights, sounds, smells, and feelings. People suf-

## Real-World Wellness

### Progressive Muscle Relaxation

*When I'm uptight, my muscles get so tense that I can't relax. What can I do to loosen them again?*

There are numerous progressive muscle relaxation activities. The exercises are frequently structured by a facilitator. Some exercises begin with the feet, hands, or face, but because of space constraints, only the relaxing of the face will be described here. You can add the other parts of the body by recording the entire process on audiotape and listening to the tape as often as desired—usually once a day or two or three times a week. Take your time (3 to 4 minutes) for each area of the body.

- Assume a comfortable position and concentrate on the instructions. You may find it beneficial to lie down or sit in a comfortable chair.
- Close your eyes.
- Allow all your muscles to relax and feel loose and heavy. Take several deep breaths.
- Wrinkle your forehead and hold for 6 seconds.
- Notice the feelings.
  - Relax; allow the forehead to become smooth.
  - Notice the feeling of relaxation.
- Frown with your eyes, forehead, and scalp and hold for 6 seconds.

- Experience the sensation of tension.
- Relax the muscles.
- Notice the feelings of relaxation.
- Keeping your eyes closed, clench your jaw and push your teeth together.
  - Hold for 6 seconds.
  - Notice the tension.
  - Relax your jaw and allow your lips to part slightly.
- Now press your tongue against the roof of your mouth and feel the tension.
  - Hold for 6 seconds.
  - Allow your tongue to return to its normal position, experiencing the sensation of relaxation.
- Now press your lips together as tightly as possible.
  - Hold for 6 seconds.
  - Relax and notice the feelings of relaxation over your lips.
- Using the same principles, gradually move through the body from the shoulders to the arms, hands, fingers, back, chest, abdomen, hips, legs, ankles, feet, and toes.

fering from a terminal illness frequently imagine scenes in which their immune system attacks or destroys their disease, or they envision themselves as healthy and disease-free. People who want to make major life changes, such as losing weight or stopping smoking, can envision themselves slim or not smoking or imagine themselves in trouble situations, such as a situation in which they are tempted to overeat or smoke. Then people can envision themselves making wise choices or not engaging in undesirable behaviors. Visualization can also be used to improve athletic performance. Tapes are available that can assist people in learning how to develop this technique.

### Biofeedback

Biofeedback, based on scientific principles, is designed to enhance the awareness of body functions—it is an educational tool. Sensory equipment demonstrates subtle body changes, such as increases or decreases in skin temperature, muscle contraction, and brain wave variations. This biofeedback, or feedback on biological pro-

cesses, enables people to become aware of what is happening in their bodies when stressed and learn how to control tensions through awareness of relaxing sensations. After a few sessions, people should begin to recognize and thereby alter their typical body responses to situations that serve as stressors for them (see Nurturing Your Spirituality: Enjoying Healthy Pleasures).

### Massage Therapy

Massage therapy has become an acceptable form of stress reduction and a healing alternative. Some people consider today's American society to be in the midst of a "touch famine." Appropriate touching is lacking, even though we recognize the need for physical interaction. Babies who are not handled can die from this type of deprivation. Although adults are not likely to respond so extremely to lack of touch, the need to be touched does not disappear with age. Research findings indicate that massage can promote physical relaxation and well-being. Certified massage therapists are licensed by the American Massage Therapy Association.[36]

## Nurturing Your Spirituality

### Enjoying Healthy Pleasures

Certain lifestyle patterns have detrimental effects on our well-being and quality of life: not exercising, smoking, drinking to excess, not wearing a seat belt, and eating poorly. However, just as important as avoiding lifestyle patterns that can negatively affect quality of life is appreciating the joys, thrills, delights, and happiness that are part of our lives. The idea is to minimize the negative and maximize the positive in our lives. Pleasure has gotten a bad name and we have become almost phobic about enjoying ourselves and having fun. In their book *Healthy Pleasures*, Sobel and Ornstein[37] point out that, even though certain negative habits and addictions are unhealthy, we also must seek to feel good mentally and emotionally. We need to seek enjoyment to enhance our

survival. Ornstein and Sobel emphasize that no better way exists to ensure healthy, life-saving behaviors than to make them pleasurable. From eating to reproduction to caring for others, pleasure can guide us to better health. Doing what feels good is often beneficial for health and survival.

A pleasurable experience can be as simple as taking time to enjoy a sunset, smelling the air after a rain shower, napping for half an hour in the afternoon, making a kind comment to a stranger or friend, or letting go of anger toward another human being. Seeking out pleasure may involve giving ourselves positive self-talks, looking for humor, and hanging out with happy people. Enjoying our gifts of pleasure is powerful medicine and can be contagious. It is cheap and effective, and its only side effect is a happy life.

### Music

The power of music is undisputed. A strong beat and rhythmic music instill in almost all people of any age the desire to respond by moving or dancing. Quiet music soothes by causing people to breathe more deeply, stilling turbulent emotions, reducing metabolic response, and calming the autonomic nervous system.

### Humor

Laughter is a powerful stress-reducing agent. A deep laugh temporarily raises pulse rate and blood pressure and tenses the muscles. After a good laugh, however, pulse rate and blood pressure go down and the muscles become more relaxed. Laughter works in two ways. Being able to laugh at a situation reminds you that life is seldom perfect or predictable. Laughing helps keep events in perspective. Laughing also works to reinforce a positive attitude. Laughing or even smiling can improve mood.

### Tai Chi

Although tai chi is an ancient form of Chinese martial arts, it differs from all other forms. Tai chi emphasizes tranquility and teaches the participant to remain calm against stressors and to harmonize with aggression and fear, rather than fight it. Further, it emphasizes internal strengths mixed with flexibility/agility rather than brute force. More than 100 positions/movements are found in tai chi's four basic philosophical concepts. The essence of each concept is

- Finding silence and solitude
- Regressing to the joys of childhood through embracing innocence, laughter, joy, and play

- Acting without forcing; moving in accordance with the flow of nature's course
- Acknowledging failure as the first step to success

Because of its philosophy, tai chi is sometimes referred to as morning meditation. There are many forms offered in the United States. Many community centers, private agencies, and universities offer various types of tai chi. The important factor is for you to find one that emphasizes the relaxation component.

### Time Management

A major contributor to stress is the pressure associated with time constraints. By effectively using time, you can eliminate a great deal of stress. For the college student, effective use of time is crucial, especially when working and attending school at the same time. Procrastination can add to stress and undermine academic work, personal relationships, and work efforts. Good time management, including appropriate prioritizing, scheduling, and completing personal responsibilities, can contribute to feelings of personal satisfaction.

Certain behaviors or habits can unnecessarily rob you of time:[38]

1. *Workaholism.* Workaholism is spending excessive amounts of time working, even though the activity may not be productive. Generally, people who engage in workaholic behavior like to work long hours and do not use time-saving techniques. They also may become overinvolved in unimportant tasks that eat away at their time, requiring them to use extra time to accomplish important tasks.
2. *Time juggling.* Time jugglers constantly overschedule themselves, often making promises to be in

more than one place at a time. This behavior often results in the neglect of important activities.

3. *Procrastination.* Procrastinators consistently put off until later things that could just as easily be done now. Some procrastinators choose the simplest of two tasks to do now to avoid the really important ones until the last possible minute, when the pressure is on.

4. *Perfectionism.* Perfectionists go beyond trying to do their best to achieve perfection. Because standards of perfection vary from one person to the next, this behavior rarely results in a sense of accomplishment, and the inability to achieve impossible goals contributes to feelings of dissatisfaction and failure.

5. *Yesism.* Yesism is the inability to tell anyone no. Extremely nice people often suffer from this condition because they don't like to disappoint others or they fear being rejected, even if saying yes ends up costing them.

Effective time management allows us to have a sense of direction and to fulfill the requirements for using time in a productive, satisfying fashion. Following are some suggestions for appropriate use of your time:

1. *Set goals.* Spend time planning your goals. Think of short-term (1 year or less) goals and long-term (1 to 3 years) goals. Ask yourself if the goals established are essential, important, or trivial. A good question is "When does this task have to be completed?" Your goals should cause you to "stretch" but not "break" as you strive to achieve them.

2. *Prioritize.* Use the 80/20 rule, which states that 80% of the reward comes from 20% of the effort. Prioritize time to concentrate your efforts on those items that will provide the greatest reward for fulfilling your short- and long-term goals. Once your priorities have been established, start with the most important tasks to be accomplished—don't procrastinate.

3. *Develop a time framework.* To help alleviate stress, establish the amount of time to be spent on each activity. Some tasks cannot be completed in a day's time. Estimate the days or weeks required to complete the task. This is especially important in accomplishing long-term goals. Allotting blocks of time each day of each week helps alleviate the pressure of completing a difficult task in a short time. For example, if a term paper is due at the end of a semester, you can spend a certain number of hours each week working on the paper. You can establish benchmarks for completing the paper and devise rewards for yourself each time you achieve a benchmark.

4. *Use a to-do list.* Two suggestions for using a to-do list are to (1) develop a list of activities each day and create priorities for accomplishing the list and (2) combine your daily list with a calendar or schedule; this allows you to see a running agenda of the important tasks to be accomplished over time. The important thing is to find a method that works for you. Don't be afraid to experiment with a variety of methods to help provide focus on your priorities.

5. *Ask for help.* If responsibilities become overwhelming, ask for help. Say no when there are too many tasks to handle. Do not feel guilty about saying no; this only adds more stress. For example, if sorority or fraternity demands are too great, either ask others to share the workload or refuse the responsibility.

6. *Be flexible.* Allow time for interruptions and distractions. Time management experts suggest planning for just 50% of your time. With 50% of your time planned, you will have the flexibility to handle interruptions and any unplanned emergency. When you expect to be interrupted, schedule routine tasks. Save larger blocks of time for your priorities.

7. *Take a break.* Every day should provide for fun, leisure, time alone, and relaxation. Make the most of every day. Schedule in time every day for yourself.

Assessment Activity 9-6 is a prioritization worksheet to help you organize your tasks. Assessment Activity 9-7 provides you with a log. Use it to record your daily activities for several days to a week. Then review it and see if you are spending your time as effectively as you thought or if you have overscheduled what you can do in 24 hours. This can provide you with a basis for devising improved time management plans.

## Exercise

Because the fight-or-flight response stimulates the body into action, exercise is a logical method of responding to that physiological command. Exercise has been found to directly affect brain chemistry. Studies have shown an increase in endorphin levels after an easy or a strenuous run. Exercise reduces exciting stress hormones by directing them into the intended metabolic responses.[39] (Endorphins are natural painkillers that help alleviate sensations of pain and stimulate a positive response from the immune system.) Exercise is a positive stressor (eustressor) and, when properly used, seems to offset the adverse effects of distress.[40] Studies have demonstrated that exercise reduces the severity of the stress response, shortens the recovery time from the stressor, and diminishes vulnerability to stress-related disease. The higher the fitness level, the more beneficial the exercise in reducing stress. (The recommended types of exercise programs are discussed in Chapter 3.)

A correctly designed exercise program produces beneficial physiological responses and can induce psychological effects that reduce anxiety, promote feelings of accomplishment, and evoke muscle relaxation.

Many people consider stretching a means of invoking feelings of relaxation, and stretching is associated with reduced tension. Moderate levels of exertion are frequently considered most beneficial for most people. (A moderate-level activity is a walk at the rate of approximately 3 miles an hour.) Excessive or addictive exercise habits can have the reverse effect and contribute to feelings of tension and irritability. When engaging in exercise as a stress-reduction technique, strive to find the level that creates the greatest sense of well-being on completion.

## Selecting a Stress-Reduction Technique

No single stress-reduction technique automatically reduces stress for everyone. People are comfortable with and enjoy different activities, and personal preference is what determines long-term use. When dealing with stress, you must first become aware that a stress response is occurring. People are frequently unaware that the reason they are always tired or irritable or have body aches is they are experiencing stress's negative effects. Second, find the stress-reduction techniques that work best for you. Usually, more than one approach is required, depending on the person and his or her type of stress response. Any technique that helps create a sense of relaxation, provides personal time, and allows you to gain control can lead to a happier, healthier, more enjoyable life. Third, the best form of stress management is the prevention of negative effects before they become unmanageable. Well-thought-out, prudent lifestyle decisions based on a knowledge of healthy behaviors and an understanding of your needs and expectations may be the best contribution you can make to your stress management plan. Finally, it is not the goal of stress-reduction strategies to overcome every stressor we face in our lives but, rather, to find effective responses to those stressors for purposes of managing our responses to them.

## Spirituality

Many of the relaxation techniques briefly described in this chapter are designed to help people cope with stress. Several of these techniques include aspects of helping to find spiritual well-being. Carl Jung, a pioneer psychologist, proposed a spiritual element to human nature. Jung's work has led to the area of study called psychospirituality—the study of the relationship between mind and soul.

Although recognized as a significant component of the wellness paradigm, the spiritual aspect is not always understood. It is becoming increasingly obvious how important our spirituality is to our total well-being.

In an attempt to grasp a difficult concept, it is essential to realize that the mind and soul are integral parts of understanding stress and finding ways to deal effectively with it. A recent trend in research has been the study of prayer, faith, and the healing/recovery of patients undergoing surgery and other medical treatments.[41]

When reviewing the concepts of wellness in Chapter 1, it becomes apparent that our spirituality is an important part of being human. Spirituality is belief in a personal relationship with a Higher Being. For members of the Christian and Jewish faiths, the higher power is God. Other people refer to their higher power by various other names. But what is spiritual health? Spiritual health is the ability to discover the purpose of our life and learn how to experience love, joy, peace, and fulfillment. Spiritual health can be further expanded to include helping ourselves and others achieve a high level of wellness. Through our spirituality we are connected to others. Our spirituality is a journey throughout our lives, and research has shown that those with strong spiritual values report more positive experiences physically, mentally, and emotionally than those reporting lesser spiritual values. One study found that men and women with strong spiritual values and beliefs were professionally successful even though they may have suffered major traumas of a psychological or physical nature.[42] The Mayo Clinic has stated that cultivating your spirituality may help uncover what's really meaningful in your life and thus enable you to focus on what is really important and let go of the unimportant things, which helps to reduce stress. Being connected creates valuable inner peace even in difficult times.[43] Spirituality seems to help buffer the negative consequences of stress by enabling a person to cope whether the stressor was physical or psychological.

## Spirituality and Religion

In some cases religion is an important part of spirituality. For this group of individuals it involves the traditions, beliefs, and practices expressing their relationship with God. Turning our attention briefly to the role of religion in reducing stress and improving quality of life, the following research has been reported:

1. People who attended religious services once a week or more lived longer than those individuals who did not.[44] Another study showed that subjects who attended church at least once a week lived 7 years longer than those who did not.[45]

2. Another study found that people who attended their places of worship weekly and prayed or studied the Bible at least daily had consistently lower blood pressure and recovered from depression more quickly than those not attending. Going to religious services seems to provide a stronger social network, improve self-esteem, and provide for better coping skills.[46]

Ray has stated that "the mind—a manifest functioning of the brain—and the other body systems interact in ways critical for health, illness, and well-being."[47]

Seaward, in his writings, points out that spiritual health is more than our religious beliefs and practices. He discusses potential characteristics, or inner resources, that help create "spiritual potential." These traits include creativity, will, intuition, faith, patience, cour-

age, love, humility, and optimism. These traits allow for specific emotional responses that enable the expansion of human potential, thus allowing for the reduction of stress in difficult emotional or physical situations. Seaward believes that "employing faith or an optimistic attitude in the face of diversity exemplifies spiritual health."[48]

For some, the religious beliefs they hold can contribute to spirituality. For others, their spirituality may be enhanced through other efforts, such as exploring their personal value systems, working on their sense of connectedness with nature, and finding a meaningful purpose for their lives. In attempting to summarize, this achieving of spiritual wellness to aid in reducing stress requires a continuing assessment of our values, our purpose in life, and how we choose to deal with conflict.

## Summary

- Stress is the nonspecific response of the body to any demands on it.
- Anything that creates stress is a stressor.
- Stressors may generate eustress (good stress) or distress (bad stress).
- The general adaptation syndrome (GAS) explains how the body responds to a stressor. The three stages of GAS are alarm, resistance, and exhaustion.
- The stress response can enhance physical and mental performance. This is referred to as the inverted-U theory.
- Whether positive or negative, a stressful event always produces a series of

neurological and hormonal messages that are sent through the body.
- The responses to stress can be physiological (cardiovascular, gastrointestinal, musculoskeletal), psychological (causing depression, anxiety, anger), or behavioral (generating an inability to work, arguments).
- The immune system can be compromised as the result of prolonged stress, resulting in increases of susceptibility to communicable diseases and chronic conditions.
- Coping is the effort(s) made to manage or deal with stress.
- Many techniques—including autogenics, deep breathing, visualiza-

tion, muscle relaxation, meditation, massage, tai chi, biofeedback, exercise, music, and humor—can help reduce stress.
- Effective time management can be a key to stress reduction.
- People's perceptions of stress are associated with self-esteem, self-efficacy, and locus of control.
- People who deal effectively with stress seem to view stressful situations as opportunities for growth, have a sense of inner purpose, and view themselves as having power over their lives.

## Review Questions

1. What is stress? What are stressors?
2. What are the stages the mind and body go through when exposed to a stressor?
3. What are some potential signals that a person is experiencing

chronic stress, and what are the possible effects?
4. What factors influence how a person perceives and copes with stress?

5. Define hardiness and how it may help a person effectively deal with stress.
6. What are some guidelines for handling stress positively?
7. Discuss various stress-reduction techniques.

## References

1. Siegel, B. S. (1988). *Love, medicine, and miracles*. New York: Perennial Library.
2. Selye, H. (1975). *Stress without disease*. New York: New American Library.

3. National Cancer Institute. (2009). *Psychological stress and cancer: Questions and answers*. Retrieved from www.cancer.gov/cancertopics/factsheet/risk/stress.

4. Hanson, P. G. (1986). *The joy of stress*. Kansas City, KS: Andrews, McMeel, & Parker.
5. Selye, H. (1978). *The stress of life* (Rev. Ed.). New York: McGraw-Hill.

y

6. Girdano, D., D. E. Dusek, & G. S. Everly. (2008). *Controlling stress and tension*. San Francisco: Pearson/Benjamin Cummings.

7. Folkman, S. (1984). Personal control and stress and coping processes: A theoretical analysis. *Journal of Personal and Social Psychology*, 46, 839.

8. American College Health Association. (2008). *American College Health Association—National College health assessment: Reference data report fall 2007 web summary*. Baltimore: American College Health Association. Available at www.acha.org/pubs_rpts.html.

9. Bovier, P. A., E. Chamot, & T. Perneger. (2004). Perceived stress, internal resources, and social support as determinants of mental health among young adults. *Quality of Life Research*, 13, 161–70.

10. Seward, B. L. (2004). *Managing stress*. Boston: Jones and Bartlett.

11. McEwen, B. S., M. J. DeLeon, & M. J. Meaney. (1999). Corticosteroids, the aging brain and cognition. *Trends in Endocrinology and Metabolism*, 10, 92–96.

12. Ibid.

13. Stefano, G., G. Fricchione, B. Slingsby, & H. Benson. (2001). The placebo effect and relaxation response: Neural processes and their coupling to constitutive nitric oxide. *Brain Research Reviews*, 35, 1–19.

14. Blonna, R. (2006). *Coping with stress in a changing world*. St. Louis: Mosby.

15. Fawzy, F. I., N. Fawzy, C. Hyur, R. Elashoff, D. Guthrie, J. Ashley et al. (1993). Malignant melanoma: Effects of an early structured psychiatric intervention, coping and affective state on recurrence and survival 6 years later. *Archives of General Psychiatry*, 50, 681–89.

16. Pert, C. (1999). *Molecules of emotion*. New York: Simon & Schuster.

17. Gelman, D., & M. Hager. (1988, November 7). Body and soul. *Newsweek*.

18. Martin, P. (1999). *The healing mind: The vital links between brain and behavior, immunity and disease*. New York: St. Martin's Press.

19. O'Leary, A. (1990). Stress, emotion, and human immune function. *Psychology Bulletin*, 108(3), 363.

20. Pellitier, K., & D. Herzing. (1988). Psychoneuroimmunology: Toward a mind-body model: A critical review. *Advances*, 5(1), 27.

21. Domar, A., & H. Dreher. (1996). *Healing mind, healthy woman: Using the mind-body connection to manage stress and take control of your life.* New York: Henry Holt.

22. Domar, A., P. Zuttermeister, & R. Friedman. (1997). *The relationship between distress and conception in infertile women.* Paper presented at the Annual Meeting of the American Society of Reproductive Medicine, Cincinnati, Ohio.

23. Greenberg, J. (2008). *Comprehensive stress management*. New York: McGraw-Hill.

24. Newman, J. (2000). C'mon get happy. *Health*, 14(6), 130.

25. Friedman, M., & R. Roseman. (1984). *Type A behavior and your heart*. New York: Alfred A. Knopf.

26. Flannery, R. B. (1987). Toward stress-resistant persons: A stress management approach to the treatment of anxiety. *American Journal of Preventative Medicine*, 3(1), 25.

27. Friedman & Roseman (1984).

28. Flannery (1987).

29. Habra, M., W. Linden, J. Anderson, & J. Weinberg. (2003). Type D personality is related to cardiovascular and neuroendocrine reactivity to acute stress. *Journal of Psychosomatic Research*, 55, 235–45.

30. Kobasa, S. (1984). How much stress can you survive? *American Health*, 5(7), 64.

31. Barefoot, J. C., et al. (1987). Predicting mortality from scores on the Cook-Medley Scale: A follow-up study of 118 lawyers. *Psychosomatic Medicine*, 49, 210.

32. National Sleep Foundation. (2002). Epidemic of daytime sleepiness linked to increased feelings of anger, stress, and pessimism. National Sleep Foundation website. Retrieved 2009, from www.sleepfoundation.org.

33. Boyce, N., & S. Brink. (2004, May17). The secrets of sleep. *U.S. News and World Report*, 136(17), 58–68.

34. Kobasa (1984).

35. Benson, H. (2000). *The relaxation response*. New York: Berkley.

36. Stoor, S. (2003). Health & fitness: The importance of physical activity for health. *Journal of Family Care*, 13, 10–13.

37. Sobel, D. S., & R. Ornstein. (1989). *Healthy pleasures*. Reading, MA: Addison-Wesley.

38. Crews, D., & D. Landers. (1987). A meta-analytic review of aerobic fitness and reactivity to psychosocial stressors. *Medicine and Science of Sports Exercise*, 19, 5114.

39. Appenzeller, D., et al. (1980). Neurology of endurance training versus endorphins. *Neurology*, 30, 418.

40. Girdano, D. A., D. E. Dusek, & B. L. Seaward. (2009). *Controlling stress and tension* (8th ed.). San Francisco: Benjamin Cummings.

41. Miller, W., & C. Thoresen. (2003). Spirituality, religion, and health: An emerging research field. *American Psychologist*, 58(1), 24–36.

42. Kirby, S., P. Coleman, & D. Daly. (2004). Spirituality and well-being in frail and nonfrail older adults. *Journal of Gerontology*, 59, 123–29.

43. Mayo Clinic Housecall. (2009). *Spirituality and stress relief: Make the connection*. Retrieved from www.mayoclinic .com/health/coping-with-stress.

44. Koenig, H., K. George, & P. Titus. (2004). Religion, spirituality, and health in medically ill hospitalized older patients. *Journal of the American Geriatric Society*, 52, 554–62.

45. Hummer, R., et al. (1999). Religious involvement and U.S. adult mortality. *Demography*, 36, 273–85.

46. Rosner, F. (2000). Therapeutic efficacy of prayer. *Archives of Internal Medicine*, 160.

47. Ray, O. (2003). How the mind hurts and heals the body. *American Psychologist*, 59(1), 29–40.

48. Seward, B. (1991). Spiritual wellness: A health education model. *Journal of Health Education*, 22(3), 166–69.

# Suggested Readings

Childre, D., & D. Rozman. (2005). *The HeartMath solution for relieving worry, fatigue, and tension*. Oakland, CA: New Harbinger Publications.

At the core of the HeartMath method of emotional regulation is the idea that by focusing on positive feelings such as appreciation, care, or compassion, anyone can create dramatic changes in his or her rhythms and lead to greater well-being. The system is interactive in nature leading users to see and experience in real time how thoughts and emotions affect their heart rhythms.

Davis, M., E. R. Eshelman, & M. McKay. (2008). *The relaxation and stress reduction workbook* (6th ed.). Oakland CA: New Hembinger Publications.

This text contains 21 chapters of excellent information on how to reduce stress. The authors describe a comprehensive collection of stress reduction techniques in a user-friendly way. A clear understanding of stress is provided, along with stress assessment instruments to assess individual sources of stress. Stress reduction techniques are provided for use and practice in reducing stress.

Freschi, Beth. (2009). *A time for relaxation, Vol 1: Guided relaxation techniques for wellness*. Amazon Digital Services.

Beth Freschi has a relaxing, calming voice. The music is extremely relaxing. Listening to the CD produces relaxation and a sense of well-being. Particularly effective is the guided imagery.

Johnson, S. (2003). *The present*. New York: Doubleday.

This book emphasizes the importance of focusing on the present; if the desire is to make the future, then we must maintain our attention to the moment, live with a purpose, and plan the future. It is easy to read and can be read in a single sitting.

Lehrer, P., R. Woolfolk, & W. Sims (Eds.) (2008). *Principles and practice of stress management*. New York: Guilford Press.

This book consists of 22 chapters, divided into three parts. Part One introduces the reader to the concept of stress and the psychology of relaxation. Part Two provides information on the various stress management techniques. Part Three discusses the applications and effects of stress man-

agement. This comprehensive book on stress provides theoretical as well as practical concrete examples.

Levin, J. (2001). *God, faith and health*. New York: John Wiley.

The author's research has established a convincing link between faith or spirituality and achieving and maintaining good health. Dr. Levin provides compelling evidence of the connection between health and a wide array of beliefs/practices, including prayer, religious service attendance, meditation, and faith in God.

Orloff, J. (2004). *Positive energy*. New York: Harmony Books.

The author provides 10 detailed prescriptions for harnessing one's "positive energy" to replace fatigue with physical and emotional vigor. The book contains many techniques/tactics to actively involve the reader in energetic transformation.

Williams, V., & R. Williams. (1999). *Lifeskills*. New York: Times Books.

This review of the research on relationships and health also describes a systematic self-help program to build better relationships and strengthen physical well-being. Eight basic life skills are described.

**Name** _____  **Date** _____  **Section** _____

# Assessment Activity 9-1

## Life Stressors

The following stress scale was developed by researchers Miller and Rahe. It includes positive and negative events, because both require adaptation. Research has confirmed that stress can have a significant impact on physical and emotional health. The total score on this self-test offers you insight into your risk for illness as a result of recent life events. Stressful changes won't necessarily harm you; the potential for damage rests in how you handle stress.

**Directions:** To determine the possible impact of various recent changes in your life, circle the "stress points" listed that you experienced during the past year.

### Health
An injury or illness that
- kept you in bed a week or more or sent you to the hospital                                           74
- did not require long bed rest or hospitalization     44

Major dental work                                     26
Major change in eating habits                         27
Major change in sleeping habits                       26
Major change in your usual type or amount of recreation  28

### Work
Change to a new type of work                          51
Change in your work hours or conditions               35
Change in your responsibilities at work
- to more responsibilities                            29
- to fewer responsibilities                           21

### Home
Major change in living conditions                     26
Change in residence
- within the same town/city                           25
- to a different town/city/state                      47

Change in family get-togethers                        25
Major change in health or behavior of family member   55
Marriage                                              50
Pregnancy                                             67
Miscarriage or abortion                               65
Addition of a new family member
- through birth of a child                            66
- through adoption of a child                         65
- through a relative moving in                        59

Spouse beginning or ending work                       46
Changes at work involving
- promotion                                           31
- demotion                                            42
- transfer                                            32

Troubles at work
- with your boss                                      29
- with coworkers                                      35
- with persons under your supervision                 35
- involving other issues or people                    28

Major business adjustment                             60
Retirement                                            52
Loss of job
- due to being laid off from work                     68
- due to being fired from work                        79

Correspondence course to help you in your work        18

### Personal and Social
Change in personal habits                             26
Beginning or ending school or college                 38
Change of school or college                           35
Change in political beliefs                           24
Change in religious beliefs                           29
Change in social activities                           27
Vacation trip                                         24
New close personal relationship                       37
Engagement to marry                                   45
Girlfriend or boyfriend problems                      39
Sexual difficulties                                   44
Child leaving home
- to attend college                                   41
- to marry                                            41
- for other reasons                                   45

Change in the marital status of your parents
- through divorce                                     59
- through remarriage                                  50

Change in arguments with spouse                       50
In-law problems                                       38
Separation from spouse
- due to work                                         53
- due to marital problems                             76

Divorce                                               96
Birth of grandchild                                   43
Death of spouse                                       119
Death of
- child                                               123
- brother or sister                                   102
- parent                                              100

### Financial
Major change in finances
- through increased income                            38
- through decreased income                            60
- through investment or credit difficulties           56

| | |
|---|---|
| Loss or damage of personal property | 43 |
| Moderate purchase | 20 |
| Major purchase | 37 |
| "Falling out" of a close personal relationship | 47 |
| Accident | 48 |
| Minor violation of the law | 20 |
| Being held in jail | 75 |
| Death of a close friend | 70 |
| Major decision about your immediate future | 51 |
| Major personal achievement | 36 |
| Foreclosure on a mortgage or loan | 58 |

**Total score:** _____

**Interpreting Your Score:** Add up your points. A total score of 250 to 500 is considered a moderate amount of stress. If you score higher than that, you may face an increased risk of illness. If your score is lower than 250, consider yourself fortunate.

**Source:** From Miller Rahe. (1997). Life changes scaling for the 1990s. *Journal of Psychosomatic Research, 43.*

# Assessment Activity 9-2

## How Stressed Are You?

**Directions:** The stress categories and stressors originally listed in Figure 9-1 on page 308 are also listed here. Underneath the stressors in each stress category is a blank. You can use this blank to rank yourself on each category and then to give yourself an overall stress rating. To rate yourself in each category, select a number from 1 to 10. A 1 indicates that you are currently experiencing no stress in that area of your life. A 10 indicates that the amount of stress you are experiencing in that area is overwhelming. This is a subjective rating and should be based on how you feel right now. After completing the assessment, note the areas currently creating difficulty for you and try to plan ways to reduce your overwhelming emotions in the next few days. Recheck your scores over the next few months to see how they change. If you chronically experience overwhelming stress in any area, you might want to seek the advice of a professional, such as a counselor or clergy.

| Physical | Social | Intellectual | Emotional | Spiritual | Environmental |
|---|---|---|---|---|---|
| Pathogens | Embarrassment | Mental fatigue | Uncontrolled anger | Guilt | Noise |
| Drugs | Teasing | Overload | Unexpressed anger | Moral conflicts | Overcrowding |
| Smoking | Ridicule | Frustration | Inability to love | Lack of purpose | Poverty |
| Lack of sleep | Arguments | Mental stagnation | Lack of love | Lack of philosophy of life | Extreme temperatures |
| Injury | Lack of social interaction | | Poor self-esteem | | |
| Sedentary lifestyle | Rejection | | | | |
| _____ | _____ | _____ | _____ | _____ | _____ |

Overall stress: _____

### Questions to Consider

1. Is the stress created from personal pressure or outside factors?

2. What changes could you make to reduce or eliminate the identified stressor(s)?

3. With whom could you discuss your feelings concerning the identified stressor(s)?

**Name** _____    **Date** _____    **Section** _____

# Assessment Activity 9-3

## Stress Style: Mind, Body, Mixed?

**Directions:** Imagine yourself in a stressful situation. When you are feeling anxious, what sensations do you typically experience? Check all that apply.

_____ 1. My heart beats faster.

_____ 2. I find it difficult to concentrate because of distracting thoughts.

_____ 3. I worry too much about things that don't really matter.

_____ 4. I feel jittery.

_____ 5. I get diarrhea.

_____ 6. I imagine terrifying scenes.

_____ 7. I cannot keep anxiety-provoking pictures and images out of my mind.

_____ 8. My stomach gets tense.

_____ 9. I pace up and down nervously.

_____ 10. I am bothered by unimportant thoughts running through my mind.

_____ 11. I become immobilized.

_____ 12. I feel I am losing out on things because I cannot make decisions fast enough.

_____ 13. I perspire.

_____ 14. I cannot stop thinking worrisome thoughts.

There are three basic ways of reacting to stress—physically, mentally, or with a combination of the two. Physical-stress-type people feel tension in the body—jitters, butterflies, the sweats. Mental types experience stress mainly in the mind—worries and preoccupying thoughts. Mixed types react with both responses in about equal measure.

Give yourself a *Mind* point if you answered yes to each of the following questions: 2, 3, 6, 7, 10, 12, 14. Give yourself a *Body* point for each of these: 1, 4, 5, 8, 9, 11, 13. If you have more *Mind* than *Body* points, consider yourself a mental stress type. If you have more *Body* than *Mind* points, your stress style is

physical. Do you have about the same number of each? You are a mixed reactor.

## Choosing a Relaxer

### Mind

If you experience stress as an invasion of worrisome thoughts, the most direct intervention is anything that will engage your mind completely and redirect it—meditation, for example. Some people find the sheer exertion of heavy physical exercise unhooks the mind wonderfully and is fine therapy. Suggestions are

| | |
|---|---|
| Meditation | Autogenic suggestion |
| Reading | Crossword puzzles |
| TV, movies | Games such as chess or cards |
| Any absorbing hobby | Vigorous exercise |
| Knitting, sewing, carpentry, or other handicrafts | |

### Body

If stress registers mainly in your body, you will need a remedy that will break up the physical tension pattern. This may be a vigorous body workout, but a slow-paced or even lazy muscle relaxer may be equally effective. Here are some suggestions to get you started:

| | |
|---|---|
| Aerobics | Progressive relaxation |
| Swimming | Body scan |
| Biking | Rowing |
| Walking | Yoga |
| Massage | Soaking in a hot bath, sauna |

### Mind/body

If you are a mixed type, you may want to try a physical activity that also demands mental rigor:

| | |
|---|---|
| Competitive sports, (racquetball, tennis, squash, volleyball, etc.) | Meditation  Any combination from the *Mind* and *Body* lists |

**Name** _____ **Date** _____ **Section** _____

# Assessment Activity 9-4

## Identification of Coping Styles

**Directions:** There are a variety of ways to deal with stress. Following is a list of positive coping behaviors. Indicate how much you currently use them to deal with stress.

| | Often | Rarely | Not at All |
|---|---|---|---|
| Listen to music | | | |
| Go shopping with a friend | | | |
| Watch television/go to a movie | | | |
| Read a newspaper, magazine, or book | | | |
| Sit alone in the peaceful outdoors | | | |
| Write prose or poetry | | | |
| Attend an athletic event, a play, a lecture, a symphony, and so on | | | |
| Go for a walk or drive | | | |
| Exercise (swim, bike, jog) | | | |
| Get deeply involved in some other activity | | | |
| Play with a pet | | | |
| Take a nap | | | |
| Get outdoors, enjoy nature | | | |
| Write in a journal | | | |
| Practice deep breathing, meditation, autogenics, muscle relaxation | | | |
| Straighten up your desk or work area | | | |
| Take a bath or shower | | | |
| Do physical labor (garden, paint) | | | |
| Make home repairs, refinish furniture | | | |
| Buy something—records, books | | | |
| Play a game (chess, backgammon, video games) | | | |
| Pray, go to church | | | |
| Discuss situations with a spouse or close friend | | | |
| Other: _____ _____ _____ | | | |

**Directions:** Following is a list of negative coping behaviors. Indicate how much you currently use them to deal with stress.

| | Often | Rarely | Not at All |
|---|---|---|---|
| Become aggressive | | | |
| Use negative self-talk | | | |
| Yell at spouse/kids/friends | | | |
| Drink a lot of coffee or tea | | | |
| Get drunk | | | |
| Swear | | | |
| Take a tranquilizing drug | | | |
| Avoid social contact with others | | | |
| Try to anticipate the worst possible outcome | | | |
| Think about suicide | | | |
| Smoke tobacco | | | |
| Chew your fingernails | | | |
| Overeat or undereat | | | |
| Become irritable or short-tempered | | | |
| Cry excessively | | | |
| Kick something or throw something | | | |
| Drive fast in your car | | | |
| Other: _____ _____ _____ | | | |

**Scoring Instructions:** Count the number of positive and negative coping techniques you use.

Number of negative techniques:_____

Number of positive techniques:_____

How often do you employ negative coping strategies?

_____

Do you use more positive than negative strategies or the reverse?_____

Do you recognize a need to change some of the techniques you are now using? If so, which ones?_____

_____

What are some ways in which you can maximize your positive coping behaviors? How can you minimize your negative ones?_____

**Name** _____  **Date** _____  **Section** _____

# Assessment Activity 9-5

## How Hardy Are You?

**Directions:**  Following are 12 items similar to those that appear on a hardiness questionnaire. Evaluating an individual's hardiness requires more than one quick test, but this simple exercise can be a good indication of your hardiness. Write down how much you agree or disagree with the following statements, using this scale:

0 = Strongly disagree
1 = Mildly disagree
2 = Mildly agree
3 = Strongly agree

_____ A. Trying my best at work makes a difference.

_____ B. Trusting to fate is sometimes all I can do in a relationship.

_____ C. I often wake up eager to start on the day's projects.

_____ D. Thinking of myself as a free person leads to great frustration and difficulty.

_____ E. I could sacrifice financial security in my work if something really challenging came along.

_____ F. It bothers me when I have to deviate from the routine or schedule I have set for myself.

_____ G. An average citizen can have an impact on politics.

_____ H. Without the right breaks, it is hard to be successful in my field.

_____ I. I know why I am doing what I'm doing at work.

_____ J. Getting close to people puts me at risk of being obligated to them.

_____ K. Encountering new situations is an important priority in my life.

_____ L. I really don't mind when I have nothing to do.

**Scoring:**  These questions measure control, commitment, and challenge. For half of these questions, a high score (agreement) indicates hardiness; for the other half, a low score (disagreement) does.

To get your scores on control, commitment, and challenge, first write in the number of your answer—0, 1, 2, or 3—above the letter of each question on the score sheet. Then add and subtract as shown. (To get your score on control, for example, add your answers to questions A and G; add your answers to B and H; and then subtract the second number from the first.)

Add your scores on control, commitment, and challenge to get a score for total hardiness. A total score of 10–18 = hardy personality; 0–9 = moderate hardiness; below 0 = low hardiness.

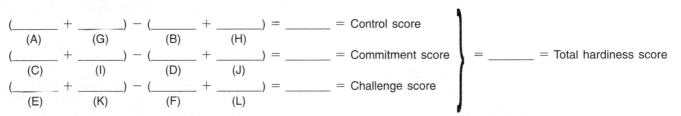

**Paths to Hardiness:**  Three techniques are suggested for becoming happier, healthier, and hardier:

* *Focusing:* Recognize signals from the body that something is wrong. Focusing increases the sense of control over plans and puts people in a psychologically better position to change.

* *Reconstructing stressful situations:* Think about a stress episode and then write down three ways the situation could have turned out better and three ways it could have been worse. Doing this helps you feel better about the way situations turn out and appreciate other coping strategies.

* *Compensating through self-improvement:* It is important to distinguish between what can be controlled and what cannot. A way to regain control is by taking on a new challenge or task to master.

Name _____    Date _____    Section _____

# Assessment Activity 9-6

## Goals and Priorities

**Directions:**   What follows is an activity designed to help establish your short-term (less than a year, a month, a week) goals and long-term (1 year or more) goals. Try to set goals that are specific, realistic, measurable, and achievable. Your goals should require effort on your part but should not cause you to burn out or fail. Your goals should give you a sense of direction. Once your short- and long-term goals have been established, determine what priorities you need to accomplish. Remember the 80/20 rule (see discussion in this chapter). Use a to-do list and establish your priorities for each day of the week. You may wish to prioritize your lists by number, letter, or color—whatever works best for you. Keep in mind the tips for time management. Be sure to schedule time for yourself regularly. It is vital to your stress management.

*Goals*

*Long-Term (1 Year or More)*

1. _____

2. _____

3. _____

Etc. _____

*Short-Term (Semester/Month)*

1. _____

2. _____

3. _____

Etc. _____

*Priorities for Next Week*

1. _____

2. _____

3. _____

Etc. _____

*Day _____ To-Do List*

   Must Do

   Important to Do

   Things I Would Like to Get Done

*Day _____ To-Do List*

   Must Do

   Important to Do

   Things I Would Like to Get Done

*Day* _____ *To-Do List*

　　Must Do

　　Important to Do

　　Things I Would Like to Get Done

*Day* _____ *To-Do List*

　　Must Do

　　Important to Do

　　Things I Would Like to Get Done

*Day* _____ *To-Do List*

　　Must Do

　　Important to Do

　　Things I Would Like to Get Done

*Day* _____ *To-Do List*

　　Must Do

　　Important to Do

　　Things I Would Like to Get Done

*Day* _____ *To-Do List*

　　Must Do

　　Important to Do

　　Things I Would Like to Get Done

Name _____   Date _____   Section _____

# Assessment Activity 9-7

## Analyzing Your Use of Time

Managing your time effectively can significantly contribute to your feeling of being in control of your life. A by-product of this sense of control is reduced stress and tension; with effective time management, you will be able to meet daily demands with less effort. The basis of change is recognizing that there needs to be a change and then determining the areas in your life that require change, so a good way to begin meeting your time management needs is to analyze how you are currently managing your time.

**Directions:**   Make several copies of this log and keep track of your time for a week. Include all your activities—including classes, meals, driving time, and conversations with friends. At the end of the day and week, rate each hour as to how important the activities that occurred during that time were. Taking time to relax, talk to friends, and be alone is considered important to total well-being and should not be discounted.

### Analyzing Your Log

1. What activities did you find to be the most productive for you? Which were the least productive? _____
_____

2. Where were your most productive activities performed? Your unproductive activities? _____   _____
_____

3. What time of day did you find to be the most productive for you   morning, afternoon, or evening? _____
_____

The analysis should be based on the full week's activities. You are looking for patterns of behavior that provide the best effects for you. You may find that you work best at home or in the dormitory in the afternoons or at the library in the evenings. Using this assessment, try to find the best patterns of achievement for you.

### Daily Log

| Time | Activities | Where | Essential, Important, or Trivial |
|------|-----------|-------|----------------------------------|
| 6:00–7:00 a.m. | | | |
| 7:00–8:00 | | | |
| 8:00–9:00 | | | |
| 9:00–10:00 | | | |
| 10:00–11:00 | | | |
| 11:00–12:00 p.m. | | | |
| 12:00 p.m.–1:00 p.m. | | | |
| 1:00–2:00 | | | |
| 2:00–3:00 | | | |
| 3:00–4:00 | | | |
| 4:00–5:00 | | | |

5:00–6:00

6:00–7:00

7:00–8:00

8:00–9:00

9:00–10:00

10:00–11:00

11:00 p.m.–12.00 a.m.

12:00 a.m.–1:00 a.m.

1:00–2:00

2:00–3:00

3:00–4:00

4:00–5:00

5:00–6:00

# Taking Charge
# of Your Personal
# Safety

## ONLINE LEARNING CENTER

Log on to our Online Learning Center (OLC) for access to these additional resources:

- Chapter key term flashcards
- Learning objectives
- Additional goals for behavior change
- Concentration game
- Self-scoring chapter quizzes
- Additional lab activities

The OLC also offers Web links for study and exploration of wellness topics. Access these links through **www.mhhe.com/anspaugh8e.**

## GOALS FOR BEHAVIOR CHANGE

- Identify and change three risky behaviors you now engage in.
- Make at least two alterations to your home environment to protect yourself and your family.
- Assess your safety precautions when participating in sports and recreational activities.
- Develop a personal safety plan for helping prevent unintentional injury.

## Objectives

After completing this chapter, you will be able to do the following:

✔ Identify potential dangers associated with unintentional and intentional injuries.

✔ List protective measures for maintaining a safe home environment.

✔ Discuss how to handle sexual harassment.

✔ Discuss the steps necessary to participate safely in recreational activities.

✔ Describe guidelines for the safe operation of a vehicle.

✔ Identify how to prepare for and deal with natural disasters.

## [ Key Terms ]

| | |
|---|---|
| acquaintance rape | rape trauma syndrome |
| carbon monoxide | road rage |
| date rape | sexual harassment |
| homicide | stalking |

This chapter follows the stress chapter for good reason. As we rush through our daily lives, one of the consequences of our high-stress, tension-filled lifestyles is accidents. Many of us experience close calls or minor mishaps during the periods when we are experiencing stress. Too often during these periods, we do not pay close attention, are careless in our behavior, or engage in behavior that puts us at greater risk for accidents or personal harm.

Statistics indicate that accidents are the leading cause of death for people between the ages of 1 and 45 years. Even in certain subgroups of this age range, where HIV has become the leading killer, accidents will still be the number two killer. College students and other young adults tend to give too little thought to their personal safety. As they participate in their daily academic and recreational activities, they encounter many potential dangers. No longer can the college campus be considered a safe haven from the violence and crime that are such significant parts of our society. Plenty of evidence indicates that people in a university environment are at significant risk for violence. You may feel safe, but that does not necessarily mean you are. This chapter explores those areas where the decisions you make can greatly influence your safety.

The first section of this chapter examines violence and intentional injury, including acquaintance/date rape, homicide, relationship violence, and hate-related crime. Included in this first section are topics related to personal safety—for example, how to be safe at the ATM, in your car, and in your apartment. The second section deals with recreation and outdoor safety. Topics discussed range from bicycling safety to avoiding road rage. The third section deals with unintentional injury, which can occur in the home during recreational activities or while driving.

## Violence and Intentional Injury

As we go about our daily activities, we are constantly conscious of violence. Acts of violence include assault, homicide (murder), sexual assault, domestic violence, suicide, and various forms of abuse. In 2008, violent crime in the United States affected 1,382,012 victims.[1] Violence has the potential to touch the lives of college students, regardless of school, gender, or ethnicity (see Assessment Activity 10-1).

### Acquaintance and Date Rape

The terms *acquaintance* and *date rape* have been brought to the national consciousness over the last 15 years. **Acquaintance rape** is forced sexual intercourse between people who know one another. **Date rape** is a form of acquaintance rape that involves forced sexual intercourse between people in a dating situation. Statistics indicate that 64% of rapes are committed by people the victims know or are dating.[2] Women were reported to be at greater risk for acquaintance/date rape if they used drugs, attended a university with high drinking rates, belonged to a sorority, and drank heavily in high school.[3]

In the college setting, poor communication is associated with behavior that results in attempts at seduction. One survey of 600 college men and women found there was substantial agreement among both genders that aggression and coercion usually occurred when one partner felt "led on" and the other did not make it clear how far she or he was willing to go.[4] One solution is for couples to learn that no really means no, regardless of the tone or hesitancy with which it is stated (see Just the Facts: Guidelines for Avoiding Acquaintance and Date Rape).

Researchers also point to a special problem on some college campuses that have strong fraternity or sorority organizations. Just because some athletic and other campus groups have condoned inappropriate actions on the part of their group members does not mean that all student social organizations are suspect. However, given the drinking, potential for intimacy, sexual teasing, and competitiveness characteristic of the house party, such gatherings sponsored by social organizations may provide social settings that encourage aggressive sexual behavior.[5] Many sorority and fraternity organizations have classes that educate members in an effort to improve mutual understanding and avoid date coercion or rape.

An important strategy in avoiding date and acquaintance rape is not to use alcohol or other drugs. Statistics indicate that 75% of male students and 55% of female students involved in rape have been drinking or using drugs when rape occurs.[6] For a discussion of Rohypnol, the so-called date rape drug, see Just the Facts: Rohypnol—Setup for Rape. Also see Chapter 11.

When a traumatic, often violent experience occurs, such as acquaintance or date rape, the victim usually experiences a great amount of enduring and substantial psychological damage. Date rape victims are particularly vulnerable because they are the victims of misplaced trust. Once the trust in a relationship is broken because of forced sex, developing new relationships becomes much more difficult for the victim.[7]

Regardless of how psychologically strong they are, most rape victims are likely to experience shock, anxiety, depression, shame, and a host of other psychosomatic symptoms. The psychological reactions following a rape are referred to as **rape trauma syndrome**. The syndrome is characterized by fear, nightmares, fatigue, crying spells, and digestive upset. Sexual function and desire

# [ JUST THE FACTS ]

## Guidelines for Avoiding Acquaintance and Date Rape

Men should observe these guidelines:

- *Know your sexual desires and limits.* Be aware of the effects of social pressure. It's okay not to "score."

- *Being turned down when you ask for sex is not a rejection of you personally.* If someone says no to sex with you, it does not mean you are being rejected personally; what is being expressed is the desire not to engage in a single sex act. Personal actions are within your control.

- *Accept the woman's decision.* Don't read other meanings into the situation; *no* means exactly that!

- *Don't assume that the way a woman dresses or flirts indicates she wants to have sexual intercourse.*

- *Don't assume that previous permission for sexual contact applies to the current situation.*

- *Avoid excessive use of alcohol and other drugs.* Alcohol and other drugs interfere with clear thinking, perception, and effective communication.

Women should observe these guidelines:

- *Know your sexual desires and limits.* Believe in your right to set limits.

- *Communicate your limits clearly.* If you are offended, say so in a firm manner and do so immediately. Say no when you mean no.

- *Be assertive.* Men sometimes interpret passivity as permission. Be direct and firm with anyone pressuring you sexually.

- *Be aware that your nonverbal actions send a message.* If you dress in a sexy manner and flirt, men sometimes assume you want to have sex. You should be able to dress as you please and flirt without its meaning anything. However, be aware of the possibility for someone to misunderstand and misinterpret your actions.

- *Pay attention to your surroundings.* Do not put yourself in vulnerable situations.

- *Trust your intuitions.* If you feel you are being pressured, you are!

- *Avoid excessive use of alcohol and other drugs.* Alcohol and other drugs interfere with clear thinking, perception, and effective communication.

may be impaired. The victim of violent sex may want her partner to be warm, tender, affectionate, and understanding, but she may not desire sexual intercourse for

# [ JUST THE FACTS ]

## Rohypnol—Setup for Rape

The drug Rohypnol (flunitrazepam) is a type of sleeping pill; it is illegal in the United States and Canada. Following is some key information about the drug:[8]

- It is produced legally in Mexico by Hoffmann-LaRoche.

- It is the most widely prescribed sedative or hypnotic in Europe.

- Manufactured illegal versions are available—the branded product seems to be preferred by illicit users.

- In the United States, it appears to be most frequently used in conjunction with alcohol, creating an enhancing (synergistic) effect.

- It is odorless and tasteless when mixed with alcohol.

- The drug seems to produce amnesia and a loss of inhibition.

- Arrests have been made in conjunction with alleged date rape involving the use of Rohypnol. Allegations are that the drug was added to women's drinks without their knowledge.

- Adverse effects can include loss of memory, impaired judgment, dizziness, and prolonged periods of blackout. Although a sedative, Rohypnol can produce aggressive behavior.

- Use is spreading among high school and college groups.

- Street names include rophies, roofies, ruffies, R2, roofenol, Roche, roachies, larocha, rope, and rib.

a long time after the rape. Sometimes lengthy counseling is necessary to help the rape victim reestablish a trusting attitude toward her relationships and sexuality.[9]

Another common psychological effect of rape is self-blame (the victim blames herself for what has occurred). The victim tends to review every aspect of the attack to understand what she could have done differently to prevent the rape. Although victims are blameless, self-accusation is common.[10] Self-blame is particularly prevalent in acquaintance or date rape because victims believe such rapes occurred because they created situations that permitted sexual coercion. Victims also tend to view their friends as being successful in the dating situation; it is common for victims to believe they are the only ones who have "failed." Rape victims tend to perceive themselves as having permitted a social occasion to turn into a painful event. Victims need the understanding of friends, family, significant others, and possibly professional counselors to help them work through these feelings.[11] Just the Facts: What to Do If You Are Raped describes the steps a rape victim should follow or be encouraged to follow as soon as possible after the assault.

The best protection against date or acquaintance rape is preparation and constant awareness that the potential always exists for unwanted sexual advances and potentially traumatic sexual experiences. Planning what to do if faced with unwanted advances and acting assertively may prevent or terminate many potentially devastating situations.

## Sexual Harassment

**Sexual harassment** includes any advances that are unwelcome along with other sexuality-related behaviors that are hostile, offensive, or degrading. Sexual harassment was identified as illegal by Title VII of the Civil Rights Act of 1964. Sexual harassment can take several forms. It can involve uninvited letters, e-mails, or telephone calls; distribution or display of materials of a sexual nature; uninvited and deliberate touching, leaning over, or pinching; uninvited sexually suggestive looks or gestures; pressure for sexual favors or dates; or sexual teasing, jokes, or remarks. Both men and women can be victims of sexual harassment, but women are more likely to be victims.

Sexual harassment can occur in the workplace, college or university, or military services. The nature of sexual harassment can take several forms.[12]

1. *Quid pro quo*—expectations to exchange sexual favors in return for some benefit. This form of sexual harassment usually involves one person holding some power over another and utilizing that power for seeking sexual bribery. An example would be a university professor suggesting that a student could get a better grade by engaging in a relationship.
2. *Hostile environment*—type of harassment involving sexual behavior that creates a hostile environment. This can be touching or looking at another in a sexually suggestive way, an uninvited request for a date, or telling of sexual jokes. It is considered hostile if the recipient finds the action offensive, even if the action was not intended to be offensive.
3. *Aggressive acts*—any overt actions such as pinching, hugging, touching, or kissing. If uninvited or unwanted, it is sexual harassment.

If any actions on the part of another are offensive, the first step is to be proactive and inform the person(s) involved of the offensive nature of the actions. Be clear as to what is offensive and the action expected to rec-

## [ JUST THE FACTS ]
### What to Do If You Are Raped

If you are raped, you should do the following:

- Call the police and tell them you were raped. Provide your location.
- Don't wash or douche before the medical exam. Take a change of clothes, but do not change until you have been examined.
- At the medical facility, you will have a complete examination. Point out any bruises, cuts, scratches, and so on.
- Tell the authorities exactly what happened. Be honest and thorough.
- Be sure you are checked for pregnancy and STDs.
- Contact the campus agency that can help with rape counseling or contact the nearest rape crisis center for counseling.

tify the situation. If this does not solve the problem then the victim should seek to inform whoever has authority over the perpetrator(s). It is important that offensive actions not be allowed to linger, since tension, stress, and anger on the part of the victim will only intensify. No one should be exposed to sexually offensive behavior, and it is the legal right of every individual not to have to tolerate it.

## Stalking

The United States Department of Justice defines **stalking** as a "pattern of repeated and unwanted attention, harassment, contact, or any other course of conduct directed at a specific person that would cause a reasonable person to feel fear."[13] Statistics indicate that 13% of college women were stalked during one 6-to-9-month period. Eighty percent of those victims knew their stalkers, and 3 in 10 college women reported being injured emotionally or psychologically from being stalked.[14] Most victims of stalking are women (78%) while 87% of the perpetrators are male. Stalking can take many forms, but the patterns of behavior include

- Repeated, unwanted, intrusive, and frightening communications from the stalker by phone, mail, and/or e-mail.
- Repeatedly leaving or sending the victim unwanted items, presents, or flowers.
- Following or lying in wait for the victim at his or her home, school, work, or other places.
- Making direct or indirect threats to harm the victim, the victim's family, or pets.
- Damaging or threatening to damage the victim's property.

- Harassing the victim through the Internet.
- Posting information or spreading rumors about the victim on the Internet, in a public place, or by word of mouth.
- Obtaining personal information about the victim by accessing public records, using Internet search services, hiring private investigators, going through the victim's garbage, following the victim, or contacting the victim's friends, family work, or neighbors.[15]

Several types of stalker profiles have been identified, but the bottom line is that to be a victim of a stalker can cause great anxiety, insomnia, social dysfunction, and severe depression. In a study that investigated female stalking victims it was found that 72.7% were verbally threatened with physical violence, and almost 46% of victims had experienced one or more violent incidents by the stalker.[16] In many stalking cases, the victim has needed counseling to help work through the psychological damage caused by the stalker.

If stalking is suspected it should be reported immediately to authorities. Additional steps are always to inform a friend where you are going and what time you expect to return, keep all apartment/dormitory doors locked, secure an unlisted telephone number or don't allow your cell phone number to be given out, have a caller ID on your cell or home phone, and always have a friend go with you when going out.

## Homicide

Murder, or **homicide**, is a crime that has been on the decline for the last several years. In 2008, murder and nonnegligent manslaughter decreased by 2.4%.[17] Still, the number of murders in the United States in 2008 was estimated at 14,180.[18]

Of this number in 2008, 6,838 were white, 6,782 black, and 560 of another race or the race was unknown. The largest group of murder victims was black males (5,752) followed by white males (4,934) and white females (1,903). As many as 3,466 of the murder victims were age 22 and under. Of this age group, almost 37% were black males. The murder weapon most frequently used was some type of firearm (9,484), and the second most frequently used weapon was a knife or cutting instrument (1,987).[19] The circumstances under which the murders occurred were robbery (924), drug-related (501), juvenile groups (711), romantic triangle (104), and rape (23).[20]

Most of us never think we might be involved in a situation where murder might occur. One needs only to think of the Ted Bundys of the world, or the disappearances of college students that occur each year. The implication for students is, first, do not put yourself in harm's way. Examples of such behavior would be making drug purchases, not locking apartment doors, using

an ATM late at night, and allowing firearms around when alcohol is present. Several of these issues are discussed in the remaining parts of this chapter.

## Relationship Violence

There are several types of violence. The first type of violence this chapter focuses on is domestic violence and the effects on any children involved in a domestic situation. The second type of violence/abuse is that found in the dating situation.

Today's families take many shapes, including single parents, blended families, and two-career families. More and more children are being left unattended while parents are either working or commuting home. Parents frequently feel overworked and children may feel neglected. The mix of related and unrelated people living in the same home can create new problems.

Domestic violence is also called spouse abuse, intimate partner abuse, battering, and partner violence. Whatever term is used, it is when an individual is in some way hurt by a person whom he or she knows. These hurts are not limited to physical harm but also include sexual and psychological abuse.[21] Authorities estimate that only about half of crimes of violence against a partner are reported. It is easy to be critical of people who do not report these crimes, but there are compelling reasons for their silence: Many women do not report abuse for fear of being killed or further injured and out of concern for the lives of any children who are part of the household. Many abused women may have little or no financial support other than the abuser, so they feel trapped. See Nurturing Your Spirituality: Learning to Communicate for some insight into the basis for some domestic violence.

Anyone, regardless of age, gender, race, or economic, educational, or religious background, can be abused. Men can be victims of abuse. However, most victims of abuse are women and are much more likely to be seriously injured. Certain groups of women seem to be at higher risk. They include women who[22]

- Are single, separated, or divorced
- Are between the ages of 17 and 28
- Abuse alcohol or other drugs or whose partners do
- Are pregnant
- Have partners who are excessively jealous or possessive

An abuser can be anyone. The abuser may be a husband, wife, boyfriend, girlfriend, or roommate. Many abusers were exposed to family violence as children. Adults who grew up in a violent home are more likely to become abusers or victims of domestic abuse. They see abuse as a normal way of life. A third of women who are physically abused grew up in a home where their mother was abused. Almost 20% were abused

# Nurturing Your Spirituality

## Learning to Communicate

Much of what occurs in relationships can be traced to how couples learn to communicate. As couples fall in love, it is important that, as they experience the wonderful, sometimes overwhelming emotions of being in love with another person, they become aware of how their communication patterns are developing. Each person brings to a relationship a different history and different perceptions and expectations. Dating couples who find that their methods of communication (or lack thereof) lead to periods of intense angry or physical confrontation, such as pushing or hitting one another, should seek to find more effective ways to communicate or, perhaps better yet, end the relationship.

Growing relationships should involve a maturing of love, care, trust, and concern. Such growth can occur only if people learn to communicate effectively and in a nonthreatening manner. Although everyone wants to avoid physically and emotionally abusive situations, learning how to understand and communicate with a person whom you care deeply about is not something that just happens. Couples must work at developing communication. The starting point is how each person views the other: No one "belongs" to someone else; no one is anybody else's property. People make choices to be with and share their lives with others and actively attempt to do so by behaving with kindness and thoughtfulness and by exhibiting a desire to grow with their partners along the journey of life. For continued personal growth, we must find ways to communicate effectively with our partners.

The starting point for good communication is mutual *trust* between partners. Honest communication requires some vulnerability. An untrustworthy partner may misuse personal, private information by mocking it, revealing it to others, or using it to justify behavior. When both partners respect and treasure verbal intimacy, trust is created.

Partners should agree on the ground rules for approaching conversations in which there is potential for disagreement. Each partner should listen carefully to what the other is saying—not to try to win the conversation, but to understand. Each person should be allowed to speak about his or her perceptions and feelings without interruption or fear of verbal or physical abuse. Each person should ask clarifying questions and attempt to repeat what the other has expressed. Anger does not lead to effective communication, and people should know when to take a time-out and move away from each other for a few minutes to allow their anger to subside.

When communicating, it is important to use *I* messages whenever possible. *I* messages convey what the speaker is feeling, not what the speaker thinks his or her partner is feeling or doing. For example, "You make me feel angry" is not an *I* message, but "*I* feel angry when you mention my family" is an *I* message. Through *I* messages, the speaker takes responsibility for his or her feelings and does not attribute them to a partner.

When communicating, it is also important to demonstrate an interest in listening and understanding. This entails maintaining eye contact and nodding or saying yes.

Finding ways to resolve conflict can improve the quality and extend the longevity of relationships. Remaining silent only fosters anger and indifference. Failing to discuss issues in a relationship merely builds walls, one brick at a time. The feelings of frustration and anger may eventually manifest in extreme verbal or physical abuse, or they may lead to indifference and loss of love.

themselves. Adults who were abused as children are more likely not to see their abuser's behavior as damaging, since they were raised in that fashion.[23]

The results of domestic abuse are not limited to physical or emotional scars. Some of the long-term effects of the abuse include

- Self-neglect or self-injury
- Depression, anxiety, panic attacks, and sleep disorders
- Alcohol and other drug abuse
- Aggression toward themselves and others
- Chronic pain
- Eating disorders
- Sexual dysfunctions
- Suicide attempts

As disgusting as domestic violence is, the impact this has on children is perhaps even more saddening. Children who either hear abuse from another room or witness actual abuse are clearly traumatized. Children in domestic abuse situations are in a situation that is detrimental to their emotional development and physical well-being. Children of domestic abuse are more likely to suffer sleeplessness, bed wetting, anxiety, and temper tantrums; to do poorly in the academic setting; and to attempt suicide. They have a higher chance of abusing alcohol or other drugs. In addition, children from abusive situations are more likely to become abusers and to abuse their own children.[24] These facts remain true whether the child was in an abusive situation or was actually abused.

There is no reason any person should have to suffer the indignity of abuse. Every person has the right to the highest possible quality of life, and no one has a right to inflict physical or psychological pain on any-

**TABLE 10-1** Examples of Abuse in the Dating Situation

| Physical | Sexual | Psychological/Emotional | Verbal | Abuse of Male Privilege |
|---|---|---|---|---|
| Punching | Unwanted touching | Humiliation | Name-calling | Making all decisions |
| Slapping | Sexual relations | Intimidation | Ridiculing | Expecting to be waited on |
| Kicking | without consent | Extreme jealousy | Insults | or pampered |
| Pulling of hair | Calling sexual names | Put-downs | Yelling | Treating another like |
| Choking | Threatening to get another | Untrustworthiness | Public humiliation | property |
| Striking with | sex partner | Blaming of partner for own | | Expecting partner to be |
| an object | Striking with an object | faults | | available at all times |
| Biting | Making fun of | Emotional withholding | | |
| Scratching | sexual activity | Stalking | | |
| Burning | | | | |
| Physical | | | | |
| confinement | | | | |

Source: Adapted from the American Bar Association. Domestic violence. www.abanet.org/domviol/typeofabuse.html.

one else. Anyone aware of an abusive situation has the moral and ethical responsibility to report the suspected abuse to authorities, so that action can be taken to protect the innocent victim and to help ensure either the punishment or rehabilitation of the abuser.

It is unfortunate that people sometimes become involved in a dating situation in which abuse occurs. Dating should be a time of having fun, getting to know a prospective mate, learning to trust and respect another, providing support, being honest, and growing more comfortable in social settings with other people. Some people may not even recognize when they have become involved in an abusive situation. Like domestic violence, dating violence can come in many forms. Abuse can be physical, sexual, psychological/emotional, verbal, or what the American Bar Association calls "abuse of male privilege."[25] Table 10-1 lists some examples of occurrences under each type of abuse.

Abusers in the dating situation use their abusive behaviors and comments to maintain control and power over the dating partner. Here is a series of questions to ask oneself when evaluating if one is in an abusive dating situation:

- Are you discouraged from pursuing your interests?
- Does he or she act extremely jealously when you talk to other people?
- Does he or she embarrass you in front of friends or make you feel stupid by calling you names?
- Has he or she forced you to do anything sexually that you didn't want to?
- Does he or she threaten you?
- Does he or she make all the decisions in the relationship?
- Does he or she control you by being bossy or giving orders?
- Does he or she make your family uneasy and concerned for your safety?

- Does he or she say it is your fault when he or she hurts you?
- Have you apologized for your partner's behavior when he or she has done something wrong to you?
- Have you been worried about upsetting your partner?

If any of these signs are present, you should examine carefully the quality of the relationship and if it is really beneficial to continue in the relationship. Remember, if marriage occurs, those little things that you think will change usually become even more of a problem—including abuse. In a healthy relationship, both partners respect each other, encourage and support the other's goals, encourage each other to have friends outside the relationship, communicate openly and honestly, trust each other, feel safe, and share in decision making.

## Hate Crimes

Hate crimes are crimes directed at people or groups because of perpetrators' hatred of their race, nationality, ethnicity, religion, or sexual orientation. In 2008, 7,783 hate-motivated criminal incidents were reported to the FBI. Of these offenses, 51.3% were motivated by racial bias; 16.7% by sexual-orientation bias; and 11.5% by ethnicity or country of origin.[26] In 2008, the majority of hate crime incidents (31.8%) occurred in or on residential properties. Seventeen percent of incidents were perpetrated on highways, on roads, in alleys, and on streets, and 11.6% of hate crimes occurred at schools or colleges.[27] Perhaps the 11.6% occurring at schools or colleges is one of the most alarming statistics, because colleges are institutions in our society that we might expect to celebrate diversity. Hate crimes can occur anywhere, but educated college students and faculty should understand the importance of tolerance and acceptance of individual differences. No person should have to suffer a diminished quality of life because of another's hatred of his or her race, religion, sexual orientation, ethnic background, nationality, or political beliefs.

## Safety at the Automated Teller Machine

Many people use automated teller machines (ATMs) to carry out various banking transactions. These machines provide a convenient way to make deposits or withdrawals in a variety of locations and at almost any time, when banks are closed, during holidays, evenings, and weekends. Over the last few years, many violent crimes have been committed at ATM sites. If you must make an ATM transaction, keep the following rules in mind at all times:

- Use the ATM during daylight hours if possible. If you must use an ATM at night, take someone with you and use a machine only in a well-lighted area.
- Before using the machine, check to make sure no one is acting suspiciously or hanging around the area. Trust your instincts if you feel uneasy. Seek a machine in another area if you sense something is not right where you are.
- Make sure no one attempts to crowd you while you are using the ATM. Take all receipts with you—do not discard your receipt nearby.
- Do not write down your personal identification number (PIN) or carry it in your billfold or purse.
- If you drive to an ATM, park in a highly visible location and under a light at night. Always lock your car and hold your keys in your hand.

- Do not assume that a drive-up ATM is free of assault potential. Always be alert to your surroundings.

## Carjacking

One of the crimes that seem to be becoming more prevalent is carjacking, a crime in which someone attempts to steal a car while the driver or owner is present. Of carjackings, 45% occur on the street and another 30% occur in parking lots or garages. A gun is used in 70% of carjackings, which makes this crime potentially violent.[28] To protect yourself against such crime and to help reduce the risk for potential assault, do the following:

- Keep the doors of your car locked at all times, even when you are in it.
- Always park in a well-lighted, busy area. Avoid parking in underground or enclosed parking because the security may be poor.
- Always check the backseat before entering your car.
- When walking to your car at night, have a friend or a security guard accompany you. Take your friend to his or her car.
- If you become lost, go to a police station or well-lighted service station for directions. Do not ask bystanders or other motorists for directions.
- If you break down on the road, raise the hood, put a white cloth on the antenna, turn on your flashers, and stay in the car. If approached, lower the window slightly and ask the person to call the

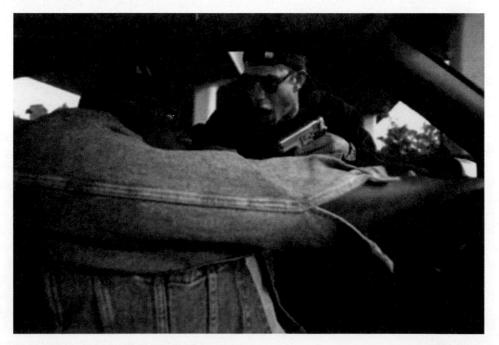

Carjacking is an increasingly frequent crime.

police if you don't have a cell phone. Do not get out of the car or accept a ride.

- If you are bumped from behind and the circumstances seem to be suspicious, stay in the car and drive to a police station or well-lighted service station and ask for help.
- Never pick up a hitchhiker.

## Apartment/Dormitory Safety

We like to think that our homes are places where we can be safe. However, within the confines of the home, dormitory, or apartment many potential hazards exist. By conducting a personal survey and remaining alert to these dangers, you can minimize many risks. Following are some suggestions for safe living in one's home (see Just the Facts: Being Safe in Our New World):

- Install smoke detectors and make sure they are in working order.
- If you are going to live above the fifth floor, make sure your fire department has the equipment necessary to reach above that level.
- Properly maintain all electrical and heating equipment.
- Plan and practice escape in case of an emergency.
- Plan alternative methods of escape in case your first-choice plan fails.
- Know how to get emergency help. Most areas of the country have 9-1-1 service, but many universities have special telephone numbers other than 9-1-1. Know your number.
- Never smoke in bed or leave lighted cigarettes unattended.
- Inspect living areas for surfaces, objects, or room design that can lead to slipping or tripping.
- Make sure all rugs have skidproof backing.
- Never overload electrical outlets.
- Do not place extension cords under rugs or where people walk.
- Never use a portable heater in an unvented area or near flammable materials.
- Keep outside doors locked at all times. Install chain locks on all doors.
- Check carefully before allowing anyone to enter.
- Look through the peephole or ask who is there before opening the door.
- Require people who claim to be maintenance workers to show identification before you allow them to enter.
- Place metal poles in the tracks of sliding doors, so that they cannot be opened unless you remove the poles.
- Be especially careful in parking garages, laundry rooms, and hallways and when entering and leaving living quarters.

# FACTS
## Being Safe in Our New World

Since the September 11, 2001, terrorism attacks on the World Trade Center in New York City and the Pentagon in Washington, D.C., many of our thoughts concerning personal safety have changed drastically. For the first time, we realize that there are dangers here in the United States; we are not immune to foreign invasion; and extremist groups can create havoc on our society psychologically, emotionally, and physically. The way we knew life prior to September 11 has probably changed forever.

The question many of us are asking is "What are we in danger of next?" Certainly, the possibility of further attacks such as those on the World Trade Center exists. We know that the threat of bioterrorism is ever present in forms of anthrax (cutaneous, intestinal, and inhalation). Other potential threats include smallpox, the plague, botulism, and viral hemorrhagic fevers, such as the Ebola virus, and chemical weapons, such as sarin, mustard gas, chlorine, phosgene, and hydrogen cyanide.

What can we do? One certainty is that fear is contagious. As a nation, we must not panic but instead must use common sense, be alert to suspicious activity, and report it to authorities. Further, we need to be alert to suspicious packages and letters. They may have characteristics such as excessive postage, incorrect titles, discoloration, odors, no return address, or excessive tape or string. If a suspicious letter or package is encountered, place it on a stable surface, leave and secure the area, wash your hands, and seek instructions from law enforcement. If you come in contact with any type of gas or chemical weapon, cover your mouth and nose and leave the area immediately. Use water to quickly rinse your eyes and skin exposed to the agent; then remove any contaminated clothing. Whatever the situation, don't panic. Certainly, we need to live our lives as normally as possible, but we must stay alert to questionable or suspicious situations and maintain a heightened sense of awareness to potential dangers.

Several useful websites provide continually updated information. Some examples are the Centers for Disease Control and Prevention, available at www.bt.cdc.gov/, the Federal Emergency Management Agency at www.fema.gov/hazard/terrorism/index.shtm, the FAA Fly Smart Guide at www.faa.gov/passengers/prepare_fly, and the National Transportation Safety Board at (See Just the Facts on Safe Air Travel – Post 9/11).

- Always tell someone where you are going, and whenever possible have a friend accompany you.
- See Just the Facts: Firearms in the Home for firearm safety guidelines.

## [ JUST THE FACTS ]
### Firearms in the Home

Many homes in the United States have firearms. If you choose to have a rifle, shotgun, or handgun, follow these guidelines for safely maintaining it:

- Keep all firearms unloaded within the home.
- Make sure firearms are locked and secured in a rack or case and have a trigger lock.
- Check to be sure a firearm is not loaded before storing it.
- Keep firearms in good working order.
- Keep your finger off the trigger when handling any firearm.
- Always point the muzzle in a safe direction (never point it at anything you do not intend to shoot).
- Store ammunition in a place separate from firearms.
- Lock the ammunition in a secure place.
- Educate all members of the household about gun safety.
- Enroll in a gun safety course if you are a new owner of a firearm.

This list is not all-inclusive, but it includes items for which you need to take responsibility. Discuss the rules for safe living with your housemates to help ensure each person's safety (see Assessment Activity 10-2). It is very important that you carry some type of insurance to protect personal property (see Real-World Wellness: Apartment and Dormitory Insurance and Just the Facts – Dealing with Diaster – Tips for Students).

## Fire Detection Devices

There are two types of devices that warn of fire: (1) heat detectors, which activate when the temperature reaches a certain point, and (2) smoke detectors, which sense the first traces of smoke and set off an alarm before toxic levels of smoke and gas are reached. Heat detectors are not recommended for the home. Smoke detectors are either photoelectric or ionization chamber detectors. Both types are effective and reliable. Both types come in battery-operated models and models that depend on household electrical current. It is advisable to have a smoke detector for each level of an apartment or a home. In placing the detector, be aware that it should (1) be on the ceiling or a sidewall 6 to 12 inches from the ceiling, (2) not be placed in the corner of a room because air does not circulate well in the corners,

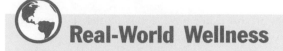

## Real-World Wellness

### Apartment and Dormitory Insurance

*I currently live in the dormitory but hope to move into a nonuniversity apartment. Do I need a rental policy? What about remaining in the dorm—do I need insurance there?*

While you are living in the dormitory, your possessions are generally covered under your parents' homeowners coverage. To be absolutely certain, you should check with your family insurance agent to confirm the type and amount of coverage. If you are not a dependent of your parents, you should check with an insurance agent to determine what coverage is available.

If you decide to move to an apartment, check with an insurance agent. Each insurance company offers slight variations, but in general good apartment/renters' insurance protects your personal property against loss or damage in the dwelling caused by fire and lighting, windstorms and hail, explosion, riot and civil commotion, aircraft, vehicles, smoke, vandalism, theft, falling objects, weight of ice or snow, glass breakage, accidental overflow of water, and accidental electrical damage to appliances. For additional costs, some insurance companies will cover computers, guns, tools, jewelry, cameras/camcorders, or money/coins/gold. Some companies will provide personal liability, which covers claims against bodily injury, sickness, disease, and accidental death of others.

The important thing is to check with an insurance specialist to determine your personal needs either when living in a dorm or when moving into an apartment.

and (3) be at least 3 feet from registers and air vents, so that drafts will not affect proper functioning.[29]

It is estimated that between 40 and 55% of fire deaths could be prevented by properly installed and well-functioning smoke detectors.

## Carbon Monoxide Detection

**Carbon monoxide** is a colorless, odorless, tasteless gas that results from incomplete combustion of carbon-containing fuels. Anywhere fuels that contain carbon are burned, there is the potential danger of death from carbon monoxide (CO) poisoning. A report by the National Center for Environmental Health (NCEH) illustrates the significance of this problem. According to the NCEH, each year more than 450 people die from exposure to carbon monoxide.[30] Motor vehicle exhausts are the leading cause of CO deaths, but deaths also result from poorly vented cooking stoves, furnaces, and ventilating systems. Death occurs when the oxygen normally found in the red blood cells is replaced by CO. Thus, to prevent CO accidents, several precautions ought to be observed: (1) Never operate a motor vehicle in an enclosed area; (2) never use charcoal in an enclosed area, such as an apartment, a garage, or the bed of a pickup with a camper top; and (3) make sure furnaces and all ductwork are inspected annually. Very small amounts of CO are potentially harmful, and anyone renting an apartment or living in a house should be aware of this danger. There are several clues you can look for to detect CO in your home. Consistently stuffy, stale, or smelly air; high humidity; moisture on the windows; no draft in the chimney; soot gathering around the outside of a furnace or fireplace; and the smell of exhaust fumes all point to the presence of CO.

Battery-operated and wired CO detectors are available. Although these detectors are usually more expensive than smoke detectors, it is recommended that all homes and apartments have at least one. Placement should be in approximately the same location as fire detectors. If a second CO detector is used, it should be placed near the heating source.

Ten percent blood level is considered the vital cutoff for exposure to carbon monoxide. CO affects children and people with smaller bodies more quickly. A healthy person can withstand a 60 to 80% CO blood level. Someone with heart disease may die at CO levels as low as 35%.[31]

# Recreational and Outdoor Safety

One of the joys of life is participating in recreational or sporting activities. To reduce stress, improve cardiovascular conditioning, and promote personal spirituality, some people find that there is nothing more satisfying than being outdoors. Regardless of the season, there are risks if personal alertness is not maintained (see Assessment Activity 10-3). Heat- or cold-related emergencies are always a potential problem. Chapter 3 discusses the prevention of these types of emergencies.

In addition to the emergencies created by extreme heat or cold, many other injuries can result from involvement in recreational activities. Some of the more common injuries are blisters, bruises, sprains, muscle cramps, nosebleeds, wounds, and sunburns. Table 10-2 provides information on how to deal with these injuries.

The list of outdoor recreational activities is almost inexhaustible, as is the potential for the unexpected to happen. As you prepare to engage in outdoor or recreational activities, be familiar with the safety rules of your endeavor, have safe and appropriate equipment for the activity, and maintain an attitude of alertness to potentially dangerous situations. Although not all-inclusive, the following rules will help keep you safe in a variety of recreational settings:

- Seek training and instruction from certified or respected instructors.
- Purchase appropriate safety equipment for the activity. Make sure your eyes and head are properly protected.
- Make sure all equipment is in proper operating order.
- Obey the laws related to your recreational pursuit.
- Begin any activity slowly and do not attempt advanced skills or actions until you are experienced enough to meet the necessary skill level.
- Stay aware of weather conditions. Always prepare for the worst possible weather.
- Never use alcohol when engaged in a dangerous recreational endeavor or during extremely hot or cold conditions. Alcohol increases the likelihood of emergency situations.
- Take a first-aid course that will prepare you to deal with a variety of unexpected situations.[32]

## Bicycling

The National Safety Council estimates that 57 million Americans ride bikes. Biking can be a highly enjoyable and, with proper precautions and common sense, safe activity. Safe biking begins with the rider. Defensive riding is the key to protecting against injury or even death. The National Safety Council reported that, in 1998, 900 bicyclists were killed and more than 70,000 cyclists suffered disabling injuries.[33] To ensure safe biking, taking precautions in traffic and wearing protective equipment are essential. Follow these guidelines for safe riding:[34]

- Always wear a helmet with a stiff outer shell designed to distribute impact and protect against sharp objects. Wear protective gloves. Wear sunglasses to reduce glare.
- Obey traffic rules. Cyclists must follow the same rules as motorists.
- Ride in single file with traffic, not against it. Watch for opening car doors, sewer gratings, soft shoulders, broken glass, and other debris.
- Use hand signals, so that drivers will know your intention to make a turn, change lanes, or stop.
- When riding at night, wear reflective clothing. During the day, wear bright, visible clothing.
- Make sure your bicycle has the proper safety equipment: a red rear reflector; a white front reflector; a red or colorless spoke reflector on the rear wheel; an amber or colorless reflector on the front wheel; pedal reflectors; a horn or bell; and a rearview mirror. A bright headlight is recommended for night riding.
- Keep a safe distance from others and never hitch a ride on another vehicle.

**TABLE 10-2** Recreational Injuries and Conditions

| Injury | Signs and Symptoms | Prevention | Treatment |
|---|---|---|---|
| Blisters | Fluid under skin | Wear shoes that fit and gloves on your hands. | Avoid breaking them; if painful, clean area, puncture, squeeze, leave skin, cover with sterile dressing. |
| Contusions (bruises) | Swelling, pain, discoloration | Wear protective equipment. | Rest; apply cold compression; bandage. |
| Sprains | Pain, tearing sensation, tenderness, loss of function, swelling | Warm up before activity; strengthen your muscles. | Apply RICE—rest, ice, compression, elevation. |
| Muscle cramps | Painful muscle contractions (legs most often affected) | Condition for the activity; warm up before the activity; strengthen your muscles. | Stretch affected muscles. |
| Nosebleeds | Bleeding from nostrils | Protect your face; moisten your nose linings in dry air or high altitude. | Pinch your nose with your fingers for 5 minutes; apply ice. |
| Wounds (skin) | Cut, bleeding skin | Wear protective equipment and clothing; inspect equipment before use. | Apply direct pressure, elevate, clean with soap and water, apply a sterile dressing. |
| Sunburns | Redness, pain, chills, blisters | Use sunscreen with a protection factor of at least 15; avoid sun exposure during peak hours. | Apply cool compresses; after pain has stopped, use a cream to keep skin moist; don't treat with oil-based products. |

- Be especially careful on wet surfaces, because stopping is much more difficult when brake pads and rims are wet. Be careful when applying the front brakes in wet conditions, because it is easy to be thrown over the front handlebars.

## Vehicle Safety

Human error accounts for nearly 85% of vehicle accidents.[35] Experts use the term *improper driving* for speeding, failure to yield right-of-way, driving left of center, incorrect passing, and following too closely.

One major cause of accidents is speed. In 13.6% of fatal motor vehicle accidents, speed is the major factor. Another persistent hazard is the use of alcohol and other drugs. Estimates are that two of five Americans will be involved in an alcohol-related crash at some point in their lives. In 2007 there were nearly 13,000 alcohol-related deaths.[36] The role that other drugs play in accidents is not clear, but a study by the National Highway Traffic Safety Administration reported that drugs other than alcohol were found in the blood samples of 18% of people killed in vehicle accidents.[37] In most cases, these other drugs were used in combination with alcohol.

Alcohol and high speeds are not the only factors that affect driving. Drowsiness is another important factor. See Real-World Wellness: Driving Drowsy for ways to minimize your risk of injury while driving your vehicle.

One of the most important factors in vehicle safety is the use of restraint systems (seat belts and air bags). The National Highway Traffic Safety Administration now requires all passenger cars and all multipurpose vehicles (jeeps, SUVs) to have dual airbags. It is estimated that 1,652 deaths and over 22,000 serious injuries could be prevented annually if nationwide seatbelt use reached 90%.[38]

For restraint systems to improve safety, they must be used properly. Children and infants should be placed in the backseat in car seats designed for their age and size. Deaths of young children have been caused by deployed air bags. Some companies have reduced the force of air bags' deployment and/or have provided drivers with the ability to disengage the passenger-side air bag. Many states have passed laws requiring that all children riding in cars be in a restraint system. All drivers transporting children should become familiar with the related state laws and be sure to use the type of car seat and restraint system recommended, according to age and size, for their child passengers. The use of restraint systems is not a luxury for adults, either. Proper restraint use is imperative to significantly improve the chances of surviving an automobile accident.

In the last few years, two other factors in vehicle safety have received a great deal of public attention. The first is the use of cell phones while driving. While cell phones are convenient and can add a measure of safety for people traveling on highways and in areas of high risk, too often cell phones are a distraction that can

## 🌐 Real-World Wellness

### Driving Drowsy

*Sometimes, when I'm driving, I seem to get really tired. What can I do to help myself remain awake and alert when driving?*

A number of conditions lead to driver drowsiness. First, today's cars and trucks have interiors with comfortable seats, are quiet and carpeted, and have temperature-regulated environments. Many vehicles also have cruise control, which can allow a driver's concentration to drift. Second, highways are constructed to eliminate sharp curves, hills, and bumps, which contributes to drowsiness while driving. Third, the repetitive patterns of oncoming light and of white and yellow lines during night driving can cause a trancelike state known as *highway hypnosis*. To prevent becoming drowsy and falling asleep behind the wheel of a vehicle, the National Safety Council offers the following tips:

- Before starting a trip, get enough sleep—at least 7 to 8 hours—the night before.

- Don't start a trip late in the day. Driving long distances is hard work, and you need to be fresh and alert.

- If possible, don't drive alone. Passengers can take turns driving and help keep each driver awake. Never allow all passengers to sleep in the vehicle at the same time.

- Avoid long drives at night because night driving increases the risk for highway hypnosis.

- Make sure the vehicle environment is cool in both the summer and winter. Turn up the radio volume and switch stations frequently; avoid soft, sleep-inducing music.

- Stay involved in the driving process—don't use cruise control. Don't allow yourself to become too comfortable. Drive with your shoulders back, your buttocks against the seat back, and your legs flexed at about a 45° angle.

- Never use alcohol when driving.

- Take frequent breaks—stop for light meals, stop at a gas station, walk in a safe area for a few minutes.

- If you feel yourself drifting off and no one else can share the driving, stop at a safe place, such as a truck stop, well-lit gas station, or rest area, and sleep for a short time; even 20 minutes will help. Always keep the doors locked.

- If you feel yourself getting drowsy, getting off the road may determine not only whether you stay awake but also whether you stay alive!

---

cause accidents. The National Safety Council recommends that drivers who do use cell phones when driving should be sure to use a phone that allows the driver to keep both hands on the steering wheel, a phone that features a microphone that can be installed on the sun visor, out of the driver's line of vision. With the upsurge in the popularity of text messaging, texting while driving has become a serious distraction to drivers. A Virginia Tech Transportation Institute study indicates that drivers are 2.8 times as likely to experience a crash while using the cell phone—but 23.2 times as likely to crash when texting.[39] Following are guidelines for car phone users:

- Safe driving should be the priority, not talking on the phone.
- Do not attempt to use the phone in heavy traffic conditions that require complete concentration.
- Program frequently called telephone numbers into speed dial to minimize the loss of concentration on driving required by dialing a bunch of numbers.
- Do not attempt to dial a number or text when the vehicle is moving. Wait for a stoplight or pull into a safe area.

- Do not attempt to take written notes while the vehicle is moving. If you need to write something down, pull off the road to a safe location.
- When using the phone, drive in the slow traffic lane in case you have to pull over.

See Just the Facts: A Distracting Factor: Cell Phone Use and Texting While Driving.

The second factor of concern for vehicle safety is overaggressive driving. The United States seems to have become a nation of rude, unthinking, aggressive drivers, manifested in what has become known as **road rage** (see Assessment Activity 10-4). According to one report, in 10 years, aggressive driving killed an average of 1,500 people each year; injured another 800,000; and cost the country roughly $24 billion in medical costs, property damage, and lost time from work.[40] The investigators believe the actual numbers were underreported because many aggressive driving crashes do not cause injuries, and in many such crashes there is not enough evidence to justify a citation. Also, aggressive driving does not always result in an accident.[41]

Men have typically been considered more aggressive drivers than have women. The National Highway Traffic Safety Administration (NHTSA) reports that aggressive drivers are more likely to be high-risk drivers, to drive impaired, to speed, and/or to drive unbuckled. Further, the aggressive drivers see their vehicles as providing a cover of anonymity; therefore, they drive more aggressively. Their behavior is characterized by running stop signs, disobeying red lights, speeding, tailgating, weaving in and out of traffic, blowing the horn, flashing their lights, and making threatening hand/facial gestures.[42] Women are now viewed as being as aggressive as their male counterparts and are increasingly displaying the aggressive driving characteristics once associated primarily with men. As a nation of road ragers, we have come to use our cars as weapons, along with tire irons, golf clubs, guns, pepper spray, and even crossbows.[43]

What we must remember, in our overaggressive commutes to our daily destinations, is to give our fellow drivers a break. It is not our responsibility to teach others how to drive. To respond with less anger to our fellow drivers, we may have to leave a few minutes early to reach our destinations; listen to quiet, relaxing music while driving; and even pretend that the person in the next car (the one possibly driving dangerously or carelessly or too slowly or stupidly) is a loved one. Each of us must assume the personal responsibility to drive in a courteous manner. Be willing to give up the right-of-way and don't take another's foolish, inconsiderate behavior personally. Some guidelines that may help prevent road rage are provided in Just the Facts: Preventing Road Rage.

## Motorcycle Safety

Motorcycles and mopeds offer several advantages over other modes of transportation. Their cost of operation is low, they consume less fuel, they take up less room on already overcrowded roads, and they provide their drivers with an often exhilarating feeling of freedom. Unfortunately, they are also two of the most dangerous transportation modes. The only protection most riders have is a helmet, and some states do not require that riders wear one. Over the last 5 years an average of 4,000 motorcyclists have been killed each year and more than 3 million more have been injured. Of fatal motorcycle crashes, 55% involve collisions with other vehicles. It has been reported that 65% of motorcycle-vehicle collisions are caused by the actions of vehicle operators and not motorcyclists.[45] The weather, malfunctioning equipment, and the surface of the road play a role in 10% of accidents. In addition, most cyclists do not receive formal training in safe riding. This becomes evident in analysis of the evasive actions of motorcycle riders. When avoidance actions are

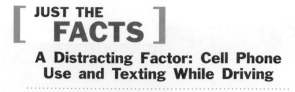

### JUST THE FACTS
### A Distracting Factor: Cell Phone Use and Texting While Driving

A formula for potential disaster is the use of a cell phone for calling or texting while driving. Talking on cell phones is a direct cause in 25% of all car accidents. One-fifth of adult drivers in the United States text while driving. In a study done by a leading insurance company, 73% of drivers surveyed talked on their cell phone when driving. The same research reported that 19% of those surveyed texted while driving. Several states have placed restrictions on use of cell phones and texting when driving. The rationale for these restrictions is clear from the data accumulated: Using a cell phone or texting while driving is a distraction and causes driver inattention. In younger drivers, driving distractions such as cell phone usage or texting contributed to 1,298 crashes in just one state in 2008. Also reported from 2002–2006, 5,715 car accidents were the result of hand-held cell phones. During the same period, 367 accidents involved the use of hands-free cell phones or Bluetooth devices. Additional data indicate that 21% of fatal car accidents involving teens were the result of cell phone usage. Researchers believe the percentage will grow by 4% per year unless behaviors can be altered in regard to texting and cell phone usage. Almost 59% of drivers between the ages of 18 and 24 text while driving. This age group reported that its number one distraction while driving is texting. Use of a cell phone or texting is risky at best. The most prudent advice is don't do it—or risk becoming one of the statistics mentioned above.

taken, 77% of those actions are improper.[46] Skidding from overbraking is the most common problem, and failure to use both brakes when attempting to avoid a collision is the second. A constant problem is the use of alcohol. Approximately 55% of motorcycle accidents involve the use of alcohol by the cyclist.[47] Finally, motorcycles present a visibility problem: Even with their headlights on, many cyclists are not seen or are overlooked by vehicle drivers.

Following are some rules of the road that make motorcycle and moped riding safer:

- Always wear a helmet. Even though some states do not require you to, you significantly improve your chances of surviving an accident on a motorcycle or moped if you wear an approved helmet.
- Helmets should meet the federal safety standards set by the Department of Transportation, indicated by the word *DOT* appearing on the helmet. Some helmets read "Approved by the Snell Memorial Foundation," which means they have passed tests even more stringent than the federal standards.

## [ JUST THE FACTS ]
### Preventing Road Rage

Following are some guidelines for reducing the incidence of road rage:[48]

- Give the other person a break.
- Do not tailgate.
- Do not let the car phone distract you.
- Do not switch lanes without signaling.
- If you are moving more slowly than most of the traffic, use the right lane.
- Do not drive in the passing lane when not attempting to pass another vehicle.
- Do not park in handicap parking if you are not disabled.
- Do not let your doors hit another person's car in a parking lot.
- Do not make obscene gestures to another motorist.
- Do not make faces at other drivers.
- Do not roll down the window and scream at other drivers.
- When confronted with an aggressive driver, slow down and back off.

- Wear gloves, boots, and heavy clothing to protect your body if you slide on the pavement, sidewalk, or gravel.
- Seek proper training in how to ride your vehicle; take a course in safe riding.
- Do not ride after drinking alcohol or taking medications that can diminish alertness or performance.
- Ride defensively. Motorcycles are harder to see, and some motorists take advantage of their superior vehicle size and weight.
- Avoid riding in the rain or other wet conditions.

## Pedestrian Safety

In their haste to get from one class to another, college students are notorious jaywalkers. Most of the time, nothing of consequence happens. However, nearly 60% of pedestrian accidents involve attempts to cross a street either at an intersection or between intersections. Usually, such accidents are the pedestrians' fault. Pedestrians make poor choices on when and where to cross streets, or they do not adequately observe traffic before attempting to cross. The student who darts suddenly from between two parked cars puts the motorist at a distinct disadvantage for seeing him or her and for stopping the vehicle. An invention of modern society, the iPod, causes users to be unaware of traffic noise and other sounds that would alert them to possible hazards or dangers.

## [ JUST THE FACTS ]
### Safe Air Travel—Post-9/11

Since the events of September 11, all of us should be prepared to take reasonable measures to protect our safety. AirSafe.com offers the following advice.[44]

1. *Be aware of your surroundings.* Take notice of any activities or situations that do not appear to be normal.
2. *Report unusual activity.* Inform authorities immediately if anything either in the airport or on the aircraft looks out of place or inappropriate.
3. *Make no assumptions about who may pose a threat.* Any person intent on violent acts against air transport can be of any age, gender, or nationality. Don't assume anything simply because of outward appearances.
4. *Stay away from suspicious circumstances.* Move away immediately from any unaccompanied packages, suspicious behavior, or unusual commotion. Notify authorities and warn others in the immediate area.
5. *Listen to the flight attendants.* If there is any kind of emergency, look to the flight attendants for guidance.
6. *Be familiar with your aircraft.* When first seated, review the written safety instructions; count the number of rows to the nearest exit. Check to see if there are seatback telephones available.
7. Have a plan for the emergency use of a wireless device. In case of an in-flight emergency, assess the situation before using any communication device. If the situation requires, use your personal wireless phone to contact someone who can help, such as the FBI. A second choice is to contact a loved one and ask him or her to call authorities.

The implication of statistics about accidents involving pedestrians is to be extremely careful when crossing a street. Remaining alert at all times, not wearing earphones, crossing only at designated crosswalks, and not entering the street from between parked vehicles are important safety precautions. When walking or jogging at night, wear light-colored clothing. Even better, wear a jacket or other apparel with reflective strips to make you visible to oncoming motorists. Statistics indicate that alcohol is a factor in 50% of fatal pedestrian accidents involving adults.[49] In this study, these adults had blood alcohol content (BAC) levels at or above 0.10 (the legal level of intoxication in most states).[50]

## [ JUST THE FACTS ]

### Dealing with Disaster—Tips for Students

Since the terrorist attack in New York and Washington on September 11, many people across the nation have had great concern for what the future may hold. If another such attack should occur, all of us may experience difficulty dealing with the event(s). Not all of us will react exactly the same, but some common responses to a terrorist attack or any other disaster are

- Disbelief and shock
- Fear and anxiety about the future
- Disorientation
- Inability to focus on schoolwork and extracurricular activities
- Apathy and emotional numbing
- Irritability and anger
- Extreme mood swings
- Feelings of powerlessness
- Eating pattern changes—overeating or loss of appetite
- Crying for "no apparent reason"
- Headaches and stomach problems

- Difficulty sleeping
- Excessive use of alcohol and other drugs

To cope with any disaster, the following suggestions are provided by the National Mental Health Association:

1. *Talk about it.* Share your feelings. Talking about a situation helps relieve stress and helps you realize that others have similar feelings.
2. *Take care of yourself.* Get plenty of rest and exercise. Do those things that are relaxing to you. Eat nutritiously and limit your viewing of media reports and images of the tragedy.
3. *Stay connected.* Call friends and family. Go home for the weekend, if possible. If you cannot visit in person, keep in touch by phone or e-mail.
4. *Do something positive.* Get involved with campus activities in response to the disaster, such as a candlelight vigil, benefit, or discussion group.
5. *Ask for help.* If you feel overwhelmed or have lingering thoughts concerning the events, talk with a friend or seek help from the college counseling center.

## Summary

- Accidents are the leading cause of death for people 1 to 25 years of age.
- Awareness of potentially hazardous situations is imperative for accident prevention.
- Acts of violence can occur anywhere and anytime. Acts of violence include assault, homicide, sexual assault, domestic violence, suicide, and abuse.
- Acquaintance rape is forced sexual intercourse between people who know one another well. Date rape is a form of acquaintance rape.
- Most rape victims suffer psychological effects, such as shock, anxiety, depression, and shame.
- Rape trauma syndrome is characterized by fear, nightmares, fatigue, crying spells, and digestive disturbances.
- Thirteen percent of college women report being stalked during one 6-to-9-month period.

- Sexual harassment can occur in the workplace, college or university, or military services.
- Sexual harassment can occur in three forms: quid pro quo, hostile environment, or through aggressive acts.
- Homicide has been declining for the last several years.
- Domestic violence can take the form of partner abuse or child abuse (physical and sexual).
- Hate crimes are crimes directed at people or groups solely because of the perpetrators' hatred of victims' sexual orientation, race, ethnicity, nationality, or religion. Nine percent of hate crimes occur at schools or on college campuses.
- Try limiting the use of ATMs to daylight hours. Never use an ATM at night alone.
- To help protect against carjacking, always lock the doors, park in a well-lighted area, and check the backseat before entering the vehicle.

- A personal survey should be conducted to determine potential hazards, danger, and risks in the home, apartment, or dormitory.
- Heat detectors and smoke detectors are the two types of devices for warning of fire. Heat detectors are not recommended for the home.
- Knowing and obeying the rules for safe participation in recreational activities are the first steps to fully enjoying a wide variety of activities.
- Common recreational injuries include blisters, bruises, sprains, muscle cramps, nosebleeds, wounds, and sunburns. A first-aid course that teaches how to manage emergencies is helpful for safe participation in recreational activities.
- Over 57 million Americans ride bikes. Defensive riding is the key to protecting against injury and death.
- Most vehicle accidents are caused by human error.

- Alcohol is involved in 39% of fatal crashes.
- All occupants of a vehicle must use a restraint system (seat belts).
- Car phones can contribute to inattention and accidents during driving.

- The United States is a nation of road ragers who commit acts of belligerence, hostility, and physical violence.
- Helmets are essential for riders of motorcycles and mopeds.

- Nearly 60% of pedestrian accidents involve jaywalking.
- A pedestrian should always remain alert, never wear earphones, and cross only at designated crosswalks.

## Review Questions

1. Identify measures to protect against rape.
2. How can rape trauma syndrome affect a victim?
3. What guidelines should men and women consider following to prevent rape?
4. Discuss wellness in relationship to homicide, abuse, and hate crimes.
5. Discuss some of the guidelines to follow to maintain a safe home environment.

6. List measures that help protect against crimes of violence, such as carjacking and ATM robberies.
7. What precautions should be taken to prevent fires and to protect oneself if a fire should occur?
8. What are guidelines for safely participating in any recreational activity?
9. What steps need to be taken to prevent hate crimes on college campuses?

10. What does the term *improper driving* connote, and what are some guidelines for safer driving?
11. Discuss measures for avoiding or dealing with road rage.
12. What would be suggestions for safely riding a motorcycle?

## References

1. Federal Bureau of Investigation. (2008). Crime in the United States. Retrieved from www.fbi.gov/ucr/cius2008/data/table_01.html.
2. Bureau of Justice Statistics Bulletin. (2008, December). 64% of female rapes in 2007 committed by non-strangers (NCJ 224390). National Crime Victimization Survey, Criminal Victimization (2007). Retrieved from www.ojp.usdoj.gov/bjs/pub/pdf/cv07.pdf.
3. Mohler-Kuo, M., G. Dowdall, M. Koss, & H. Wechsler. (2004). Correlates on rape while intoxicated in a national sample of college women. *Journal of Studies on Alcohol*, 65(1), 37–45.
4. Copenhaver, S., & E. Gaverhola. (1991). Sexual victimization among sorority women: Exploring the link between violence and institutional practices. *Sex Roles*, 24, 31–42.
5. Payne, W. A., & D. B. Hahn. (2002). *Understanding your health* (7th ed.). New York: McGraw-Hill.
6. Fisher, B., F. Cullen, & M. Turner. (2000). *The sexual victimization of college women*. Washington, DC: United States Department of Justice.
7. National Institutes of Health. (2009). Retrieved from www.nlm.nih.gov/medlineplus/ency/article/001955.htm.
8. Federal Bureau of Investigation. (2006). Tips for parents—the truth about club drugs. Retrieved from www.fbi.gov/hq/ood/opca/outreach/clubdrugs/clubdrug.htm.
9. Fisher et al. (2000).
10. Ibid.
11. Kelly, G. (2006). *Sexuality today*. New York: McGraw-Hill.
12. Ibid.
13. United States Department of Justice. (2009). About stalking. Retrieved from www.ojp.usdoj.gov/nij/topics/crime/stalking/welcome.htm.
14. Fisher et al. (2000).
15. United States Department of Justice. (2004). Stalking. COPS—Problem-oriented guides for police, problem-specific guides series. (No. 22). Retrieved from www.cops.usdoj.gov/files/RIC/Publications/e12032163.pdf.
16. Ibid.
17. Federal Bureau of Investigation. (2008). Crime in the United States. Retrieved from www.fbi.gov/ucr/cius2008/data/table 12.html.
18. U.S. Department of Justice. (2009). Federal Bureau of Investigation, Criminal Justice Information Services Division; Expanded homicide data, table 1. Retrieved from www.fbi.gov/ucr/cius2008/offenses/expanded information/data/shrt-able 01.html.
19. U.S. Department of Justice. (2009). Federal Bureau of Investigation, Criminal Justice Information Services Division; Expanded homicide data, table 9. Retrieved from www.fbi.gov/ucr/cius2008/offenses/expanded_information/data/shrt-able_09.html.
20. Ibid.
21. Mayo Clinic. (2004). Domestic abuse: Help is available. Retrieved from www.mayoclinic.com/health/domestic-violence/WO00044.
22. Ibid.
23. National Coalition Against Domestic Violence (NCADV). (2007) Retrived from www.ncadv.org/files/DomesticViolenceFactSheet(National).pdf.
24. Mayo Clinic (2004).
25. Ibid.
26. U.S. Department of Justice. Federal Bureau of Investigation. (2008). 2008 Hate crime statistics. Retrieved from www.fbi.gov/ucr/hc2008/incidents.html.
27. Ibid., table 10.
28. Bever, D. L. (2001). *Safety: A personal focus* (4th ed.). St. Louis: Mosby.
29. Ibid.
30. National Center for Environmental Health. (2009). Carbon monoxide poisoning. Retrieved from http://ephtracking.cdc.gov/showCarbon-MonoxideLanding.action.
31. Ibid.
32. Bever (2001).
33. National Safety Council. (2003). *Accident facts: 2003 edition*. Chicago: National Safety Council.

34. National Safety Council. (2009). Safe bicycling fact sheet. Retrieved from www.nsc.org/news_resources/Resources/Documents/Safe_Bicycling.pdf.

35. American College of Emergency Physicians. (2009). Alcohol and driving. Retrieved from www.acep.org.

36. Ibid.

37. National Safety Council (2009).

38. National Highway Traffic Safety Administration. (2009, May). Traffic safety facts. Research note DOT HS 811 140. Retrieved from www-nrd.nhtsa.dot.gov/Pubs/811140.PDF.

39. Virginia Tech Transportation Institute. (2009). Cell phones and driver distraction. Press Release. Retrieved from www.VTnews.VT.edu/article/2009/07/2009.S11.html.

40. Bowles, S., & P. Overberg. (1998, November 23). Aggressive driving: A road well-traveled. *USA Today*.

41. National Safety Council. (2004).

42. American College of Emergency Physicians. (2008). Aggressive driving fact sheet. Retrieved from www.acep.org.

43. Bowles & Overberg (1998).

44. Air Safe. (2004). Tips for travel under increased hijack threats. Retrieved from www.airsafe.com/events/war/safetips.htm.

45. National Highway Traffic Safety Administration. (2007). Action plan to reduce motorcycle fatalities. Retrieved from www.nhtsa.dot.gov.

46. Ibid.

47. ACEP (2009).

48. Bever (2001).

49. Parmet, S. (2006). Pedestrian safety. *Journal of American Medical Association, 288*, 17. Retrieved October 14, 2006, from www.jama.com.

50. National Highway Traffic Safety Administration. (2007). Traffic safety facts. *Pedestrians* (DOT HS 810 994).

# Suggested Readings

Berg, D. (2009). *The ultimate guide to home security*. The complete guide to locks, alarms, cameras, security systems, and secret bookcase door plans designed to protect homeowners and their valuables. A Kindle e-book by Amazon.com.

This full color e-book is packed with information, hardware and systems designed for homeowners to help protect against home burglary. Includes all the basics along with proven tips so you can easily transform your home from a burglary target to a sanctuary for your family and property. Information is provided on which locks are best and how to obtain the best window or door security. Book also includes sections on skylights, garage and shed security, attached garages, alarm systems, panic buttons, wireless alarm systems, and much more.

Mueller, J. (2005). *Savvy guide to home security*. Indianapolis: Indy-Tech Publishing.

The text discusses home security in a general way. The book covers all forms of intrusion detection as well as fire and smoke protection. Excellent information provided to help identify security needs for an apartment or a house.

Patire, T. (2003). *Tom Patire's personal protection handbook: Absolutely everything you need to know to keep yourself, your family, and your assets safe*. New York: Three Rivers Press.

This publication provides a great amount of material on how to protect against robberies, assault, and accidents at home, on the job, and while traveling. The text provides commonsense advice on dozens of topics ranging from physical confrontation to preventing identity theft. The book also contains easy-to-learn nonviolent tactics that can be used when one is feeling threatened.

Rawls, N., & S. Kovach. (2002). *Be alert, be aware, have a plan: The complete guide to personal safety*. New York: Lyons Press.

This book provides advice on how to protect oneself and one's family in any situation. The text provides excellent information on protecting children, dealing with stalkers, violence in the workplace, and traveling safely.

Robinson, F. (2003). *It didn't happen*. Boston: Custom Multimedia Creations.

This book is based on a true story involving a young woman who graduated from college with honors and became a rising star in her profession. After her involvement with a coworker who gave her liquid ecstasy (GHB), her association with the coworker and exposure to ecstasy almost ruined her life and left her with amnesia. It took her almost 10 years to find the answers to what had happened to her.

# Assessment Activity 10-1

## Encounters of the Dangerous Kind

Unfortunately, our everyday lives seem to be associated with many aspects of violence. This activity is designed to help you determine how at risk you are for such violence as carjacking, ATM robbery, gang violence, domestic violence, rape, and even homicide. This survey will ask you to think about some issues and situations that can have dangerous, life-threatening consequences.

**Directions:** Indicate whether each statement is always, sometimes, or never true for you.

| General Safety Considerations | Always | Sometimes | Never |
|---|---|---|---|
| I am aware of my surroundings. | _____ | _____ | _____ |
| I tell someone where I am going when leaving my home. | _____ | _____ | _____ |
| I am careful about providing personal information and daily schedule information to people I do not know. | _____ | _____ | _____ |
| I vary my daily routine and walking patterns. | _____ | _____ | _____ |
| If I walk at night, I walk with others. | _____ | _____ | _____ |

### Carjacking

| | Always | Sometimes | Never |
|---|---|---|---|
| I look in the backseat before entering my car. | _____ | _____ | _____ |
| I survey the location before parking, stopping, or getting into or out of my car. | _____ | _____ | _____ |
| I keep my car doors locked. | _____ | _____ | _____ |
| I have a plan of action if my car should break down. | _____ | _____ | _____ |
| I check my mirrors and scan ahead for potential dangers. | _____ | _____ | _____ |
| I avoid driving alone at night. | _____ | _____ | _____ |

| General Safety Considerations | Always | Sometimes | Never |
|---|---|---|---|
| I avoid dangerous areas that have a reputation for being high-risk areas. | _____ | _____ | _____ |
| If hit from behind, I travel to the nearest police station, motioning to the person who hit me to follow. | _____ | _____ | _____ |
| If I notice anyone loitering near my car, I do not go near it but go to a safe place and call the police. | _____ | _____ | _____ |

### ATM Safety

| | Always | Sometimes | Never |
|---|---|---|---|
| I avoid using an ATM at night. | _____ | _____ | _____ |
| I attempt to take someone with me when going to use an ATM. | _____ | _____ | _____ |
| I look for suspicious people or activity before entering an ATM area. | _____ | _____ | _____ |
| If I drive to an ATM, I park under a light in a highly visible area. | _____ | _____ | _____ |
| I remember my PIN number. | _____ | _____ | _____ |
| I take all receipts with me. | _____ | _____ | _____ |
| Even if using a drive-up ATM, I survey the area carefully. | _____ | _____ | _____ |

### Violence, Rape, and Homicide

| | Always | Sometimes | Never |
|---|---|---|---|
| I avoid dangerous areas of my city or campus. | _____ | _____ | _____ |
| I watch my alcohol intake carefully when at parties. | _____ | _____ | _____ |
| I do not drink alcohol on a first date. | _____ | _____ | _____ |
| I avoid arguments or potentially violent situations after drinking alcohol. | _____ | _____ | _____ |

I refuse to be with anyone who seems to be violent. _____ _____ _____

I do not strike or allow myself to be struck by another person. _____ _____ _____

I do not allow myself to be around anyone who has a gun and is drinking alcohol or using other drugs. _____ _____ _____

I break off a verbally or physically abusive relationship. _____ _____ _____

**Scoring:** In each section of the survey, give yourself 3 points for each time you checked the "always" column and 2 points for each check in the "sometimes" column. Give yourself 0 points for any checks in the "never" column. Although not scientific, the following point scheme may help you assess your total risks. Even though your score may reflect a high level of safety, make sure to examine each section for too many "sometimes" or "never" answers, which could indicate you are at serious risk.

| | |
|---|---|
| 87–81: | You are probably safe if you continue to observe current precautions. |
| 80–70: | You may have some areas to reexamine and change. |
| 69 and below: | You may be engaging in some behaviors that require significant change. |

**Name** _____   **Date** _____   **Section** _____

# Assessment Activity 10-2

## How Safe Is Your Home?

**Directions:** This activity is designed to help you assess the safety of your living environment—apartment, dormitory, or house. Indicate whether each statement is or is not true for you or if you are unsure about it. A scale is provided at the end of the assessment.

| General Concerns | Yes | No | Not Sure |
|---|---|---|---|
| I have homeowners or renters insurance. | ___ | ___ | ___ |
| I have personal liability insurance. | ___ | ___ | ___ |
| There is at least one smoke detector per floor (including the basement). | ___ | ___ | ___ |
| There is a carbon monoxide detector on each floor. | ___ | ___ | ___ |
| All detectors are in working order. | ___ | ___ | ___ |
| There is at least one fire extinguisher in the house. | ___ | ___ | ___ |
| I know (and my housemates know) the location and operation of the fire extinguisher. | ___ | ___ | ___ |
| Electrical outlets are never overloaded. | ___ | ___ | ___ |
| There is a rehearsed plan of escape from the house. | ___ | ___ | ___ |
| Everyone in the household knows how to protect himself or herself in a fire emergency. | ___ | ___ | ___ |
| Emergency phone numbers are posted near every phone. | ___ | ___ | ___ |
| All guns are safely stored with trigger locks engaged. | ___ | ___ | ___ |

**Entryways and Windows**

| | Yes | No | Not Sure |
|---|---|---|---|
| Doors and windows are locked at all times. | ___ | ___ | ___ |
| There are deadbolts on all the doors. | ___ | ___ | ___ |
| I use the peephole before allowing anyone to enter. | ___ | ___ | ___ |
| Strangers are not allowed to enter without first showing identification. | ___ | ___ | ___ |
| There are safety bar locks on all the sliding doors. | ___ | ___ | ___ |

| Surface, Hallways, and Stairs | Yes | No | Not Sure |
|---|---|---|---|
| There are slip-proof floor coverings on all floors. | ___ | ___ | ___ |
| There is sufficient lighting in halls, stairs, and entryways. | ___ | ___ | ___ |
| Electrical outlets are childproofed. | ___ | ___ | ___ |
| Halls, stairs, and entryways are clear of obstacles. | ___ | ___ | ___ |

**Kitchen**

| | Yes | No | Not Sure |
|---|---|---|---|
| Surfaces are clean and free of dangerous objects and substances. | ___ | ___ | ___ |
| Sharp objects are properly stored. | ___ | ___ | ___ |
| There are skid-proof floors and throw rugs. | ___ | ___ | ___ |
| I position panhandles safely while cooking. | ___ | ___ | ___ |
| All food-preparation surfaces are clean. | ___ | ___ | ___ |
| Household cleaning agents and other dangerous products are kept in a safe location. | ___ | ___ | ___ |

**Bathroom**

| | Yes | No | Not Sure |
|---|---|---|---|
| Electrical appliances are not near sinks or tubs. | ___ | ___ | ___ |
| There is a bath mat or nonskid strips in each tub. | ___ | ___ | ___ |
| Toilets are clean and free of mildew and bacteria. | ___ | ___ | ___ |
| Drugs and other dangerous products are kept out of reach of children. | ___ | ___ | ___ |
| Drugs and other products are stored in their original containers. | ___ | ___ | ___ |

**Living Room and Den**

| | Yes | No | Not Sure |
|---|---|---|---|
| Electrical cords are placed in safe locations and do not trail across the floor. | ___ | ___ | ___ |
| Unused outlets are covered. | ___ | ___ | ___ |
| Rugs are secured with skid-proof backing. | ___ | ___ | ___ |

**Bedroom and Nursery**

Smoke and carbon monoxide detectors are installed and working. ___ ___ ___

There are night lights in the room or adjoining hallway. ___ ___ ___

There is no high threshold to trip over. ___ ___ ___

Unused electrical outlets are covered. ___ ___ ___

**Scoring:** Although this assessment is designed only to be a thought-provoking activity, the following scale may help increase awareness of the potential dangers within your house. Give yourself 1 point for each "yes" answer. Give yourself 0 points for each "no" or "not sure" answer:

39–34:  Good score, but stay alert.
33–28:  Check carefully for potential hazards.
27 and below:  Significant risks; changes are necessary.

**Name** _____   **Date** _____   **Section** _____

# Assessment Activity 10-3

## Recreational Safety—How Safe Are You?

**Directions:** This activity is designed to assess your susceptibility to accidents and events when participating in recreational activities. Indicate whether each statement is always, sometimes, or never true for you. Skip over the activities in which you never participate.

| General Considerations | Always | Sometimes | Never |
|---|---|---|---|
| I seek proper instruction before participating in a recreational activity. | ____ | ____ | ____ |
| I take a safety class for each new recreational activity. | ____ | ____ | ____ |
| I use appropriate safety equipment. | ____ | ____ | ____ |
| All my equipment is in excellent working order. | ____ | ____ | ____ |
| I do not use alcohol or other drugs when engaging in a recreational activity. | ____ | ____ | ____ |
| I can swim well enough to save myself in a given situation. | ____ | ____ | ____ |
| I know the basic first aid and CPR for a given situation. | ____ | ____ | ____ |
| I can effectively deal with heat and cold emergencies. | ____ | ____ | ____ |
| I use sunscreen when in the sunlight. | ____ | ____ | ____ |
| I obey rules, laws, and regulations related to my activity. | ____ | ____ | ____ |
| I am aware of weather conditions when engaging in my activity. | ____ | ____ | ____ |

### Bicycling

| | Always | Sometimes | Never |
|---|---|---|---|
| I obey traffic rules and follow the same rules as motorists. | ____ | ____ | ____ |
| I use hand signals to inform others of my intentions. | ____ | ____ | ____ |
| I wear a helmet. | ____ | ____ | ____ |

| General Considerations | Always | Sometimes | Never |
|---|---|---|---|
| I wear a helmet with the following features: | | | |
| • A stiff outer shell designed to distribute impact and protect against sharp objects | ____ | ____ | ____ |
| • An energy-absorbing liner 1/2 inch thick | ____ | ____ | ____ |
| • A chin strap and fastener | ____ | ____ | ____ |
| • Lightweight, cool, and comfortable clothing | ____ | ____ | ____ |
| At night I wear brightly colored, reflective clothing. | ____ | ____ | ____ |
| I ride in single file with traffic, not against it. | ____ | ____ | ____ |
| I remain alert to holes, sewer gratings, soft shoulders, broken glass and other debris, and people opening car doors. | ____ | ____ | ____ |

### Motorcycling

| | Always | Sometimes | Never |
|---|---|---|---|
| I wear a helmet (regardless of state laws). | ____ | ____ | ____ |
| I wear boots, gloves, and heavy clothing to protect my skin when riding. | ____ | ____ | ____ |
| I keep abreast of safety techniques and regulations through proper training. | ____ | ____ | ____ |
| I avoid riding in wet or icy weather. | ____ | ____ | ____ |
| I do not take drugs or drink alcohol when riding. | ____ | ____ | ____ |
| I ride defensively, giving up the right-of-way. | ____ | ____ | ____ |

### Boating and Personal Watercraft (PWC)

| | Always | Sometimes | Never |
|---|---|---|---|
| I know the latest rules of operation for a power boat. | ____ | ____ | ____ |
| I do not operate a boat while drinking alcohol or intoxicated; I do not ride in a boat operated by someone who is or has been drinking alcohol. | ____ | ____ | ____ |

| General Considerations | Always | Sometimes | Never |
|---|---|---|---|
| I wear a personal flotation device (PFD) when in a boat. | ___ | ___ | ___ |
| I make sure I have an observer when water skiing or operating a watercraft pulling a skier. | ___ | ___ | ___ |
| I am alert to changing weather conditions. | ___ | ___ | ___ |
| I do not ride or operate a PWC without wearing a securely fastened PFD. | ___ | ___ | ___ |
| I do not drink alcohol when operating a PWC. | ___ | ___ | ___ |
| I look in all directions when operating a PWC. | ___ | ___ | ___ |
| I do not jump the wakes of boats. | ___ | ___ | ___ |
| I remember that, when I release the throttle, the PWC cannot be steered or controlled. | ___ | ___ | ___ |
| I cruise an area to check for hazards before skiing, operating a PWC, or operating a boat at increased speed. | ___ | ___ | ___ |

**In-Line Skating**

| | Always | Sometimes | Never |
|---|---|---|---|
| I wear protective equipment (helmet, elbow and knee pads, light gloves, wrist guards). | ___ | ___ | ___ |
| I practice stopping, turning, and making general movements on the skates before skating on streets. | ___ | ___ | ___ |
| I am skilled at skating backward. | ___ | ___ | ___ |
| I can safely stop by using the heel stop, T-stop, or power stop. | ___ | ___ | ___ |
| My skates fit me properly. | ___ | ___ | ___ |
| I obey all traffic laws. | ___ | ___ | ___ |
| I am watchful of pedestrians, cyclists, and autos when skating. | ___ | ___ | ___ |
| I do not pass other skaters or pedestrians without alerting them. | ___ | ___ | ___ |
| I inspect my equipment before skating. | ___ | ___ | ___ |

**Skateboarding**

| | Always | Sometimes | Never |
|---|---|---|---|
| I wear protective equipment (helmet, elbow and knee pads, light gloves, wrist guards). | ___ | ___ | ___ |

| General Considerations | Always | Sometimes | Never |
|---|---|---|---|
| I wear slip-resistant shoes. | ___ | ___ | ___ |
| My skateboard has a slip-resistant surface. | ___ | ___ | ___ |
| I inspect my board prior to riding. | ___ | ___ | ___ |
| I do not ride in the street. | ___ | ___ | ___ |
| I do not skate in crowds of nonskateboarders. | ___ | ___ | ___ |
| I obey the laws about where and where not to skate. | ___ | ___ | ___ |
| I know and practice how to fall. | ___ | ___ | ___ |
| I do not hitch a ride from a car, a bicycle, or another vehicle. | ___ | ___ | ___ |

**Firearms**

| | Always | Sometimes | Never |
|---|---|---|---|
| Gun safety is a high priority. | ___ | ___ | ___ |
| I obey the gun possession laws in my state. | ___ | ___ | ___ |
| My guns are in proper operating condition. | ___ | ___ | ___ |
| I consider every gun to be loaded. | ___ | ___ | ___ |
| I keep the safety on until ready to shoot. | ___ | ___ | ___ |
| I keep the gun barrel pointed down. | ___ | ___ | ___ |
| When stored, my gun has a trigger lock on it. | ___ | ___ | ___ |
| I do not store a loaded gun. | ___ | ___ | ___ |
| I do not handle a firearm when drinking or intoxicated. | ___ | ___ | ___ |
| I target practice only at approved ranges. | ___ | ___ | ___ |

**Assessment:** This activity is designed to help you assess your behavior when participating in a variety of activities. Evaluate your participation in any of your activities. Any check in the "never" or "sometimes" column means that precautions should be taken to correct the situation. Safe participation in any activity requires careful planning—not doing so can place you at serious personal risk. Following are some questions to consider:

1. What needs to be done to correct each of the "sometimes" or "never" items?

2. What are the potential consequences of not taking corrective action(s)?

3. Are you endangering others through your present behaviors?

**Name** _____   **Date** _____   **Section** _____

# Assessment Activity 10-4

## Road Rage and You

**Directions:**   The best way to avoid problems and conflicts when driving is to prohibit yourself from becoming an aggressive driver. Following is a series of questions designed to help you determine how prone you are to provoking rage in other drivers. Indicate how often you adhere to each driving safety guideline.

| | Rarely/ Never | Sometimes | Often | Always |
|---|---|---|---|---|
| I give the other driver the benefit of the doubt when there is confusion about who has the right-of-way. | _____ | _____ | _____ | _____ |
| I practice driving courteously. | _____ | _____ | _____ | _____ |
| I try to leave early, so I don't feel pressure to drive aggressively. | _____ | _____ | _____ | _____ |
| I do not block the passing lane. | _____ | _____ | _____ | _____ |
| I use my horn sparingly. | _____ | _____ | _____ | _____ |
| I do not make or return obscene gestures. | _____ | _____ | _____ | _____ |
| I use my signal when switching lanes. | _____ | _____ | _____ | _____ |
| I do not tailgate or talk on my car phone when driving. | _____ | _____ | _____ | _____ |
| If I am moving slowly, I pull over to allow traffic to pass. | _____ | _____ | _____ | _____ |
| I do not stop in my car to talk to another driver or pedestrian. | _____ | _____ | _____ | _____ |
| I do not allow my door to hit another parked car when I'm exiting or entering my car. | _____ | _____ | _____ | _____ |
| I avoid using my high beams in the city or when there is oncoming traffic. | _____ | _____ | _____ | _____ |

**Points to Ponder:**   Consider the following questions:

1. As you reflect on the items in the list, what are the driving situations that anger you the most?

2. How do you handle these situations? What could you do to handle them better?

3. How many of the statements in the list reflect your driving habits? What might you do to improve your current patterns of behavior?

4. In your opinion, what should be done about aggressive driving?

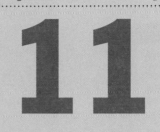

# Taking Reponsibility for Drug Use

## ONLINE LEARNING CENTER

Log on to our Online Learning Center (OLC) for access to these additional resources:

- Chapter key term flashcards
- Learning objectives
- Additional goals for behavior change
- Concentration game
- Self-scoring chapter quizzes
- Additional lab activities

The OLC also offers Web links for study and exploration of wellness topics. Access these links through **www.mhhe.com/anspaugh8e.**

## GOALS FOR BEHAVIOR CHANGE

- Make more informed decisions about alcohol, tobacco products, and other drugs.
- Assess your personal attitudes about drugs and drug use behavior.
- Discontinue any risky behaviors related to drug use.
- Develop a personal safety plan for your use of alcohol.

## Objectives

After completing this chapter, you will be able to do the following:

✔ Identify reasons why people use drugs.
✔ Define specific terms associated with drugs and drug use.
✔ Explain how drugs are classified.
✔ Describe the dangers associated with the use of various drugs.

---

### [ Key Terms ]

| | |
|---|---|
| addictive behavior | mainstream smoke |
| alcohol | marijuana |
| binge drinking | narcotics |
| caffeine | nicotine |
| caffeine toxicity | passive smoking |
| cocaine | psychoactives |
| depressants | reward deficiency |
| designer drugs | syndrome |
| drug | sidestream smoke |
| inhalants | stimulants |

Quality of life is a frequently used term that refers to the "how" of life—how well you live, how healthy you are, how much you are able to accomplish your goals, and how happy you are. The primary determinants of quality of life are the decisions you make that affect your life either positively or negatively. As suggested by this book, a high quality of life balances the physical, mental, emotional, social, and spiritual needs of a person for optimal health, satisfaction, and enjoyment. Achieving this goal means making intelligent choices—ones that contribute to your well-being—both for the moment and for your future. To make informed choices, you must have accurate information and you must understand that your actions have consequences. The decisions you make are cumulative. As time goes on and as you age, the consequences of previous decisions, actions, habits, and modes of behavior increasingly affect the way your body and your mind function. The emphasis of much of this book is on personal behaviors, such as exercise, weight maintenance, proper nutrition, and the prevention of disease through lifestyle. Other factors and decisions also influence your quality of life.

This chapter deals with drugs. Drug use or nonuse can strongly affect your health and quality of life. Drugs used for treatment, cure, prevention, or relief of pain or disease are categorized as medicines. Many people are alive because of the therapeutic effect of drugs used to prevent or manage disease and maintain health. However, not all drugs are used as medicines. When usage involves reasons other than medicinal, even if usage is considered recreational, the potential exists for tragic consequences. Understanding potential problems can help you make wiser decisions about drug use.

## Reasons for Drug Use

A **drug** is any substance that kills organisms (such as bacteria and fungi) in the body or that affects body function or structure.[1] A drug has also been defined as "any substance, natural or artificial, other than food, that by its chemical or physical nature alters structure or function in the living organism."[2] (Other terms that may be important for understanding drugs are listed in Just the Facts: Understanding Drug Terminology.) People use drugs for many reasons. Some need drugs for health reasons—to maintain a normal life or to alleviate symptoms or complications of diseases or other conditions. Others indulge in drugs to alter their moods. Researchers have identified several reasons people use drugs:[3]

- *Medicinal purposes:* Medicines are used for a wide range of purposes—from reducing symptoms of the cold and flu or treating headaches to lowering blood pressure or cholesterol to extend life and maintain quality of life. People who suffer from chemical imbalances, such as with bipolar disorder or depression, would be unable to live normal lives without the availability of certain drugs. Methylphenidate (Ritalin), commonly used illegally as a stimulant, is also used to treat adults and children who have attention-deficit disorder. When used in this capacity, Ritalin frequently helps such people focus on and complete tasks—something difficult for these people to do without medical intervention. Medicines, although dangerous even under a physician's supervision if misused or prescribed incorrectly, are invaluable to many for maintenance of an active, positive lifestyle.

- *Recreational/social facilitation:* People frequently use drugs with the belief that they will lessen the tension associated with social encounters. Marijuana and alcohol are particularly popular in social situations. Potential dangers of using drugs for this purpose include mental dependency on the drug and an inability to cope with social events without using the drug.

- *Sensation seeking:* Some people enjoy taking risks. For them, drugs fulfill the need for excitement and adventure. Others turn to drugs out of boredom or a feeling of inadequacy in their lives. Unfortunately, when they become tolerant to the drug or they do not find the type of "high" they were looking for, users frequently turn to increasingly dangerous drugs or to increased doses to provide equivalent or more exciting thrills.

- *Religious or spiritual factors:* Throughout history, people have used drugs to enhance their spirituality or to achieve spiritual states of awarenesses. Too often in these situations, the drug becomes the object of worship. Though many people have tried, the spiritual realm has not been achieved through the use of mind-altering drugs.

- *Altered states:* Drugs are sometimes used to increase the intensity of a mood or create a state of euphoria. Some people attempt to enhance physical performance or stimulate artistic creativity. Evidence indicates that perceptions of improved abilities induced by drugs are false.

- *Rebellion and alienation:* The use of drugs can be a deliberate act of rebellion against social values, especially the values of parents or society. Many people who experience extreme pressures and have difficulty coping turn to drugs as an escape. These people include college-age stu-

# [ JUST THE FACTS ]

## Understanding Drug Terminology

Following are possibly unfamiliar terms that are useful for understanding the effects of substances:

- *Addiction:* Compulsive, uncontrollable, chronic dependence on a drug or drugs to the degree that severe emotional, mental, or physiological reactions occur; a desire to use drug(s) contrary to legal and/or social prohibitions

- *Alcohol:* Generally refers to grain alcohol or ethanol as opposed to other forms of alcohol that are too toxic for ingestion

- *Antagonistic:* Opposing or counteracting

- *Binge drinking:* Consuming five or more drinks in a row for males and four in a row for women

- *Dependence:* The need to continue using a drug for physical and/or psychological reasons

- *Designer drugs:* Illegally manufactured psychoactive drugs similar to controlled drugs on the FDA's schedule

- *Drug:* Any substance, except food, that upon entering the body alters its function

- *Drug abuse:* The excessive and pathological use of a drug that has dangerous side effects

- *Drug misuse:* The use of a drug for purposes other than intended

- *Effective dose:* The amount that produces the desired effect

- *Habit:* As pertains to drug use, a patterned, regular, and possibly involuntary involvement with a particular drug

- *Lethal dose:* The amount capable of causing death

- *Medicines:* Drugs used to prevent illness or to treat the symptoms of an illness

- *Narcotic:* A morphinelike substance that relieves pain and induces a stuporous state.

- *Over-the-counter (OTC) drugs:* Nonprescription drugs

- *Physical dependence:* A physiological need for a drug

- *Polyabuse:* The use of multiple drugs

- *Potentiating:* An exaggerated drug response obtained when two drugs are taken together; a much greater effect is obtained than when either drug is taken separately

- *Prescription drugs:* Drugs obtained only by order of a physician or dentist

- *Psychoactive:* Affecting mood and/or behavior

- *Psychological dependence:* An emotional or a mental need to use a drug

- *Synergistic:* A combined effect greater than the sum of the individual effects when two or more drugs are used at the same time; the combination produces an exaggerated effect or a prolonged drug action

- *Therapeutic index:* The difference between the minimum amount of a drug needed for a therapeutic effect and the minimum amount that has a toxic concentration or effect

- *Toxic dose:* The amount that produces a poisonous effect

dents facing academic pressure and increased personal freedom.

- *Peer pressure and group entry:* People who have a great desire to feel accepted socially often use drugs to demonstrate their sameness with other members of their group. People claim to use drugs to feel accepted, to imitate people they admire, and to attempt to create an identity or project a specific image. Self-esteem seems to be a vital component. People with high self-esteem see themselves as competent, successful, self-sufficient, accepting, outgoing, and well rounded. People with low self-esteem tend to feel isolated and unloved and have a reduced capacity for joy or self-fulfillment. To overcome these sensations and perceptions, many people turn to drugs.

- *Curiosity:* Many people first experiment with drugs out of curiosity—the desire to see what using the drug feels like or what the attraction is for chronic users. Although curiosity is normal and healthy in many circumstances, the primary problem associated with experimentation with drugs out of curiosity is the inability to know how a drug will affect any one person. Whereas one person may consider the effects of a drug pleasurable, someone else may have a different, even fatal, reaction. Most people try alcohol during their lives. For most people, this creates no problem; they can choose to use it or not use it. For some people, however, one act of curiosity about alcohol can result in the disease of alcoholism.

## [ JUST THE FACTS ]

### What's the Cause of Addiction?

*Addiction* has been defined as "a condition characterized by the compulsive abuse of a drug or drugs."[4] In other words, addiction is a pathological relationship with a substance that has life-damaging potential. Following are some theories about addiction:

- The spectrum of addictions ranges from alcohol and tobacco to behavior such as eating and working.

- The causes of addiction are complex and interrelated. A number of interacting variables may contribute to the development of addiction.

- Variables that may contribute to addiction include genetics, family influences, friends, life events, social and cultural values, availability, and personality.

- Studies indicate that some inherited traits may lead to alcoholism.[5] For instance, alcoholics may have an inherited inability to determine their levels of intoxication when drinking alcoholic beverages.

- Studies have found that addictive, impulsive, and compulsive disorders may have a common genetic origin.[6] These disorders may result from the failure

of cells to signal molecules in the brain's reward system, so that the brain is unaware of certain sensations of pleasure or success. This failure is viewed as a type of sensory deprivation of the brain's pleasure mechanisms. The manifestation of this disorder is referred to as **reward deficiency syndrome.**

- Personality type, temperament, and attitudes may also contribute to drug use and addiction.

- Personality traits associated with drug abuse include rebelliousness, resistance to authority, independence, and low self-esteem. In addition, people who abuse drugs seem to have a high tolerance for deviance in others, place a low value on education and religion, display low levels of competence in task performance, have low degrees of obedience, and have an underdeveloped sense of diligence.[7]

- Because innumerable circumstances, factors, and conditions influence personality and predisposition to addiction, it has not yet been determined whether predetermination of addiction is chemical, genetic, or psychological.

---

The reasons any person uses drugs are usually not easily categorized. (List yours in Assessment Activity 11-2.) Most drug use situations depend on personality, experience, perceptions of the environment, and expectations (see Just the Facts: What's the Cause of Addiction?).

## What Causes Addiction—a Model

A variety of models are used to explain why addiction develops. The disease model of addiction, also known as chemical dependency, has been favored for many years. According to this model, alcoholics are medical patients who need treatment rather than condemnation. Today most experts purport to rely on the *biopsychosocial model of addiction.* According to this theory, addiction is due to the interaction of different individual and social pathologies, as well as biochemical and genetic factors. The primary factors addressed in the biopsychosocial model include biological, environmental, psychological, and social interaction elements. This model incorporates the majority of theories that have been used in an attempt to explain addiction and is considered the most comprehensive

and holistic body of theory and practice today. This more holistic approach allows for the frequent outcome of most treatment, which is relapse, and addresses this issue through psychological vulnerability assessments while incorporating other factors to explain why one person becomes alcoholic and another one doesn't—even if both are from the same genetic and social family. The following are the basic tenets of the theory.

Studies investigating genetic influences toward addiction indicate a strong tendency to run in families. In several studies, children of parents who were drug-addicted were much more likely to engage in drug-taking behaviors than were the children of nonaddicted parents.[8,9] The correlation remained consistent even if the children did not live with their addicted parents.

Oakley Ray states that "no genetic physiological or biochemical marker has been found that strongly predicts alcoholism or any other addiction."[10] However, researchers who believe in biological causes of addiction have found that addicted people metabolize mood-altering substances differently than nonaddicted individuals. Some studies have found that adult children of alcoholics have abnormal concentrations of

**TABLE 11-1**  Addictive Behaviors

| | |
|---|---|
| Compulsion | Excessive preoccupation/obsession with a behavior or preoccupation with the need to perform it |
| Loss of control | Loss of the ability to control an action or a behavior; inability to block the impulse to engage in a behavior |
| Escalation | More of an activity is needed in order to produce a desired effect. This requires more time and frequently more monies directed toward the behavior. |
| Denial | Inability or refusal to see or comprehend that a behavior is destructive or the extent of its destructiveness |
| Negative consequences | Serious negative consequences, including academic, family/personal relationships, health, legal, and financial |

neurotransmitters that affect mood (endorphins, enkephalins, norepinephrine, and serotonin). Theoretically, abnormal levels of these hormones cause mood disorders, which lead individuals to seek mood-altering drugs.[11]

Psychological makeup has been considered a contributing factor for a long time. People have even spoken of the "addictive personality," indicating that certain behaviors tend to be found in people who become addicted to alcohol or other drugs. Individuals who become addicted tend to have lower self-esteem and seek positive reinforcement from others. They may also be having more trouble managing life events (fewer coping skills) in a positive way and want someone else to solve their problems rather than reacting more aggressively to situations.

Social learning theory states that people learn by watching others and that much **addictive behavior** (behavior that is excessive, compulsive, and psychologically and physically destructive) is learned. The tendency for addictions to run in families could be due to the behavior children learn about how to spend their spare time or what to do when faced with a difficult or traumatic situation. If the family of origin tends to drink or use other drugs, then the child learns the same behavior.

In general, children who feel unloved or insecure or who feel as if they cannot "be themselves" or are abused are more likely to engage in addictive behaviors. Throughout life, when people are faced with traumatic or extremely difficult situations, such as the loss of a spouse, addictive behaviors are more likely to surface.

Habit and addiction are not the same. Addiction is defined by continued involvement in a behavior in spite of ongoing negative consequences. Examples of addictive behaviors are listed in Table 11-1.

## Drug Classification

Drugs can be classified in a number of ways. For example, they can be classified according to legality (legal or illegal), whether their effects are primarily physiological or psychological, or whether their use has more medicinal benefits or a greater potential for abuse. The last system is based on the Controlled Substance Act of 1970, which classifies **narcotics** and other dangerous drugs. The system contains five classifications called *schedules*. Schedule I drugs have no medical use and a high potential for abuse (such as heroin and LSD); schedule II through V drugs have approved medicinal uses with varying potentials for abuse and significant psychological and physical dependence. Excluded from this classification system are two of the most deadly drugs found in modern society: alcohol and tobacco products.

Drugs are also classified according to the physiological effect they have. Categories include stimulants, depressants, hallucinogens, narcotics, and inhalants. Two other types are also important. Designer drugs are manufactured to mimic the effects of drugs found in the previously mentioned categories, and marijuana, or cannabis, is difficult to classify but is usually included as a hallucinogen. Depending on the dose, marijuana can mimic a variety of substances found in other categories. The following is a list of drug categories and the effects they have on the body:

- *Stimulants:* **Stimulants** speed up the central nervous system, producing an increase in alertness and excitability. Examples are amphetamines, **cocaine,** crack cocaine, methamphetamines, and drugs such as Ritalin and phentermine (Ionamin).
- *Depressants:* Also known as *sedatives* and *tranquilizers,* **depressants** slow down the central nervous system, causing a feeling of relaxation. Examples of the depressant drugs are barbiturates; methaqualone (Quaaludes, or "quad"); and tranquilizers such as diazepam (Valium), chlordiazepoxide HCl (Librium), and meprobamate (Miltown).
- *Psychoactives:* **Psychoactives** can alter feelings, moods, and/or perceptions. Marijuana is classified as a psychoactive drug but can exhibit effects similar to those of stimulants, depressants, and narcotics. Some examples of psychoactive drugs

are lysergic acid diethylamide (LSD), mescaline, peyote, phencyclidine (PCP), and psilocybin.

- *Narcotics:* Narcotics are powerful painkillers. They also produce pleasurable feelings and induce sleep. The narcotic drugs include codeine, heroin, methadone, morphine, opium, and substances such as oxycodone (Percodan), propoxyphene (Darvon), pentazocine (Talwin), and difenoxin (Lomotil).
- *Inhalants:* **Inhalants** are volatile nondrugs that cause druglike effects if inhaled. Examples are glue and gasoline. Some, such as nitrous oxide and amyl nitrate, have medical uses.
- *Designer drugs:* **Designer drugs** are drug analogs (newly synthesized products that are already outlawed or for which no law yet exists) of amphetamines, methamphetamines, narcotics, and hallucinogens manufactured in illegal laboratories to mimic controlled substances. They are often more powerful and less predictable than the drugs they imitate. The number and variations of designer drugs available are increasing rapidly.

Currently, three main types of illegal synthetic analog drugs are available: (1) analogs of phencyclidine (PCP); (2) analogs of synthetic narcotic analgesics, such as Demerol; and (3) analogs of amphetamines and methamphetamines. Perhaps one of the best-known analogs in the third category is MDMA, known as *ecstasy* or *Adam.* It is widely used in the college setting as a euphoriant.[12]

## Commonly Abused Substances

This section briefly examines some of the most well-known and frequently used drugs—caffeine, alcohol, tobacco products, designer drugs, club drugs, cocaine, and marijuana. This section is not intended to be all-inclusive. A wide range of other substances are potentially dangerous if misused or abused. Because these drugs are so frequently used, it is important for you to understand their positive and negative effects, so that you can make decisions based on information rather than myth.

### Caffeine

**Caffeine** is probably the most commonly used drug in American society. The average American adult consumes 280 mg of caffeine daily.[13] Caffeine is a stimulant that speeds heart rate, temporarily increases blood pressure, and disrupts sleep. It also relieves drowsiness, helps in the performance of repetitive tasks, and improves work ability.[14] Negative effects include insom-

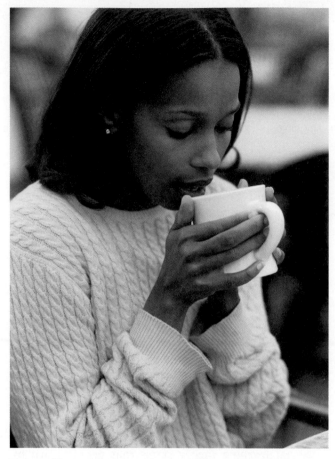

Today, millions of Americans ingest caffeine in some form.

nia, anxiety, heart dysrhythmias, gastrointestinal complaints, dizziness, and headaches.

The active ingredient in caffeine belongs to a group of drugs with similar structures known as *xanthines.* Xanthines include a substance found in cocoa beans, which are used to make chocolate, and in tea leaves. In the past, caffeine consumption was thought to cause birth defects, breast-feeding problems, cardiovascular disease, cancer, and fibrocystic breast disease. Current research has found no substantial association with these conditions.[15] However, pregnant and nursing women should consume no more than two cups of coffee a day and should consume tea and caffeinated soft drinks only in moderation (less than 300 mg per day).[16] Furthermore, women who suffer from premenstrual syndrome (PMS) should eliminate caffeine. Research has indicated that women who drink one-half to four cups (25 to 200 mg) of caffeinated tea a day are twice as likely to suffer PMS symptoms as are women who drink none at all.[17]

Most adults can consume relatively low doses of caffeine (the equivalent of two to three cups of coffee per day) safely. Approximately 10% of the adult population experiences *caffeinism,* a condition in

# [ JUST THE FACTS ]

## What Products Contain Caffeine and How Much?

| Item | Milligrams of Caffeine | |
| --- | --- | --- |
| | Typical | Range* |
| **Coffee (8-oz. cup)** | | |
| Brewed, drip method | 85 | 65–120 |
| Instant | 75 | 60–85 |
| Decaffeinated | 3 | 2–4 |
| Espresso (1-oz. cup) | 40 | 30–50 |
| **Teas (8-oz. cup)** | | |
| Brewed, major U.S. brands | 40 | 20–90 |
| Brewed, imported brands | 60 | 25–110 |
| Instant | 28 | 24–31 |
| Iced (8-oz. glass) | 25 | 9–50 |
| **Some soft drinks (8 oz.)** | 24 | 20–40 |
| **Energy drinks (8 oz.)** | 65 | 33–500 |
| **Cocoa beverage (8 oz.)** | 6 | 3–32 |
| **Chocolate milk beverage (8 oz.)** | 5 | 2–7 |
| **Milk chocolate (1 oz.)** | 6 | 1–15 |
| **Dark chocolate, semisweet (1 oz.)** | 20 | 5–35 |
| **Baker's chocolate (1 oz.)** | 26 | 26 |
| **Chocolate-flavored syrup (1 oz.)** | 4 | 4 |

*Due to brewing method, plant variety, brand, and so on.

which frequent high dose use causes psychological and physical problems. Doses as low as 250 mg per day can produce restlessness, nervousness, excitement, insomnia, flushed face, diuresis, muscle twitching, rambling thoughts and speech, and stomach complaints. Doses greater than 1 gram per day can cause muscle twitching, rambling thoughts and speech, heart dysrhythmias, and motor agitation. Higher doses can cause ringing in the ears and flashes of light.[18] (See Just the Facts: What Products Contain Caffeine and How Much? for caffeine amounts found in various products.)

Soft drinks can be a substantial source of caffeine intake, particularly the products labeled as energy drinks. Retail sales of energy drinks increased 54% from 2002 to 2006. Caffeine levels in energy drinks can range from 50 mg to a whopping 505 mg per can or bottle. Caffeine levels are not always listed on the labels of these drinks, and many manufacturers avoid regulated limits on caffeine in food products by identifying their product as a dietary supplement.[19] Energy drinks are frequently marketed as performance enhancers, but caution must be exercised when using these products to avoid what is known as **caffeine toxicity**. High levels of caffeine may actually impact performance negatively and cause tremors, nausea, dizziness, and chest pain. Extreme caution should be exercised when combining energy drinks with alcohol consumption.[20]

## Alcohol

**Alcohol** use is pervasive. Alcohol is a drug generally deemed socially acceptable. Nevertheless, no other drug causes so much physical, social, and emotional damage to people and their families. People drink alcoholic beverages in many situations and for many reasons. They drink when they are among friends and when they are upset or depressed. People drink to spark romantic feelings, to put themselves at ease in social situations, and to celebrate special occasions. In addition, people drink because their role models drink and because the advertising industry has convinced them that alcohol contributes to self-enhancement. Unfortunately, the devastation associated with alcohol is often not mentioned. Table 11-2 (page 374) summarizes the short- and long-term effects of the drug. Because society has labeled alcohol appropriate and

**TABLE 11-2** Effects of Alcohol Use

| Number of Drinks* | Blood Alcohol Concentration (BAC) | Effect(s) | System/Organ | Health Risks |
|---|---|---|---|---|
| | **Short-Term or Immediate** | | **Long-Term** | |
| 1–2 | 0.00–0.05 | Usually relaxation and euphoria; decrease in alertness | Breast | 50% higher risk for cancer in women who drink any alcohol; 100% increase for women having three or more drinks per day |
| 2–3 | 0.05–0.10 | Exaggerated feelings and behavior; emotional instability; increased reaction time and diminished motor coordination; impaired driving; a legally drunk designation in most states | Cardiovascular | High blood pressure; irregular heartbeat; chest pain/angina; myocardial infarctions; damage to coronary arteries |
| 4–5 | 0.10–0.15 | Loss of peripheral vision; highly impaired driving ability; unsteady walking/standing | General gastrointestinal | Risk for mouth, tongue, throat, esophageal, stomach, and liver cancer; pancreatitis; malnutrition; digestive impairment |
| 5–10 | 0.15–0.30 | Significant impairment of sensory perceptions; slurred speech; decreased sensitivity to pain; difficult and staggering walk | Immune system | Lower resistance to infectious diseases |
| | | | Liver | Hepatitis; cirrhosis |
| | | | Pancreas | Interference with insulin production |
| 10+ | > 0.30** | Stupor or unconsciousness; anesthetization; possible death at levels greater than 0.35 | Small intestine | Interference with or prevention of absorption of proteins, iron, calcium, thiamine, and vitamin $B_{12}$ |
| | | | Stomach | Bleeding from irritation, ulcers |
| | | | Muscular system | Destruction of muscle fibers |
| | | | Nervous system | Destruction of brain cells; interference with neurotransmitters; slowing of reaction time |
| | | | Reproductive system | Impotence; decreased testosterone production; fetal alcohol syndrome; miscarriage |

*1 drink = 12 oz. beer, 6 oz. wine, 1 oz. hard liquor.

** > greater than

even necessary for some occasions, abstinence may seem unrealistic for many people.

As with many drugs, there are times and places where medicinal and health reasons are cited for alcohol use. Current research suggests that moderate amounts of alcohol may help reduce the risk for heart disease. The possible benefits and pleasures of the use of alcoholic beverages do not eradicate the dangers that result from misuse or abuse, however (see Assessment Activity 11-1). Nearly half of annual traffic deaths are caused by accidents involving alcohol consumption. This figure does not include permanent physical injuries and emotional damages caused by alcohol-induced traffic accidents and deaths, nor does it include the increased number of violent acts associated with alcohol intoxication. Drinking of alcohol, if

it occurs, ought to be approached responsibly, with recognition of the potential for harm to self and others. Real-World Wellness: Responsible Drinking provides suggestions for responsible drinking.

Although there are several types of alcohol, the intoxicating agent in all alcohol drinks is ethyl alcohol, a colorless liquid with a sharp, burning taste (see Just the Facts: How Much Alcohol Is in Beer, Wine, and Other Drinks?). The percentage of alcohol in a beverage is measured by its proof, twice the percentage of alcohol. A beverage that is 40% alcohol has a proof of 80. The blood alcohol concentration (BAC) is the percentage of alcohol content in the blood. This percentage determines the alcohol's effect on a person (Table 11-2). The more quickly the alcohol is absorbed, the quicker the BAC increases.

## Real-World Wellness

### Responsible Drinking

*I enjoy an occasional drink, and I often invite friends to my home to celebrate holidays and special events. How can I make sure I'm drinking and hosting parties responsibly?*

Following are suggestions to help each person be a responsible drinker and host:

- Drink slowly; never consume more than one drink per hour.
- Eat while drinking, but do not eat salty food.
- When mixing drinks, measure the amount of alcohol; never just pour.
- Serve and choose nonalcoholic drinks as an alternative.
- As host, always serve the guests or hire a bartender. Do not have an open bar or serve someone who is intoxicated.
- Stop using or serving alcohol 1 hour before a party is over.
- Don't drink and drive. Have a nondrinker drive or call a cab.

Alcohol enters the bloodstream quickly from the stomach and even more quickly from the small intestine. In the stomach, food inhibits absorption of alcohol. Food does not affect absorption in the small intestine.[21]

## [ JUST THE FACTS ]

### How Much Alcohol Is in Beer, Wine, and Other Drinks?

Did you know that all of the following contain the same amount of alcohol? Each contains the equivalent of 3 ounces of pure alcohol. A 160-pound person who consumed these amounts within a 2-hour period would be considered legally intoxicated in most states:

- Six 12-oz. glasses of beer
- 15 ounces of fortified wine (about two glasses)
- 24 ounces of table wine (about four glasses)
- Six servings of liquor (1.3 oz. of 80 proof)
- One measure of vermouth
- One jigger (1.5 oz.) of whiskey

Following are some other factors that affect the rate of absorption and effect of alcohol:

- *Rate of consumption:* How quickly is the beverage consumed? Large amounts of alcohol quickly consumed expose the brain to higher peak concentrations, altering perceptions and response times.
- *Type of beverage:* Beer and wine contain substances that slow the rate of absorption; thus, the effects are experienced more slowly than are the effects of drinking distilled spirits, even when the same amount of alcohol is consumed. Carbonated beverages added to liquor speed absorption, but diluting them with water slows the process.
- *Body weights:* Body weight and body composition do not influence the rate of absorption, but they do influence the effects of alcohol. More weight and/or more muscle mass (muscle with more fluid volume than fat) results in a greater distribution of the alcohol, lowering its concentration in the body and weakening its effects.
- *Tolerance to alcohol:* Some people seem to remain sober, while others react quickly to the same amount of alcohol. One drink for a novice may have the same effect as three drinks for a more experienced drinker. This indicates that the experienced drinker's body has adapted to the alcohol at the cellular level and is encouraging increased consumption. Tolerance consists of an increase in the rate of alcohol absorption metabolism as well as a reduced response to the drug. It is the reduced response that is frequently associated with physical and psychological dependence. Increased tolerance to alcohol can also result in a decreased response to other drugs, specifically other central nervous system depressants.

Alcoholism is a disease in which a person loses control over drinking. According to a definition approved by the National Council on Alcoholism and Drug Dependence and the American Society of Addiction Medicine, alcoholism is a "primary, chronic disease with genetic, psychosocial, and environmental factors influencing its development and manifestations. The disease is often progressive and fatal."[22] An alcoholic is a person who suffers from the disease of alcoholism. For alcoholics, alcohol increasingly becomes the focus of life, and family, social, work, or school responsibilities become less important and are eventually disrupted by the desire and need for alcohol. Some alcoholics make this transition rapidly, whereas others maintain the appearance of being social drinkers for many years. Unfortunately, predetermining who will have trouble with alcohol is impossible. Alcoholism crosses all social and economic barriers and can affect everyone from

# Wellness for a Lifetime

## Alcohol and Tobacco Use Among Young Women

At one time, it was thought that alcohol-related problems occurred more often in men than women. Now mounting evidence indicates that women—especially young women—are drinking more. This fact is reflected in the increased number of admissions of younger women to treatment centers.[24] Women who are alcoholics often drink for reasons different from those that prompt men to abuse alcohol, and some of the consequences of drinking are different between the genders. Smoking, too, poses special risks for women, especially those who are pregnant. Here are some of these gender differences:

- More women than men who abuse alcohol can identify a specific triggering event that prompted them to start drinking, such as a death, a divorce, a job change, or the departure of a child from home.
- Women tend to begin abusing alcohol later in life than men do and to progress more quickly in their abuse pattern.
- Women are prescribed more mood-altering drugs than men are and are thus at greater risk for drug interactions and cross-tolerance.
- Alcoholic women are less likely than men are to have a family support system to aid them in their recovery attempts.
- Women alcoholics tend not to receive as much social support as men do during their treatment for and recovery from alcoholism.
- Women tend to have more financial problems than men do, which makes entry into a treatment program more difficult.[25]

Here are some alcohol- and tobacco-related effects of concern to parents and couples considering pregnancy:

- The children of pregnant women who drink are at a high risk for fetal alcohol syndrome (FAS), which causes a variety of birth defects, including abnormal eye alignment, nose and jaw irregularities, cleft palate, joint defects, heart defects, and inadequate brain development. FAS has been reported in children of women who drank as little as 30 milliliters of alcohol per day (about two mixed drinks, three bottles of beer, or two glasses of wine). Thus it is recommended that women abstain from drinking any alcohol during pregnancy.
- Babies born to mothers who smoke have a lower average birth weight and length and have a smaller head circumference.[26]
- Infants born to mothers who smoke are more likely than children born to nonsmokers to die from sudden infant death syndrome (SIDS).[27]
- Smoking during pregnancy may cause hyperactivity in children.

Finally, men and women who smoke should know the following:

- Smoking by both men and women is associated with premature facial wrinkling.
- Osteoporosis (loss of calcium from the bones) is associated with smoking.

---

clergy, medical doctors, high school students, and college students to professors.

Women who are alcoholics face unique problems, and women who use alcohol or tobacco during pregnancy put their children at risk of developing certain health problems. The rate of alcoholism is increasing among younger women (see Wellness for a Lifetime: Alcohol and Tobacco Use Among Young Women).

There is no single accepted reason any person becomes an alcoholic. Most researchers think that a variety of events, genetic tendencies, and situations working together result in alcoholism for some people. The medical model of alcoholism includes biological, or genetic, explanations of abuse. It views alcohol abuse as uncontrollable because of physiological differences between alcoholics and nonalcoholics. Research seems to link alcoholism to an inherited susceptibility, or predisposition, for the disease:[23] Children of alcoholic parents are four times more

likely to become alcoholics even when raised by nonalcoholics.

Treatment for alcoholism is often long term (see Just the Facts: The 12-Step Program). The course of treatment usually occurs in three stages: (1) detoxification (eliminating the alcohol from the body), (2) medical care (attending to any health-related problems), and (3) the changing of long-term behavior (helping the recovering alcoholic overcome long-established drinking patterns and destructive behaviors). Several sources provide long-term medical and psychological support to people with alcohol or other drug problems.

Alcoholics remain alcoholics for life, regardless of whether they drink. Recovering alcoholics must therefore be careful about any products they consume, including medicines and mouthwashes, which sometimes contain alcohol. Currently, an estimated 10 million adults and 3 million adolescents under the age of 18 are alcoholics.[28]

## [ JUST THE FACTS ]

### The 12-Step Program

Twelve-step programs remain the basis of most addiction recovery programs. The first step in all 12-step programs is the individual's admitting that he or she is powerless over alcohol, and step 2 is seeking a higher power to help him or her get the strength needed to change. The 12-step program states that successful treatment and change require six principles of change:[33]

1. Believing you can change is the key to change.
2. The type of treatment is less critical than individual commitment to change.
3. Brief treatments can change behaviors as successfully as longer interventions.
4. Life skills can be the key to licking addiction.
5. Repeated efforts are critical in change.
6. Improvement without abstinence counts.

While Alcoholics Anonymous says abstinence is vital, this approach says getting better counts and that most people will not succeed the first time they try to quit. What do you think?

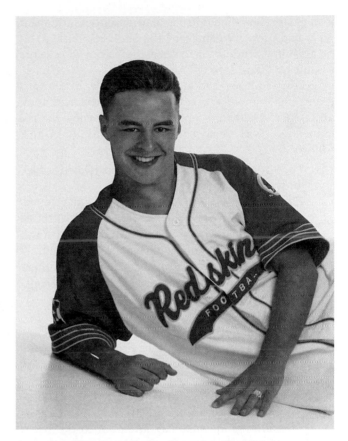

Jason Alan Bitter was killed on November 19, 1994, by a drunken driver who crossed the center line. The offender's BAC was .36, more than three times the legal limit in Missouri. Dina Khoury-Hager was also killed in the crash. Both were 17 years old and would have graduated from college in 1999.

Alcohol use has been demonstrated to have a strong association with crime and violence. Data clearly indicate that homicide is more likely to occur in a situation in which drinking has occurred.[29] In the same study, all incidents of spouse and child abuse were correlated with drinking. A Canadian study found that at least 42% of violent crimes involved alcohol.[30] In addition, 75% of suicide attempts involved alcohol use.[31]

As explained in Chapter 10, alcohol and driving can be a lethal combination. Alcohol is linked to at least half of all highway fatalities, and this figure includes only crashes involving drivers classified as legally intoxicated. Finally, in single-vehicle fatal wrecks occurring on weekend nights, the driver is legally intoxicated almost 70% of the time.[32]

### Binge Drinking Among College Students

**Binge drinking** is defined as consuming five or more drinks in a single session for men and four or more for women at least once within the previous 2 weeks. According to a national survey conducted by the Harvard School of Public Health, nearly half of college students surveyed drank four or five drinks in the 2 weeks preceding the survey.[34] Another study reported that 39% of college women binge drank within a 2-week period before the survey.[35] In a multicampus survey, American Indian or Alaska Native students reported the highest percentage of binge drinking in a 2-week period (58%), followed by whites (23.8%), not Hispanic or Latino (22.6%), and black or African Americans (18.4%).[36]

For a discussion of how much alcohol is contained in various types of alcoholic drinks, review Just the Facts: How Much Alcohol Is in Beer, Wine, and Other Drinks? on page 375.) This information is alarming in light of the number of deaths in the last few years caused by binge drinking during fraternity or campus rituals. Problems associated with student binge drinking include residence hall damage, fights, sexual assault, and drunken driving. The greater a student's alcohol use, the poorer his or her academic performance.[37] The most distressing fact is that binge drinking too often causes unnecessary deaths of drinkers, their friends, and other innocent victims. Consider these facts: Seventy-five percent of students reporting for a study on binge drinking indicated adverse consequences as a result of another student's binge drinking. Seventy-one percent had sleep or study interrupted; 57% had to take care of an intoxicated student; 36% had been insulted or humiliated; 23% had a serious argument; 16% had property damage; 11% had been pushed, hit, or assaulted; and 1% had been the victim of a sexual assault or "date rape."[38]

Many colleges and universities have begun programs that emphasize responsible, rather than total, abstinence. Guidelines published for reducing the risk associated with heavy or binge drinking are as follows.

1. *Pace your drinking.* Allow time between drinks and sip the drink.
2. *Do not drink every day.* Tolerance is developed and a person must increase the amount of alcohol consumed before effects are noticed. BAC is still rising even though effects are unnoticed.
3. *You decide when to drink.* Do not allow others or situations to determine your drinking. Drink on your terms.
4. *Consider alternating nonalcoholic drinks with those containing alcohol.* Drink a soft drink without alcohol every other drink or drink plain orange juice every other drink.
5. *Don't drink on an empty stomach.* Food with fats and/or protein slow the absorption of the alcohol.
6. *Measure the alcohol.* Pay attention to the size of containers. Do not provide kegs of beer or use larger wine, beer, or shot glasses. Do not participate in "chugging" contests or other drinking games.
7. *Avoid using energy drinks or high-caffeine products while drinking.* The buzz from caffeine can disguise the effects of the alcohol.
8. *Don't drink for more than 1 hour.* Decide what nonalcoholic drink you are going to drink after the hour.
9. *Learn how to calculate your BAC.* Know how many drinks are allowed within your hour period.
10. *If you are a female, drink less.* Women become more intoxicated than men after drinking the same amount of alcohol, even when differences in body weight are taken into account. Women have proportionately less water in their bodies than men; thus, women become more highly concentrated in BAC.
11. *Avoid taking over-the-counter (OTC) or prescription medications.* More than 100 medications interact with alcohol. If you are taking any OTC or prescription drugs, ask your doctor or pharmacist whether you can safely drink alcoholic beverages.

Fortunately, most college students moderate their drinking after their college years. However, about 12%

are unable to control their drinking and continue to abuse alcohol. You should weigh carefully the potential harmful consequences of alcohol use and abuse before partaking in binge or heavy drinking.

## Tobacco Products

All tobacco products, including cigarettes, cigars, pipes, and smokeless tobacco (snuff and chewing tobacco), contain the drug **nicotine**. Nicotine is an addictive substance and an alkaloid poison. It affects the body by increasing heart and respiratory rates, elevating blood pressure, increasing cardiac output and oxygen consumption, and constricting the bronchi (the two main branches of the trachea that lead to the lungs). A person inhales nicotine when smoking a tobacco product. Nicotine in smokeless tobacco is absorbed through membranes of the mouth and cheek.

Smoking is directly or indirectly responsible for various conditions and diseases. Some components of cigarette smoke are known as *carcinogens* (substances that cause cancer or foster the growth of cancer cells). Nicotine, tar, and carbon monoxide are found in cigarette smoke. The tar in tobacco is a black, sticky, dark fluid composed of thousands of chemicals. Many of the chemicals found in tar are cancer-causing. Carbon monoxide is a deadly gas emitted in the exhaust of cars and in burning tobacco. The carbon monoxide level in cigarette smoke is 400 times greater than what is considered safe in industrial settings. Carbon monoxide binds to hemoglobin more readily than oxygen does, interfering with the ability of blood to transport oxygen to the body. Carbon monoxide impairs the nervous system and increases the risk for heart attacks and strokes.

The addictive nature of nicotine has come under substantial public scrutiny. Some experts consider nicotine to be as addictive as cocaine and other drugs. Tobacco is considered the leading preventable contributor to disease and early death in the United States (from heart disease and cancer, specifically) and is listed as a primary risk factor for heart disease by the American Heart Association. Cigarettes are responsible for 442,000 deaths annually.[39] Because of the health risks and because of what many view as an effort by tobacco companies to intentionally increase nicotine addiction to increase the sales of cigarettes, some people suggest that tobacco should be made an illegal drug.

### Secondhand and Sidestream Smoke

**Passive smoking** is the inhalation by a nonsmoker of what is known as *secondhand cigarette smoke* from the environment. Smokers inhale what is known as **main-**

stream smoke; passive smokers most frequently inhale **sidestream smoke,** which results from burning tobacco products (the end of the lighted tip of a cigarette, cigar, or pipe).[40] Because it is not filtered by either a cigarette filter or the smoker's lungs, sidestream smoke contains higher concentrations of carbon dioxide and carbon monoxide. For each pack of cigarettes smoked indoors by a smoker, a nonsmoker in the vicinity passively smokes the equivalent of three to five cigarettes.[41] Research shows that nonsmokers living with smokers have a 20% higher mortality rate than do the non-smoking partners of nonsmokers. The bottom line about passive smoking is that there is no safe level of exposure to tobacco smoke.

### Cigars and Pipes

In the hope of avoiding the dangers associated with cigarette smoking, some smokers have turned from cigarettes to cigars or pipes. Since pipe and cigar smokers don't inhale, they do seem less likely to develop lung and heart disease. However, pipe and cigar smokers have a much higher risk of developing mouth, larynx, and esophageal cancers because they hold the nicotine and tars from their tobacco products in their mouths instead of inhaling them. Furthermore, when a cigarette smoker switches to cigars or a pipe, he or she tends to continue to inhale and, thus, to remain at the same risk for lung and heart disease while the risk of other cancers increases.[42]

### Smokeless Tobacco Products

Smokeless tobacco products consist of snuff and chewing tobacco. Snuff is a finely shredded or powdered tobacco sniffed by the user, allowing nicotine to be absorbed through the mucous membranes of the nose and mouth. Chewing tobacco consists of loose-leaf tobacco mixed with molasses or other flavors and pressed into what are called *plugs* or twisted into rope-like strands. This material is then placed between the gums and cheek or lower lip, where the nicotine is absorbed. In 2003, about 3% of U.S. adults used smokeless tobacco; this represents 7% of adult men and 1% of women.[43]

Smokeless tobacco is not a safe alternative to cigarettes. It contributes to the development of periodontal (gum) disease, which can result in bleeding gums, loss of teeth, staining of teeth, and tooth decay. Periodontal disease is less significant than the oral cancers that may be caused by frequent contact of the cells of the gums and cheek with the carcinogenic agents in the tobacco. Two early danger signs of such cancers are leukoplakia (white spots) and erythroplakia (red spots), which indicate precancerous conditions; they should be evaluated by a physician imme-

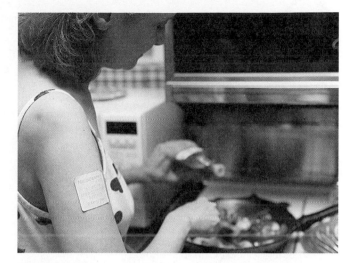

Many people have used nicotine patches to help them quit smoking. If you're a smoker, have you considered trying the patch?

diately. If treatment is delayed, cancer can quickly spread to the jaw, neck, brain, and digestive and urinary systems.[44]

### Clove Cigarettes

Some people smoke clove cigarettes, sometimes called bidis (pronounced "bee-dees"), as an alternative to regular cigarettes. Clove cigarettes usually consist of 60% tobacco and 40% clove buds. Clove cigarettes generate even more nicotine, tar, and carbon monoxide than do regular cigarettes, so the dangers are even greater. Tests have shown that clove cigarettes have 2–3 times more tar and nicotine than other American cigarettes. Some users have developed serious lung and respiratory illnesses.[45]

### Advantages of Quitting

Smoking is an extremely strong addiction. To quit completely, many people require the help of trained professionals (see Real-World Wellness: Charting a Plan to Quit Smoking or Stop Using Tobacco Products on page 380 and Real-World Wellness: Choosing a Smoking Cessation Aid on page 381). Although quitting is difficult, the health benefits gained far outweigh the problems. When people stop smoking, their risk of developing heart disease and some kinds of cancer (if not already present in the body) eventually decreases to that of nonsmokers; in other words, some of the effects of smoking are reversible (see Figure 11-1, page 380). Real-World Wellness: Choosing a Smoking Cessation Aid includes products that can help control cravings and stop smoking.

## Real-World Wellness

### Charting a Plan to Quit Smoking or Stop Using Tobacco Products

*I've tried several times to quit smoking, but I'm still lighting up. This time I want to be prepared. Is there a plan I can follow that will help me quit for good?*

The *Mayo Clinic Health Letter* offers the following suggestions:[46]

- *Set a date.* Make the date reasonably soon. Make a list of reasons you want to quit.

- *Start stopping before you reach the date.* Taper off the number of cigarettes you are currently smoking. Choose a milder brand.

- *Make your plans known.* Tell a friend, your family, and colleagues of your plans. Ask for their support.

- *Take it one day at a time.* Get up every morning and decide not to smoke that day. Focus your attention on that day only.

- *Change your routine.* Avoid or change situations in which you have previously smoked.

- *Alter your surroundings.* Start new activities, such as exercising or needlepoint.

- *Time the urge.* Identify when your urge to smoke is the strongest. Being prepared will help you resist.

- *Use substitutes.* Substitutes can include gum, celery, carrots, and pickles.

- *Prepare a daydream.* Have a pleasant daydream ready to help fight off the desire to smoke. This can be an image of yourself without a cigarette in a situation you find highly desirable.

- *Use relaxation techniques.* Deep breathing or progressive muscle relaxation can help.

- *Stay busy.* Find ways to keep yourself and your mind occupied, so you do not miss smoking or having a cigarette in your hand.

- *Practice positive thinking.* Tell yourself, "I can make it." Remember that you can do it.

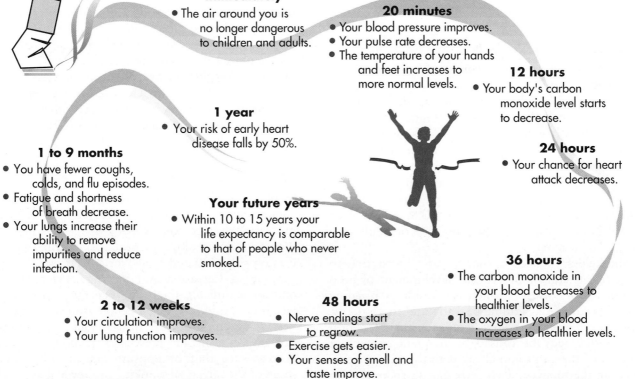

**Your first year as a nonsmoker**

**Immediately**
- The air around you is no longer dangerous to children and adults.

**20 minutes**
- Your blood pressure improves.
- Your pulse rate decreases.
- The temperature of your hands and feet increases to more normal levels.

**12 hours**
- Your body's carbon monoxide level starts to decrease.

**24 hours**
- Your chance for heart attack decreases.

**1 year**
- Your risk of early heart disease falls by 50%.

**1 to 9 months**
- You have fewer coughs, colds, and flu episodes.
- Fatigue and shortness of breath decrease.
- Your lungs increase their ability to remove impurities and reduce infection.

**Your future years**
- Within 10 to 15 years your life expectancy is comparable to that of people who never smoked.

**36 hours**
- The carbon monoxide in your blood decreases to healthier levels.
- The oxygen in your blood increases to healthier levels.

**2 to 12 weeks**
- Your circulation improves.
- Your lung function improves.

**48 hours**
- Nerve endings start to regrow.
- Exercise gets easier.
- Your senses of smell and taste improve.

**FIGURE 11-1** Health Benefits of Quitting Smoking

Quitting smoking results in benefits that begin immediately and become more significant the longer a person stays smoke-free.

## Real-World Wellness

### Choosing a Smoking Cessation Aid

*I've been smoking since my freshman year in high school, and I'm about to graduate from college and enter the workforce. I'd like to quit, but I'm confused about all the smoking cessation products available. How do I choose the one that's best for me?*

Several tools are available to help smokers wean themselves off cigarettes. These smoking cessation aids can be purchased over the counter (OTC) or with a doctor's prescription. The dosages for both versions can vary widely. For this reason, it is probably better to seek a prescription version, which will be targeted more specifically to your needs. Read the following information about three commonly used methods, and then talk to your doctor to choose the one best suited to your needs.

• *Nicotine-containing gum:* Nicotine gum requires immediate smoking cessation. The dosage is 2 to 4 mg of nicotine per piece of gum. When used under a physician's guidance, the success rate is about 40%. Chewing the gum may cause mouth ulcers and nausea in some people, and the product should not be used by pregnant or nursing women. Initial doses of the chewing gum cost about $50, and weekly refills cost about $30.

• *Transdermal patches:* The patch is designed to aid smoking cessation by relieving nicotine withdrawal cravings. Two types are available: a step-down version and a single-dose version. The single-dose version provides the same milligrams of nicotine in each dose (15 mg). The step-down version provides different levels of nicotine for various periods after cessation, theoretically reducing the amount of nicotine available as the person is weaned away from the drug. The step-down method is designed to ease withdrawal by making the symptoms less severe and withdrawal more gradual. The patches contain 15 to 21 mg of nicotine a day for the first weeks. After 4 to 12 weeks, the dosage is reduced to 10 to 14 mg a day. A final set of patches used for 2 to 4 weeks contains 5 to 7 mg of nicotine. Single-dose patches eliminate the step-down effect. Used alone, both versions of the patch seem to be less than 25% effective. When used with the prescription medication mecamylamine, however, the effectiveness rate rises to 40%. The patch can cause skin irritation, redness, and irregular heart rate in some users. The cost is about the same as for nicotine-containing gum.

*Nicotrol*TM *inhaler:* A federal advisory panel to the FDA has endorsed a prescription inhalation device that is an alternative to chewing gum and transdermal patches. The Nicotrol inhaler is meant to simulate cigarette smoking. The device has a mouthpiece with a nicotine plug attached to it. Seventy to 80 puffs on the inhaler provide the amount of nicotine in 10 puffs on a regular cigarette. Having the inhaler to handle may help smokers who miss having something to do with their hands while providing a low level of nicotine to ease cravings.

## Illegal Drugs

### Designer Drugs/Club Drugs

Designer drugs resemble those controlled by the Food and Drug Administration (FDA); that is, they act like known drugs but have a different chemical composition. Probably the two best-known designer drugs currently being used are *China white,* an analog of heroin, and *ecstasy.* Ecstasy is an analog of the amphetamines and hallucinogens under FDA control since 1985. Designer drugs appear so rapidly that it is difficult or impossible to restrict sales. Poor quality control and combinations with other, often poisonous, substances can result in neurological damage or death. Brain damage is often caused by a single dose.

Club drugs are among a group of drugs used by teens and young adults who are part of a bar, rave, or trance scene. Raves and trances are generally nightlong dances, often held in warehouses. Not everyone attending these events uses drugs, but those who do are attracted to the low cost, the seemingly increased stamina, and the intoxicating highs said to increase the rave or trance experience.[47]

The drugs of concern are MDMA (ecstasy), Rohypnol, GHB, and ketamine. Researchers are finding that critical parts of the brain are showing changes from the use of these drugs. When used in higher doses, most of these drugs can cause a sharp increase in body temperature, which leads to muscle breakdown, cardiovascular incidents, and kidney failure.[48]

## MDMA (Ecstasy)

MDMA is a chemical substance that combines methamphetamines with hallucinogenic (LSD-like) properties. Ecstasy is the street name for MDMA. Other names include Adam, X-TC, hug, beans, love bug, clarity, and lover's speed. Ecstasy is a combination of several illicit drugs. Because so many different recipes are used to make ecstasy, the risk for death and permanent brain damage is heightened. The drug works primarily by affecting nerve cells that produce serotonin, one of several chemicals transmitting signals from one nerve to the next. Ecstasy causes nerve cells to release all the stored serotonin at once and then keeps it from being reabsorbed, further increasing the concentration in the synapse. The result can lead to long-term or permanent damage to those areas of the brain critical to thought, memory, and pleasure.[49] The aftermath of use can include a depressive hangover, sometimes called "Terrible Tuesday." Other psychological effects are confusion; sleep problems; severe anxiety; paranoid thinking; enhanced mental and emotional clarity; sensations of floating; and violent, irrational behavior. These problems can occur during and sometimes days or weeks after taking MDMA. Some reported physical effects of the drug include muscle tension, involuntary teeth clenching, blurred vision, hypertension, loss of control over voluntary body movements, tremors, kidney failure, heart attack, stroke, seizures, and malignant hyperthermia (increased body temperature).[50]

Additionally, animal research has shown that long-term use of MDMA has led to neurotoxicity with damage to serotonin nerve terminals. This damage was evident 6 to 7 years after the animals' consumption of the drug. Granted, similar results have not been demonstrated in humans, but with the plethora of animal research available, it is clear that MDMA is not a safe drug for human consumption.[51] Unfortunately, in 2008 an estimated 2.1 million people in the United States ages 12 and older used MDMA in a given 30-day period of time. The good news in this statistic is that it represents a 1% decrease in use from 2008.[52]

## Rohypnol

Rohypnol, a trade name for flunitrazepam, has been a serious concern for several years because of its abuse in date rape (see Chapter 10). When mixed with alcohol, Rohypnol incapacitates its victims and prevents them from resisting sexual assault. Slang names for the drug include rophies, roofies, roach, and rope. The drugs (alcohol and Rohypnol) produce a form of amnesia, in which individuals may not remember events they experienced while under the effects of the drugs. Further, Rohypnol may be lethal when mixed with alcohol or other depressants.[53] Abuse of two other similar drugs appears to have replaced Rohypnol abuse in some regions of the country. These are clonazepam (Klonopin in the United States) and alprozolom, marketed as Xanax.

## GHB

GHB (gamma-hydroxybutyrate) has been abused in the United States for euphoric, sedative, and anabolic (bodybuilding) effects. It is a central nervous system depressant that was widely available over the counter in health food stores during the 1980s and until 1992. It was purchased mostly by bodybuilders to aid in muscle building and fat reduction. Street names include liquid ecstasy, soap, easy lay, and Georgia home boy. GHB is difficult to distinguish from water. Coma and seizures can occur with abuse and, when it is combined with methamphetamines, there appears to be an increased risk for seizure, nausea, and difficulty breathing. Withdrawal effects include insomnia, anxiety, tremors, and sweating. The drug is sold over the Internet and is available in some workout gyms, rave night clubs, gay male parties, and college campuses, as well as on the street. The duration of the drug is short, but it may cause unconsciousness when mixed with alcohol.[54]

## Ketamine

Ketamine is an anesthetic approved for both human and animal use in medical settings. Over 90% of the drug sold legally is used for practice of veterinary medicine. ketamine can be injected or snorted. On the street, it is known as special K or vitamin K. At high doses, ketamine can cause delirium, amnesia-impaired motor function, high blood pressure, depression, and potentially fatal respiratory problems. Certain doses can cause dreamlike states and hallucinations. Because of these last characteristics, it has become common in club and rave scenes and has been used as a date rape drug.[55]

## How to Protect Yourself from Being a Victim of Designer Drugs/Club Drugs

If you go to parties or clubs and drink alcohol, you are at increased risk for becoming a victim of date rape drugs. GHB has been used most in California, Texas, Georgia, and Florida. Rohypnol has been used extensively across the South, but it has been most used in Texas, where it is popular among high school students.

There are behaviors you can use to help defend yourself. If you are at a party or club, never leave your drink unattended. Cover it with your hand in between sips (not gulps) to discourage anyone from tampering with it. Even if you are not drinking an alcoholic drink, use caution. Go out with friends you can trust and watch out for each other. Double date instead of going alone. At a party, accept a drink only in a closed can or container. Never drink from punch bowls or drink anything that tastes or smells strange. If drinking a mixed drink, make sure you watch the bartender prepare it. Always be aware of your surroundings (don't get so incapacitated that you cannot do this; that is, drink moderately, so you can keep your wits about you) and trust your instincts. If you feel ill, do not wait to get help but seek out a safe person you can trust (*never* a stranger or someone whom you do not know very well).

## Cocaine

At one time, **cocaine** was considered the drug of upper-class America. Unfortunately, the use of cocaine and its derivative, crack, is now epidemic. In 2007, the National Survey on Drug Use and Health (NSDUH) estimated that 2.1 million persons reported using cocaine in the last month, and 610,000 were current crack users. The highest rate of cocaine use was by adults aged 18 to 25 years.[56]

A powerful stimulant, cocaine is derived from the leaves of the South American coca shrub and ground into a crystalline powder. The most common methods of using the drug are snorting it, liquefying it and then injecting it, and freebasing (smoking). When snorted, the white powder is sniffed up through the nose. The most potent and expensive method of cocaine use is freebasing. The drug is usually smoked in a water pipe because this provides faster absorption into the bloodstream.

Crack is relatively easy to make and fairly inexpensive to buy. At $10 to $15 a dose, crack is the form of cocaine most prevalent on the streets. When snorted, crack reaches the brain in about 5 minutes. When injected or smoked, the drug takes effect in only a few seconds.

The use of cocaine produces feelings of well-being, euphoria, and extreme exhilaration. Mental alertness seems to increase. Blood vessels constrict, causing heart rate and blood pressure to rise. Cocaine is rapidly metabolized by the liver. Snorting cocaine results in a 5- to 15-minute "high," and the effects of crack last 20 to 30 minutes. Psychological and physical dependency on crack develops rapidly because of the brief period of stimulation. The feelings of exhilaration experienced while under the influence of the drug are quickly followed by depression.

The physical consequences of cocaine use are extreme and highly dangerous. Cocaine use can cause headaches, exhaustion, shaking, blurred vision, nausea, impaired judgment, hyperactivity, loss of appetite, loss

of sexual desire, and paranoia that can lead to violence. Snorting cocaine can destroy the septum in the nose. Freebasing may damage the liver and the lungs; fluid buildup in the lungs caused by freebasing has resulted in death. Cocaine can initiate strokes, bleeding in the brain, heart attacks, irregular heartbeat, and sudden death.[57]

Cocaine addiction is extremely difficult to overcome. Addiction researchers currently believe a broad-based treatment program, including medical, psychiatric, pharmacological, and psychosocial elements, is the most successful.

## Marijuana

In the 1960s, **marijuana** became a cultural phenomenon, the symbol of one generation's disregard for or anger with another. The marijuana found on the streets at that time, however, lacked the potency of current crops. The crossbreeding of more potent varieties, improved cultivation, and the use of different parts of the plant all contribute to increased levels of delta-9-tetrahydrocannabinol (THC), the major psychoactive drug found in marijuana. Some marijuana currently grown in the United States rivals the previously stronger varieties of Mexico, Jamaica, and other areas. The THC percentage of *Cannabis sativa* (the Indian hemp plant from which marijuana is derived) in plants grown in the United States can range from 2% to as high as 7%. A variety of marijuana known as *sinsemilla*, made from the buds of flowering tops of female plants, can have a potency as high as 24%.[58] The higher the percentage of THC, the more potent the drug. Marijuana is composed of the dried leaves and flowering tops of the cannabis plant. Hashish, which has stronger effects, is processed from the resin of the plant. The resin is either dried and pressed into cakes or sold in liquid form called *hash oil*. Marijuana is used more extensively than hashish in the United States.

It is estimated that each year there are 2.6 million new marijuana users. In 2008, 25.8 million Americans age 12 and older used marijuana at least once in the month prior to being surveyed. In 2002, marijuana was the third most commonly abused drug mentioned in hospital emergency department visits in the United States.[59]

More than 400 known chemicals constitute marijuana. More than 60 of these are *cannabinoids*, chemicals found only in cannabis. THC is the cannabinoid that appears to be most responsible for the sensations experienced by marijuana users. Cannabinoids are different from other drugs in that they are fat-soluble rather than water-soluble; they have a decided affinity for binding to fat in the human body. Although other drugs enter and then leave the body within relatively short periods, marijuana tends to attach to fatty organs, such as the gonads and brain, and remain.[60] A single ingestion of THC may require up to 30 days to be eliminated from the body.

Marijuana can be eaten in baked goods, such as brownies, but the effects tend to be less predictable. Because it better controls the amount ingested, smoking is generally a more efficient and powerful technique for achieving the desired effect. When inhaled, THC reaches the brain in as little as 14 seconds. Hashish is so concentrated that a single drop can equal the effects of an entire marijuana joint (cigarette). Cannabis products are difficult to classify but are considered hallucinogens by many researchers.

Small doses or the short-term use of marijuana creates sensations of euphoria and relaxation often accompanied by hunger or sleepiness. Time seems to slow, and the senses appear heightened. Memory of recent events, physical coordination, and perceptions may be impaired. Students, for example, may have difficulty remembering events that occurred when they were high. Even with small amounts of marijuana, driving ability can be affected. Physiologically, heart rate speeds up and certain blood vessels become dilated, which may create problems for people with any types of heart problems. One study indicated that an abuser's risk of heart attack more than quadruples in the first hour after smoking marijuana.[61] Some users experience anxiety, panic, and paranoia. In rare cases or with stronger doses, people may suffer from a sense of depersonalization, image distortion, and hallucinations. Chronic use seems to lead to behavior changes that in some people may be permanent. Lack of motivation or interest in activities unrelated to drug use is one result. Use by teenagers leads to impaired thinking, poor reading comprehension, and reduced verbal and mathematical skills.

All the long-term effects of marijuana use have not been determined. This is partly because of the lesser potency of marijuana used previously. In addition, people vary greatly in their responses to the drug. Chronic users may experience psychological dependence and need increased doses as tolerance develops. Very heavy users experience withdrawal symptoms of restlessness, irritability, tremors, nausea, vomiting, diarrhea, and sleep disturbances.[62]

Physically, marijuana appears to be more carcinogenic than tobacco. Known carcinogens occur in larger amounts in marijuana, and when marijuana is smoked, the smoke is held in the lungs. Cannabis smoke contains more tar than does tobacco smoke. Marijuana use quickly affects pulmonary function adversely, and long-term use causes cellular changes in the lungs. People who have angina pectoris (chest pains associated with heart disease) may be significantly at risk because more oxygen is required during marijuana use.

Marijuana binds readily to hemoglobin, reducing the amount of oxygen carried to the heart and other tissues.

Many people consider cannabis an aphrodisiac. Over time it has the opposite effect, depressing the sex drive and causing impotence. Regular male users show a decrease in sperm count and reduced motility of sperm. Proportionately, more sperm appear abnormally shaped, a phenomenon associated with lessened fertility. In women, THC blocks ovulation. Pregnant women who smoke marijuana frequently use other drugs, all of which have a detrimental effect on the fetus. Marijuana also depresses the immune system.[63]

Therapeutic use is still being explored. At this time, the most promising application seems to be as an antinausea drug for chemotherapy patients. Glaucoma patients may have access to and may use marijuana to reduce intraocular pressure (pressure within the eye).[64]

Marijuana is an illegal drug. As with alcohol and all other drugs, the way a person reacts to marijuana or is most adversely affected by it cannot be predicted. People do not begin use with the intention of having a drug become the focus of their lives, but some ultimately allow the drug to control them. Marijuana is a drug with that potential.

## Other Drugs of Concern

The drugs discussed in the following sections have been abused for many years. Unfortunately, some that had become less popular seem to be reappearing, along with a dangerous new generation of illicit drugs. All illegal drugs have quality-control problems: Because there is no federal regulation of these drugs and because people involved in the transportation and distribution of illegal drugs are not always concerned about purity or quality, dangerous and even poisonous substances may be added to drugs. Also, it is frequently impossible to determine the potency of a drug. A very pure form of a drug can easily be lethal for a person who has been using a less potent form.

### Heroin

Heroin is a narcotic synthesized from morphine. This drug induces a strong sensation of euphoria but quickly leads to physical and psychological dependency. The physical tolerance for heroin develops rapidly. Because heroin is usually injected, addicts often share needles, which increases the risk of contracting diseases such as AIDS and hepatitis. Experts fear the younger generation may become addicted to heroin through a substance called *moonrock*—a mixture of heroin and cocaine that can be injected, smoked, or snorted. Heroin is used in this way to reduce the paranoia and depression that follow a cocaine high. Heroin use is considered to be on the rise. Recent studies have suggested a shift from injecting heroin to snorting or smoking. This trend seems to have resulted from the misconception that these forms are safer.[65]

Heroin use has remained stable among junior high and high school groups according to research conducted in 2005. Usage for 8th, 9th, and 10th graders was reported at 1.5% for all three grades. More potent forms of heroin are available that allow the user to experience a more pronounced effect by snorting it instead of injecting it, which people may be reluctant to do in part because of fear of HIV transmission. In addition, many users believe that smoking or snorting heroin, unlike injecting it, is nonaddicting—obviously this is not true.[66] Users may not realize they are becoming addicted because they may function normally for some time after starting to use the drug before their behavior changes significantly enough for friends and family to become aware of their use.

## Methamphetamine (Crank)

Methamphetamine is a potent stimulant that can cause uncontrollable manic behavior or paranoid thinking. The most current use of this drug is as crystal methamphetamine, or *ice*. Methamphetamines are chemically related to amphetamines. Although crystal methamphetamine has been touted as a safe alternative to cocaine, evidence indicates otherwise. Recent headlines told about a father who, under the influence of methamphetamine, decapitated his son. Overdoses are often fatal, and the drug is extremely addictive. In many areas of the United States, the use of ice is a widespread problem. In many rural areas, the drug is manufactured because of the ease of preparation. Crank labs are especially found in the midwestern states of middle Illinois, Michigan, and Ohio.[67]

## Lysergic Acid Diethylamide (LSD)

LSD is a hallucinogenic drug that has become more popular, especially among the upper class. The substance induces altered perceptions of shapes, images, time, self, and sound. Although the effects of the drug are primarily emotional and sensory, users may experience increased heart rate and blood pressure, dry mouth, nausea, dizziness, and other physiological changes. Tolerance to the drug develops quickly with frequent use, and occasionally users experience long-term reactions like flashbacks (hallucinogen persisting perception disorder) or mild to moderate psychosis.[68]

## Phencyclidine (PCP)

PCP was originally intended for use as a surgical anesthetic for humans. However, the drug was determined unsuitable for this purpose because of its unusual and undesirable effects on patients.[69] Also called *angel dust, ozone, wack,* and *rocket fuel,* PCP provokes a variety of unpredictable responses in users. These reactions include feelings of unreality, depersonalization, confusion, depression, anxiety, aggressive and violent behavior, acute or permanent psychosis, and coma. At high doses, PCP causes dramatic changes in blood pressure, respiration, and pulse rate. This severe reaction may cause nausea, vomiting, blurred vision, and dizziness. Users often fail to experience sensations of pain and report feeling uncoordinated in their movements. Classified as a hallucinogen, PCP has been used as an additive to cocaine, a combination that multiplies the toxic effects of both drugs.

## Over-the-Counter Drugs

An area of drug use that is sometimes overlooked and assumed to be safe is the use of over-the-counter drugs (OTCs). The power of OTCs is often underestimated. As with all drugs, the ultimate responsibility for the correct use of OTC drugs rests with each person. Because OTCs are readily available, abuse is a possibility. OTCs may potentiate the effects of prescription drugs, herbs, vitamins, alcohol, or other OTCs, especially when not taken according to directions. OTCs can cause physiological damage to various body structures; symptoms range from disorientation to kidney or liver damage. Following are some guidelines for safe use of OTCs:[70]

- Always know what you are taking and the product's active ingredients.
- Know the drug's effects (including its undesired ones) and possible side effects. Be sure you understand how the drug is supposed to work.
- Read and heed warnings and cautions concerning the use of the product.
- Don't use any OTC product continuously for more than 2 weeks. If the problem for which you are taking the drug persists, consult your physician.
- Be particularly cautious if you are also taking any prescription drugs, because serious interactions can occur.

**Nurturing Your Spirituality**

### Finding Alternatives to Drug Use

The best treatment for any alcohol or other drug abuse problem is to prevent it. Adolescents and college-age students need attractive alternatives to drugs, such as participation in organizations or groups that fulfill in safe, constructive ways their need for camaraderie, acceptance, and group involvement. These organizations or groups can be developed around athletics, recreational activities, career development, or service opportunities. Involvement in enjoyable and meaningful activities tends to discourage drug use by providing a strong reinforcement system that helps people feel good about themselves and their abilities. All people, young and older, need a positive group atmosphere that fosters self-esteem, develops participants' ability to help others, and provides role models who pursue selfless, achievement-oriented goals.

At the college and university level, students aged 25 and younger may be faced with an autonomy never before experienced when they leave home to go to school. They are faced with the fact that no one is standing over them to ensure their attendance at and productivity in school, at work, or in other areas. Their decision-making power is increased as well as is the pressure to conform to peer standards, many of which they are encountering for the first time. This newfound freedom sometimes requires a continuation of prevention education and activities that direct them toward positive activities and behaviors. University administrators should seek to make such programs highly visible within the institutions they serve. It is helpful for everyone connected with a college or university to demonstrate positive behaviors concerning the prevention of drug and alcohol abuse on campus. This may require

that the president not serve alcoholic beverages at receptions and that faculty actively discourage binge drinking and other dangerous forms of drinking and be willing to engage in activities outside the classroom that involve positive alternatives to alcohol and other drug use. Another important component of any alternative program is a strong peer education network, in which student leaders promote a healthy campus life by discouraging alcohol and other drug abuse and related problems, such as property destruction, violence, and sexual assault.

Other prevention-oriented programs are recreational activities, such as hiking, camping, and canoeing, and leadership challenge courses, such as rope courses and Outward Bound experiences. The programs should offer diverse opportunities that appeal to a wide variety of student interests. Art exhibits; musical events; movie or book clubs; and community service programs, such as Humanity for Mankind, can all offer further opportunities for students to engage in personally and socially beneficial activities. Having mentors assigned to incoming first-year students and holding group discussions of various problems associated with collegiate life, perhaps with mandatory attendance by first-year students, may also be helpful. In addition, the college or university should emphasize to students that the purpose of higher education is to gain the experience and expertise to better serve one's family, community, and country. To truly accept responsibility for their lives, all people need to understand and accept responsibility for their behavior and recognize that alcohol and other drug use never offers a long-term solution to personal, emotional, or spiritual difficulties.

---

- If you have any questions about an OTC product, consult a pharmacist.
- If you don't need a drug, don't use it.
- Three types of drugs are misused or abused most often:
  - *Opioids*, prescribed for pain relief.
  - *Central nervous system depressants,* and drugs prescribed for anxiety or sleep problems often referred to as sedatives or tranquilizers.
  - *Stimulants,* prescribed for attention-deficit hyperactivity disorder (ADHD) and narcolepsy, a sleep disorder.

### A Final Thought

To develop a high level of wellness, you must address the issue of drug use. Drugs prescribed as medicine can promote quality of life, but unwise use severely diminishes quality of life. Alcohol continues to be the most abused drug among college students. Perhaps as people become more aware of the dangers associated with alcohol and drug use, a smaller percentage of college students will use them (see Nurturing Your Spirituality: Finding Alternatives to Drug Use).

# Summary

- People use drugs for a variety of reasons, including for recreational or social enjoyment, to seek novel sensations, to enhance religious or spiritual experiences, to alter consciousness, to rebel or alienate oneself from society, and to submit to peer pressure.
- Drugs are commonly classified in a variety of ways, including according to their physiological effects.
- Caffeine is probably the most commonly used drug in the United States. It is a stimulant that speeds heart rate, increases blood pressure, and can cause insomnia.
- Caffeine in energy drinks can range from 50 mg to over 500 mg per can or bottle.
- Energy drinks are marketed as performance enhancers, but some individuals experience tremors, nausea, dizziness, and chest pain. This is referred to as caffeine toxicity.
- Alcohol is a socially acceptable drug that is a major source of physical and emotional damage and death.
- The blood alcohol concentration (BAC) of ethyl alcohol is affected by the rate of consumption, the type of alcoholic beverage being consumed, and the drinker's body weight and tolerance to alcohol.
- Binge drinking often occurs on college campuses and can lead to property destruction, sexual assault, and even death.
- Alcoholism is a disease in which a person loses control over drinking.
- Determining who will become an alcoholic is impossible because alcoholism crosses all social, economic, gender, educational, and racial lines.
- Nicotine is an addictive drug contained in tobacco. The tars found in tobacco are carcinogenic agents.
- No tobacco product is safe. Cigarettes, cigars, pipes, and smokeless products all pose threats to health.
- Carbon monoxide, formed when tobacco is smoked, interferes with the body's ability to transport oxygen and increases the risk for heart attack and stroke.
- Sidestream smoke has a higher concentration of tar and nicotine than the smoke inhaled by the smoker.
- Clove cigarettes contain even more nicotine and carbon monoxide than do regular cigarettes.
- Cocaine use has become epidemic in the United States. Cocaine can be snorted, injected, or freebased (smoked).
- The primary psychoactive ingredient in marijuana is delta-9-tetrahydrocannabinol.
- Carcinogens can be found in more potent levels in marijuana than in tobacco.
- Hashish is more potent than regular marijuana. Sinsemilla is a form of marijuana that can have a potency as high as 24%.
- Short-term effects of marijuana use include euphoria and perceptual impairment. Some people experience anxiety, a sense of depersonalization, and hallucinations.
- Some drugs, such as heroin, methamphetamine (crank), and LSD, have been abused in our society for many years.
- The newest form of methamphetamine is ice, which is smokable and more addictive, potent, and destructive than crack cocaine.
- Heroin use has been increasing among college and high school students.
- Designer drugs are analogs of controlled substances. They are more powerful, less pure, and have less predictable effects than do controlled substances.
- OTC drugs must be used carefully to avoid psychological and physiological problems.

# Review Questions

1. What are some reasons people choose to use drugs?
2. Discuss the ways in which drugs can be classified.
3. What are the positive and negative effects of caffeine use?
4. What factors affect a drinker's blood alcohol concentration (BAC)?
5. How can a person practice responsible drinking?
6. What are some potential effects of long-term alcohol use?
7. Discuss the risks of using any tobacco product.
8. Discuss the specific benefits of quitting smoking.
9. Why is heroin use increasing among high school and college students?
10. What makes cocaine such a dangerous drug?
11. What factors should you consider before using any OTC product?

# References

1. Pinger, R., W. Payne, D. Hahn, & E. Hahn. (1998). *Drugs: Issues for today.* Dubuque, IA: WCB/McGraw-Hill.
2. Ksir, C., C. Hart, & O. Ray. (2006). *Drugs, society, and human behaviors* (10th ed.). New York: McGraw-Hill.
3. Blum, K., & J. Payne. (1991). *Alcohol and the addictive brain.* New York: Free Press.
4. Ibid.
5. National Institute on Drug Abuse. (2001). Genetic factors in drug abuse and dependence. In *The biobehavioral etiology of drug abuse,* edited by H. W. Gordon & M. D. Glantz. Research Monograph, 159. Duarte, CA.
6. Blum, K., G. Cull, E. Braverman, & D. Comings. (1996). Reward deficiency syndrome. *American Scientist,* 84, 132–45.

7. National Clearinghouse for Alcohol and Drug Information. (2004). *Mind over matter—the brain's response to hallucinogens*. Rockville, MD: U.S. Government Printing Office.

8. National Institute on Drug Abuse (2001).

9. Morse, R. M., & D. K. Flavin. (1992). The definition of alcoholism. *Journal of the American Medical Association, 268*, 1012–14.

10. Ksir et al. (2006).

11. Blum & Payne (1991).

12. Hanson, G., & P. J. Venturelli. (2002). *Drugs and society* (7th ed.). Boston: Jones and Bartlett.

13. Juliano, L. M., & R. R. Griffiths. (2004). A critical review of caffeine withdrawal: Empirical validation of symptoms and signs, incidence, severity, and associated features. *Psychopharmacology, 176.*

14. Chawla, J., & A. Suleman. (2009). Neurologic effects of caffeine. Retrieved January 19, 2010, from http://emedicine.medscape.com/article/1182710-overview.

15. National Institutes of Health—Medline Plus. (2009). Caffeine in the diet. Retrieved from www.nlm.nih.gov/medlineplus/ency/article/002445.htm.

16. Ibid.

17. Rossignol, A. M. (1985, November). Caffeine-containing beverages and premenstrual syndrome in young women. *Am J Public Health, 75*(11), 1335–37. Retrieved January 9, 2010, from www.ncbi.nlm.nih.gov/pmc/articles/PMC1646701/.

18. Hansen & Venturelli (2002).

19. Chad J., A. Reissig, C. Eric, A. Strain, & R. R. Griffiths. (2009, 1 January). Caffeinated energy drinks—A growing problem. *Drug and Alcohol Dependence, 99*(1–3), 1–10.

20. Ibid.

21. Carroll, C. R. (2001). *Drugs in modern society* (5th ed.). Dubuque, IA: Wm. C. Brown.

22. Morse, R. M., & D. K. Flavin. (1992). The definition of alcoholism. *Journal of the American Medical Association, 268*, 1012–14.

23. National Institute on Drug Abuse. (1998). Biological vulnerability to drug abuse. Research Monograph 89. Retrieved from www.drugabuse.gov/pdf/monographs/download89.html.

24. Ikonomidocou, C., et al. (2000). Ethanol-induced apopototic neuro degeneration and the fetal alcohol syndrome. *Science, 287*, 1056–60.

25. American Academy of Pediatrics. (1998). *AAP releases new findings on teen and underage drinking*. Washington, DC: American Academy of Pediatrics.

26. Ibid.

27. Ibid.

28. Morse & Flavin (1992).

29. National Clearinghouse for Alcohol and Drug Information (2004).

30. Ksir et al. (2006).

31. Pinger et al. (1998).

32. Ksir et al. (2006).

33. Ibid.

34. Wechsler, H., et al. (1998). Changes in binge drinking and related problems among American college students between 1995 and 1997. *Journal of American College Health, 45*, 57–68.

35. National Institute on Alcohol Abuse and Alcoholism. (2003). Underage drinking: A major public health challenge. *Alcohol Alert, 59.*

36. Substance Abuse and Mental Health Services Administration (SAMHSA). Office of Applied Studies. (2005). *Binge drinking among underage persons. The national survey on drug abuse report*. Retrieved from www.drugabusestatistics.samhsa.gov.

37. Lyall, K. (1999). *Binge drinking in college: A definitive study in binge drinking on American college campuses: A new look at an old problem*. Report supported by the Robert Wood Johnson Foundation. Princeton, NJ: Robert Wood Foundation.

38. Alcohol Policies Project Center for Science in the Public Interest. (2006). Fact sheet: Binge drinking on college campuses. Retrieved from www.cspinet.org/booze/collfact/.htm.

39. American Cancer Society. (2009). Cancer facts and figures 2008. Atlanta, GA: American Cancer Society.

40. Mayo Clinic. (2008). Secondhand smoke: Avoid dangers in the air. Retrieved from www.mayoclinic.com/health/secondhand-smoke/CC00023.

41. Ibid.

42. MacKay, J., M. Eriksen, & O. Shafey. (2006). *The Tobacco Atlas* (2nd ed.). Atlanta, GA: American Cancer Society.

43. Ibid.

44. Pinger et al. (1998).

45. Action on Smoking and Health. (2001). Herbal cigarettes not safe. Retrieved from www.no.smoking.org/jan02/01-03.01-2.html.

46. Mayo Clinic. (2010). Quit smoking: Proven strategies to help you quit. Retrieved from www.mayoclinic.com/health/quit-smoking/SK00056.

47. National Institute on Drug Abuse. (2009). Retrieved from www.drugabuse.gov/infofacts/Clubdrugs.html.

48. Ibid.

49. National Institute on Drug Abuse. (2009). MDMA (ecstasy). Retrieved from www.drugabuse.gov/infofacts/ecstasy.html.

50. Ibid.

51. National Institute on Drug Abuse (2006).

52. Ibid.

53. National Institute on Drug Abuse. (2009). Rohypnol and GHB now covered with club drugs, fact sheet. Retrieved from www.drugabuse.gov/infofacts/Clubdrugs.html.

54. Ibid.

55. National Institute on Drug Abuse Research Report Series. (2009). Cocaine: Abuse and addiction. Retrieved from www.nida.nih.gov/DrugPages/Cocaine.html.

56. National Institute on Drug Abuse. (2009). Cocaine. Retrieved from www.drugabuse.gov/ResearchReports/Cocaine/cocaine.html.

57. Ibid.

58. Ksir et al. (2006).

59. Substance Abuse and Mental Health Service Administration. (2003). *National survey on drug abuse—Annual report*. Washington, DC: U.S. Government Printing Office.

60. Ksir et al. (2006).

61. Mittleman, M., et al. (2001). Triggering myocardial infarction by marijuana. *Circulation, 103*(23), 2805–09.

62. Ksir et al. (2006).

63. Ksir et al. (2006).

64. Ibid.

65. National Institute on Drug Abuse Research Report Series. (2005). Heroin: Abuse and addiction. Retrieved from www.drugabuse.gov/ResearchReports/heroin/heroin.html.

66. Ibid.

67. National Institute on Drug Abuse Research Report Series. (2006). Methamphetamine: Abuse and addiction. Retrieved from www.drugabuse.

gov/ResearchReports/Methamph/
Methamph.html.
68. National Institute on Drug Abuse Research Report Series. (2001). Hal-

lucinogens and dissociative drugs. Retrieved from www.drugabuse.gov/ResearchReports/hallucinogens/hallucinogens.html.

69. Ksir et al. (2006).
70. Hansen & Venturelli (2002).

## Suggested Readings

DeSena, J., J. Schaler, & J. Gerstein. (2003). *Overcoming your alcohol, drug and recovery habits: An empowering alternative to AA and 12-step treatment.* Tucson, AZ: Sharp Press.

This text is a self-help guide for those who have gone through Alcoholics Anonymous, Narcotics Anonymous, and other formal 12-step addiction treatments to overcome self-destructive beliefs and attitudes.

Gately, I. (2003). *Tobacco: A cultural history of how an exotic plant seduced civilization.* New York: Grove Press.

This text provides an excellent look at the complex history of tobacco from the time of Columbus to the present day. It is provocative and interesting reading.

Nakken, C. (1996). *The addictive personality: Understanding the addictive process and compulsive behavior.* Center City, MN: Hazelden.

This book examines genetic factors tied to addiction, cultural influences on addictive behavior, the progressive

nature of the disease, and the steps necessary for a successful recovery.

Owens, F. (2006). *The fabulous rise and murderous fall of the club culture.* New York: Broadway Books.

The book provides an overview of the notorious world of clubs and raves in the 1990. The author describes a coterie of hustlers, drug dealers, and "scene makers." Ultimately what is described is the personal harm and brokenness of the experience.

Prentiss, C. (2007). *The alcoholism and addiction cure.* Malibu, CA: Power Press.

The book is an excellent resource for anyone dealing with addiction or for anyone who knows someone dealing with addiction. A thought-provoking book that helps the reader examine his or her life.

Ruden, R. (2002). *The craving brain: A bold new approach to breaking free from drug addiction, overeating, alcoholism, and gambling* (2nd ed.). New York: Perennial.

This book offers an interesting comment concerning addiction. The author states that the roots of addiction are found in our genes and builds a solid foundation for his beliefs.

Sanders, B. (2006). *Drugs, clubs, and young people.* Burlington, VT: Ashgate Publishing.

The book offers insight into behaviors at raves and clubs. The book raises concerns surrounding young people who attend clubs and who use club drugs. Thoughtful presentation on sociological components of young people involved with the club lifestyle.

Walters, S., & J. Baer. (2006). *Talking with college students about alcohol.* New York: Guilford.

Provides readily applicable guidelines for helping deal with the alcohol problems on today's campuses. The text provides resources and practical advice helping students and administrators confront the problem.

**Name** _____ **Date** _____ **Section** _____

# Assessment Activity 11-1

## Do You Have a Drinking Problem?

Many self-tests have been published for people to use to determine whether they are alcoholics or have drinking problems. None can provide a definite diagnosis; deciding whether someone should seek help is usually a complex, subjective matter. One of the most popular printed self-tests appeared in a "Dear Abby" advice column, and it is offered here as a guide. If these questions seem to indicate that you or a friend needs to seek help, you should visit a counselor, psychologist, or physician experienced in the assessment of chemical dependency.

**Directions: Check all that apply.**

_____ 1. Have you ever decided to stop drinking for a week or so but lasted for only a couple of days?

_____ 2. Do you wish people would stop nagging you about your drinking?

_____ 3. Have you ever switched from one kind of drink to another in the hope that this would keep you from getting drunk?

_____ 4. Have you had a drink in the morning in the past year?

_____ 5. Do you envy people who can drink without getting into trouble?

_____ 6. Have you had problems connected with drinking during the past year?

_____ 7. Has your drinking caused problems at home?

_____ 8. Do you ever try to get "extra" drinks at a party because you did not get enough to drink?

_____ 9. Do you tell yourself you can stop drinking anytime you want, even though you keep getting drunk when you don't mean to?

_____ 10. Have you missed days at work (or school) because of drinking?

_____ 11. Do you have blackouts?

_____ 12. Have you ever felt that your life would be better if you did not drink?

If you checked four or more of these items, you should seek the guidance of a specialist in chemical dependency or seek help directly through Alcoholics Anonymous (AA) or a similar organization. It is acceptable to go to an open AA meeting, listen to what is being said, and decide for yourself if the program would be useful to you.

**Name** _____   **Date** _____   **Section** _____

# Assessment Activity 11-2

## What Are Your Reasons for Drug Use?

**Directions:** In the following table are listed various drugs and products that can affect your life either positively or negatively. Think about how you view each product and what the long-term and short-term conse- quences of use might be. You might wish to consult other sources to help you determine possible effects. In the last column, explain briefly why you choose to use or to refrain from using the drug or product.

| Drug | Possible Negative Effects | Possible Positive Effects | Reasons for Using or Not Using |
|---|---|---|---|
| Caffeinated drinks (tea, coffee, cola) | | | |
| Alcohol | | | |
| Cigarettes | | | |
| Pipe or cigar | | | |
| Cocaine (any form) | | | |
| Marijuana (any form) | | | |
| Designer drugs (any form) | | | |
| Heroin | | | |
| Over-the-counter medications | | | |

### Points to Ponder

1. Which drugs do you view positively?

2. Are you unsure of your feelings about any substance? If so, why?

3. What potential is there for abuse or misuse of any of the drugs (even those you have positive feelings about)? If so, what is the potential source of problems?

**Name** _____   **Date** _____   **Section** _____

# Assessment Activity 11-3

## Why Do You Smoke?

This assessment is designed to provide you with a score on each of six factors that describe many people's feelings toward smoking. Three of these factors represent the *positive* feelings people get from smoking. The fourth is the *reduction of negative feelings*, such as a decrease in tension or anxiety. The fifth factor concerns a "craving" for smoking, which represents a dependence on cigarettes. The final factor is *habit* smoking, which takes place in an absence of feeling, or when smoking is purely automatic.

Circle the number that most accurately describes how you feel about each statement.

|   |   | Always | Frequently | Occasionally | Seldom | Never |
|---|---|:---:|:---:|:---:|:---:|:---:|
| A. | I smoke cigarettes to keep myself from slowing down. | 5 | 4 | 3 | 2 | 1 |
| B. | Handling a cigarette is part of the enjoyment of smoking it. | 5 | 4 | 3 | 2 | 1 |
| C. | Smoking cigarettes is pleasant and relaxing. | 5 | 4 | 3 | 2 | 1 |
| D. | I light up a cigarette when I feel angry about something. | 5 | 4 | 3 | 2 | 1 |
| E. | When I have run out of cigarettes, I find it almost unbearable until I get them. | 5 | 4 | 3 | 2 | 1 |
| F. | I smoke cigarettes automatically without even being aware of it. | 5 | 4 | 3 | 2 | 1 |
| G. | I smoke cigarettes to stimulate me, to perk myself up. | 5 | 4 | 3 | 2 | 1 |
| H. | Part of the enjoyment of smoking a cigarette comes from the steps I take to light up. | 5 | 4 | 3 | 2 | 1 |
| I. | I find cigarettes pleasurable. | 5 | 4 | 3 | 2 | 1 |
| J. | When I feel uncomfortable or upset about something, I light up a cigarette. | 5 | 4 | 3 | 2 | 1 |
| K. | I am very much aware of the fact when I am not smoking a cigarette. | 5 | 4 | 3 | 2 | 1 |
| L. | I light up a cigarette without realizing I still have one burning in the ashtray. | 5 | 4 | 3 | 2 | 1 |
| M. | I smoke cigarettes to give me a "lift." | 5 | 4 | 3 | 2 | 1 |
| N. | When I smoke a cigarette, part of the enjoyment is watching the smoke as I exhale it. | 5 | 4 | 3 | 2 | 1 |
| O. | I want a cigarette most when I am comfortable and relaxed. | 5 | 4 | 3 | 2 | 1 |
| P. | When I feel "blue" or want to take my mind off cares and worries, I smoke cigarettes. | 5 | 4 | 3 | 2 | 1 |
| Q. | I get a real gnawing hunger for a cigarette when I haven't smoked for a while. | 5 | 4 | 3 | 2 | 1 |
| R. | I've found a cigarette in my mouth and didn't remember putting it there. | 5 | 4 | 3 | 2 | 1 |

**Source:** U.S. Department of Health and Human Services, Public Health Service. (2004). Publication No. (CDC) 75-8716.

Write the number you have circled after each statement in the corresponding spaces that follow. Add the scores down each column to get your totals. For example, the sum of your scores for A, G, and M gives you the total score for the first column.

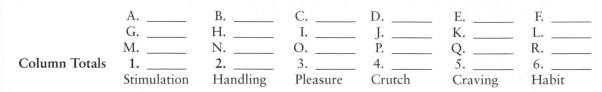

| | | | | | |
|---|---|---|---|---|---|
| A. _____ | B. _____ | C. _____ | D. _____ | E. _____ | F. _____ |
| G. _____ | H. _____ | I. _____ | J. _____ | K. _____ | L. _____ |
| M. _____ | N. _____ | O. _____ | P. _____ | Q. _____ | R. _____ |
| **Column Totals** 1. _____ | 2. _____ | 3. _____ | 4. _____ | 5. _____ | 6. _____ |
| Stimulation | Handling | Pleasure | Crutch | Craving | Habit |

In this test, a score of 11 or above on any factor indicates that smoking is an important source of satisfaction for you. The higher your score (15 is the highest), the more important a particular factor is in your smoking and the more useful the discussion of that factor can be in your attempt to quit. If you do not score high on any of the six factors, more than likely you do not smoke very much or have not been smoking for very many years. If so, giving up smoking—and staying off—should be easy.

The following categories describe motivations for smoking and suggest alternative activities to meet those needs.

1. **Stimulation**

   If you score high or fairly high on this factor, you are one of those smokers who is stimulated by the cigarette—you feel that it helps wake you up, organize your energies, and keep you going. If you try to give up smoking, you may want a safe substitute, such as a brisk walk or moderate exercise, whenever you feel the urge to smoke.

2. **Handling**

   Handling things can be satisfying, but there are many ways to keep your hands busy without lighting up or playing with a cigarette. Why not toy with a pen or pencil? Or try doodling. Or play with a coin, a piece of jewelry, or some other harmless object.

3. **Accentuation of Pleasure—Pleasurable Relaxation**

   It is not always easy to determine whether you use the cigarette to feel *good*—that is, get real, honest pleasure out of smoking (Factor 3)—or to keep from feeling *bad* (Factor 4). About two-thirds of smokers score high or fairly high on *accentuation of pleasure,* and about half of those also score as high or higher on *reduction of negative feelings.* Those who do get real pleasure out of smoking often find that honest consideration of the harmful effects of their habit is enough to help them quit. They substitute social and physical activities and find they do not seriously miss their cigarettes.

4. **Reduction of Negative Feelings, or "Crutch"**

   Many smokers use cigarettes as a kind of crutch in moments of stress or discomfort. But the heavy smoker, the person who tries to handle severe personal problems by smoking many times a day, is apt to discover that cigarettes do not help in dealing with problems effectively. When it comes to quitting, this kind of smoker may find it easy to stop when everything is going well but may be tempted to start again in a time of crisis. Again, physical exertion or social activity may serve as useful substitutes for cigarettes, even in times of tension.

5. **"Craving" or Dependence**

   Quitting smoking is difficult for the person who scores high on this factor. For the addicted smoker, the craving for a cigarette begins to build up the moment the cigarette is put out, so tapering off is not likely to work. This smoker must go "cold turkey." If you are dependent on cigarettes, it may be helpful for you to smoke more than usual for a day or two, so that the taste for cigarettes is spoiled. Then isolate yourself completely from cigarettes until the craving is gone.

6. **Habit**

   If you are smoking out of habit, you no longer get much satisfaction from your cigarettes. You just light them frequently without even realizing you are doing so. You may find it easy to quit and stay off if you can break the habit patterns you have created. Cutting down gradually may be quite effective if there is a change in the way the cigarettes are smoked and the conditions under which they are smoked. The key to success is to become aware of each cigarette you smoke. This can be done by asking yourself, "Do I really want this cigarette?" You may be surprised at how many you do not want.

You must make two important decisions: (1) whether to go without the satisfactions you get from smoking or find an appropriate, less hazardous substitute activity and (2) whether to cut out cigarettes all at once or taper off. Your scores on this test should guide you in making these decisions.

Name _____   Date _____   Section _____

# Assessment Activity 11-4

## How Much Does Smoking Cost You?

Cost of 1 pack of cigarettes:          _____
Number of packs per day you smoke: + _____
     *Cost per day*
Seven days per week:
        7 × _____ = _____
          (cost per day)    (cost per week)
52 weeks per year:
       52 × _____ = _____
         (cost per week)    (cost per year)

A pack of cigarettes is constantly increasing in price. Based on the current price of a pack of cigarettes, calculate the cost for a week and then the cost for a year. If you weren't spending money on cigarettes, what would you like to do with this money?

**Name** _____  **Date** _____  **Section** _____

# Assessment Activity 11-5

............................................................................................................

## Drug Diary

Each day for 2 weeks, record every drug you take on the following forms. Include any prescription and over-the-counter drugs as well as alcohol, nicotine, caffeine, and street (illicit) drugs. Record the exact type and amount of the drug taken and the setting in which you took the drug. Also make note of your mood (angry, happy, depressed, bored, etc.) at the time you used the drug. Finally, make note of your stress level at the time using the following level designations: 1. very relaxed; 2. low stress; 3. moderate stress; 4. very stressed. For this exercise to be a useful tool, you must be honest.

An example of a completed daily record follows.

**DATE:** Friday, December 4, 2004

|  | Type | Amount | Setting/Mood | Stress |
|---|---|---|---|---|
| Prescription | Birth control pill | 1 | Home | 1 |
| Over-the-counter | Tylenol | 2 | School/headache | 3 |
| Caffeine | Coffee | 1 cup | Home | 2 |
|  | Pepsi | 16 oz. | School—lunch | 2 |
| Nicotine | —— |  |  |  |
| Alcohol | Beer | 4 | Party | 2 |
| Steroids | —— |  |  |  |
| Street drugs | —— |  |  |  |

**DATE:**

|  | Type | Amount | Setting/Mood | Stress |
|---|---|---|---|---|
| Prescription |  |  |  |  |
| Over-the-counter |  |  |  |  |
| Caffeine |  |  |  |  |
| Nicotine |  |  |  |  |
| Alcohol |  |  |  |  |
| Steroids |  |  |  |  |
| Street drugs |  |  |  |  |

**DATE:**

|  | Type | Amount | Setting/Mood | Stress |
|---|---|---|---|---|
| Prescription |  |  |  |  |
| Over-the-counter |  |  |  |  |
| Caffeine |  |  |  |  |
| Nicotine |  |  |  |  |
| Alcohol |  |  |  |  |
| Steroids |  |  |  |  |
| Street drugs |  |  |  |  |

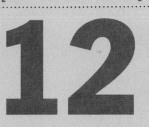

# Preventing Sexually Transmitted Infections

## ONLINE LEARNING CENTER

Log on to our Online Learning Center (OLC) for access to these additional resources:

- Chapter key term flashcards
- Learning objectives
- Additional goals for behavior change
- Concentration game
- Self-scoring chapter quizzes
- Additional lab activities

The OLC also offers Web links for study and exploration of wellness topics. Access these links through **www.mhhe.com/anspaugh8e.**

## GOALS FOR BEHAVIOR CHANGE

- Make choices regarding your personal sexual behavior.
- Practice safer sex if you have chosen to be sexually active.
- Take responsibility for the potential consequences of your sexual behavior.
- Learn how to talk with your partner about your sexual history.

## Objectives

After completing this chapter, you will be able to do the following:

- ✔ Discuss the difference between being HIV positive and having AIDS.
- ✔ Identify the signs and symptoms of various STDs.
- ✔ Evaluate the risks of having multiple sex partners.
- ✔ Discuss the meaning of having a monogamous relationship.
- ✔ Identify safer sex practices.

## [ Key Terms ]

abstinence
acquired immunodefi-
    ciency syndrome (AIDS)
chlamydia
cunnilingus
fellatio
genital warts
gonorrhea
hepatitis B

herpes
human immunodeficiency
    virus (HIV)
safer sex
sexually transmitted infec-
    tions (STIs)
syphilis
viral hepatitis

exuality is a lifelong part of a person's life, affecting and being affected by relationships, anatomy, behaviors, thoughts, and values. Sexual behavior is only one aspect of sexuality.

Decisions concerning sexual behavior have many far-reaching consequences. These choices can enhance or severely diminish feelings of well-being. Sex can be wonderful and fulfilling but may also cause serious problems. This chapter examines some of the **sexually transmitted infections (STIs)** that can result when people engage in behavior that puts them at risk. The chapter also identifies how to avoid contracting and spreading STIs. The chapter examines viral, bacterial, and other common STIs and infections.

## Safer Sex

This book discusses the various components of optimal wellness. Sexual behavior can have a strong positive or negative impact on physical and emotional health (see Assessment Activity 12-1). Making decisions concerning sexual behavior is not easy (see Nurturing Your Spirituality: Making Decisions About Sex). If people (whether heterosexual or homosexual) choose to have multiple sexual partners, they must realize that, each time a sexual act occurs, the potential sexual histories of two people are brought together. Even though it may be the first experience for one, the other partner may have had sex with three other people. In this case, the person for whom it is the first experience is essentially exposed to the sexual histories of four others. The diseases or infections of any of those four people may be brought to the present relationship (see Assessment Activity 12-2).

Unfortunately, people are not always honest about their past relationships. For many reasons, they may not tell the truth about the number of past partners or about the frequency of condom use. The potential for dishonesty in others makes the prevention of STIs a personal responsibility for everyone.

Some people choose abstinence. **Abstinence** means voluntarily refraining from all sexual acts—which includes practicing sexual activities that involve vaginal, anal, or oral stimulation or penetration. People choose abstinence for a number of reasons, most frequently moral or religious. Abstinence is the only way that STIs can be avoided and the possibility of pregnancy eliminated. This is an area that must be discussed with one's partner. It is difficult to accomplish abstinence if both partners are not in agreement.

A second frequent choice is to have sexual contact within a monogamous (involving only one long-term partner) relationship. Monogamy obviously is dependent on both partners' willingness to maintain a monogamous relationship. Monogamy may be a choice

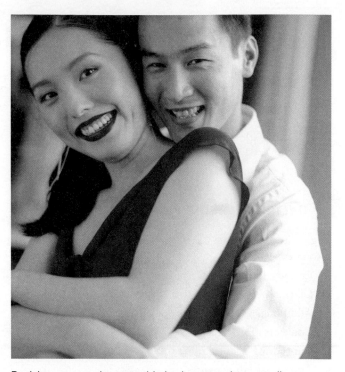

Decisions concerning sexual behavior can enhance wellness.

for two people who have never had sexual intercourse with anyone else or for two people who have had sex partners in the past but have decided to limit their future sexual practices to those they share with each other. Having sex with only one uninfected and faithful partner is as effective in preventing STIs (not pregnancy) as abstinence—if it is practiced consistently by both partners. However, even with monogamy, precautions are necessary to prevent unwanted pregnancies.

People embarking on a monogamous relationship who have had partners in the past need to discuss their sexual histories as well as their commitment to the present relationship. This commitment may involve a willingness to be tested for possible STIs (see Real-World Wellness: Communicating with Your Partner About STIs on page 404). Some STIs take time to manifest, so testing for them may have to be done several times over a period of years. Assuming that the people involved are committed to monogamy and are honest about their sexual histories, monogamy can protect against the spread of STIs.

In modern society, many relationships are not of long duration, and the practice of *serial monogamy* is common. Serial monogamy is monogamy for as long as a relationship is intact; for the duration of their relationship, two partners have sex only with each other. Because relationships may be of relatively brief duration (ranging from weeks to years) and each partner may then seek new partners, the risk with serial monogamy for contracting and spreading an STI is significant.

# Nurturing Your Spirituality

## Making Decisions About Sex

Everyone must decide at some point whether to engage in sexual activity. For some people, the decision is ongoing. Even after having a sexual experience, a person must decide whether to have sex with the first partner again, to have sex with another person, or not to have sex. Having sex *is* always a choice, unless rape or abuse is involved.

People sometimes change their minds about wanting to have sex. A person may have sex with someone once or many times and then decide to refrain from having sex with that person again. Some people decide to wait to have sex until they are married or until their financial, social, or emotional circumstances change. Some decide to change their sexual behavior to be more closely aligned with moral, ethical, or religious beliefs.

Why do people change their minds about sex? The decision to refrain from further sexual intercourse is sometimes referred to as *secondary virginity*. Couples choosing to engage in sex must make sure that their choice fits with their value systems and understand that they are emotionally, socially, and financially responsible for the results of their decisions. Before initiating sexual intercourse, couples should discuss the following:
- Their thoughts and feelings about sexual activity
- Whether sexual intercourse fits their moral and ethical codes
- Willingness to practice safer sex to protect themselves as well as to deal with the potential pregnancy created as the result of their decision

What considerations are important when deciding whether to have sex? Reasons for having or not having sex are varied. Some couples may believe their feelings are strong enough for one another that sex would seal their commitment to the relationship. Others may decide that if two people love one another it is OK to have sex. Some people engage in sexual activity because they see it as a way to be popular or as evidence that they are attractive. Some people have sex because they think everyone else is and that not to have sex would make them outsiders.

(Not everyone is having sex! Many people, young and old, choose to abstain until marriage or some other long-term commitment.)

Some people choose to refrain from having sex until marriage because they view sex outside marriage as morally wrong. Another reason for abstinence is a desire to get to know one's partner well (which takes time) before sex. Having sex may alter expectations and the nature of a relationship; some people do not have sex because they don't want their relationship to change. If the physical component of a relationship is emphasized over other aspects, partners may find it difficult to get to know each other well. Many people choose to abstain because they do not want to risk unwanted pregnancy; STIs; or the financial, emotional, and social responsibility of having sex. Some say that not having sex allows them to know themselves better and to figure out what they are looking for in a potential mate. Still others say that not having sex reduces the stress in their lives, freeing them from worries about problem pregnancies and STIs.

How do you decide whether to have sex? It is vitally important to know what your values are and to do only what furthers your total wellness. If you are choosing to have sex because of peer pressure or fear of being alone, then you are not acting out of a wellness perspective. If you are having sex for what you consider to be valid reasons and you are truly comfortable with your decision, then having sex may be an overall positive experience for you. Young adults often fail to realize that, during the next few years, they will be going through many changes as they move from home and from school out into the work world. These changes will alter their self-perceptions and their values. Making the wrong decision now may put that future in jeopardy. Taking time to consider behaviors carefully is crucial, because the regret of an unwanted pregnancy or a lifelong STI can be life altering or even fatal.

What factors will affect your decision to have or not have sex?

---

A third choice is to have sex with more than one partner but to practice **safer sex.** There is no such thing as *safe* sex with multiple partners, but steps can be taken to help ensure *safer* sex. Regardless if you are heterosexual or homosexual, or male or female, you can follow certain practices to limit your exposure to STIs. The starting point for safer sex is using some of the guidelines outlined in Real-World Well-

ness: Communicating with Your Partner About STIs on page 404. Anyone who is sexually active with multiple partners should be checked every 3 to 6 months for possible STIs. It is often the case that people, especially women, who are not disease-free are asymptomatic (have no symptoms);[1] no persons should let their lack of symptoms lull them into assuming they are disease-free.

## Real-World Wellness

### Communicating with Your Partner About STIs

*My partner and I have been very close to having sex on several occasions. I am very worried about contracting an STI. I really don't know much about my partner's sexual history. How do I open the discussion or ask the questions concerning safer sex practices? How do I find out if there is anything I should be aware of in this person's past?*

The decision about whether to have sex is extremely important. Considerations include the possibility of contracting an STI, the potential for an unwanted pregnancy, and the psychological and emotional ramifications of intimate contact, should the relationship end. Sex represents a psychological, physical, emotional, and financial commitment to another person. Don't be reluctant to bring up the topic of safer sex. The ability to discuss important issues is a sign of personal and social maturity. The following are some suggestions on ways to introduce the topic. What others can you suggest?

- "I feel that we both are thinking about sex, but before I make a final decision, I have some concerns I'd like to discuss with you."
- "I've always practiced safer sex in the past and, if we're going to have sex, I think it's important for us to use condoms."

- "What type of protection do *you* have if we decide to have sex? This is the type of protection *I* have."
- "I know if you really care about me you'll be willing to use a condom."
- "Before this relationship goes any further, I want to ask you about your sexual history and our plans for practicing safer sex."
- "I really like you and I hope we can have a more intimate relationship at some point. But I think there are some important things we should talk about first."
- "You're so sexy that sometimes I just get carried away when I'm close to you. Why don't we have a quiet dinner together to discuss our sexual past and what we want from this relationship?"

You can probably think of even better ways to approach a conversation concerning sex. What is important to remember is that sex can be a wonderful emotional and physical experience, but it's not worth dying for.

Following are some practices for people who are straight or gay that represent either safer sex, possible safe practices, or unsafe practices:

*Safer Practices*

- Hugging
- Kissing (not deep or French kissing)
- Petting
- Watching erotic videos, reading erotic books, and so on
- Masturbation (solo or mutual unless there are sores, lesions, and/or abrasions on the genitalia or hands)

*Possibly Safer Practices*

- Deep, French kissing, unless there are sores in the mouth
- Vaginal intercourse with a latex condom
- **Fellatio** (oral stimulation of the penis) with a latex or polyurethane condom
- **Cunnilingus** (oral stimulation of the clitoris and vaginal opening) with a latex dental dam, unless a female partner is menstruating or has a vaginal infection

- Anal intercourse with a latex condom, but there is a great amount of disagreement concerning the safety of this practice even with a condom—this is the riskiest sexual behavior

*Unsafe Practices*

- Vaginal or anal intercourse without a latex condom
- Fellatio or cunnilingus without a condom or latex dental dam
- Oral-anal contact
- Contact with blood, including menstrual blood
- Taking semen in the mouth
- Sharing a vibrator or other sex toys without washing them between uses[2]

See Just the Facts: Effective Condom Use.

## Sexually Transmitted Infections (STIs)

Each year in the United States it is estimated that more than 19 million new infections occur.[3] Approximately 25% of new cases occur among teenagers. Fifty per-

[ **JUST THE**
**FACTS** ]
**Effective Condom Use**

Condoms can be effective in protecting against STIs if used properly:

- Use one every time you have sexual intercourse or oral sex involving a penis.

- Use only latex or polyurethane condoms.

- Put the condom on before any contact with the vagina.

- When the condom is on the penis, there should be about ½ inch of space left at the condom tip to hold the ejaculate.

- Withdraw the penis soon after ejaculation. Hold the base of the condom firmly against the penis as it is withdrawn, so the condom does not come off.

- Use foam, spermicide, or a female condom in combination with a condom.

- Check for possible breaks immediately after the use of any condom.

- Always use a water-based lubricant, such as K-Y jelly. Vaseline or other oil-based lubricants can cause the condom to break down and become ineffective.

- Never reuse a condom.

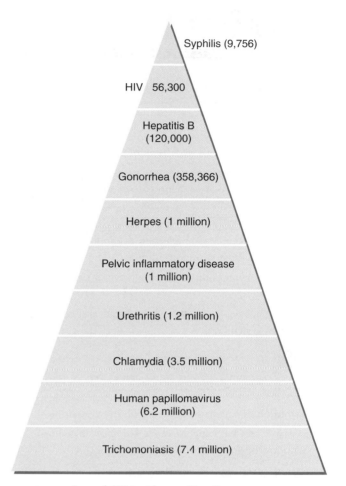

**FIGURE 12-1**   Annual STI Incidence–New Cases

**Source:** National Institute of Allergy and Infectious Diseases (2006).
Available online at *http://www.niaid.nih.gov*

cent of STI cases occur in people between the ages of 15 and 24.[4] Another particularly disturbing fact is that young women under 24 years of age may be at more risk for STIs than are older women because the cells of the cervix in young women are immature and more easily infected.[5] An important component of these statistics is that a large number of STI cases go unreported because many are asymptomatic (particularly in women) or because they are treated by a private physician and never reported. Consequently, the estimated 19 million may reflect a vast underreporting of the number of cases. The estimates for annual STI incidence are shown in Figure 12-1.

## Viral Diseases

### Human Immunodeficiency Virus and Acquired Immunodeficiency Syndrome

Damage to the immune system as a result of infection with **human immunodeficiency virus (HIV)** leads to a complex of rare diseases called **acquired immunodeficiency syndrome (AIDS).** The Centers for Disease Con-

trol and Prevention (CDC) lists two conditions to be used in diagnosing AIDS. These are an HIV seroconversion (the development of evidence of antibody response to a disease) and a blood T-cell count below 200 cells per millimeter, regardless of other specific symptoms that may or may not be present.[6] A normal range of T-cells is 800 to 1,000. In the presence of these two conditions, some other conditions may be used to diagnose AIDS. These conditions fall into several categories and are presented in Just the Facts: Conditions Used to Diagnose AIDS on page 406.

People infected with HIV may experience a variety of symptoms or may appear to be quite healthy. A small percentage of HIV-positive people seem to have been able to suppress and survive HIV infection for more than 20 years without developing AIDS. The reason for this is not understood by experts. It has been suggested that suppressor compounds formed by the immune system cells may be responsible. However, even people with no obvious symptoms can transmit HIV to others. The indicators of possible HIV infection include persistent diarrhea,

## [ JUST THE FACTS ]

### Conditions Used to Diagnose AIDS

The following are some conditions besides HIV seroconversion and low T-cell counts used to diagnose AIDS:

*Opportunistic Infections (Infections That Take Advantage of a Weakened Immune System)*

- *Pneumocystis carinii* pneumonia (PCP)—a type of lung disease caused by a protozoan or fungus, usually not harmful to humans
- Tuberculosis—either *Mycobacterium avium-intracellulare* (MAI) or *Mycobacterium tuberculosis* (TB); MAI is the most common among AIDS patients
- Bacterial pneumonia—caused by several common bacteria
- Toxoplasmosis—a disease of the brain and central nervous system

*Cancers*

- Kaposi sarcoma, a cancer that causes red or purple blotches on the skin
- Lymphomas, cancers of the lymphatic system
- Invasive cervical cancer—more common in women who are HIV positive

*Other Conditions*

- Wasting syndrome, which involves persistent diarrhea, severe weight loss, and weakness
- AIDS dementia, impairment of mental function, mood changes, and impaired movement as a result of HIV infection of the brain

*Other Infections*

- Candidiasis (also called thrush), a fungal infection that affects the vagina, mouth, throat, and lungs
- Herpes, a common viral STI
- Cytomegalovirus, a virus that, in AIDS patients, can lead to brain infection, infection of the retina, pneumonia, or hepatitis

dry cough, and shortness of breath; fatigue; skin rash; swollen lymph nodes (neck, armpits, groin); candidiasis (infection of the skin or mucous membranes, usually localized in skin, nails, mouth, vagina, or lungs); unexplained fever or chills; night sweats (over several weeks); and unexplained weight loss of 10 pounds or 10% of body weight in less than 2 months. Women may experience these symptoms as well as abnormal Pap smears, persistent vaginal can-

didiasis, and abdominal cramping as a result of pelvic inflammatory disease (PID). These infections are a result of HIV infection and are caused by immunodeficiency, but they are not AIDS (see Wellness for a Lifetime: HIV and AIDS Pose Special Risks to Women and Their Children).

The reason some people develop AIDS rapidly and others do not is not known. Factors that may contribute to the advancement of the condition are weakening of the immune system through other infections, alcohol or other drug abuse, poor nutrition, and stress.[7] The longer the virus is in the system, the greater the chances of developing AIDS. In one study spanning 6 years, 30% of the participants with the virus developed AIDS, 49% displayed symptomatic HIV infections, and 21% remained free of symptoms. All these people could continue to spread the disease.[8] Another problem is the rapid development and emergence of new drug-resistant strains of HIV.[9]

Two types of HIV have been identified.[10] Almost all cases of HIV in the United States are a virus known as HIV-1. Another type of virus, HIV-2, is found mainly in West Africa and appears to take longer than HIV-1 to damage the immune system. The virus replicates inside human cells and is transmitted by blood, blood products, semen, vaginal secretions, and breast milk. HIV is an extremely fragile virus in that it does not survive in air and can be destroyed readily by soap and water, household bleach, and chlorine used in swimming pools. Just the Facts: How HIV Is and Is Not Transmitted explores transmission in greater detail.

The HIV virus attacks the helper T-lymphocytes, specifically the T-4 cells, possibly the most critical element in the body's immune system. HIV attaches to the part of the T-cell that recognizes viral infections and blocks its ability to react to them. Over time, HIV may even multiply and destroy T-cells, leaving the body more defenseless against invasion by opportunistic organisms that can lead to illness and eventually death.[14,15,16]

In the United States, whether through homosexual or heterosexual contact, anal intercourse is still the most prevalent means of spreading HIV infection. This may be because this activity increases the likelihood of making small tears that facilitate the spread of the virus from semen to blood. Vaginal and oral sex are also considered highly dangerous.[17] Sharing needles among drug users and having sex with an IV drug user are high-risk activities. Sex with a prostitute is a significant risk factor. Anyone who has had multiple sexual partners during the last 5 to 10 years is at risk because there is no way of knowing the sexual histories of all the sex partners of one's multiple sex partners. People who are not sexually active are not at risk. People in

## Wellness for a Lifetime

### HIV and AIDS Pose Special Risks to Women and Their Children

In 2007, women represented almost 26% of all AIDS cases reported.[11] Most women are infected through the use of injected drugs or through sex with infected partners. Activities that put women at high risk include being a partner of an injected-drug user or of a gay or bisexual man and having multiple sex partners. Although lesbians with HIV are in a small minority, they can and do contract HIV in the same ways as heterosexual women. Lesbians who share sex toys without first washing and cleaning them are at greater risk for HIV than are those who practice safer sex.

Heterosexual women are at greater risk of contracting HIV from an infected man than are non-HIV-positive men from HIV-positive women. Women are more susceptible to HIV infection because they have more surface area of contact in the vagina, and the tissue there is softer and more easily scratched or torn. Further, semen is often ejaculated directly into the uterine and cervical canal. Semen normally contains 10 to 100 times more migratory lymphocytes than does cervical mucus, thus placing more virus in the area for potential infection.[12]

Women tend to be diagnosed at a later stage in the HIV process than are men, and they have almost a 30% greater chance than men do of dying before they have an AIDS-defining condition.[13] Because female physiology is different from male physiology, women need to participate in clinical trials to ensure that new experimental drugs and therapies work for them as effectively as they do for men. Several studies are under way that investigate gender-specific differences in disease progression, complications, and treatment.

A pregnant woman has about a 30% chance of passing the virus to her newborn. The Centers for Disease Control and Prevention has recommended HIV testing for all pregnant women. HIV transmission from mother to infant can be reduced from almost 25% to 1% when both the HIV-positive mother (predelivery) and infant (postdelivery) are provided treatment combined with cesarean section. An HIV-positive mother can infect her newborn by breast-feeding. The exact risk for this form of transmission is not known, but the risk can be completely avoided through the use of formula as opposed to breast milk.

## [ JUST THE FACTS ]

### How HIV Is and Is Not Transmitted

Following are possible means of transmission of HIV and some activities that, contrary to misinformed opinion, do not transmit HIV.

#### How HIV Is Transmitted

*Sexual Activity*

- Homosexual, between men
- Heterosexual, from men to women and women to men

*Blood*

- Through needle sharing among intravenous drug users
- Through transfusions of blood and blood products
- To health care workers through a needle stick, an open wound, or mucous membrane exposure
- Through injection with an unsterilized needle (including needles used in acupuncture, medical injections, ear piercing, and tattooing)

*Childbirth*

- Intrauterine (within the uterus)
- Peripartum (during labor and delivery)

#### How HIV Is Not Transmitted

- Through food and water
- Through sharing of eating and drinking utensils
- Through shaking or holding hands
- Through use of the telephone
- Via a toilet seat
- Via insects
- In whirlpools or saunas
- Through coughing or sneezing
- Via domestic pets
- Through an exchange of clothing
- From swimming in a pool
- Through bed linens

using heterosexuals in the United States doubled during the 1990s.[18]

AIDS is a preventable disease, and education is still the best defense. People who have sex outside a monogamous relationship and those who share needles from intravenous drugs are still at extremely high risk for infection.

monogamous relationships in which neither partner has an STI or has used IV drugs are considered safe. It is estimated that HIV infections among non-drug-

## [ JUST THE **FACTS** ]
### Preventing the Spread of AIDS[6]

The spread of AIDS can be stopped by preventing the transmission of the HIV virus from one person to another. This means eliminating direct sexual contact with infected people and not using contaminated needles. Recommendations to reduce the possibility of becoming infected include the following:

- Practice abstinence or mutual monogamy.

- Always use protection (that is, latex condoms) if having sex with multiple partners or with people who have multiple partners.

- Do not have unprotected sex with people with AIDS, those who engage in high-risk behavior, or those who have had a positive test for the AIDS virus.

- Avoid sexual activities that might cut or tear the rectum, vagina, or penis.

- Do not have sex with prostitutes.

- Do not use IV drugs or share needles. Refrain from having sex with IV drug users.

HIV is spread through intimate sexual contact; through transfusion of blood from an infected individual; and from an infected mother to her fetus during the prenatal period, the birth process, or breast-feeding (see Just the Facts: Preventing the Spread of AIDS). In no case has HIV been spread through casual contact—this includes close contact between family members or friends and infected adults or children. Very few health care professionals working with AIDS patients have contracted the disease, and their infection was caused by rare mishandling of blood. The AIDS virus is not transmitted from toilet seats, foods, beverages, or social kissing. The virus is found in small amounts in tears and saliva, although transmission through these mediums is undocumented.

Probably no other infectious disease has taken or is taking such a devastating toll on Americans. It is estimated in 2007 that 1.1 million persons were living with HIV. Of this number, 74% were males and 26% were female. In 2004, 6,025 AIDS cases were estimated in children under the age of 13.[11] Further, the CDC reported that 5% of AIDS cases were among people 13 through 19 years of age.[20] From 2001 to 2004, 10,457 people with AIDS in the United States had died.[21] In 2007, the estimated death count from AIDS was 14,561 in the United States and the District of Columbia. The cumulative estimated number of deaths of people with AIDS in the United States was

583,298 people. This estimated number included 557,902 adults and adolescents and 4,891 children under age 13.

### Testing for HIV

Several tests are currently being used to detect HIV. The EIA (enzyme immunoassay) is the antibody test initially used. If the EIA result indicates that the patient has HIV, one of two possible tests should be administered for confirmation: Western blot or an immunofluorescence assay (IFA) technique. Antibodies may develop within 2 months or may take up to 36 months to develop.[22] Usually, Western blot results are clearly either HIV positive or negative. If there is an inconclusive Western blot test, the person should be retested in 6 months. A polymerase chain reaction (PCR) test can detect the genetic material of HIV rather than the antibodies to the virus. The HIV in the blood can be identified within 2 to 3 weeks of infection. Home tests are now available for over-the-counter use. The home tests are much less invasive, since a finger lancet is used to collect a few drops of blood. The sample is placed on blotter paper and mailed to a laboratory, which then performs the test to determine if the sample is positive or negative. The person then telephones the lab for the results. The results are discussed with a counselor if the HIV test is positive. Home tests are now available that use saliva to test for HIV. The test results can be interpreted in just a few minutes. Any positive HIV home test should be followed up with one of the aforementioned tests for HIV. Remember, anyone who tests positive is infected with HIV and can transmit the infection. Although not always reliable, two other tests are now available for use in diagnosis.[23] Currently the Food and Drug Administration has approved four rapid antibody tests for use. These are tests that can be administered in a matter of minutes. Medical authorities feel that by using tests that can provide a quick diagnosis, HIV-positive individuals can begin proper care. Two of these tests are approved for use at point-of-service sites outside the traditional laboratory. All four tests are visually interpreted and cost between $14 and $25.

### Treatment of HIV and AIDS

At present, no cure exists for HIV and AIDS, which results in a multitude of infections leading to death. It is essential that treatment begin as soon as possible after the diagnosis. Currently, 26 drugs have been approved for treating HIV-infected individuals. They fall into the following categories:[24]

- *Reverse transcriptase (RT) inhibitors*. RT inhibitors interfere with HIV's ability to make copies of itself. There are two main types of RT inhibitors, and they work differently. *Nucleoside and nucleotide inhibitors* provide faulty DNA building blocks, halting the DNA chain that the virus uses to make copies of itself. Nonnucleoside RT inhibitors bind RT so the virus cannot carry out its copying function.

- *Protease inhibitors (PI).* Protease inhibitors interfere with the protease enzyme that HIV uses to reproduce copies of itself.
- *Fusion inhibitors.* This is the newest class of antiretroviral drugs, which are substances used to kill or inhibit the multiplication of retroviruses such as HIV. They act by interfering with the virus's ability to fuse or invade cells.

Table 12-1 lists the current drugs available for treatment.

The recommended treatment for HIV is a combination of three or more medications in a regimen called highly active antiretroviral therapy (HAART). Each HAART regimen is tailored to the individual patient.[25] However, dangerous side effects seem to accompany this type of therapy, including diabetes, abnormally high cholesterol and triglyceride levels, shrinking limbs, and the bizarre appearance of disfiguring deposits of fat on parts of the body. In July 2006 the federal government approved the first HIV treatment that put a triple drug cocktail into a once-a-day pill. This represents a tremendous breakthrough since, even with the many new drugs developed over the past few years, treatment still required taking several pills a day. In the early days of treating AIDS, a regimen of 20–30 drugs was required. This new once-a-day drug is to be sold as Atripla and includes doses of three drugs now sold in the United States. This drug is very expensive but should help prevent patients from missing doses and keep the virus from rebounding and becoming resistant to treatment.[26]

Even with this dramatic improvement, the AIDS crisis is far from over. Although some patients appear virus-free, it has been demonstrated that discontinuing therapy will increase the amount of HIV found in the blood. Even with all the advancements, the best protection for those choosing to be sexually active is education and the practice of safer sex.

Currently no HIV vaccines exist to prevent infection or disease. A great deal of research is being done on the possible development of vaccines. The task is made difficult because of HIV's ability to mutate and thus avoid developing immune system recognition. In fact, many HIV-positive individuals may carry several versions of the virus.[27]

AIDS is the most deadly of all STDs, but it is preventable. With education, wisdom, and reduction in high-risk behaviors, AIDS can be prevented (see Just the Facts: Preventing the Spread of AIDS). Information on AIDS can be obtained through various sources (see Just the Facts: AIDS and HIV Sources of Information on page 410).

## Herpes

**Herpes** is caused by the herpes simplex virus (HSV). The most common strains are herpes simplex-1 (HSV-1) and herpes simplex-2 (HSV-2). Type 1 is usually

---

**TABLE 12-1**  Drugs Approved for HIV Infections

| Nucleoside/Nucleotide RT Inhibitors | Nonnucleoside RT Inhibitors | Protease Inhibitors | Fusion Inhibitors | Multiclass Combination Products |
|---|---|---|---|---|
| Retrovir (zidovudine, AZT)* | Viramune (Nevirapine)* | Invirase (saquinavir-HGC) | Fuzeon (enfuvirtide)* | Atripla |
| Videx (didanosine, ddI)* | Rescriptor (delavirdine) | Norvir (ritonavir)* | | |
| Hivid (zalcitabine, ddC) | Sustiva (efavirenz)* | Crixivan (indinavir) | Selzentry | |
| Zerit (stavudine, d4T)* | | Viracept (nelfinavir)* | | |
| Epivir (lamivudine, 3TC)* | | Fortovase (saquinavir-SGC) | | |
| Combivir (AZT and 3TC) | | Agenerase (amprenavir)* | | |
| Ziagen (abacavir)* | | Kaletra (lopinavir and ritonavir)* | | |
| Trizivir (AZT + 3TC + abacavir) | | Lexiva (fosamprenavir) | | |
| Viread (tenofovir) | | Aptivus (tipranavir) | | |
| Emtriva (emtricitabine) | | Reyataz (atazanavir) | | |
| Epzicom (abacavir/lamivudine) | | | | |
| Truvada (tenofovir/emtricitabine) | | | | |

*Pediatric approved.

**Source:** United States Department of Health and Human Services. (2009). Antiretroviral drugs. www.aidsinfo.nih.gov/drugs/.

[ **JUST THE** ]
**FACTS**
### AIDS and HIV Sources of Information

Contact the following organizations for information about HIV and AIDS:

**CDC National AIDS Hotline**

(800) 342-2437

Free information on HIV and AIDS available in several languages

**CDC National AIDS Clearinghouse**

(800) 458-5231

www.cdcnpin.org

Information on services and education services; copies of Public Health Service publications available

**Linea Nacional de SIDA**

(800) 227-8922

Twenty-four-hour hot line that provides information and referrals in Spanish for HIV and AIDS

**HIV Insite Gateway to AIDS Knowledge**

www.ashastd.org/nah/sida

Information concerning prevention, education, treatment, and clinical trials

Local health departments also offer valuable information concerning HIV and AIDS.

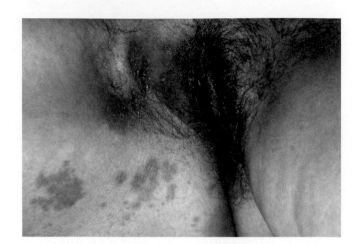

A severe herpes infection.

confined to congenital areas in the form of cold sores or fever blisters. It is a common form of herpes but is not categorized as an STI. Type 2 generally causes lesions on and around the genital areas and is an STI. However, through either direct or indirect contact, type 1 can affect the genital area and type 2 can produce sores in the mouth. The common sites for type 1 and type 2 can thus be reversed. Estimates indicate that 45 million people in the United States are infected with genital herpes.[28]

Type 2 herpes usually appears as a single blister or a series of painful blisters on the penis or inside the vagina or cervix. The blisters may also be present on the buttocks and thighs and in the groin area. Following a short prodromal period (time interval between the earliest symptoms and appearance of actual disease) of tingling, discomfort, or itching, small red lesions appear. This phase is followed by the formation of a small blister filled with clear fluid. This fluid is highly contagious. The infection usually lasts 1 to 3 weeks and then abates, but it does not leave the body. The virus retreats to the nerve endings, where it remains dormant. Herpes can become active again without any warning; that is, the disease may be recurrent. Menstruation, stress, trauma to the skin (such as too much sunlight), lack of sleep, and poor nutrition seem to trigger recurrences. Recurrences are generally less severe and of shorter duration than the initial episode.[29]

Genital herpes is acquired by sexual contact. It was once believed that herpes could be transmitted only when the virus was active and causing symptoms, such as the presence of blisters or sores. It is now known that the virus can be spread even when there are no symptoms.[30] Research does indicate that the risk for transmission is greatest among couples during the first 3 months of a sexual relationship. Estimates are that half of couples transmit within this period, indicating the possibility that partners develop a natural immunity to the virus over time.[31]

Men do not seem to experience any major long-term complications from herpes. Women, however, may be faced with the possibility of cancer of the cervix and infection of their newborns during the birth process. Any woman with a history of herpes should have an annual Pap smear test. Physicians attending the pregnancy of a woman with a history of herpes should be informed, so that the course of the pregnancy can be monitored. If herpes becomes active or the physician feels the baby would be at risk through a vaginal birth, caesarean section delivery (surgical removal of the fetus through the abdominal wall) is often used. Additional hazards of herpes infection are herpes encephalitis, in which the virus invades the brain, and herpes keratitis, or eye infection. These two conditions are rare and can be treated effectively with antiviral drugs.

Three antiviral prescription drugs are available for treating herpes. Acyclovir (brand name Zovirax, now available as a generic) promotes healing and helps suppress future outbreaks. Two newer drugs, valacyclovir and famciclovir, are similar to acyclovir but are designed to make higher levels of the drug's active ingredient available to the body. Some physicians prescribe a course of suppressive therapy with one of these drugs, which keeps herpes from recurring in up to 90% of patients. Patients must start taking the drugs at the first hint of symptoms. This therapy works only as long as the drug is taken, and if the drug is stopped there may be recurrences.[32] Warm compresses, sitz baths, and aspirin may help relieve discomfort. There is some evidence that zinc and vitamins C and A can enhance the immune system's response to herpes.

## Hepatitis B

Hepatitis is an inflammation of the liver caused by one or more viruses. There are five distinct types of **viral hepatitis:** hepatitis A, hepatitis B (*formerly serum hepatitis*), hepatitis C, hepatitis E, and hepatitis D.

**Hepatitis B** is considered the most serious of the five types of hepatitis. It has an incubation period of between 45 and 160 days. The symptoms of hepatitis B include vomiting, abdominal pain, loss of appetite, and jaundice (an excess of a bile pigment in the blood that causes the skin to look yellow). Some infected people do not develop the worst symptoms of the disease but experience mild, flulike illness without jaundice. (This group does not usually seek treatment but still can transmit the infection to others.) However, the CDC estimates that approximately 25% of carriers suffer chronic symptoms, and these people are at the greatest risk for one of the most serious consequences of infection, cirrhosis of the liver. Cirrhosis is a degenerative disease in which liver cells are damaged and scarred, with the eventual outcome of death or the necessity of liver transplantation. All carriers of hepatitis B are at greater risk of developing primary liver cancer than are noncarriers. At one time, hepatitis B was spread primarily through tattoo needles, the sharing of needles by drug users, and transfusions of contaminated blood. Today, it is more commonly spread through body secretions, including sweat, breast milk, and semen. A vaccine has been developed to immunize against the disease.

Viral hepatitis is a type of liver injury. Most patients with hepatitis recover without serious problems. However, serious scarring of the liver or even death may occur. In some cases of hepatitis B, the person with the disease becomes a chronic carrier or can develop chronic progressive hepatitis, which eventually leads to liver failure. There is a vaccine against hepatitis B.

It is recommended that all infants through adults receive the vaccine.[33]

## Human Papillomavirus Infection (HPV)

Warts on the genitalia, around the anus, in the vagina, and on the cervix are called **genital warts,** or *condyloma*. These warts are caused by the human papillomavirus (HPV). There are more than 100 forms of HPV. Experts postulate that this condition is the third most prevalent STI. It is also estimated that 6.2 million people are infected annually. At least 20 million people in the United States are already infected.[34] Genital warts most commonly involve people between the ages of 15 and 24.

Genital warts are cauliflower-like. In moist areas, they are soft and either pink or red. On dry skin, they are usually yellow-gray and hard. The warts are transmitted sexually and generally appear 1 to 6 months after exposure. There are 30 distinct varieties of HPV, some of which have been specifically linked to cervical cancer and cancers of the rectum, vulva, skin, and penis. The warts appear most often on the shaft of the penis, the vulva, the vaginal wall, the cervix, and the perineum.[35] They may also be found in the anal area of both sexes and are associated with anal intercourse with an infected partner. Cryosurgery (freezing) is the treatment of choice, although electrocautery (burning) and use of the topical agent podophyllin also are successful methods of treatment. Podophyllin should not be used during pregnancy or on warts in the cervical area. If the infected person has had a variety of partners, the genitalia of all partners should be examined, so that treatment can be initiated if appropriate.

There is now available a highly effective vaccine for the prevention of several types of HPV. The HPV viruses protected against are those responsible for 70% of cervical cancers and 90% of genital warts.

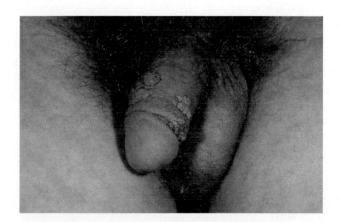

Genital warts are the result of human papilloma virus.

The vaccine is called Gardasil. At this time it has not proven to provide complete protection against infection from other HPV types.[36] Thus far, no serious side effects have been shown to be caused by the vaccines. The most common problems have been brief soreness and other local symptoms at the injection site. These problems are similar to ones commonly experienced with other vaccines. Studies are currently being conducted to determine how long immunity is provided by the vaccine and if a possible booster vaccination might be needed.[37]

# Bacterial Diseases

## Chlamydia

**Chlamydia** is the most common STI in the United States, with an estimated 2.8 million new cases each year. In 2007, 1,108,374 chlamydia infections were reported to CDC.[38] The causative agent is the bacterium *Chlamydia trachomatis*. Chlamydia is frequently found with other STIs, such as herpes, and it may be contracted through oral, anal, and vaginal intercourse. Approximately 75% of women and 50% of men have no symptoms. Most people infected with chlamydia are not aware of their infections and therefore do not seek medical help.[39] If symptoms do appear, it is usually within 1–3 weeks of the exposure.

In men the infection is usually manifested by inflammation of the urethra (urethritis). Infected men generally experience a burning sensation during urination and possibly a mild discharge.

Symptoms in women include vaginal discharge, intermittent vaginal bleeding, and ill-defined discomfort or pain on urination. Infected mothers may pass the infection to their babies during the birth process. This may result in conjunctivitis in the baby or a more serious condition known as *chlamydial pneumonia*.

When left untreated, chlamydia can lead to arthritis and can damage the heart valves, blood vessels, and heart muscle. In men the condition can also lead to sterility. In women the disease can infect the uterus, fallopian tubes, and upper reproductive areas, producing the chronic condition pelvic inflammatory disease, or PID. This scarring of the fallopian tubes by PID causes sterility and an increased risk for ectopic pregnancy (a condition in which the embryo is implanted outside the uterus). Women infected with chlamydia have a three- to fivefold increased risk of acquiring HIV, if exposed.

Most of the time, chlamydia is treated with an antibiotic, such as azithromycin, which requires taking for only 1 day. Doxycycline is taken for 7 days but is widely prescribed. Other drugs used include tetracycline, erythromycin, and ofloxacin. These drugs are taken orally for 1 to 3 weeks. Taking the full course of medication is extremely important because relapse can occur. All sexual partners should be treated, or the disease can be passed among them.[40] All sex partners should refrain from sexual intercourse until all have been treated and retested.

## Gonorrhea

In 2007, 355,991 cases of **gonorrhea** were reported, making it the second most prevalent STI.[41] Gonorrhea is caused by the bacterium *Neisseria gonorrhoeae*, which attacks the mucous membranes of the penis, vagina, rectum, throat, and eyes. The disease is spread by vaginal, oral, and rectal contact.

Gonorrhea produces symptoms in 80% of men. The symptoms appear 2 to 30 days (an average 3 to 5 days) after contact with the bacteria and include a thick, milky discharge from the penis and a painful, burning sensation on urination. These signs should cause men to seek medical treatment immediately. Untreated gonorrhea can result in sterility.

The symptoms in women are discharge and burning on urination, but they may be so mild that they are unnoticed. The bacteria can survive in the vagina and other areas of the female reproductive system for years. During this time, women can infect any sex partners and their fetuses if they become pregnant. The baby's contact with the bacteria during childbirth can lead to an eye infection, resulting in blindness. Untreated gonorrhea can lead to PID, the leading cause of sterility in women. In both men and women, rectal anal oral gonorrhea may go unnoticed. The disease can develop into a serious infection, resulting in arthritis; meningitis;

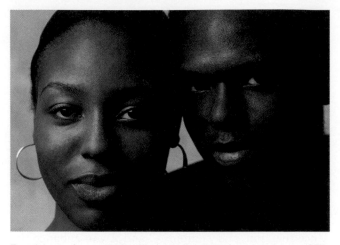
Practicing safer sex helps diminish the risk of contracting an STD.

skin lesions; and liver, heart, brain, and spinal cord problems. Symptoms of rectal infection in both men and women may include discharge, anal itching, soreness, bleeding, or painful bowel movements.[42]

Gonorrhea is diagnosed either by obtaining a smear from the penis or cervix or by doing a urine test. Physicians commonly treat for chlamydia as well when gonorrhea has been diagnosed. This dual therapy can be most cost-effective because the cost of treatment is less than the cost of testing. Most gonococci in the United States can be cured with doxycycline and dzithromycin; therefore, cotreatment might hinder the development of antibiotic-resistant strains of gonorrhea.[43] Over the last two decades, four types of antibiotic-resistant strains have developed and new antibiotic or combination drugs must be used to cure the infection.[44] Gonorrhea can be completely cured, although there is no immunity to the disease. If a person has multiple sex partners, medical help and advice must be sought regularly.

## Syphilis

Syphilis is caused by a corkscrew-shaped bacterial spirochete called *Treponema pallidum*. Kissing, oral-genital contact, and intercourse are the most common forms of transmission. The spirochete dies quickly when exposed to air, so primary entry to the body is through a break in the skin. Once in the bloodstream, it exists in a variety of organs and mimics the symptoms of many major chronic diseases. Because of this ability to mimic other diseases, it is referred to as *the great imitator*.

One interesting fact concerning syphilis is that some HIV infections seem to be exacerbated by it. The lesions caused by syphilis seem to help the HIV virus seep into or out of the body. Not everyone who has sex with a person who is HIV positive becomes infected, but if either partner also has primary or secondary syphilis, the risk of transmission increases sixfold.[45] There are four stages of syphilis.

### Primary Syphilis

The initial sign of primary syphilis is a lesion called a *chancre*, located at the site of entry of the pathogen. The incubation period ranges from 10 to 90 days (an average of 21 days) before symptoms appear. The chancre varies from the size of a pinhead to the size of a dime. Even though the chancre may look painful, it is not and may go unnoticed. If the lesion occurs on the labia, vagina, or rectum, it can easily remain undetected. The chancre remains for 3 to 6 weeks. In 90% of women and 50% of men, the chancre is difficult to identify.[46]

### Secondary Syphilis

From 4 to 12 weeks after the chancre disappears, the symptoms of secondary syphilis may appear. Symptoms include headaches, swollen glands, low-grade fevers, skin rash, white patches on the mucous membranes of the mouth and throat, hair loss (alopecia), arthritis pain, and large sores around the mouth and genitals. These sores contain the bacteria responsible for syphilis, and contact with them can spread the disease. Symptoms may be mild or severe, and in rare instances no symptoms appear. If left untreated, symptoms usually run their course, lasting anywhere from a few days to several weeks. The pathogen remains active in the body even with the absence of symptoms and will reappear later—perhaps as long as 20 years after the initial infection.

### Latent Syphilis

During latent syphilis, there are few or no clinical signs that the disease exists, although the spirochetes are invading the various organs and systems of the body, including the brain, heart, and central nervous system. The spirochetes multiply relentlessly and begin to destroy the tissues, bones, and organs. At this stage, a person is not contagious.

### Tertiary Syphilis

From 15 to 20 years after the onset of latent syphilis, the disease progresses to its most devastating stage. Tertiary syphilis can cause heart damage, central nervous system damage, blindness, deafness, paralysis, and psychosis. Death from the effects of this stage of syphilis is probable.

Penicillin is the preferred drug for treating syphilis. People who are penicillin-sensitive are placed on other antibiotics, such as tetracycline or erythromycin. For an individual who has had syphilis less than a year, a single dose will cure the disease. Larger doses are needed for those who have had the disease longer than a year.[47,48] Antibiotics can kill the pathogen at any stage, but any damage incurred cannot be reversed. People with syphilis commonly have other STIs, such as gonorrhea and chlamydia, thereby requiring greater doses of antibiotics.

## Other Common STIs

In addition to the STIs mentioned, there are several others that have potential for harm. Table 12-2 lists several other common STIs.

**TABLE 12-2**　Other Common STIs

| STI Causative Agent | | Symptoms | Treatment |
|---|---|---|---|
| Candidiasis (yeast infection) | A fungus (*Candida albicans*) that can be transmitted through sexual coitus or an imbalance of the acidity of the vagina | White, "cheesy" discharge; irritation of vaginal and vulva tissue | Vaginal cream or suppositories, such as miconazole (Monistat) |
| Chancroid | A bacterium (*Haemophilus ducreyi*) that can be contracted through a lesion or its discharge | Cluster of small bumps or blisters on the genitals or around the anus that rupture and ulcerate | Antibiotics, such as erythromycin |
| Granuloma inguinale | A bacterium (*Calymmatobacterium granulomatis*) that can be contracted through contact with a lesion or its discharge | Painless red bumps or sores in the groin that ulcerate and spread | Antibiotics, such as tetracycline or doxycycline |
| Nongonococcal urethritis (NGU) | A bacterium (mostly *Chlamydia trachomatis*) that can be transmitted during coitus | Inflammation of the urethra; for men, discharge and irritation during urination; for women, possible mild discharge of pus from the vagina or no symptoms | Antibiotics, such as tetracycline, doxycycline, or erythromycin |
| Pediculosis (crabs) | *Phthirus pubis* (pubic lice) | Intense itching in the genital area | Shampoos, such as those with lindane solution (Kwell) |
| Pelvic inflammatory disease (PID) (women only) | Untreated chlamydia or gonorrhea; may lead to infertility or arthritis | Low abdominal pain, bleeding between menstrual periods, persistent low fever | Penicillin or other antibiotics |
| Trichomoniasis (trich) | A protozoan parasite (*Trichomonas vaginalis*) contracted through sexual intercourse; can be spread by towels, toilet seats, or bathtubs used by an infected person | White to yellow discharge with an unpleasant odor | Anti-infectives, such as metronidazole (Flagyl) |

# Summary

- The only way to completely avoid acquiring an STI is to abstain from sex or to have sex in a purely monogamous relationship.
- Practicing safer sex helps reduce the possibility of contracting an STI. The use of condoms is associated with decreased risk.
- The human immunodeficiency virus (HIV) attacking the immune system causes a complex of rare diseases called acquired immunodeficiency syndrome (AIDS).
- Although no cure exists for AIDS, some of the latest combinations of drugs seem to be prolonging life and reducing the HIV content in the body.
- Genital herpes is a viral disease characterized by lesions around the

genital area. The disease can recur at any time and represents a serious threat to women by increasing their risk for cancer of the cervix. Three drugs are used to treat the disease (acyclovir, valacyclovir, and famciclovir).
- Viral hepatitis is an injury to the liver. There are several types of hepatitis. Hepatitis B is perhaps the most serious.
- Genital warts, or condyloma, are caused by the human papillomavirus (HPV) and have been linked to some cancers.
- Chlamydia is caused by a bacterium that produces the most common STI in the United States. Untreated, it can cause arthritis, sterility, damage

to the heart and blood vessels, and ectopic pregnancies.
- Gonorrhea is the second leading STI. It can lead to sterility in both men and women. The symptoms are often unnoticed by women.
- Syphilis is a bacterial disease that has four stages. The stages are primary, secondary, latent, and tertiary.
- Several other STIs that have damaging potential are candidiasis, chancroid, granuloma inguinale, nongonococcal urethritis (NGU), pediculosis, pelvic inflammatory disease (PID), and trichomoniasis.

# Review Questions

1. How can people accept responsibility for their sexual behavior?
2. What makes HIV an extremely dangerous infection?
3. What precautions can you take to protect against the spread of AIDS?
4. What are the various kinds of viral hepatitis, and how are they spread?
5. Discuss why HPV is more dangerous for women than for men.
6. Why does chlamydia represent a serious problem?
7. Why is gonorrhea a more serious problem today than it was just a few years ago?
8. List and explain the four stages of syphilis.
9. Discuss some other common STIs.
10. If one STI is present, why may it be necessary to get treatment for more than one?

# References

1. Strong, B., C. DeVault, & S. B. Werner. (1999). *Human sexuality—diversity in contemporary America* (3rd ed.). Mountain View, CA: Mayfield.
2. San Francisco AIDS Foundation. (2006). Reducing the risk of getting HIV from sexual activities. Retrieved from www.sfaf.org/aids101/sexual.html.
3. Centers for Disease Control and Prevention. (2007). Trends in reportable sexually transmitted diseases in the United States, 2007. Retrieved from www.cdc.gov/std/stats/htm.
4. Centers for Disease Control and Prevention. (2007). Sexual and reproductive health of persons aged 10–21 years—United States 2002–2007. *Mortality and Morbidity Weekly Report, 58*(SS06),1–58
5. Pallella, F. L., et al. (1998). HIV outpatient study investigation. Declining morbidity and mortality among patients with advanced human immunodeficiency virus infections. *New England Journal of Medicine, 338*(13), 853.
6. Ibid.
7. CDC (2007). Trends.
8. Cox, F. D. (1999). *The AIDS booklet* (5th ed.). Boston: WCB/McGraw-Hill.
9. CDC (2007). Trends.
10. Wikipedia. (2009). HIV. Retrieved from http://enWikipedia.org/wiki/HIV.
11. Centers for Disease Control and Prevention. (2009). HIV/AIDS in the United States 2007. Retrieved from http://cdc.gov/hiv/resources/focTsheets/print.htm.
12. Centers for Disease Control and Prevention. (2009). Sexually transmitted diseases treatment guidelines—2009. *Mortality and Morbidity Report, 51*,RR-6.
13. Strong et al. (1999).
14. CDC (2007). Trends.
15. Wikipedia (2009).
16. Nevid, J. S. (1995). *Choices: Sex in the age of STDs*. Boston: Allyn & Bacon.
17. Notes from the Twelfth World AIDS Conference, Geneva, Switzerland. 26 June–12 July 1998. Retrieved from www.mhhe.com/hper/health/personal-health/aidsnotes.mhtml.
18. Centers for Disease Control and Prevention. (2006). HIV/AIDS surveillance report 2002. *Mortality and Morbidity Weekly Report, 14*, 1–40.
19. CDC (2009). HIV/AIDS.
20. Ibid.
21. Centers for Disease Control and Prevention. (2009). Basic Statistics—2007. Retrieved from http://cdc.gov/hiv/surveillance/basic.htm ddaids.
22. Centers for Disease Control and Prevention. (2006). Guidelines for treatment of sexually transmitted diseases. Retrieved from www.cdc.gov/wonder/STD/STD98TG.
23. National Institute of Allergy and Infectious Diseases. (2006). HIV vaccines—questions and answers. Retrieved from www.niaid.hig.gov/factsheets/treat-hiv.htm/publications/vaccine/faqhivadvoctes.htm.
24. National Institute of Allergy and Infectious Diseases. (2009). Treatment of HIV infection. Retrieved from www.niaid.nih.gov/factsheets/treat-hiv.htm.
25. Ibid.
26. National Institute of Allergy and Infectious Diseases. (2009). HIV/AIDS treatment. Retrieved from www3.n121d.nih.gov.
27. NIAID (2009).
28. Centers for Disease Control and Prevention. (2009). *Genital herpes—CDC factsheet.* Retrieved from www.cdc.gov/std/
29. National Women's Health Resource Center. (2008). Health topics—genital herpes. Retrieved from www.healthywomen.org.
30. National Women's Health Resource Center. (2008). Treatment of genital herpes. Retrieved from www.healthywomen.org.
31. Ibid.
32. Ibid.
33. Centers for Disease Control and Prevention. (2009). Hepatitis factsheet. Retrieved from www.cdc.Gov/std/Hepatitis/STDFact-Hepatitis.htm.
34. National Institute of Allergy and Infectious Diseases. (2009). Human papillomavirus and genital warts. Retrieved from www.naid.nig.gov.
35. Ibid.
36. National Institute of Allergy and Infectious Diseases. (2009). Human papillomavirus (HPV) and genital warts. Retrieved from www3.naid.nih.giv/topics.
37. Ibid.
38. Centers for Disease Control and Prevention. (2009). Chlamydia. Retrieved from www.cdc.Gov/std/Chlamydia/STDFact-chlamydia.htm.
39. Ibid.
40. Ibid.

41. Centers for Disease Control and Prevention. (2009). Gonorrhea. Retrieved from www.cdc.Gov/std/Gonorrhea/STDFact-gonorrhea.htm.
42. Ibid.
43. Ibid.
45. Ibid.
44. National Institute of Allergy and Infectious Diseases. (2009). Syphilis. Retrieved from www.niaid.nih.gov/factsheets/htm.
45. Ibid.
46. Ibid.
47. Ibid.
48. Ibid.

## Suggested Readings

Centers for Disease Control and Prevention. (2006). *Sexually transmitted diseases*. Atlanta, GA: Alternate Treatment Guidelines 2006.

This replaces the 1998 *Guidelines for Treatment*. It was developed by CDC staff members after consultation with a group of experts on the treatment of STDs.

Larson, L. (Ed.) (2009). *Sexually transmitted disease sourcebook* (4th ed.). Detroit, MI: Ominigraphic Publishing.

Excellent resource book that contains all the symptoms and treatment of nearly all of the sexually transmitted infections. The latest research on treatments and vaccines is discussed. Resources for additional help are provided for those living with various STIs.

Shilts, R. 1987. *And the band played on: Politics, people, and the AIDS epidemic*. New York: St. Martin's Press.

This classic book, written by a gay man with AIDS, expresses the author's views about the political aspects of AIDS and the difficulties in receiving treatment.

**Name** _____    **Date** _____    **Section** _____

# Assessment Activity 12-1

## Making a Decision

The decision to have sexual intercourse is a major one. Many factors affect this decision, and many factors will be affected by it. People engage in sexual activity for a variety of reasons that are often unrelated to love and that often disregard the consequences of that behavior.

**Directions:** Listed here are factors that may influence your decision to engage in sexual activity. Rank each

of these factors as to how they affect your behavior now and when you are in a situation in which you have to make a decision. Answer as truthfully as possible—you do not need to submit this activity to your instructor.

| Factor | Not Important | Slightly Important | Important | Very Important | Extremely Important |
|---|---|---|---|---|---|
| Risk for AIDS | | | | | |
| Risk for other STD | | | | | |
| Risk for pregnancy | | | | | |
| Sexual history of partner | | | | | |
| History of partner with regard to IV drug use | | | | | |
| Biological gratification (physical sensations) | | | | | |
| Need for money | | | | | |
| Desire to be accepted by partner or social or cultural group | | | | | |
| Chance to reduce stress or to get mind off other problems | | | | | |
| Intense need to feel loved or cared for | | | | | |
| Desire to show commitment to a relationship | | | | | |
| Desire to express love for partner | | | | | |
| Monogamous nature of relationship | | | | | |
| Desire for a variety of partners | | | | | |
| Chance to feel desirable | | | | | |
| Chance to prove sexual prowess | | | | | |

Consider asking your potential partner to also take this assessment as a basis for discussion. As you assess your responses, note the factors that are important to you in making this decision.

What are the most important factors? _____

_____

_____

Does the person you are considering having sex with have any history, behaviors, or other qualities that you consider to be negative in terms of your decision to have sex? What are they? _____

_____

_____

How important are these histories, behaviors, and other qualities to you? _____

_____

_____

How severe are the potential consequences of your or your partner's ideas and/or actions? _____

_____

_____

**Name** _____   **Date** _____   **Section** _____

# Assessment Activity 12-2

## Are You at Risk for a Sexually Transmitted Disease?

**Directions:** Review each of the following sexual behaviors listed. If you engage in any of the listed activities, assess your personal risk of contracting a sexually transmitted disease through that activity by checking the appropriate line.

There is no risk for activity 1. The risk is low for activity 2. The risk is high for activities 3, 4, 5, and 6.

After reviewing the different categories of activities, are there areas of concern for you?

| Activity | Risk | Precautions |
|---|---|---|
| 1. _____ No sex | No risk: There is virtually no chance of getting an STD. | No precautions are necessary. |
| 2. _____ Sex with only one partner | Low risk: If both partners have no other sex partners and no disease, there is almost no risk of getting an STD. | Remain monogamous. |
| 3. _____ Sex with a variety of partners | High risk: Each time there is another partner, the risk increases. | Choose partners carefully, use condoms and spermicides, wash after sex, do not douche, and urinate after sex. |
| 4. _____ Sex with a partner who has sex with a variety of partners | High risk: The more partners, the greater the risk an STD will be transmitted. | Be aware of symptoms. |
| 5. _____ Sex with someone who is or has been an IV drug user | High risk: If needles are shared, the risk is great, particularly of getting AIDS and hepatitis B. | Know the social and sexual history of your partner. |
| 6. _____ Oral sex | High risk. | Know your partner; do not engage in oral sex if you do not know the history of your partner. |

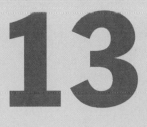

# Understanding Cancer and Diabetes

## ONLINE LEARNING CENTER

Log on to our Online Learning Center (OLC) for access to these additional resources:

- Chapter key term flashcards
- Learning objectives
- Additional goals for behavior change
- Concentration game
- Self-scoring chapter quizzes
- Additional lab activities

The OLC also offers Web links for study and exploration of wellness topics. Access these links through **www.mhhe.com/anspaugh8e.**

## GOALS FOR BEHAVIOR CHANGE

- Identify and change two behaviors that put you at risk for cancer.
- Begin an exercise program for preventing cancer as well as promoting overall wellness.
- Regularly perform the self-examinations for cancer described in this chapter.
- Identify your personal risk factors for the cancer and diabetes discussed in this chapter.
- Select strategies for the prevention of cancer and diabetes.

## Objectives

After completing this chapter, you will be able to do the following:

✔ Define cancer.
✔ Identify the various types of cancer.
✔ List the signs and symptoms of the various types of cancer.
✔ Identify ways of protecting against various cancers.
✔ Discuss treatments for cancer.
✔ Differentiate between Type 1 and Type 2 diabetes mellitus.

## [ Key Terms ]

| | |
|---|---|
| basal cell carcinoma | leukemia |
| benign | lymphoma |
| cancer | metastasis |
| carcinogens | oncogene |
| carcinoma | sarcoma |
| diabetes mellitus | squamous cell carcinoma |

**T**his chapter focuses on two conditions that are detrimentally affected by lifestyle. If precautions are taken against the onset of cancer and diabetes, their impact on the body may be lessened or even avoided.

## Cancer

Probably no disease strikes more fear in people than cancer. The term **cancer** refers to a group of diseases characterized by uncontrolled, disorderly cell growth. It is the second leading cause of death.

In 2008, almost 565,650 Americans were expected to die of cancer, over 1,500 people a day.[1] Since 1999 cancer has been the leading cause of death in the United States for people under 85 years of age.[2]

Death rates for many major cancers have leveled off or declined over the past 50 years. Still the lifetime risk for men getting cancer is 1 in 2 while the lifetime risk for women is 1 in 3. Lifetime risk is the probability that a person over their lifetime will develop or die from cancer.[3] For many types of cancers, 85% of people will be alive 5 years after diagnosis and considered cured. Others, however, who survive for 5 years may still show evidence of cancer.[4] *Cured* means that a patient has no evidence of disease and has the same life expectancy of a person who never had cancer. Although it strikes more frequently with advancing age, cancer causes the deaths of more children than any other disease (see Wellness for a Lifetime: Children and Cancer). The chances of developing cancer can be reduced by assuming control of your daily behaviors and activities (see Just the Facts: Tips for Cancer Prevention; see also Assessment Activity 13–1).

Cell growth is controlled by deoxyribonucleic acid (DNA) and ribonucleic acid (RNA) in the nucleus of each cell in the body. If the nuclei lose the ability to regulate and control this growth, cellular metabolism and reproduction are disrupted and a mutant cell is produced that varies in form, quality, and function from the original. When a mass of these cells develops, it is considered a neoplasm, or tumor. It may be malignant (cancerous) or **benign** (noncancerous). A benign tumor will not spread throughout the body. It is enclosed by a membrane, which prevents it from invading other tissues. A benign tumor is not life-threatening unless it is in an area that interferes with normal functioning. A malignant tumor is the most dangerous tumor because it has a tendency to spread from its original location to other parts of the body, which can make it life-threatening. Cancer cells can crowd out normal cells, invade surrounding tissue, and move through the lymphatic or circulatory system to infiltrate other areas of the body. (The lymphatic system is a network of nodes and vessels that drains fluid from tissues and returns it to the bloodstream. It is also part of the body's immune system.) The process by which cancerous cells spread from their original site (primary site) to another location (sec-

# Wellness for a Lifetime

### Children and Cancer

Despite its rarity, cancer is the chief cause of death by disease in children under the age of 15. Cancer is a devastating event, particularly when the diagnosis occurs in children. The overwhelming emotional and psychological trauma associated with cancer affects not only the child but also brothers, sisters, parents, and other relatives. If there is any good news to report, it is that mortality rates have declined 57% since the 1970s. St. Jude Children's Research Hospital, the only cancer research center in the world devoted solely to children, reports that, since 1962, the survival rates for various childhood cancers have risen significantly.

As researchers move slowly toward providing cures and increasing life expectancy of children affected by cancer, we can all hope that, one day, we will know of children dying from cancer only through reading about them in textbooks. For more information about childhood cancers, visit the following website: **www.stjude.org**.

|  | *Now* | *1962* |
|---|---|---|
| • Acute lymphoblastic leukemia | 94% | 4% |
| • Hodgkin lymphoma (cancer of the lymph nodes): | 90% | 50% |
| • Non-Hodgkin lymphoma (malignant tumor): | 85% | 7% |
| • Retinoblastoma (cancer affecting the eyes): | 95% | 75% |
| • Neuroblastoma (cancer of the nervous system): | 55% | 10% |
| • Wilms tumor (cancer of the kidney): | 90% | 50% |
| • Osteosarcoma (bone cancer): | 65% | 20% |
| • Rhabdomyosarcoma (cancer affecting the muscles): | 70% | 30% |

## [ JUST THE FACTS ]

### Tips for Cancer Prevention

More than 200 studies demonstrate a strong association between diets high in fiber, vegetables, and fruits (five to nine servings a day).[5] Observe the following guidelines to improve your chances of avoiding cancer:

*What to Do*

- Eat more broccoli, cauliflower, and brussels sprouts. Eat more cabbage-type vegetables, such as cabbages and kale. These vegetables protect against cancers of the colon, rectum, stomach, and lung.
- Add more high-fiber foods to your diet. Eat more peaches, strawberries, potatoes, spinach, tomatoes, wheat and bran cereals, rice, popcorn, and whole-wheat bread. Fiber protects against cancer of the colon.
- Choose foods containing vitamin A. Eat more carrots, peaches, apricots, squash, and broccoli. Fresh foods are the best sources and are far better than vitamin pills. Vitamin A protects against cancers of the esophagus, larynx, and lung.
- Choose foods containing vitamin C. Eat more grapefruit, cantaloupe, oranges, strawberries, red peppers, green peppers, broccoli, and tomatoes. These help fight cancers of the esophagus and stomach.
- Practice weight control. Exercise and eat foods low in calories. A good exercise for most people is walking. Obese people have a high chance of getting cancers of the uterus, gallbladder, breast, and colon. Check with your doctor before you start an exercise program or a special diet.
- If female, perform monthly breast exams, and get annual mammograms after age 40. Males should get annual digital and prostate-specific antigen (PSA) exams after age 50 (40, if African American or with a family history). Males over age 16 should perform monthly testicle exams. Males and females over age 50 should get annual colon cancer checks.[6]

- Certain cancers are related to infectious diseases. Hepatitis B virus (HBV), human papillomavirus (HPV), the human immunodeficiency virus (HIV), and *Helicobacter pylori* (*H. pylori*) are associated with certain types of cancer. Many of these cancers could be prevented by behavioral changes, vaccines, or antibodies.[8]

*What to Avoid*

- Avoid fat. Eat lean meat, fish, and low-fat dairy products. Cut extra fat off meats and skin poultry before cooking. Avoid pastries and candies. A high-fat diet increases the chance of getting cancer of the breast, colon, and prostate. Calories loaded with fat cause weight gain.
- Avoid salty foods. Stay away from nitrite-cured and smoked foods. Bacon, ham, hot dogs, and salt-cured fish are examples. People who eat these foods have a greater chance of getting cancer of the esophagus and stomach.
- Avoid smoking. Smoking is the main cause of lung cancer. Pregnant women who smoke harm their babies. Parents who smoke at home cause breathing and allergy problems for their children. Chewing tobacco can cause cancers of the mouth and throat. Pick a day to quit, and call the American Cancer Society for help.
- Avoid alcohol in excess. If you drink a great deal, you may get cancer of the liver. It is worse to smoke and drink. This increases the chances of getting cancers of the mouth, throat, larynx, and esophagus.
- Avoid too much sun. The sun causes skin cancer and other damage to skin. Use a sunscreen. Wear long sleeves and a hat between 11 a.m. and 3 p.m. Do not use indoor sunlamps, visit tanning parlors, or take tanning pills. Be alert for changes in a mole or sore that does not heal. If changes occur, go to a doctor.

ondary site) is called **metastasis.** The ability of cancerous cells to metastasize makes early detection critical. Table 13–1 on page 424 describes the types of cancer and where they are most often found.

## Causes and Prevention

Cancer is caused by both external factors (chemicals, diet, radiation, viruses, pollutants, etc.) and internal factors (hormones, immune conditioning, and inherited mutations). Any combination of these factors may initiate or promote carcinogenesis—the development of

cancer cells. Ten or more years often pass between exposures or mutations and the detection of cancer.[7]

Although the causes of cancer are not clearly understood, correlations have been found between cancer and everything from genetic factors to exposure to the sun's radiation. Many **carcinogens** (cancer-causing agents) trigger the development of cancer. (Table 13–2 on page 424 contains a list of substances known to be carcinogenic.)

An inherited tendency for cancer has been theorized for years. Everyone seems to have genes that may cause cancer, but not everyone gets cancer. In most

**TABLE 13-1**　Types of Cancer and Most Common Sites

| Type | Most Common Site | Method of Spread |
|---|---|---|
| Carcinoma | Tissues covering body surfaces and lining the body cavities are the most common locations. Sites include the breast, lungs, intestines, skin, stomach, uterus, and testes. | Lymphatic and circulatory systems |
| Sarcoma | The connective system is most commonly affected. Sites include bones, muscle, and other connective tissue. | Circulatory system |
| Lymphoma | The condition develops in the lymphatic system, infectious regions of the neck, armpits, groin, and chest. Hodgkin disease is an example. | Lymphatic system |
| Leukemia | The blood-forming tissues, bone marrow, and spleen are particularly affected. | Circulatory system |
| Adenocarcinoma | Cancer evolving from the endocrine glands. | Circulatory system |
| Melanoma | A type of skin cancer arising from the melanin-containing cells of the skin. If not diagnosed early, it is a very deadly type of cancer. | Circulatory system |
| Neuroblastoma | Most often a childhood cancer involving the central nervous system. | Nervous system |

cases, environmental factors activate the cancer. A good example of the interplay between genetic and environmental factors is found in cigarette smoking. Approximately 87% of lung cancers occur in cigarette smokers,[9] but only 15% of smokers develop lung cancer. Why not the other 85%? The 15% who develop cancer are thought to be susceptible to the disease on the basis of their genes. If they had not activated the cancer genes by smoking, they probably would not have contracted the disease.

A gene that causes cancer is called an **oncogene**. Within a tiny segment of DNA is an area that can be activated to form an oncogene. All cells have normal regulatory genes, called *proto-oncogenes*. A variety of genetic mutations, viral infections, or other carcinogens cause these normal genes to lose their ability to replicate themselves in a normal genetic fashion. If the gene that is miscopied is one that controls specialization, replication, repair, or tumor suppression, the result is a cancer-producing gene. Unless it is activated,

**TABLE 13-2**　Factors That Can Cause Cancer

| Carcinogen | Site of Cancer | Comments |
|---|---|---|
| Alcohol | Liver, larynx, pharynx, breast, esophagus | Heavy drinking increases the risk for cancer, especially when accompanied by cigarette smoking or use of chewing tobacco. |
| Smoking | Lungs, mouth, pharynx, larynx, bladder, esophagus | Smoking accounts for about 30% of cancer deaths. It is considered the number one carcinogen in the United States and the most preventable cause of death. It is responsible for 87% of lung cancer deaths. |
| Ultraviolet radiation | Skin | Almost all skin cancers are sun related. |
| Ionizing radiation | Blood-forming tissues, lungs | Excessive exposure to radiation increases cancer risk. Excessive radon exposure increases the risk for lung cancer. |
| Smokeless tobacco | Mouth, larynx, pharynx, esophagus | Oral cancer risk increases with the use of chewing tobacco and snuff. |
| Estrogen | Endometrium (uterus), liver, breast | Oral contraceptives increase the risk for liver cancer. Estrogen treatment to control menopausal symptoms increases the risk for cancer and heart disease. |
| Industrial agents | | Industrial chemicals and agents, such as nickel, chromate, asbestos, and vinyl chloride, increase the risk for various cancers. |
| Dietary fat | | High consumption of dietary fat is related to cancers of the colon, prostate, and pancreas; replacing fat with complex carbohydrates provides protection against several cancers (see Chapter 6). |

**Source:** American Cancer Society. (2009). *Cancer prevention and early detection facts and figures 2009.* Atlanta, GA: American Cancer Society.

however, it will never cause cancer. If an oncogene is formed, it acts with other oncogenes to produce abnormal cells that can replicate and spread.

Suppressor genes also play a role in cancer. Suppressor genes, which exist in normal cells, control cell growth. If suppressor genes mutate, cells are permitted to grow unrestrained.

Another explanation of cancer is an error in cell duplication on the basis of chance alone. Several trillion new cells are formed each year, and perfect duplication does not occur with each new cell formation. When an abnormal cell develops, the immune system recognizes it as a rogue cell and attacks it. Every cancer cell needs to be killed because almost all cancers arise from a single cancer cell. Cancer develops as a result of the immune system's failure to clear the body of cancer cells. This is one reason the immune system is receiving considerable attention from cancer researchers.

The development of cancer is a process that generally takes years. By stopping this process at any step, the deadly potential of cancer is ended. After the cancer process is initiated, due to environmental or genetic causes, several things must happen. The cancer cells have to grow and reproduce; the immune system must fail to recognize the cancer and leave it alone; and the new tumor must eventually find a way to "feed" itself by forming new blood vessels to supply itself with blood (a process called angiogenesis).[10]

Much research appears to link psychological states with the prevalence of disease in certain people. People with positive, involved attitudes who view life's challenges as opportunities for personal growth seem to have fewer diseases and recover from them more often. People who feel lonely and depressed and lack appropriate social support are more cancer-prone than are their mentally healthy counterparts.[11]

Emotional factors, such as stress, lack of social support, and the inability to express and cope with the range of emotions brought on by a frightening diagnosis of cancer, have been linked to the progression of cancer. Several studies have reported that patients who participate in support groups while receiving standard medical care live significantly longer than do those receiving medical care alone. Conversely, cancer patients who are socially isolated have poorer survival rates than do those with more social connections.[12] This doesn't suggest that stress and social isolation cause cancer. It does suggest a significant correlation between emotion and the progression of cancer once the disease is established. Many experts believe that a person's emotional state may somehow bolster the body's natural cancer-fighting power.

Although some of these concepts are controversial, it is generally accepted that substances such as tobacco, tobacco smoke, alcohol, asbestos, herbicides, and pesticides are carcinogens. Scientists believe that more than 80% of cancers are associated with lifestyle factors that are easily controlled—diet, smoking, and exposure to the sun.[13] Almost two-thirds of cancer deaths are attributed to diet and tobacco. According to a 20-year study of 115,195 healthy women ages 30 to 55, one-third of cancer deaths are caused by excessive weight.[14] The American Cancer Society estimated that in 2006 about 170,000 cancer deaths were caused by tobacco use.[15] Scientific evidence suggests that about one-third of the 564,830 cancer deaths expected in 2008 would be related to nutrition, inactivity, and obesity, and thus could have been prevented.[16] (Chapter 6 provides guidelines for cancer prevention as related to diet; Chapter 8 provides guidelines for weight maintenance.)

One of the major carcinogens may be sun radiation—more specifically, excessive exposure to the ultraviolet (UV) rays of the sun. People who spend hours in the sun without protection have an increased risk for skin cancers. UV light peaks from 10 a.m. to 2 p.m. (11 a.m. to 3 p.m. during daylight savings time). Avoiding sun exposure during these hours can cut UV light exposure by up to 60%. Most major newspapers now include the UV index as a routine part of the weather report. Many of the more than 1 million basal and squamous skin cancers and 621,480 melanomas that were expected to be diagnosed in 2008 could have been prevented by protection from the sun's rays. Using tanning beds also increases the risk for skin cancer.

Finally, the herpes viruses have been connected with cancer of the cervix. Viruses may be involved in the development of some forms of leukemia, Hodgkin disease, and Burkett lymphoma. The exact role of viruses in causing cancer is not known, but they may provide an opportunistic environment for cancer development. Other researchers have suggested that it is a combination of factors, in which the virus may play a part, rather than the virus itself that causes cancer.

## Cancer Staging

Staging is the process of determining how far cancer has spread. Staging is extremely important since it is a vital step in determining what types of treatment will be used. Staging also provides the physicians and the health care team with the prognosis of the cancer. There are several systems for staging, but a procedure called TNM is most commonly used. The system provides three key pieces of information:

T—Describes the size of the tumor and if cancer has spread to other tissue and organs

N—Describes how far the cancer has spread to nearby lymph nodes

M—Determines if cancer has metastasized to other organs of the body

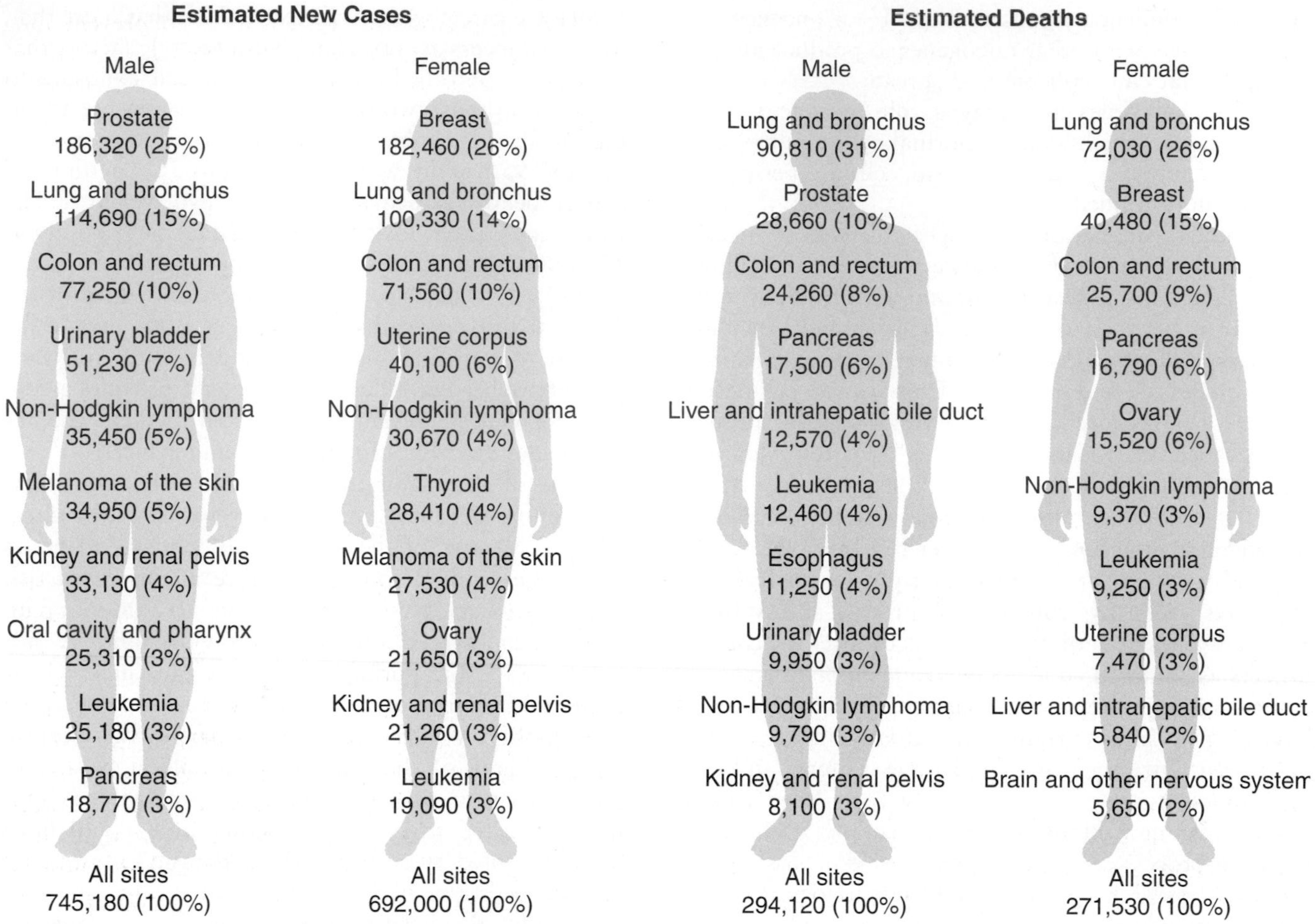

## Estimated New Cases

### Male

Prostate
186,320 (25%)

Lung and bronchus
114,690 (15%)

Colon and rectum
77,250 (10%)

Urinary bladder
51,230 (7%)

Non-Hodgkin lymphoma
35,450 (5%)

Melanoma of the skin
34,950 (5%)

Kidney and renal pelvis
33,130 (4%)

Oral cavity and pharynx
25,310 (3%)

Leukemia
25,180 (3%)

Pancreas
18,770 (3%)

All sites
745,180 (100%)

### Female

Breast
182,460 (26%)

Lung and bronchus
100,330 (14%)

Colon and rectum
71,560 (10%)

Uterine corpus
40,100 (6%)

Non-Hodgkin lymphoma
30,670 (4%)

Thyroid
28,410 (4%)

Melanoma of the skin
27,530 (4%)

Ovary
21,650 (3%)

Kidney and renal pelvis
21,260 (3%)

Leukemia
19,090 (3%)

All sites
692,000 (100%)

## Estimated Deaths

### Male

Lung and bronchus
90,810 (31%)

Prostate
28,660 (10%)

Colon and rectum
24,260 (8%)

Pancreas
17,500 (6%)

Liver and intrahepatic bile duct
12,570 (4%)

Leukemia
12,460 (4%)

Esophagus
11,250 (4%)

Urinary bladder
9,950 (3%)

Non-Hodgkin lymphoma
9,790 (3%)

Kidney and renal pelvis
8,100 (3%)

All sites
294,120 (100%)

### Female

Lung and bronchus
72,030 (26%)

Breast
40,480 (15%)

Colon and rectum
25,700 (9%)

Pancreas
16,790 (6%)

Ovary
15,520 (6%)

Non-Hodgkin lymphoma
9,370 (3%)

Leukemia
9,250 (3%)

Uterine corpus
7,470 (3%)

Liver and intrahepatic bile duct
5,840 (2%)

Brain and other nervous system
5,650 (2%)

All sites
271,530 (100%)

**FIGURE 13-1** Cancer Incidence and Death by Site and Sex—2008 Estimates

The figure excludes basal and squamous cell skin cancer and in situ carcinomas except urinary bladder.

SOURCE: American Cancer Society, Surveillance Research, 2008.

Letters or numbers after the T, N, and M provide details about each of the three factors. A tumor classified as T1, N0, M0 is one that is very small, has not spread to the lymph nodes, and has not metastasized.[17]

## Cancer Sites

The American Cancer Society reports each year on the incidence and number of deaths from cancer for a variety of sites (Figure 13–1). Skin cancer is the most common cancer. More than 1 million people are diagnosed annually with **basal** and **squamous cell carcinoma.** Almost all of these are considered sun-related cases.[18] Fortunately, most skin cancers are highly curable. For both genders, the cancer that kills most often is lung cancer. Excluding basal cell and squamous cell carcinomas, the breasts are the most prevalent cancer site for women, and the prostate is the leading cancer site for men. Fifty-nine percent of cancer deaths among males are from four primary sites—bronchus, colon and rec-

tum, prostate, and pancreas. Sixty-two percent of female cancer deaths occur from five sites—lung, breast, colon, pancreas, and ovary.[19] For any cancer, early detection is imperative (see Assessment Activity 13–2). If cancer is diagnosed while it is still localized, the cure or survival rate may be 90% or higher for some cancers, such as skin, colon, and rectum cancers.[20]

## Cancers of Concern to Everyone

### Lung Cancer

Although breast cancer and prostate cancer receive the most attention in the United States, lung cancer is the leading cause of cancer death in the United States[21] and throughout the world.[22]

Lung cancer is the most common cause of cancer-related deaths in both men and women. An estimated 159,390 deaths were expected to occur in 2009.[23] There are two main types of lung cancer. They are small cell lung cancer and non-small cell lung cancer (NSCLC). About 10 to 15% of all lung cancers are small cell type.[24,25] Eighty-five to 90% of lung cancers are non-small cell cancers. There are three subtypes of NSCLC, each of them differing in size, shape, and chemical makeup. The three types of squamous cell carcinoma adenocarcinoma, and large cell carcinoma. A third type of lung cancer is carcinoid tumors, which are slow growing and can usually be cured by surgery. One important concept to keep in mind is cancer which begins at other sites (e.g., the breasts) and metastasizes to the lungs is still not lung cancer, but remains breast cancer in definition.

Lung cancer is more difficult to detect and thereby more deadly than other, even more frequently occurring types of cancer. Lung cancer is one of the most preventable forms of cancer, because the vast majority of cases are directly associated with lifestyle—smoking cigarettes. All cancers caused by cigarette smoking are 100% preventable.

The incidence of lung cancer is highest among people who started smoking cigarettes at an early age and those who smoke the most cigarettes daily. Tobacco products cause more than 80% of lung cancer.[26] The single best prevention of lung cancer is never to smoke. Passive, or involuntary, smoke also contributes significantly to lung cancer. A person who lives or works with smokers significantly increases his or her risk of developing lung cancer, even if choosing to not smoke. Symptoms of lung cancer typically include a persistent cough, blood in the sputum, chest pain, recurring pneumonia, and bronchitis.

The bad news about lung cancer is that early diagnosis tends to be rare. Regular X-rays of the lungs and checkups for blood in the sputum seem to be ineffective means of early detection, perhaps because of the altered appearance and function of lung cells from smoking. By the time most lung cancers are detected, either the cancer is not treatable because of widespread metastasis or the treatment is limited to ensuring a short-term extension of life. New studies are under way to determine whether a particular type of CT scan may find lung cancers early. Five-year survival rates following diagnosis of lung cancer are between 7 and 12%, which is low.

The colorless, odorless gas radon has been somewhat inconsistently associated with increased risk for lung cancer.[27] People living in areas designated high in radon should have their homes measured. Asbestos inhalation has also been associated with lung cancer. Marijuana cigarettes have more tar than regular cigarettes. Many of the cancer-causing substances in tobacco are also found in marijuana. However, because marijuana is an illegal substance, it is difficult to gather data on its effects on the body.[28]

Although the absolute best ways to prevent lung cancer are not smoking, not living with a smoker, not working in a smoking environment, ensuring that radon levels in the home are safe, and avoiding asbestos, substantial evidence exists for the role of diet in lung cancer prevention.[29,30] A diet high in whole fruits and vegetables seems to protect against lung cancer. Smokers who regularly consume much produce (fruits and vegetables) seem to have reduced incidence. While regular consumption of whole fruits and vegetables does not ensure that a smoker (or anyone else) will not get cancer, especially lung cancer, there is convincing evidence that a healthy diet provides some protection.

## Colorectal Cancer

Colon cancer and cancer of the rectum rank as the third leading causes of cancer deaths in the United States.[31] When detected early, 90% of localized colorectal cancers can be cured. Once the cancer has spread, however, this chance drops to only 10%.

A family history of colon cancer doubles the risk, but family history accounts for only 10 to 15% of colon cancers.[32] People with a family history need to be extra vigilant and participate in regular screenings, but so do people with family histories of benign polyps (growths) in the colon. Any change or increases in constipation or chronic constipation suggest the need for follow-up screening for abnormal growths. Consuming large numbers of calories may increase colon cancer risk.[33] Symptoms of colorectal cancer include a change in bowel habits, chronic abdominal discomfort, sudden weight loss, lack of appetite, or rectal bleeding. Long-term survival rates are much higher when potential cancers are detected before symptoms develop. Detection of colorectal cancer can frequently be accomplished via screenings.

Identification of polyps is a primary screening method. The occurrence of polyps in the colon and rectum does not mean a person will develop cancer. In cases in which the polyps do become cancerous, the length of time from initiation to cancer may be 5 to 10 years.[34] The type of screening test used depends on the age of the person as well as family and personal history. Anyone over age 50, even without a family history of the disease, should be tested.

Anyone can undertake prevention of colorectal cancer. Diet is believed to be the primary cause for its development. The National Cancer Institute, the American Cancer Society, and the American Institute for Cancer Research recommend a diet high in vegetables (especially cruciferous vegetables) and fiber and low in fat.[35] Regular physical activity and maintenance of recommended body weight are also probably preventive. Long-term (15 years or more) ingestion of the B vitamin folate may reduce the risk for colon cancer. Recent studies suggest that 81 mg of aspirin (the lowest observable amount that produced desirable results) may also have a protective effect against colon cancer.[36] Although aspirin is a drug with side effects, some potentially life-threatening, it may also be beneficial for people at elevated risk who can tolerate it. However, aspirin as a preventive should never be taken without prior consultation with a physician. People who smoke have a 30 to 40% greater probability of developing colorectal cancer than do nonsmokers.[37]

## Stomach, Liver, and Pancreatic Cancer

### Stomach Cancer

Stomach cancer, except for cancer of the upper part of the stomach (which may be associated with obesity), has steadily declined in the United States and other developed countries. This decrease seems to be strongly linked to the availability of refrigeration, eliminating the need for salt as a preservative. Refrigeration also provides year-round availability of fresh fruits and vegetables, linked to decreased risk. The popular interest in green tea consumption may prove beneficial in reducing the risk for stomach cancer. Diets high in salt, smoked food, and pickled vegetables probably increase the risk for stomach cancer. However, the survival rate for all people with stomach cancer is about 23%. The reason for this is that diagnosis usually occurs at an advanced stage of the disease. Smokers have double the rate of stomach cancer of nonsmokers. The major non-lifestyle cause of stomach cancer is infection with the *Helicobacter pylori* bacteria.[38]

Most types of stomach cancer can be prevented by diet. Although the numbers of cases are declining, stomach cancer still ranks among the top 10 cancer killers in the United States. Symptoms are nonspecific, and diagnosis at early stages is not usual.

### Liver Cancer

Liver cancer is relatively uncommon in the United States and other developed countries. No effective treatment exists for it; the 5-year survival rate is only 6%. Many liver cancers are lifestyle-related. The primary risk factor for liver cancer is infection with hepatitis B or hepatitis C viruses. The major method of transmission for these viruses is the sharing of needles or sexual contact.[39] Research suggests that hepatitis B can also be transmitted by sharing a rolled paper used for snorting cocaine or other drugs.[40] Regular, heavy (more than moderate) consumption of alcohol, leading to cirrhosis and a condition known as *alcoholic hepatitis,* is closely associated with the development of liver cancer.[41] Ingestion of aflatoxins (a type of food mold) from contaminated food has been demonstrated to produce liver

cancer, particularly among people in developing countries,[42] but it tends to be rare in the United States.

### Pancreatic Cancer

Pancreatic cancer, lesser known than the cancers mentioned previously, ranks among the leading five causes of cancer death in the United States. Pancreatic cancer does not seem to get the publicity of many other types of cancer, yet it is extremely deadly and very difficult to diagnose. Researchers are currently investigating tests for detecting pancreatic cancer. There is currently a test that looks at changes in pancreatic fluids as a result of the DNA changes in what is known as the K-ras oncogene. The change in this oncogene alters the regulation of pancreatic cell growth.[43] An estimated 42,470 new cases were expected in the United States in 2009, with 35,240 cases resulting in death.[44] No effective method exists to screen or diagnose this cancer. Imaging tests can help find precancerous changes called dysplasia.[45] Occasionally, depending on where the tumor originates, jaundice may occur while the tumor is in an early stage. Even so, the 5-year survival rate is only 4%. Little is known about pancreatic cancer except that smoking increases the risk. Because the pancreas is related to digestion and absorption, speculation is that diet affects the development and course of this cancer, but no specifics are known at this time.

### Leukemia and Lymphoma

**Leukemia** and **lymphoma** (Hodgkin disease and non-Hodgkin lymphoma) are two of the most frequent childhood cancers, but they strike more adults than children every year. Leukemia occurs in adults nearly 10 times more often than in children. Leukemias can be divided into four main types, which include acute (AML), chronic myeloid (LMC), acute lymphocytic (ALL), and chronic lymphocytic (CCC).[46] The causes of leukemia are largely unidentified, although people with genetic abnormalities, such as Down syndrome, experience it more frequently. Excessive exposure to certain chemicals, such as benzene, or infection with the retrovirus HTLV-I also places people at elevated risk. The symptoms resemble those of many other conditions, so they are frequently overlooked initially. They include fatigue, paleness, weight loss, repeated infections, easy bruising, and nosebleeds or other hemorrhages. Children usually experience the onset of these symptoms abruptly, but adults with chronic leukemia progress slowly and exhibit few symptoms.

Early, appropriate diagnosis is the key to long-term survival for leukemia. Depending on the type of leukemia and stage of diagnosis, 5-year survival rates may be as high as 68% for adults and 86% for children.[47]

Lymphoma is a condition in which a tumor composed of lymphoid tissue occurs. The two most general categories of lymphoma are Hodgkin disease and non-

Hodgkin lymphoma, which includes all types of lymphoma other than Hodgkin. Hodgkin disease rates have declined, especially in the elderly, but cases of non-Hodgkin lymphoma have nearly doubled since the 1970s. Causes involve reduced immune function and exposure to infectious agents via organ transplants or viruses such as HIV (human immunodeficiency virus) or Epstein-Barr. Herbicides and other chemicals may influence the development of the disease. Lifestyle habits, such as smoking and excessive drinking of alcohol, may increase risk. These lifestyle factors are not strongly linked to the development but being obese may increase the risk for non-Hodgkin lymphoma.

The symptoms of lymphoma include enlarged lymph nodes, itching, fever, night sweats, anemia, and weight loss. The fever may come and go over periods of weeks or months. Survival rates vary greatly, according to the type of disease and stage at diagnosis but can be as high as 53 to 91% after 5 years.[48]

## Skin Cancer

The most frequently occurring types of cancer are skin cancers. Skin cancers fall into three main categories: basal cell carcinoma, squamous cell carcinoma, and melanoma. Of the three categories, melanoma is by far the most deadly.

### Basal Cell Carcinoma

Basal cell **carcinoma** is the most common skin cancer and, along with squamous cell, is responsible for approximately 1 million cases of skin cancer a year.[49] Basal cell carcinoma occurs in the outermost skin layers and tends to spread by widening rather than by growing deeper into the skin. The cancer develops into a central sore, which crusts over and bleeds but does not go away.[50] Basal cell carcinoma grows slowly and rarely spreads to other parts of the body.

### Squamous Cell Carcinoma

The second most common type of skin cancer is squamous cell. Squamous cell carcinoma grows faster than basal cell cancer but still grows fairly slowly and can metastasize to other parts of the body. Typically, a squamous cell skin lesion is a firm, red, painless nodule.[51] Both basal cell and squamous cell carcinomas are usually the result of overexposure to sunlight. They occur on a part of the body that has been exposed to the sun.

### Malignant Melanoma

Although it is the least common type of skin cancer, about 75% of skin cancer deaths are due to malignant melanoma. The American Cancer Society estimated that 68,720 new melanomas would be diagnosed in 2009. All skin cancers, but especially malignant melanoma,

have increased in number in recent years, so that the current lifetime risk of developing malignant melanoma is about 1 in 50 for whites, 1 in 100 for blacks, and 1 in 200 for Hispanics.[52] Although the use of sunscreens with an SPF of 15 or higher seems to reduce the number of basal and squamous cell skin cancers, it does not appear to decrease the risk for melanoma.[53] Genetics is a strong factor in getting malignant melanoma, but it does not explain the explosive increase in the disease that has occurred in the last few decades. Melanoma often grows on parts of the body that are rarely exposed to the sun (such as the buttocks or feet) and does not increase in incidence among people whose occupations require them to spend long hours in the sun (such as farmers). Melanoma appears to be more highly associated with intermittent sun exposure and blistering sunburns occurring early in life (before age 15).

All adults are susceptible, but particularly those with the following risk factors:

- A family history of melanoma
- A personal history of one or more severe sunburns as a child
- Fair skin and many freckles, blonde or red hair, and light eyes
- Occupational exposure to industrial radiation or certain chemicals
- Consumption of medications that increase sensitivity to ultraviolet light

People with these factors should check their entire bodies regularly for any change in the size or color of a mole or other spot; any scaling, oozing, or bleeding from a bump or nodule; pigmentation spreading beyond its border; and a change in sensation, itchiness, tenderness, or pain. Any skin growth that bleeds or crusts should be seen by a physician (Figure 13–2).[54,55]

Knowing the ABCDs of skin cancer can help people identify melanoma during the early stages when it is still highly treatable (with a 95% 5-year survival rate):

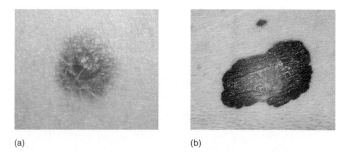

(a)                                    (b)

**FIGURE 13-2** Comparison of Nonmalignant and Malignant Skin Growths

(a) A normal mole. Note its symmetrical shape, regular borders, even color, and relatively small size (about a half centimeter). (b) A malignant melanoma. Note its asymmetrical shape, irregular borders, uneven color, and relatively large size (about 2 centimeters).

- *Asymmetry:* If you drew an imaginary line through the center of the mole or pigmented area, the two halves would be shaped differently.
- *Border:* Most normal moles are regularly shaped and their outside borders are regularly shaped. If a border appears to have scalloped edges or to be poorly defined in areas or uneven, it is not normal.
- *Color:* A mole should be one color. Variation in color—differing shades of black, brown, tan, red, or some combination of colors—or an intensely black color indicates a problem and need for further investigation.
- *Diameter:* A mole or pigmented area greater than 6 mm (the size of a pencil eraser) should be looked at by a specialist.

As with all cancers, the first line of defense is prevention. Because most skin cancers are directly related to overexposure to the sun's ultraviolet rays, take caution to limit this exposure. Although the use of sunscreen (with an SPF of 15 or higher) may not prevent malignant melanoma, it does decrease the incidence of basal and squamous cell skin cancers. Newer sunscreens block a wider range of ultraviolet rays and may prove to reduce even melanoma over time.[56] Children particularly should always wear sunscreen when playing outside to prevent the blistering sunburn associated with melanoma later in life. The sun's rays are the strongest between 10 a.m. and 2 p.m. (even on cloudy days) and direct exposure at that time should be avoided, even with a sunscreen. Protective clothing, such as hats, long-sleeve shirts, long pants, and ultraviolet-protecting sun-

## Real-World Wellness

### Are Tanning Devices Hazardous to Your Health?

*I want to be tan this summer and thought I would get a head start by using a tanning bed. Is it safe for me to do so?*

Sunlight produces two types of ultraviolet radiation: ultraviolet A (UVA) and ultraviolet B (UVB). UVB is 1,000 times more likely to cause burns than is UVA. Because it penetrates the skin more deeply, UVA radiation causes the skin to tan or burn more slowly. A small amount of UVB radiation, however, can cause skin damage.

Most tanning devices (for example, sunlamps) give off either mostly UVA or UVB radiation. Newer UVA sunlamps give off as much as 10 times more UVA than is received from the sun or given by older UVB sunlamps. Although exposure to UVA sunlamps is less likely to cause burns of the skin and eyes, UVA radiation in high doses may increase the risks for skin cancer and premature skin aging. Studies also suggest that skin cancer is exacerbated when people combine tanning in the sun with tanning by sunlamps. Here are some facts concerning tans and tanning devices:

- *Skin cancer* risks increase each time the skin is exposed to UV radiation.
- *Burns* of the skin and eyes may occur.
- *Photosensitivity* means being extra sensitive to UV radiation as a result of using or consuming various substances that may cause allergic reactions, severe skin burns, itchy and scaly skin, and rash. Examples of photosensitizing products are soaps, shampoos, makeup, birth control pills, antibiotics, antihistamines, diuretics, and tranquilizers.

- *Cataracts,* an eye condition in which the lens becomes cloudy, may develop as a result of unprotected exposure to UVA and UVB radiation. For this reason, it is required that tanning devices have labels warning users to wear protective eyewear.
- *Premature skin aging,* in which the skin becomes dry, wrinkled, and leathery, is one of the most noticeable signs of repeated UV exposure.
- *Blood vessel damage and reduced immunity* may result from exposure to UV radiation.
- People who have red or blond hair and blue eyes, are fair-skinned, have freckles, and sunburn easily are at highest risk for skin damage. If you burn and do not tan in sunlight, you will probably burn and will not tan using sunlamps.
- A UVA tan offers some protection against further UV damage—about the same as an SPF of 2 or 3. Even with a dark tan, UV damage continues to accumulate.
- Sunscreens are not recommended for tanning indoors except to protect parts of your body you do not want to tan (for example, the lips). Sunscreens do not prevent UVA allergic-type reactions of photosensitive people.
- Always wear special goggles that block UV radiation, avoid using photosensitizing products, avoid tanning if your skin never tans, and follow the manufacturer's recommended time of exposure for your skin type.[57]

glasses (too much sun can lead to cataracts or melanoma in the eyes), should be worn. Avoid tanning booths and sunlamps (see Real-World Wellness: Are Tanning Devices Hazardous to Your Health?). No matter how dark a person's skin is, he or she becomes darker when exposed to the sun. Although the risk is greatly reduced for darker-skinned people, anyone can get skin cancer.

## Oral Cancer

Oral cancers are cancers of any part of the oral cavity, including the lip, tongue, mouth, and throat. Oral cancer occurs more than twice as often in males than in females. This is because the risk factors of cigar and pipe smoking and the use of smokeless tobacco are practiced much more frequently by men than by women. Cigarette smoking and excessive consumption of alcohol (both on the rise among women) are also considered risk factors. Wiser lifestyle choices (choosing not to use tobacco products and reducing the consumption of alcohol) could practically eliminate oral cancers.

## Cancers That Can Affect Women

### Breast Cancer

The rate of cures for breast cancer has increased significantly over the last decade (see Just the Facts: Drugs and Breast Cancer Treatment). In addition, women's groups and public and private health agencies have done an excellent job of getting the word out about early detection and have supported efforts for improved treatment for all age groups. These efforts have led to a decline in cancer deaths, except in women over 50

### [ JUST THE FACTS ]
#### Drugs and Breast Cancer Treatment

The drug tamoxifen has received a great deal of coverage in the press about its use as an anticancer drug. As with all drugs, tamoxifen has side effects. These side effects can be deadly, and use of the drug should be carefully considered. Tamoxifen has also been used as a cancer preventive among women at high risk (which can include any woman over 60 years of age, as well as younger women with several factors, including breast cancer in first-degree relatives). Other drugs that seem to reduce the rate of invasive breast cancer are raloxifene (a drug used to prevent bone loss); taxol, as a treatment in even late-stage cancer; and herceptin, which seems to delay progression of late-stage cancer.[59] Good news emerges almost daily about treatment for breast cancer. Early detection can result in a complete recovery.

years of age. However, surgeries and other treatments associated with breast cancer can still be devastating. Although breast cancer is relatively rare in men, about 1,910 men were diagnosed with it in 2009.[58]

One in nine women who live to age 85 will develop breast cancer. Being over the age of 60 automatically places a woman in a high-risk category. Mutation in the genes known as *BRCA1, BRCA2* (also referred to as p53 suppressor genes) accounts for the development of breast cancer in some women. The *BRCA* gene is a tumor suppressor gene. When it is mutated, it no longer functions to suppress abnormal growth. Most DNA mutations related to breast cancer occur in single breast cells during a woman's life rather than having been inherited.[60] A woman with a mother or sister who has had breast cancer has double the risk of getting breast cancer. This risk is particularly high if the cancer occurred in the relative before menopause, if it involved both breasts, or if it affected more than one first-degree relative (for example, a mother and sister or two sisters) or other close relatives in several generations.

Still, most cases of breast cancer cannot be explained because most women have at least one risk factor. Other

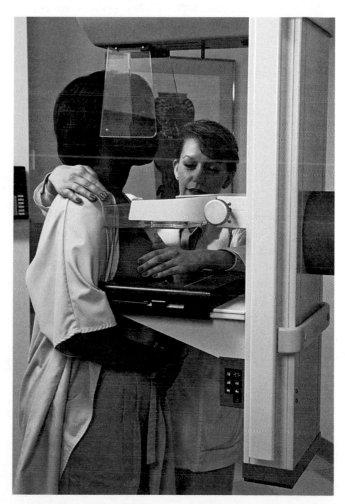

Mammography is important in the early detection of breast cancer.

risk factors include early menarche (before age 12), late menopause (after age 55), recent use of oral contraceptives or postmenopausal estrogens, and never having had children or having given birth to a first child after age 30.[61] The role of lifestyle factors remains somewhat nebulous. Although breast cancer is worldwide, a strong cultural relationship exists between diet, especially high fat intake, and cancer. The reasons for this relationship have not been established.[62] Other factors related to the incidence of breast cancer are alcohol intake (women who have 2 to 5 drinks daily have about 1½ times the risk of women who are nondrinkers); weight gain, particularly following menopause; and physical inactivity.[63] No studies have conclusively linked cigarette smoking to breast cancer. Research is building that suggests smoking does increase the risk. What is known is that smoking affects overall health and increases the risk of developing many other types of cancer.

Early detection is the best means of reducing mortality (see Just the Facts: Cancer-Related Checkup Guidelines). The 5-year survival rate for localized cancers is 96%. Localized spread of the cancer lowers that survival rate to 76%, and distant metastasis yields only a 21% 5-year survival rate.[64] Eighty percent of breast cancers are found by the affected women through self-examination. Monthly self-examination remains the primary way to find small, localized cancers, especially in young women (see Just the Facts: Breast Self-Examination on page 434). Mammograms are useful tools but are more useful for detection in older women whose breast tissue is less dense. Even the best mammogram misses 10% of tumors, because breast tissue extends beyond the area X-rayed in a mammogram. Examinations by qualified physicians are helpful in detecting breast cancer, but most examinations occur only on an annual or biannual basis. The time lapse between such exams provides aggressive, fast-growing tumors with time to spread to surrounding tissue or lymph nodes.

Symptoms include a tumor that may feel like a piece of gravel or hard nodule. The tumor will not enlarge and shrink in size from month to month. Other symptoms include thickening, swelling, dimpling, scaling, pain, and tenderness of the nipple or discharge from the nipple. Breast cancer can occur at any age, even in very young women. Anyone (male or female) detecting these symptoms should consult a physician without delay. Usually breast pain results from benign conditions and is not the first symptom of breast cancer.

### Uterine Cancer

Uterine cancers can occur either in the cervix (cervical cancer, or cancer in the neck of the uterus) or in the endometrium (endometrial cancer, or cancer of the lining of the uterus). Cervical cancer is closely linked to sexual behavior, especially through transmission of the human papillomavirus. Because of its close association with sexual activity (sex at an early age, multiple partners, a partner who has had multiple partners, multiple pregnancies, and a history of sexually transmitted diseases, such as herpes and genital warts), many experts considered it a sexually transmitted disease. However, this is not the only reason people develop this cancer. As women have participated more frequently in annual Pap smears and preventive reproductive health, the number of deaths from cervical cancer has declined significantly (70% decrease).[65] Smoking seems to increase the risk for the disease. Prevention involves following safer sex practices (see Chapter 12), not smoking, and having regular Pap smears.

The symptoms include abnormal vaginal bleeding or spotting or discharge. Late symptoms include pain. When diagnosed early, invasive cervical cancer is one of the most treatable cancers, with a 5-year survival rate of 91%. Regular Pap smears after age 18 or after sexual activity is initiated (no matter how young) can detect early, abnormal cells or localized cancers. Women should have regular Pap smears for the rest of their lives.

The lining of the uterus is the endometrium. Endometrial cancers occur in the upper, broader portion of the uterus, as opposed to in the narrower opening (the cervix). Endometrial cancer is more common among women over the age of 50, following menopause.

## [ JUST THE FACTS ]

### Cancer-Related Checkup Guidelines

Listed here are checkup guidelines to help healthy people with early cancer detection. These are guidelines and not rules. They apply only if none of the following seven warning signs is present:

C   hange in bowel or bladder habits
A   sore that does not heal
U   nusual bleeding or discharge
T   hickening or lump in breast or elsewhere
I   ndigestion or difficulty swallowing
O   bvious change in wart or moles
N   agging cough or hoarseness

# [ JUST THE FACTS ]

## Screening Guidelines For the Early Detection of Cancer in Asymptomatic People

| Site | Recommendation |
|------|----------------|
| Breast | • Yearly mammograms are recommended starting at age 40. The age at which screening should be stopped should be individualized by considering the potential risks and benefits of screening in the context of overall health status and longevity.<br>• Clinical breast exam should be part of a periodic health exam about every 3 years for women in their 20s and 30s and every year for women 40 and older.<br>• Women should know how their breasts normally feel and report any breast change promptly to their health care providers. Breast self-exam is an option for women starting in their 20s.<br>• Screening MRI is recommended for women with an approximately 20%–25% or greater lifetime risk of breast cancer, including women with a strong family history of breast or ovarian cancer and women who were treated for Hodgkin disease. |
| Colon & rectum | Beginning at age 50, men and women should begin screening with 1 of the examination schedules below:<br>• A fecal occult blood test (FOBT) or fecal immunochemical test (FIT) every year<br>• A flexible sigmoidoscopy (FSIG) every 5 years<br>• Annual FOBT or FIT and flexible sigmoidoscopy every 5 years*<br>• A double-contrast barium enema every 5 years<br>• A colonoscopy every 10 years<br>*Combined testing is preferred over either annual FOBT or FIT, or FSIG every 5 years, alone. People who are at moderate or high risk for colorectal cancer should talk with a doctor about a different testing schedule. |
| Prostate | The PSA test and the digital rectal examination should be offered annually, beginning at age 50, to men who have a life expectancy of at least 10 years. Men at high risk (African American men and men with a strong family history of 1 or more first-degree relatives diagnosed with prostate cancer at an early age) should begin testing at age 45. For both men at average risk and high risk, information should be provided about what is known and what is uncertain about the benefits and limitations of early detection and treatment of prostate cancer so that they can make an informed decision about testing. |
| Uterus | **Cervix:** Screening should begin approximately 3 years after a woman begins having vaginal intercourse, but no later than 21 years of age. Screening should be done every year with regular Pap tests or every 2 years using liquid-based tests. At or after age 30, women who have had three normal test results in a row may get screened every 2 to 3 years. Alternatively, cervical cancer screening with HPV DNA testing and conventional or liquid-based cytology could be performed every 3 years. However, doctors may suggest a woman get screened more often if she has certain risk factors, such as HIV infection or a weak immune system. Women aged 70 and older who have had 3 or more consecutive normal Pap tests in the last 10 years may choose to stop cervical cancer screening. Screening after total hysterectomy (with removal of the cervix) is not necessary unless the surgery was done as a treatment for cervical cancer.<br><br>**Endometrium:** The American Cancer Society recommends that at the time of menopause all women should be informed about the risks and symptoms of endometrial cancer and strongly encouraged to report any unexpected bleeding or spotting to their physicians. Annual screening for endometrial cancer with endometrial biopsy beginning at age 35 should be offered to women with or at risk for hereditary nonpolyposis colon cancer (HNPCC). |
| Cancer-related checkup | For individuals undergoing periodic health examinations, a cancer-related checkup should include health counseling and, depending on a person's age and gender, might include examinations for cancers of the thyroid, oral cavity, skin, lymph nodes, testes, and ovaries, as well as for some nonmalignant diseases. |

American Cancer Society guidelines for early cancer detection are assessed annually in order to identify whether there is new scientific evidence sufficient to warrant a reevaluation of current recommendations. If evidence is sufficiently compelling to consider a change or clarification in a current guideline or the development of a new guideline, a formal procedure is initiated. Guidelines are formally evaluated every 5 years regardless of whether new evidence suggests a change in the existing recommendations. There are 9 steps in this procedure, and the "guidelines for guideline development" were formally established to provide a specific methodology for science and expert judgment to form the underpinnings of specific statements and recommendations from the Society. These procedures constitute a deliberate process to ensure that all Society recommendations have the same methodological and evidence-based process at their core. This process also employs a system for rating strength and consistency of evidence that is similar to that employed by the Agency for Health Care Research and Quality (AHCRQ) and the US Preventive Services Task Force (USPSTF).

# [ JUST THE FACTS ]

## Breast Self-Examination

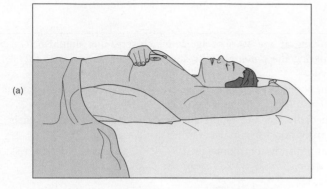
(a)

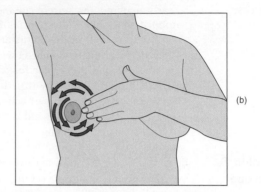
(b)

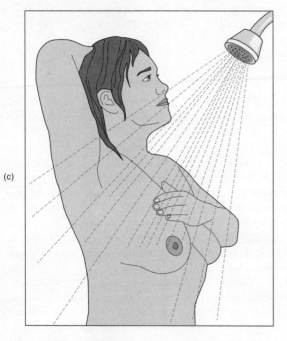
(c)

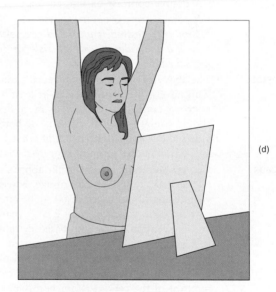
(d)

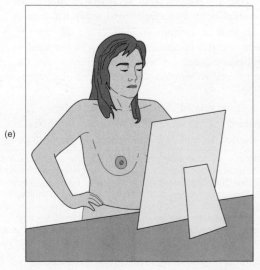
(e)

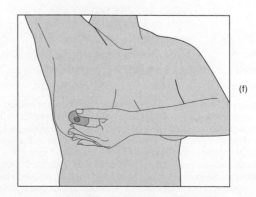
(f)

*continued*

## [ JUST THE FACTS ]

JUST THE FACTS
*continued*

Following are the proper techniques for examining the breasts.

1. Lying in bed, place a pillow under one shoulder to elevate and flatten the breast. Examine each breast using the opposite hand, first with your arm under your head and again with your arm at your side (a).
2. Make small, circular motions with the flat pads (not the tips) of your fingers (b).
3. Examine your breasts in concentric circles from the rims inward toward the nipples. Feel for knots, lumps, thickenings, indentations, and swellings. Be sure to include the armpit (b).
4. Wet, soapy skin makes it easier to feel lumps. Keep one hand overhead and examine each breast with the opposite hand while you are in the shower (c).
5. In front of a large mirror, stand with your arms relaxed at your sides. Examine your breasts for swelling, dimpling, bulges, retractions, irritations, and sores or changes in mole or nipple color, texture, or orientation. Repeat with the arms extended and again with your arms clasped behind your head (d).
6. Repeat the inspection in step 5 while contracting your chest muscles: first clasp your hands in front of your forehead, squeezing your palms together; then place your palms flat on the sides of your hips, pressing downward. This highlights the bulges and indentations, which may signal the growth of tumors (e).
7. Bend forward from the hips, resting your hands on your knees or two chairbacks. Use a mirror to examine your breasts for normal irregularities and abnormal variances; both are pronounced in this position.
8. Squeeze your nipples to inspect for secretions and discharge (f).
9. Report any suspicious findings to your doctor without delay.
10. Supplement your self-examination with a breast examination by your doctor as part of a regular physical examination and cancer checkup.

---

Increasing evidence points to high levels of the hormone estrogen as contributing to the course of the disease. This is because estrogen causes the lining of the uterus to grow, which can lead to a premalignant condition that can lead to invasive cancer.

Risk factors include being overweight (extreme obesity), diabetes, high blood pressure, early menarche (before age 12), late menopause (after age 52), never giving birth, and receiving unopposed estrogen replacement therapy. Those with risk factors should check with their gynecologists.[66]

### Ovarian Cancer

Ovarian cancer is difficult to diagnose, having few symptoms until reaching an advanced stage. Ovarian cancer is the ninth most common cancer in women and the fifth cause of cancer death in women.[67] Five to 10% of ovarian cancers are inherited, meaning that family history and mutations in the same genes that are related to breast cancer (*BRCA1* and *BRCA2*) serve as potential markers. Symptoms are frequently vague and include cramping, discomfort, distention of the abdomen resulting from fluid buildup, diarrhea or constipation, gas, and a feeling of incomplete emptying of the bladder. Full-term pregnancies and breast-feeding, as well as the use of oral contraceptives, seem to reduce the risk. A high-fat diet seems to increase the risk. Fertility drugs that stimulate ovulation may be associated with increased risk.

Although considered a relatively rare cancer, late diagnosis can be deadly. If found in stage I, the cure rate is about 90%. The risk for ovarian cancer increases with age and peaks in the late 70s.[68]

## Cancers That Can Affect Men

### Testicular Cancer

About 8,400 men and boys, usually ages 15 to 34, are diagnosed with testicular cancer per year. These cancers are very treatable. Testicular cancer is painless and asymptomatic, but it is detectable by self-examination. Every boy old enough to be in high school and every man should do a monthly self-exam until reaching the age of 40 (see Just the Facts: Testicular Self-Examination on page 436). Signs of possible testicular cancer include any lump, enlargement, or hardening of either testis. Any changes should be followed up with an examination by a physician. Undetected, the disease can spread to the lymph nodes and beyond. Early detection results in a high cure rate.[69]

## [ JUST THE FACTS ]

### Testicular Self-Examination

Cancer of the testes (the male reproductive glands) is one of the most common cancers in men 15 to 34 years of age. It accounts for 12% of cancer deaths in this group. The best hope for early detection of testicular cancer is a simple, 3-minute monthly self-examination. The best time is after a warm bath or shower, when the scrotal skin is most relaxed.

Roll each testicle gently between the thumb and fingers of both hands. If you find any hard lumps, or nodules, see your doctor promptly. The lumps, or nodules, may not be malignant, but only a doctor can make the diagnosis.

After a thorough physical examination, your doctor may perform X-ray studies for the most accurate diagnosis.

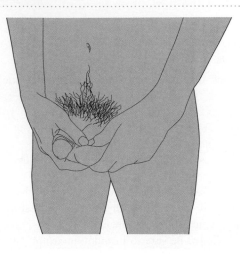

### Prostate Cancer

Most men who live long enough will have some evidence of prostate cancer. The second leading cause of cancer death among men, prostate cancer has a 100% cure rate when diagnosed while localized (58% of prostate cancers). Improvement in diagnosis has resulted from a blood test for prostate-specific antigen (PSA test). The PSA test, in combination with a digital (manual) rectal exam (DRE), has made prostate cancer much easier to detect at earlier stages. There has been some research indicating that the PSA test could still miss some prostate cancer, however.

Men at elevated risk include African Americans (who have incidence and death rates twice as high as those of white men), increasing age (PSAs and DREs should be annual events in men over age 50; prostate cancer is rare in young men), and men with family histories of prostate cancer. Dietary fat intake may also be a factor. African American men and those with family histories should begin annual checkups at age 40.

The symptoms for prostate cancer tend to be nonspecific and similar to those of a condition known as *benign prostate hypertrophy*. They include weak or interrupted urine flow; inability to urinate; difficulty starting or stopping urine flow; frequent need to urinate, especially at night; pain or burning on urination; and continuing pain in the lower back, pelvis, or upper thighs.[70]

### Treatment

The best treatment for cancer is prevention by leading a wellness lifestyle. Even with a family history, it is impossible to determine at this time who will get cancer. Taking appropriate lifestyle measures may make the difference.

Eating a healthy diet high in fruit, vegetable, and grain products; exercising regularly; avoiding tobacco products and excessive alcohol consumption; performing self-exams accurately and regularly; and getting screenings as recommended can save lives. Screenings that result in accurate diagnoses are vital. When detected while still local, prostate and thyroid cancers are considered 100% "curable" (the patient is still living with no signs of cancer at 5 years). The cure rate for melanoma and ovarian cancer, when diagnosed early, is 95%; breast cancer is 96%; and testicular cancer is 99%.[71]

Traditional cancer treatment has involved the use of surgery, radiation, chemotherapy, or some combination of these three. Today, these more traditional approaches are being combined with new, experimental approaches. At the same time, traditional methods are being continuously refined, and every year, more experimental methods are being used. New treatments for cancer are being tested every day.

## Types of Treatment

### Surgery

Cancers are often treated surgically. A surgeon removes the malignant tissue and some additional normal tissue. Current surgical techniques focus on removing less surrounding normal tissue than before and combining surgery with chemotherapy and/or radiotherapy. Surgery is used most often with breast, skin, gastrointestinal tract, female reproductive organ, prostate, and testicular cancers. Surgery may be used for curative, diagnostic, or staging (determines how far the cancer has spread) purposes. Sometimes surgery is used to remove some, but not all, of the tumor because too much damage to surrounding organs would occur.

## Chemotherapy

Chemotherapy is the use of drugs and hormones to treat cancers. More than 100 drugs are currently used for chemotherapy. These drugs may be used either alone or in combination with other drugs in treatments.[72] Some of the most important advances in the treatment of cancer have been in the area of chemotherapy. Most chemotherapeutic agents work by destroying the cancer cells' ability to carry out cell division and replication. Unfortunately, chemotherapy influences all cell division, even in healthy cells that need to divide to function normally. As a result, people having chemotherapy often have side effects, some of which can be dangerous. These side effects include suppression of the immune system, diarrhea, and hair loss.

Newer drug therapies take a different approach. New types of drugs include antigrowth drugs that block the body's signals that promote cancer cell growth (called antigrowth drugs); drugs that cause the cancer cells to self-destruct; antiangiogenesis drugs that cut off the cancer cells' blood supply; and drugs that "coordinate" radiation dosages with monoclonal antibodies (molecules specifically engineered to fit into the receptacles on certain cells) that target specific cancer cells. These drugs have much fewer and less severe side effects than traditional chemotherapies. Chemotherapies may be administered by pill or liquid, chemo shots, or intravenous (IV) injections into the veins.

## Antiangiogenesis Therapy

Antiangiogenesis therapy is the use of drugs to stop cancerous growths from developing new blood vessels. This type of therapy is one of the most promising treatments to come out of research in recent years. Since all parts of the body and every cell within those structures, including cancerous tumors, require a regular supply of blood to survive, antiangiogenic drugs prevent the formation of new blood vessels in the cancerous growths. Currently, there are more than 50 compounds that interfere with the reproduction of the blood vessels. Significant advantages of these drugs are that they have only mild side effects, as opposed to the devastating side effects of other treatments. When combined with chemotherapy, an increase in length of life has been achieved; but, unfortunately, the present group of antiangiogenic drugs cannot bring about a cure.[73]

## Radiotherapy

Radiotherapy is the use of radiation to destroy cancer cells or their reproductive mechanisms, so that they can-

not replicate. As a result of radiation, side effects, such as diarrhea, itching, and difficulty swallowing, can occur. However, as the ability to plan more carefully the preciseness of focus, length of exposure, and time of treatment has improved, the damage to noncancerous cells and the potential side effects have decreased.

## Bone Marrow and Peripheral Blood Stem Cell Transplants

Bone marrow is the spongy tissue that makes blood cells. Part of this process is making disease-fighting cells that are part of the immune system. Our blood cells start out as immature cells called *stem cells*. Stem cells are found primarily in bone marrow, where they produce blood cells.

There are three basic types of stem cell transplants. Where the stems are taken (the source) from determines the type. The three types are as follows:[74]

1. *Syngeneic SCT.* This is a very rare type of transplant because the donor is an identical twin.
2. *Allogeneic SCT.* This type of transplant comes from another individual whose tissue best matches the patient. The donor may or may not be a family member. There is a national registry where potential donors can be identified.
3. *Autologous SCT.* The patients act as their own donor. The stem cells are taken (called harvesting) from either the patient's bone marrow or his or her circulatory blood. After treating the stem cells with an extremely high dose of chemotherapy or radiation, they are frozen. This is called purging and is done to reduce the number of cancer cells. Unfortunately, the purging may kill many of the stem cells. This type of transplant is used to treat lymphomas and myeloma.

Until the new bone marrow starts making new white blood cells (approximately 6 weeks), the patient is prone to infections, nosebleeds, bleeding gums, bruising, and pneumonia. The worst case is that the transplant can fail to function.

## Immunotherapy

Immunotherapy is the use of a variety of substances to trigger a person's immune response, which then attacks malignant cells or keeps them from becoming active. Currently immunotherapy has a fairly small role in fighting cancer.[75] There are two main types of immunotherapy. One type is active immunotherapy. Active immunotherapy stimulates the body's own immune defenses to fight the cancer. The second type is passive immunotherapy. These types of immunotherapy use immune system components to fight the cancer. Most immunotherapies being used target one type of cancer cell.

## Nurturing Your Spirituality

### Living Well with Cancer

Chemotherapy and other drug treatments offer potentially life-saving solutions for cancer patients. But does the cure lie solely in the doctor's office? Perhaps not. Research indicates that spiritual practices may increase a cancer patient's chance of survival and enhance his or her quality of life.

Scientists are studying how the mind affects the neurological and immune systems.[77] This discipline, known as *psychoneuroimmunology,* is of great interest to cancer researchers. For example, participation in support groups has been shown to increase the life expectancy of people with cancer. The results of a study reported by Johns Hopkins University are striking: "Women with breast cancer who took part in a support group lived an average of eighteen months longer (a doubling of the survival time following diagnosis) than those who did not participate. In addition, all the long-term survivors belonged to the therapy group."[78]

Although support groups do not improve physical health, they seem to provide a camaraderie that contributes to overall wellness. Belonging to groups such as prayer circles also plays a beneficial role in recovery. Support groups offer patients a sense of connectedness that promotes wellness. Conversely, social isolation—lack of a support network of friends and family—seems to increase the likelihood of death.[79] Although the extent of its influence is unknown, the nurturing of cancer patients' spiritual side as well as care for their physical health seems to help in the effort to maintain wellness.

Cancer vaccines have shown promise in several clinical trials. A few have reached late stages clinical trials. Cancer vaccines are thought of as active immune therapies because they attempt to involve a person's own immune system to attack the cancer cells.

### Gene Therapy

It is now believed that most cancers are the result of changes in several genes. Genes are passed on to children from their parents. Genes determine the color of our eyes, hair, and body shape, to name just a few characteristics. Genes also carry the tendency to develop diseases such as cancer. Researchers now know that cancer is the result of gene mutations. Research is proceeding at a rapid pace in many areas. It is speculated that in the future, gene therapy may be used to add healthy genes to cells where there are abnormal or missing genes; stop oncogenes; add genes to make cancer cells unstable and more susceptible to treatment; and stop genes that play a role in forming new blood vessels.[76] The formation of blood vessels allows tumors to grow.

### Complementary Therapies

New technologies enhance the diagnosis and treatment of cancer. Magnetic resonance imaging (MRI) and computered tomographic (CT) scanning help detect and map hidden tumors. Bone marrow transplantation is now a treatment option for select patients with leukemia and lymphoma.

Other approaches that have been used or are under investigation as alternatives to conventional treatment or as methods to use in conjunction with traditional therapies are acupressure, acupuncture, herbs, vitamins (for prevention and free radical removal), biofeedback (monitoring body functions to control body functions), homeopathy (use of extremely small doses of toxic substances), reflexology (massaging certain areas of the feet), therapeutic touch (redirecting the "life forces" of the body), and visualization (envisioning a cure happening). Some of these alternative methods have been proven to help in the treatment process. Others seem to do nothing. Others are still being investigated (see Nurturing Your Spirituality: Living Well with Cancer). Some may become part of more traditional treatments. None of these approaches are substitutes for the medical approaches to treatment.

Today, more than ever, there is hope for anyone with cancer. Cancer trials are ongoing, and new drugs are constantly being developed. Even the most deadly cancers have new treatments being tested. As more is learned about cancer, more will be done to stop its deadly attack on the human body.

## Diabetes Mellitus

**Diabetes mellitus** is a group of diseases resulting from one of the following situations: The body doesn't make insulin, the body doesn't make enough insulin, or the body doesn't use insulin properly. Diabetes is characterized by high levels of blood glucose resulting from defective insulin production or use. See Just the Facts: How Diabetes Affects the Body, p. 440.[80] People with diabetes experience an abnormality in the way their bodies use glucose (blood sugar); this results from the deficient production of insulin by the pancreas or from resistance of the body's tissues to the action of insulin.[81] The blood may contain ample glucose (blood sugar), but without enough insulin available for use, the glucose cannot move from the bloodstream into the cells, where it is needed for fuel. As a result, people with diabetes cannot use the energy they consume, and high glucose levels build up in the blood and urine, leading to a condition known as *hyperglycemia* (high blood sugar). Large amounts of sugar in the urine require additional water, so that the sugar can be diluted for elimination. The body's increased need for water leads to a depletion of the body's water stores, causing excessive thirst and frequent urination. When the body becomes unable to completely break down glucose as a source of energy, fat must be used. Fat is metabolized differently than glucose, and its breakdown is incomplete when glucose is not available. Incomplete metabolism causes an excess amount of chemicals called *ketone bodies* to build up in the body. The buildup of ketones is used to perform the functions that glucose would perform under normal conditions (supplying energy), but the excess amounts of ketone bodies disrupt the body's chemical balance, altering the blood's chemistry and making it more acidic. Acidic conditions in the body are extremely hazardous.

Diabetes can be a serious disorder. The symptoms include excessive thirst; increased urination; hunger; a tendency to tire easily; wounds that heal slowly; blurred vision; and frequent skin, vaginal, and urinary tract infections. Dehydration and the buildup of ketones can cause ketoacidosis (the accumulation of ketones) and nausea, vomiting, abdominal pain, lethargy, and drowsiness. Ketoacidosis often leads to severe sickness, coma, and even death. Of equal significance is that prolonged periods of elevated glucose levels disrupt normal enzyme and membrane functions.[82] Chronic complications that may result are eye disease, kidney disorders, painful nerve and muscle symptoms, and decreased circulation. Diabetes is a leading cause of foot and leg amputations. Diabetes can also produce impotence in men and increased risk for heart disease and heart attacks in both genders.

The prevalence of diabetes in the United States is 23.6 million people or 7% of the population. Of this number, 5.7 million people are unaware that they have diabetes. Approximately 19 per 100,000 children and adolescents have Type 1 diabetes. Type 2 diabetes affects about 5.3 per 10,000 children and adolescents.[83] Prevalence is becoming more common in American Indians, African Americans, and Hispanics. Rates are also increasing in white adolescents, but not at the same rate as that of the previously mentioned groups. Most researchers are attributing these alarming increases to sedentary lifestyles, overweight, and the poor nutritional habits of adolescents.

## Type 1 Diabetes

Diabetes consists of two diagnostic categories. *Type 1 diabetes* occurs most commonly in children and young adults, although it may develop at any age. Type 1 is an autoimmune disease in which the body produces antibodies that attack and damage its own cells—in this case, the insulin-producing cells of the pancreas.[84] The symptoms may be sudden and sometimes progress rapidly, requiring quick intervention to prevent death. People with Type 1 diabetes produce little or no insulin and require insulin injections to function. Before insulin was discovered, the average life span for a person with Type 1 diabetes was 2 years after diagnosis. Properly treated, these people now live almost as long as the general population.

## Type 2 Diabetes

*Type 2 diabetes* is the most common type and is found primarily in people over the age of 40. Scientists believe that it is strongly linked to genetic factors. If an identical twin develops Type 2 diabetes, the other most likely will as well. People with Type 2 either develop a resistance to insulin activity or experience insufficient insulin action. Their bodies are usually capable of producing adequate amounts of insulin—something a person with Type 1 diabetes cannot do. The difficulty in Type 2 diabetes is that body cells become resistant to insulin at the receptor sites (the place where insulin attaches to the cell). There are several types of tests to diagnose diabetes. The most common test is the fasting glucose test. An individual is considered to have Type 2 diabetes if his or her fasting glucose value is above 125 mg/dL on at least two tests.[85] Type 2 is linked strongly to obesity. Almost 80% of diabetics with Type 2 are overweight at the time of diagnosis.[86]

## Causes

Type 1 diabetes is an autoimmune disease. This means the body's immune system attacks a part of the body that is well. In Type 1 diabetes, the body produces antibodies that attack and damage the area of the pancreas that produces insulin. Initially, the ability to produce insulin is impaired, but eventually, usually in less than a year, little or no insulin is produced. The onset is usually before age 35 and often in childhood. Type 1 diabetes is sometimes associated with a viral infection within the insulin-producing cells, resulting in the inability to produce insulin.[87]

Heredity plays a role in Type 2 diabetes. In a study of 218 people with Type 2 diabetes, 66% reported at least one relative with diabetes, and 46% reported at least two relatives with diabetes. Patients whose mothers had diabetes were twice as likely to develop the disease than were those whose fathers had diabetes.[88]

Obesity also is an important factor (see Just the Facts: Preventing and Controlling the Effects of Diabetes). Not

## [ JUST THE FACTS ]

### How Diabetes Affects the Body

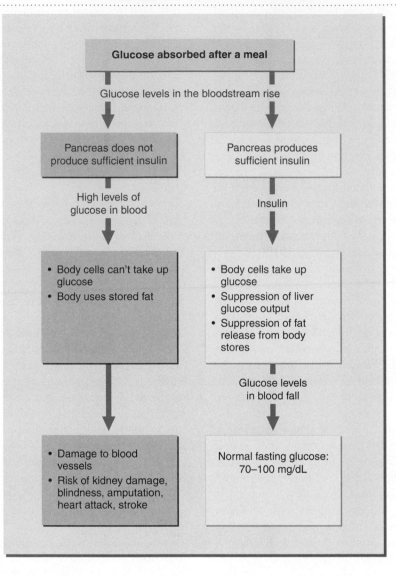

Glucose absorbed after a meal

Glucose levels in the bloodstream rise

| Pancreas does not produce sufficient insulin | Pancreas produces sufficient insulin |

High levels of glucose in blood / Insulin

- Body cells can't take up glucose
- Body uses stored fat

- Body cells take up glucose
- Suppression of liver glucose output
- Suppression of fat release from body stores

Glucose levels in blood fall

- Damage to blood vessels
- Risk of kidney damage, blindness, amputation, heart attack, stroke

Normal fasting glucose: 70–100 mg/dL

all people who are obese develop diabetes, but 90% of people with diabetes are overweight. Tumors of certain endocrine organs, such as the pituitary gland, adrenal glands, and pancreas, can all interfere with or destroy insulin production. Taking corticosteroids, used to treat asthma or arthritis, may result in latent diabetes.[89]

## Prediabetes

Prediabetes is a condition that raises the risk of developing Type 2 diabetes.[90] This condition exists when blood glucose levels are higher than normal but are not high enough for a diagnosis of diabetes. Prediabetes is sometimes referred to as impaired fasting glucose (IFG) or impaired glucose tolerance (IGT), depending on the test used to identify the condition. Individuals with predia-

betes are at a higher risk of developing Type 2 diabetes, heart disease, and stroke. An important point is that the progression from prediabetes to Type 2 diabetes is not inevitable. Research has indicated that, with weight loss and increased exercise, the progression to Type 2 can be delayed or prevented and that blood glucose levels may return to normal.[91] It is estimated that as many as 20 million people may have prediabetes.

## Gestational Diabetes

Gestational diabetes is Type 2 diabetes that occurs in some women during pregnancy. It is more common among obese women and those with a family history of the disease. The condition must be normalized to prevent complications in the infant. After pregnancy, 5 to

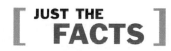

## Preventing and Controlling the Effects of Diabetes

Several lifestyle behaviors can significantly reduce the likelihood of developing Type 2 diabetes:

- Maintaining normal weight
- Exercising regularly
- Not smoking
- Maintaining blood pressure levels or treating high blood pressure
- Maintaining normal blood lipid levels
- Eating a low-fat, high-fiber diet

10% are found to have Type 2 diabetes and those who have had gestational diabetes have a 20 to 50% chance of developing Type 2 diabetes in the next 10 years.[92]

## Exercise and Diabetes

The need for exercise for the individual with diabetes is the same as that for anyone without the condition. The American Diabetes Association recommends a total of 30 minutes a day at least 5 days a week. The exercise routine for a diabetic should incorporate the same components as for a nondiabetic. It should include an aerobic component, strength training, and flexibility exercises.

Exercise lowers blood sugar levels by reducing the body's resistance to insulin. Cells become more sensitive to insulin and more capable of absorbing glucose. The effect is lower levels of circulating blood sugar. This benefit of exercise, however, lasts for only 24 hours, which means exercise must be done every day. Regular activity doesn't seem to have the same dramatic effect on Type 1 diabetes, but it does lower the amount of insulin needed and the risk for cardiovascular disease.[93] (See Just the Facts: Advances in Treating Diabetes.)

There are several precautions a diabetic must take when engaging in an exercise program. A physician should be consulted to ensure that there are no exercise activities that would be contraindicated. An exercise stress test may be recommended to determine how the heart reacts to exercise. It is essential that the exerciser learn how his or her blood glucose responds to exercise. Checking the glucose level before and after exercise can demonstrate the benefits of exercise. If the blood glucose is above 300, exercise can elevate it even higher; thus, caution should be used when engaging in exercise.

## JUST THE FACTS

## Advances in Treating Diabetes[95]

### Medications

There are new classes of blood-glucose-lowering drugs. Those drugs are sulfonylureas, meglitinides, biguanides, alpha-glucosidase inhibitors, and thiazolidinediones. Each class of drugs increases insulin, slows absorption of blood sugar, or makes the body more sensitive to the effects of insulin.

### New Types of Insulin

Newer types of insulin more closely mimic natural insulin. Newer types of insulin are absorbed more quickly and prevent glucose levels from rising too high after meals. One type is long-acting and requires only one injection a day. Researchers are hopeful that the long-acting varieties will enable more consistent blood sugar control over an entire day.

### Methods of Delivering Insulin

The most common method of delivering insulin is with either a syringe or an insulin pen. Now available are insulin pumps, which provide a continuous supply through a tiny needle implanted under the skin, eliminating the need for shots. Other delivery systems being experimented with include skin patches, nasal sprays, and oral inhalers.

### More Efficient Methods of Monitoring Glucose

The FDA has approved the first device that combines a glucose meter, insulin pump, and a dosing calculator. There also are new devices that use lasers and electrical currents to monitor blood glucose levels without having to prick a finger to obtain a blood sample.

### Islet Cell Transplant

Islet cells are found in the pancreas and produce insulin. In Type 1 diabetes, when these cells are destroyed, diabetes develops. Researchers have developed a method to implant new islet cells in the liver. Although still experimental, this procedure is showing promise and may eventually lead to a cure for Type 1 diabetes. Better drugs to prevent rejection and new surgical techniques are eliminating many of the past problems with such transplants.

### Pancreas Transplants

This procedure is usually reserved for people under age 45 and with Type 1 diabetes. Unfortunately, not all transplants are successful; however, when a successful transplant occurs, the need to take insulin is eliminated. But there is a need to take immune-suppressing drugs, which may lead to serious side effects.

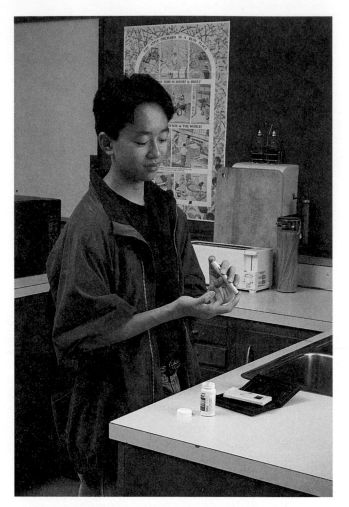

To manage their condition successfully, people with Type 1 diabetes must periodically test their blood glucose level.

For those with Type 1 diabetes when the glucose level is above 250 and ketones are present in the urine, exercise should be avoided.

For the diabetic exerciser, avoiding low blood glucose (hypoglycemia) also is important. Sometimes eating a snack before exercising or adjusting medications will alleviate any problems with hypoglycemia. Blood glucose should be checked during exercise if symptoms, such as nervousness or shakiness, are noticed. If the blood glucose is 70 or below, fruit juice, a soft drink, or glucose tablets can be used to raise the glucose level.[94] There should always be snacks and water available during exercise. Lastly, it is imperative that a medical ID tag be worn, in case an emergency does occur.

## Treatment

Although there is no cure for diabetes, the disease can be controlled by diet, exercise, drugs, and/or insulin. People with Type 1 must have insulin injections, usually several a day, and they must manipulate dosage levels according to dietary and activity levels (see Just the Facts: American Diabetes Association [ADA]

Guidelines for Diabetes Screening). Self-administered blood glucose tests help them monitor blood sugar levels and determine the appropriate insulin dose. Good blood sugar control reduces the risk for the complications associated with Type 1 diabetes.

Many people with Type 2 diabetes can control their blood glucose by following a careful diet, exercising, losing weight, and taking oral medication. People with Type 2 may find it necessary to take medication to control their cholesterol and blood pressure. Of adults with diagnosed diabetes, 13% take both insulin and oral medication, 14% take insulin only, 16% take oral medication only, and 57% take neither insulin nor oral medication.[96] Losing weight helps lower insulin resistance, enabling the body to make more efficient use of the insulin available. Nutrition guidelines developed by

## Wellness for a Lifetime

### Are Illness and Chronic Disease Inevitable as We Age?

As the population of the United States continues to age, chronic conditions are becoming increasingly common. The largest group of maturing adults, known as *baby boomers*, were born after World War II, between 1946 and 1964. Are they doomed to develop age-related conditions? Will you or someone close to you inevitably have to face a chronic condition or disease associated with aging?

The answer for all age groups is a resounding NO. We may have genetic predispositions of which we should be aware; however, we can embrace the concepts of wellness, including maintaining an active lifestyle, eating properly, not smoking, and controlling stress. By doing so, we may

be able to delay the onset of many chronic conditions, diminish their severity, or prevent the factors that cause them. The earlier we begin to practice positive behaviors, the greater the likelihood of healthy outcomes.

All people can make health-related choices that enhance their well-being and that of their families and communities. It is imperative that we accept responsibility for improving our lives. Regardless of age, we are empowered through our attitudes and actions to create a high quality of life. Wellness is a journey, not a destination, filled with opportunities for joy, happiness, learning, and making the most of each day.

the American Diabetes Association (ADA) dispel the notion of a diabetic diet that is good for everyone with the disease. For example, the previous emphasis on sugar consumption has given way to an emphasis on carbohydrate consumption.[97] The total amount of carbohydrate, regardless of its source, is what affects blood sugar levels.[98]

Many of the complications associated with diabetes are preventable or treatable, but diagnosis and proper treatment are necessary (see Wellness for a Lifetime: Are Illness and Chronic Disease Inevitable as We Age?). Neglect of diabetes and its complications may result in early death (see Just the Facts: Major Complications of Diabetes).

## JUST THE FACTS

### Major Complications of Diabetes

**Coronary heart disease (CHD)**
People who are middle-aged and have diabetes are 2 to 4 times more likely to die of CHD than people without diabetes of similar age. CHD and heart attack risk can be reduced by controlling cardiovascular risk factors: lose weight (if needed); quit smoking; exercise regularly; eat a low-fat, high-fiber diet; and, if necessary, use medication to control blood pressure and cholesterol levels.

**Dental disease**
Gum disease can lead to tooth loss and occurs more frequently in people with diabetes. You can reduce this risk simply by brushing and flossing teeth at least twice daily. Visit the dentist at least twice a year, and keep an eye out for the early signs of gum disease, including gum redness, swelling, tenderness and bleeding, and bad breath.

**Foot problems**
If you've had diabetes for a while, you must make every effort to avoid or quickly treat athlete's foot, blisters, calluses, infections, and other foot problems. If not treated, the most minor injuries can eventually lead to infections and amputation because they can go unnoticed (due to nerve damage) or fail to heal properly (due to poor blood circulation). Be sure your doctor examines your feet regularly, especially if you notice inflammation or injury.

**Kidney disease**
Neuropathy (nerve damage) occurs in 30 to 40% of people with Type 1 diabetes and in 20% of those with Type 2. This can lead to kidney failure. The best preventive measure is tight blood glucose control. High blood pressure and a poor cholesterol profile should be treated with lifestyle changes and/or drug therapy. Decreasing your intake of dietary protein is also helpful.

**Nerve damage**
Neuropathy (nerve damage) occurs in 60 to 70% of people with diabetes, often with no symptoms. Tight blood glucose control can delay the onset of peripheral neuropathy (nerve damage to the extremities) or slow its progression. Peripheral neuropathy is more common in smokers, so quitting is key to helping prevent this complication.

**Peripheral arterial disease (PAD)**
The risk of developing PAD (atherosclerosis in the leg arteries that impairs blood flow and increases the risk of foot problems and amputations) is doubled or tripled by both diabetes and smoking. Using the same measures that reduce the risk of CHD can help prevent PAD.

**Skin problems**
Increased skin infections and other skin problems are common in people with diabetes. Good skin hygiene

JUST THE FACTS
*continued*

is essential: Keep skin clean; use lotion (except between toes) and, if needed, a humidifier to prevent dryness; avoid hot showers and baths; use moisturizing soaps and mild shampoos and wash minor cuts promptly with soap and water, then cover them with dry, sterile dressings. Tell your doctor about more serious skin injuries or abnormalities.

## Stroke

The risk of stroke is increased 2 to 4 times in people with diabetes. To reduce your risk, follow the same measures used to prevent CHD, such as treating high blood pressure and elevated cholesterol levels, losing weight, quitting smoking, exercising regularly, and eating a low-fat, high-fiber diet.

## Vision loss

The leading cause of blindness among Americans is diabetic retinopathy. Diabetes also raises the risk of glaucoma and cataracts. Fortunately, most people with diabetes can avoid eye problems, or minimize them, by controlling blood glucose, treating high blood pressure, quitting smoking, visiting an ophthalmologist at least once a year, and watching for signs of trouble, such as blurriness, eye pain or pressure, redness, or any other vision changes.

Source: Adapted from *Johns Hopkins white papers: Diabetes.* 2009. Baltimore: Johns Hopkins Medical Institutions.

# Summary

- *Cancer* refers to a group of disorders characterized by uncontrolled, disorderly cell growth.
- Cancer is the second leading cause of death, and one in four Americans will eventually develop one or more of the 100 different forms.
- There are two types of tumors, or neoplasms. A malignant (cancerous) tumor can spread or metastasize (move from one location to another), while the second type of tumor, called benign, cannot.
- Cancer is caused by either external factors (chemicals, diet, radiation, viruses, pollutants) or internal factors (hormones, immune, inherited).
- A carcinogen is anything that triggers the development of cancer.
- A gene that enables cancer to develop is called an oncogene.
- Exercise has been found to help prevent colon, breast, and prostate cancers.
- Passive smoke (smoke from other people's tobacco products) is dangerous to the nonsmoker by increasing the risk of developing cancer.
- Colon and rectum cancer, when detected early, are very curable. Colon cancer is associated with family history, constipation, and high calorie consumption. Diet is believed to be the primary cause.
- Leukemia is cancer of the blood-forming mechanisms, involving the white blood cells. It strikes both children and adults.

- Lymphoma is cancer of the lymphoid tissue. The two types of lymphoma are Hodgkin's disease and non-Hodgkin's lymphoma. Non-Hodgkin's includes all lymphomas except Hodgkin's.
- The three types of skin cancer are basal cell, squamous cell, and melanoma. Basal and squamous cell cancers are treatable. Melanoma, although most deadly, is treatable if detected early. Exposure to the sun's ultraviolet light is most responsible for causing the three types of skin cancer.
- The ABCDs of skin cancer are helpful in identifying melanoma: A = Asymmetry; B = Borders uneven; C = Color (different shades of brown or black); D  Diameter greater than 6 mm.
- Oral cancer affects the lip, tongue, mouth, and throat. Risk factors are cigar and pipe smoking and the use of smokeless tobacco.
- A woman with a mother or sister with breast cancer has double the risk for breast cancer. Early detection is the best means of reducing mortality.
- Breast self-examination and mammograms are useful tools for preventing breast cancer.
- Uterine cancers can occur either in the cervix or in the endometrium. Cervical cancer is closely associated with sexual behavior, especially through transmission of the human

papillomavirus. Smoking seems to increase the risk.
- Testicular cancer is painless and asymptomatic but is detectable by self-examination. Early detection results in a high cure rate.
- Prostate cancer is the second leading cause of cancer death among men. The PSA and a digital rectal exam have made prostate cancer much easier to detect at earlier stages. These should be done annually after age 50. Symptoms include weak urine flow, inability to urinate, frequent need to urinate, painful or burning urination, and continuing pain in the lower back or upper thighs.
- Cancer is treated through the use of surgery, chemotherapy, radiotherapy, immunotherapy, antiangiogenesis, and stem cell transplantation.
- Diabetes mellitus is a group of diseases with one of the following symptoms: The body doesn't make insulin, it doesn't make enough insulin, or it doesn't use insulin properly.
- The two major categories of diabetes are Type 1 and Type 2.
- Type 1 diabetes usually occurs early in life and requires insulin injections because the pancreas loses its ability to produce insulin.
- Type 2 diabetes occurs most often in people over 40 years of age who do not exercise and are obese.

# Review Questions

1. Describe the process by which cancer cells develop.
2. What characteristics differentiate cancer cells from other cells?
3. Discuss lifestyle factors that may contribute to the development of cancer.
4. Explain the concept of oncogenes.
5. What role does exercise play in the prevention of various cancers? What mechanisms seem to be aiding in the prevention of these cancers?
6. Differentiate among the three types of skin cancer.
7. Describe the conventional methods of treating cancer.
8. Explain the difference between Type 1 and Type 2 diabetes.
9. Describe the main symptoms of diabetes.
10. What are the most serious potential complications of uncontrolled diabetes?

# References

1. American Cancer Society. (2009). *Cancer prevention and early detection facts and figures 2008.* Atlanta, GA: American Cancer Society.
2. American Cancer Society. (2008). What is cancer? Retrieved from www.cancer.org.
3. Ibid.
4. Margolis, S., & J. M. Samet. (2008). *The Johns Hopkins white papers: Early detections and preventions of cancer.* Baltimore: Johns Hopkins Medical Institutions.
5. Margolis & Samet (2008).
6. Ibid.
7. Ibid.
8. American Cancer Society. (2008). What is cancer?
9. International Agency for Research on Cancer. (2002). *Tobacco smoke and involuntary smoking.* IARC Monograph 83. Lyon, France: IARC Press.
10. ACS (2008). What is cancer?
11. Margolis & Samet, 2008.
12. Ibid.
13. American Institute for Cancer Research. (2001). JAMA findings on diet and breast cancer misunderstood, experts say. *AICR Science News, 20,* 1–2.
14. American Cancer Society. (2004). *Jesse Harris Cancer Answer Week* (leaflet).
15. ACS (2006). *Cancer prevention.*
16. Ibid.
17. American Cancer Society. (2009). *Cancer facts and figures 2008.* Atlanta, GA: American Cancer Society.
18. Ibid.
19. Ibid.
20. ACS (2008). What is cancer?
21. American Cancer Society. (2009). Cancer facts and figures. Atlanta, GA: American Cancer Society.
22. American Cancer Society. (2009). What causes cancer? Cancer reference information. Retrieved from www.cancer.org.
25. American Cancer Society, (2009). What causes cancer?
26. ACS (2009). What causes cancer?
27. ACS (2008). What is cancer?
28. Ibid.
29. Consumer Reports on Health (1998). Fruits and vegetables: Nature's best protection. *Consumer Reports, 10* (6), 1.
30. American Cancer Society. (2006). *What causes colorectal cancer?* Atlanta, GA: American Cancer Society.
31. Ibid.
32. Margolis & Samet (2008).
33. Ibid.
34. ACS (2006). *What causes colorectal cancer?*
35. ACS (2009). *Cancer prevention.*
36. Margolis & Samet (2008).
37. ACS (2009). *What causes colorectal cancer?*
38. American Cancer Society (2006). What are the risk factors for stomach cancer? Reference information. Retrieved from www.cancer.org.
39. American Cancer Society. (2009). What are the risk factors?
40. Ibid.
41. Ibid.
42. Ibid.
43. American Cancer Society, (2009). How is pancreatic cancer found? Retrieved from www.cancer.org.
44. American Cancer Society. (2009). How many people get pancreatic cancer? Retrieved from www.cancer.org.
45. Ibid.
46. American Cancer Society. (2009). Detailed quick; Leukemia. Retrieved from www.cancer.org.
47. Ibid.
48. American Cancer Society. (2009). How is non-Hodgkin's lymphoma staged? Retrieved from www.cancer.org.
49. Ibid.
50. Mosby. (2005). *Mosby's dictionary of medicine, nursing, and health professionals* (7th ed.). St. Louis: Mosby.
51. Ibid.
52. American Cancer Society. (2009). How many people get melanoma skin cancer? Retrieved from www.cancer.org
53. American Cancer Society. (2009). Can melanoma be prevented? Retrieved from www.cancer.org.
54. Ibid.
55. Editors. (1997). Health news: Evaluating melanoma risk. *New England Journal of Medicine, 3* (8), 1–2.
56. ACS (2009). Can melanoma be prevented?
57. University of California at Berkeley. (1998). Casting a shadow on sunscreens. *UC Berkeley Wellness Letter, 14*(9), 2.
58. American Cancer Society. (2009). What are the key statistics about breast cancer in men? Reference information. Retrieved from www.cancer.org.
59. American Cancer Society. (2009). What are the risks for breast cancer? Retrieved from www.cancer.org.
60. ACS (2009). What causes breast cancer?
61. Ibid.
62. ACS (2009). *Cancer prevention.*
63. Ibid.
64. Ibid.
65. American Cancer Society (2009). Uterine sarcoma—detailed guide. Retrieved from www.cancer.org.
66. Ibid.

67. American Cancer Society. (2009). Ovarian cancer. Retrieved from www.cancer.org.
68. Ibid.
69. American Cancer Society. (2009). Testicular cancer. Retrieved from www.cancer.org.
70. American Cancer Society. (2009). Prostate cancer. Retrieved from www.cancer.org.
71. Ibid.
72. American Cancer Society. (2009). What is chemotherapy? Retrieved from www.cancer.org.
73. American Cancer Society. (2009). Antiangiogenesis treatment. Retrieved from www.cancer.org.
74. American Cancer Society. (2009). Types of stem cell transplants. Retrieved from www.cancer.org.
75. American Cancer Society. (2009). Type of immunotherapy? Retrieved from www.cancer.org.
76. American Cancer Society. (2009). Gene therapy. Retrieved from www.cancer.org.

77. Mayo Health Clinic. (1999). Mind of malignancy? Attitude and cancer survival. Retrieved from www.mayo-health.org.
78. Johns Hopkins University. (1999). Overview of NIH Office of Alternative Medicine Fields of Practice: Mind/Body Control. Retrieved from www.intelihealth.com.
79. Ibid.
80. Centers for Disease Control and Prevention. (2007). National diabetes fact sheet. Retrieved from www.cdc.gov/diabetes/pubs/factsheets.html.
81. Margolis, S., & C. D. Saudek. (2009). *The Johns Hopkins white papers: Diabetes mellitus.* (2009). Baltimore: Johns Hopkins Medical Institutions.
82. Margolis, S. (2001). *The Johns Hopkins consumer guide to medical tests.* New York: Rebus.
83. National Diabetes Information Clearinghouse (NDIC). (2009). National diabetes statistics. Retrieved from http://diabetes.niddk.nih.gov.
84. Margolis & Saudek (2009).

85. National Diabetes Clearinghouse (2009).
86. Margolis & Saudek (2009).
87. CDC (2009).
88. Margolis & Saudek (2009).
89. Ibid.
90. NDIC (2009).
91. Ibid.
92. Ibid.
93. Nieman, D. (1999). Exercise testing and prescription—a health-related approach (4th ed.). Mountain View, CA: Mayfield.
94. Margolis & Saudek (2009).
95. Ibid.
96. NDIC (2009).
97. American Diabetes Association. (2009). Making healthy food choices. Retrieved from http://www.diabetes.org.
98. Ibid.

## Suggested Readings

Dyer, D. (2004). *A dietitian's cancer story: Information and inspiration for recovery and healing from a three-time cancer survivor.* Washington, DC: American Cancer Society.

This book is used by thousands of cancer survivors as they search for strategies for improving their quality of life.

Kirkendoo, A. (2004). *The end of cancer.* Miami, FL: Lysmata.

This book is not about a magic bullet but, rather, a new way of thinking about and attacking cancer.

The author brings together highly specialized topics in the areas of cancer research and molds items into a unified theory that makes a great deal of sense.

Link, J., M. James, C. Waisman, & C. Forstoff. (2003). *The breast cancer survival manual: A step-by-step guide for women with newly diagnosed breast cancer* (3d ed.). New York: Owl Books.

This is a comprehensive book on everything concerning the topic of breast cancer, including how breast cancer is characterized, the factors affecting prognosis, diet, exercise, and how to manage the psychological component of the disease.

Ruderman, N., J. Devlin, & S. Schneider. (2006). *Handbook of exercise in diabetes.* Alexandria, VA: American Diabetes Association.

This book provides a comprehensive exercise program for the prevention and treatment of diabetes. It contains data on the effects of exercise on blood glucose and metabolism, treatment plans, and information on how exercise affects the many conditions associated with diabetes.

# Assessment Activity 13-1

## Are You Practicing Cancer Prevention?

Listed here are several common cancers and the significant risk factors for each. As you look at each risk factor, determine whether you should increase or decrease that factor. If the factor does not apply to you or your lifestyle, leave the I/D column blank.

| Cancer | Smoking | | Fruit and Vegetable Consumption | | Exercise | | High Fat Percentage | | Smokeless Tobacco Use | | Meat Consumption | | Obesity | | High Alcohol Consumption | |
|---|---|---|---|---|---|---|---|---|---|---|---|---|---|---|---|---|
| | RF | I/D | RF | I/D | RF | I/D | RF | I/D | RF | I/D | RF | I/D | RF | I/D | RF | I/D |
| Lung | + | | + | | | | | | | | | | | | | |
| Colon and rectum | | | I | | ✓ | | ✓ | | | | ? | | ? | | | |
| Breast | | | ✓ | | ✓ | | ? | | | | | | ✓ | | ✓ | |
| Prostate | | | ✓ | | | | | | | | ? | | ✓ | | | |
| Stomach | ✓ | | ✓ | | | | | | | | | | | | | |
| Kidney | + | | | | | | | | | | | | ✓ | | | |
| Esophagus | + | | ✓ | | | | | | + | | | | | | ✓ | |
| Oral | + | | ✓ | | | | | | + | | | | | | ✓ | |
| Larynx | + | | ✓ | | | | | | + | | | | | | ✓ | |

RF = Risk factor.

I/D = Increase or decrease?

 + = Solid body of evidence suggests a link between this lifestyle factor and cancer.

 ✓ = Many studies suggest a plausible link between this lifestyle factor and cancer.

 ? = Some research suggests a connection; the jury is still out.

### Follow-Up Questions

1. Are you following a more positive lifestyle for the prevention of cancer?
2. How many lifestyle factors do you need to increase? Decrease?
3. What would you say are your main strengths in the effort to prevent cancer?
4. What are your greatest risk factors for cancer?

**Name** _____   **Date** _____   **Section** _____

# Assessment Activity 13-2

## Cancer Early Detection Inventory

This inventory was developed to help in the early detection and treatment of cancer. It presents common symptoms for various cancer sites. If you have symptoms, check with your physician. The chances are that you will not have cancer, but any symptoms suggest a potential problem with your health—it is wise to be safe and consult your physician.

**Directions:** For each cancer site, check any of the symptoms you experience.

### Bladder

1. Blood in urine? _____
2. Unusual change in bladder habits? _____
3. Discomfort during urination? _____
4. Change in flow during urination? _____
5. Urge to urinate more frequently? _____

### Bone

1. Pain in the bone or joint? _____
2. Swelling in the bone or joint? _____
3. Unusual warmth in the bone or joint? _____
4. Protruding veins along the bone or joint? _____

### Breast

1. Thickening or lump in the breast? _____
2. Lump under the arm? _____
3. Thickening or reddening of the skin of the breast? _____
4. Puckering or dimpling of the skin of the breast? _____
5. Nipple discharge? _____
6. Inverted nipple, if nipple was previously erect? _____
7. Persistent pain and tenderness of the breast? _____
8. Unusual changes in the nipple and surrounding skin? _____
9. Benign breast lumps? _____

### Colon and Rectum

1. Continuous constipation or diarrhea? _____
2. Rectal bleeding? _____
3. Change in bowel habits? _____
4. Increase in intestinal gas? _____
5. Abdominal discomfort? _____

### Lung

1. Unusual cough? _____
2. Shortness of breath? _____
3. Sputum streaked with blood? _____
4. Chest pain? _____
5. Recurring attacks of pneumonia or bronchitis? _____

### Lymphatic System

1. Painless enlargement of a lymph node or cluster of lymph nodes? _____
2. Profuse sweating and fever? _____
3. Weight loss? _____
4. Unexplained weakness? _____
5. Unusual itching? _____

### Oral

1. Sore in the mouth that does not heal? _____
2. Lump or thickening that bleeds easily? _____
3. Difficulty in chewing or swallowing food? _____
4. Sensation of something in the throat? _____
5. Restricted movement of the tongue or jaw? _____
6. Poor oral hygiene? _____

### Prostate

1. Weak or interrupted flow of urine? _____
2. Inability to urinate or difficulty in starting urination? _____

3. Need to urinate frequently, especially at night? _____

4. Blood in urine? _____

5. Urine flow that is not easily stopped? _____

6. Painful or burning urination? _____

7. Continuing pain in lower back, pelvis, or upper thighs? _____

**Skin**

1. Obvious change in wart or mole? _____

2. Unusual skin condition? _____

3. Chronic swelling, redness, or warmth of the skin? _____

4. Unexplained itching? _____

5. Overexposure to the ultraviolet rays of the sun? _____

**Testes**

1. Enlargement and change in the consistency of the testes? _____

2. Dull ache in the lower abdomen and groin? _____

3. Sensation of dragging and heaviness? _____

4. Difficulty with ejaculation? _____

**Thyroid**

1. Lump or mass in the neck? _____

2. Persistent hoarseness? _____

3. Difficulty in swallowing? _____

4. Overexposure to head and neck X-ray treatments? _____

**Uterus and Cervix**

1. Irregular bleeding? _____

2. Unusual vaginal discharge? _____

3. Positive Pap smear, class 2 to 5, some signs of abnormality? _____

4. Recurring herpes simplex virus? _____

5. Fibroid tumors of the uterus? _____

**Application:** Carefully evaluate any statement you have checked. If the symptom appears severe (such as blood in the stool), see a physician immediately. However, nonsevere symptoms (such as pain in a joint) may be observed for a short period to see if there is improvement. Never wait longer than 2 weeks to see a physician if the symptom persists.

1. How many symptoms have you checked? _____

2. How serious do these symptoms seem? _____

_____

3. Should you see a physician now or wait? _____

_____

# Assessment Activity 13-3

## Are You at Risk for Diabetes?

**Directions:**   Check the appropriate column in response to the following questions to assess your probability of having diabetes. The more questions that you answer with a yes, the higher the probability you have of becoming diabetic.

Taken alone, any yes answer does not necessarily indicate you are diabetic. However, if you have answered yes more than five times, consult your physician for a urine test.

|  | Yes | No |
|---|---|---|
| 1. Is there a history of diabetes in your family? | ____ | ____ |
| 2. Do you tire quickly or seem always to be fatigued? | ____ | ____ |
| 3. Do you urinate frequently? | ____ | ____ |
| 4. Are you constantly thirsty? | ____ | ____ |
| 5. Is your vision blurry? | ____ | ____ |
| 6. Have you suddenly lost weight? | ____ | ____ |
| 7. Are you overweight? | ____ | ____ |
| 8. Do you eat excessively? | ____ | ____ |
| 9. Do your wounds heal slowly? | ____ | ____ |
| 10. Is your skin frequently itchy? | ____ | ____ |

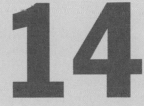

# Becoming a Responsible Health Care Consumer

## ONLINE LEARNING CENTER

Log on to our Online Learning Center (OLC) for access to these additional resources:

- Chapter key term flashcards
- Learning objectives
- Additional goals for behavior change
- Concentration game
- Self-scoring chapter quizzes
- Additional lab activities

The OLC also offers Web links for study and exploration of wellness topics. Access these links through **www.mhhe.com/anspaugh8e.**

## GOALS FOR BEHAVIOR CHANGE

- Apply criteria for determining whether health information is valid, reliable, and based on scientifically controlled studies.
- Identify specific strategies for enhancing communication with your physician.
- Determine the diagnostic tests and immunizations appropriate for your age, gender, and health status.
- Find a specific online newsgroup or patient support group that might be helpful to you.

## Objectives

After completing this chapter, you will be able to do the following:

✔ Explain how to evaluate the accuracy, validity, and reliability of health information.

✔ Discuss the criteria for determining when, where, and how to choose health care.

✔ Describe the functions and purposes of the major components of a physical examination.

## [ Key Terms ]

absolute risks
allopathic medicine
alternative medicine
complementary medicine
contraindications
defensive medicine
diagnostic laboratory tests
direct-access testing (DAT)
double-blind study
epidemiologic studies
false negative
false positive
hospitalist
iatrogenic condition
immunizations
implied consent
informed consent
integrative medicine
medical reconciliation

periodic examinations
personal health record (PHR)
placebo
polypharmacy
primary care physician
provocative effect
relative risks
reliability
risk factor
scientifically controlled studies
selective health examinations
self-care
statistical relationship
statistical significance
validity

**T**raditionally, Americans have had a rather passive attitude toward health care. Whether taking medicine, purchasing health care products, undergoing surgery, or having a diagnostic test administered, people have operated as if following orders. Fortunately, this attitude is changing. People are viewing themselves as active participants in their health care. They are asking questions, placing demands on *health care providers* (people and/or facilities that provide health care services), getting second opinions, and sometimes even refusing treatments. People realize that they must assume more responsibility for safeguarding their health. With this responsibility, however, comes the challenge of knowing what one can and should do for oneself. The purpose of this chapter is to lay the groundwork to enable you to become an informed, active participant in the health care marketplace.

## Understanding Health Information

The first and perhaps most difficult challenge for consumers is to make sense of the health information explosion. Many popular magazines regularly print health articles, newspapers often devote entire sections to medicine, the publications of health newsletters abound, television programs feature numerous health stories, and thousands of scientific, health-related studies are published daily. Interest in health information appears to have reached an all-time high.

The availability of so much health information has drawbacks; the major drawback is that so much of the information is confusing, sometimes even contradictory. Even medical experts have trouble separating fact from fiction. It is not unusual for a new finding to be headlined one day and completely refuted the next. For some people, the seemingly endless contradictions and medical flip-flops lead to an attitude that, carried to the extreme, completely disregards new developments and information, even those with life-saving potential. Two examples illustrate this point. For years eggs have been on everyone's list of foods to be avoided because they are high in cholesterol and increase the heart disease risk of many Americans. The assumption was that dietary cholesterol from egg yolks caused high blood cholesterol. However, recent evidence from the Physician's Health Study, a landmark study that began in 1982, suggests the warning that eggs are bad for heart health is unfair and misrepresents the truth. Except for men with diabetes, researchers found that men who ate up to six eggs a week did not increase their risk of dying or having a heart attack or stroke.[1] Experts conclude that the consumption of an egg a day does not contribute to health problems. Why the change? One possible explanation: It is saturated fat in the diet,

more than cholesterol in the diet, that raises blood levels of cholesterol and leads to atherosclerosis, heart attacks, and stroke. This was not known when eggs were first linked to heart disease. For egg lovers, this provides some flexibility in egg consumption but it comes with a caveat: The study focused on one egg a day, and not indiscriminate consumption of eggs. Moderation still rules.

Another nutrition-related example is coffee. For years common thinking held that the caffeine in coffee elevated blood pressure, increased heart rate, constricted blood vessels, and increased heart attack and stroke risk. In addition, other substances in coffee were linked to cancer, bone density loss, and diabetes. The more coffee consumed, the greater the risk of a host of health problems. However, now the health research community associates health benefits with coffee consumption. Coffee drinkers do better on memory tests and other cognitive tests than coffee abstainers. Caffeine is anti-inflammatory and as such may protect against Alzheimer disease, an inflammation in the brain, dementia, and Parkinson disease.[2] It may also reduce the risk of contracting diabetes.[3] The benefits of coffee consumption led one health editor to conclude: "Recent studies have elevated coffee to health-drink status."[4] How can this flip-flop in medical opinion be explained? Were early messages about coffee and caffeine consumption wrong? Yes and no. Yes, the caffeine in coffee is a stimulant that produces a number of measurable changes in the body, but no, coffee consumption by itself doesn't tell the whole story. Now we know the substances in coffee may offer antioxidant and anti-inflammatory benefits in ways that protect us from some diseases.

Will today's knowledge about the risks and benefits of eggs, coffee, and countless other health claims be obsolete tomorrow? Possibly; but even if this happens, such claims are likely to have served as an important building block for the medical truths of tomorrow. Much of what is known about health and medicine is like this. Rather than giving up on medical advice even if it is sometimes contradictory, the challenge for most people is to keep an open mind and realize that health information is constantly evolving. The truth is rarely clearly black or white. It is helpful to remember the following quote from a prominent health editor: "Science proceeds by one good study at a time. There's never a direct, final answer because our information keeps increasing. So consumers and doctors often need to make tough decisions amid incomplete, changing, and contradictory information."[5]

Given the mixed messages about health, it is perhaps a good idea to adopt a somewhat skeptical attitude, especially toward extreme and sensational health claims. The First Amendment to the U.S. Constitution,

## [ JUST THE FACTS ]

**Headlines and Medical Contradictions**

Consider four contradictory headlines regarding multivitamin supplements: "Multivitamins: Simple Health Insurance," "Multivitamins Don't Work," "Multivitamins Linked to Better Survival," and "Multivitamins Backfire." By themselves, these headlines suggest that multivitamins are both good and bad for us. What are laypeople to believe? Should we throw away our multivitamins—or, instead, do we stock up on them? One of the most frustrating predicaments associated with the explosion of new information regarding health matters is the barrage of contradictory information. This is especially true in the area of nutrition.

It's helpful to remember that journalists and editors often highlight unusual findings in headlines for the simple purpose of grabbing your attention. The goal is to sell newspapers, magazines, or in the case of the Internet or television, advertising time and space. Researchers, on the other hand, typically view each new study as one piece of a large puzzle and are well aware that the latest finding may not stand the test of time. It is the substance of the evidence, not the latest headline, that should influence our thinking about health issues.

Often what seems like a medical contradiction is a shift in emphasis for scientists. To the casual reader, it may appear as a reversal in thinking. In reality, it may not be. It becomes more complex, requiring researchers to refine the message. In the case of multivitamins, the main issue may turn out to be a person's overall eating habits and the interaction of foods with vitamin supplements. Or, it could be a person's age or health status, or some other combination of factors. Time and more research will tell.

which guarantees freedom of the press, also guarantees Americans the right to publish health-related nonsense. The more you read, generally the more contradictions you will uncover (see Just the Facts: Headlines and Medical Contradictions). This should not make you feel uncomfortable; to the contrary, it should make you realize that medicine is still as much art as science.

## Guidelines for Evaluating Health Information

Adhering to the guidelines that follow should help your search for correct health information.

### Avoid Jumping to Conclusions

Most health misinformation is based on facts, not lies. The problem is that facts get exaggerated and sometimes lead people to wrong conclusions.

A good example involves screening for breast cancer. For a long time, the American Cancer Society has recommended mammography screening (X-ray examination of the breast) annually for women starting at age 40. It is an accepted and routine practice in many doctors' offices. In 2010, a U.S. government advisory panel questioned this practice and advised against routine, automatic mammography screening for all women. The rationale for this recommendation is that mammography screening often produces false positives, which leads to more tests and in some cases unnecessary medical procedures, including surgery. So, if you are a woman in your forties, what are you to do? What are you to believe? Avoid jumping to the conclusion that mammography screening is no longer recommended, or that it is bad advice to continue with this screening. It may not be necessary for you, but then again, in your particular situation it may be not only good advice but also life saving. For this reason, the best conclusion is to consult with your physician. There are just too many variables to draw one single conclusion that is appropriate for everyone. Much of the health information and medical advice we are exposed to is like this. By being aware that the truth of most health issues is not simple, the tendency to oversimplify and overgeneralize health information can be thwarted. (See page 478 for recommendations on mammography screening.)

### Remember That Health Discoveries Take Time

Health discoveries often make their way into media headlines, but a cardinal rule of science is that findings must be replicable. Health information based on a dramatic discovery is not usually considered valid unless it is confirmed in several follow-up studies or experiments.

### Beware of Headline Reading

Newspaper, magazine, and television headlines are intended to arouse your curiosity primarily for one purpose: to make you buy or watch. A headline might cleverly capture the essence of a story or it might present a partial truth that leads to wrong conclusions. A common media strategy is to sensationalize a story by crafting a headline that contradicts conventional wisdom. Newspapers tend to feature headlines and report scientific results that convey "bad news."[6] Consider several examples: "Snacking Promotes Weight Loss," "Mammograms Increase Health Risks," "Live Longer, Eat Soy," "Beware of Prostate Exams." These headlines are fraught with possible deceptions. They may represent the results of isolated studies that run against mainstream medical thought. They may serve as punchlines for stories based on studies with many shortcomings. Or they may actually represent new trends in thinking supported by a medical consensus. The only way to know for sure is to become a well-informed, discriminating consumer of information the way you are a consumer of products, goods, and services. This is not easy because there is a big difference between how scientific studies are conducted and how their findings are reported in the popular press. Authors of a recent landmark report on obesity claim that the media do not report enough of the nuances or caveats of studies, and, as a result, end up providing misinformation to the public.[7] In another report, authors analyzed the media reports on a major medical meeting and concluded that the newspaper and broadcast stories were so overstated or lacking in basic information and context as to be worthless—or even worse, dangerously misleading.[8] The challenge for consumers is to avoid the tendency toward headline reading and to apply the criteria for determining if health information is both valid and reliable.

## Apply the Criteria for Determining Validity and Reliability of Health Information

Health information that can be trusted is based on studies that are valid, reliable, and reported in a way that includes research and statistics in their proper context. When assessing validity and reliability, know the type of study that serves as the basis for new information. Knowing the meanings of the following terms will help put new information in a proper context.

### Validity

In health research, **validity** means *truthfulness*. If a study is designed and conducted properly, its findings are likely to be valid. For example, a new cancer cure that is based on an experiment involving a special breed of mice in a laboratory falls far short of being generalizable, and valid, to cancer patients. Controlled experiments conducted on animals in a laboratory setting may produce promising results in treating various diseases, including cancer, but that doesn't mean these results apply to something as complex as cancer in humans.

### Reliability

**Reliability** is another key criterion for evaluating health information. It is the extent to which health claims can be consistently verified. If a claim is reliable, it can be demonstrated to occur consistently in study after study. The test of time is perhaps the ultimate criterion for evaluating the trustworthiness of new information.

### Statistical Significance

Researchers and reporters often use the term **statistical significance** to give meaning and credibility to findings. For example, in one study a group of college students who ate breakfast every morning before going to class did better in school than a comparison group who skipped breakfast. The differences were reported to be statistically significant. Does this mean that the differences between the two groups were large, maybe equivalent to a full letter grade? Does this mean that breakfast is the key to academic success? *Statistical significance* means that the probability that a study's findings are due to chance alone is less than 5%. That is, in 95 of 100 times, similarly designed studies would yield similar results. If the differences between two groups are not statistically significant, they may be due to chance findings and might not show up again if a study is repeated. While statistical significance implies probability and therefore is a highly valued result, it is important to remember that it does not imply largeness. For example, students in the breakfast group might consistently outperform the breakfast skippers by 1 point, and this 1-point gain might be statistically significant. But, is it large enough to really make a difference? Because so many studies are performed, some studies that yield statistically significant results eventually prove to be wrong. Consequently, it takes hundreds of studies, many of them conflicting, to create a consensus on a particular health issue. Any health claim worth considering should be based on numerous studies or experiments conducted over many years.

### Statistical Relationship

**Statistical relationship** refers to the extent to which two or more variables or events are associated with each other. Much health literature is based on research involving statistical relationships or associations. For example, it is well known that a statistical relationship exists between the consumption of salt and high blood pressure for some people. In other words, an increase in salt intake is accompanied by an increase in blood pressure. Conversely, a drop in salt intake is associated with a decrease in blood pressure. This is helpful information, but does it mean that high salt intake causes high blood pressure? No. If this were true, then all Americans who eat too much salt would have high blood pressure. The mistake many people make is to conclude that one event in a statistical relationship causes the other. Relationships are important and helpful clues to health, and they provide a basis for better understanding health risks. However, they cannot and do not establish cause and effect.

## Provocative Effect

**Provocative effect** refers to the tendency to adopt or practice a behavior as a result of being asked about it. It occurs in many types of research but recently emerged as a controversial issue in survey research on drug use. When asking students about their prior use of drugs, researchers learned that drug use increased after the administration of the survey.[9,10] Although the increased use applied only to people at risk for drug use, concerns about potential harm surfaced. Studies involving other issues produced similar results. For example, college students who were asked about skipping classes and drinking cut class and drank more.[11] According to the researchers, "any time you are asking about risky behaviors, there is a chance that merely asking will activate a positive attitude for those who already have a positive inclination toward the behavior."[12] Stated another way, it's akin to the "power of suggestion." The provocative effect appears to apply also to healthy behaviors. For example, people exercised more after they were asked how much they exercise.[13]

Survey research does not purport to change attitudes or behavior. Rather, its goal is to report on attitudes and behaviors. But when people respond to questionnaires, they often think and talk about a topic in a way that changes attitudes and behaviors.[14] When you are reading the health literature, the provocative effect is another factor to consider before drawing conclusions based on survey research and questionnaires.

Survey researchers are exploring ways to minimize negative health behaviors associated with survey research and maximize positive health behaviors. Possible applications are as diverse as health itself.

## Risk Factor

The term **risk factor** refers to health habits and/or practices that increase the risk of getting certain diseases. The emphasis in Chapter 2, for example, is on those risk factors related to heart disease. Risk factors may be reported in terms of absolute risks or relative risks. **Absolute risks** indicate the actual number or percentage of people affected by a risk factor. **Relative risks** indicate the number or percentage of people affected by a risk factor in relation to or comparison with something else. Relative risks are often cited in the media because they are more impressive and make better headlines than absolute risks. But relative risks are also more misleading than absolute risks. For example, consider the following headline: "Bicycle Deaths Quadruple Auto Deaths on College Campus." The basis for the headline was a study that reported that the risk for death from bicycling to school increased 100% over the previous year, whereas deaths caused by driving to school increased by only 25%. The reporter incorrectly concluded that bicycling is four times riskier (relative risk) than driving. What is missing is information about baseline risk. If the baseline risk of deaths from bicycling is 1 in 1,000, a 100% increase raises it to 2 in 1,000. If the baseline risk for driving to school is 400 in 1,000, then a 25% increase boosts the risk for death by 100 to 500 in 1,000. Driving to school then turns out to be 250 times riskier (absolute risk) than bicycling to school, a complete reversal of the meaning of the headline. Although this example is hypothetical, it serves as a reminder of the importance of inquiring about the chances of getting a disease in the first place before drawing conclusions regarding risk factors, diseases, and death.

Risk factors are also often reported out of context. Even if they are reported fairly and accurately, they still are sometimes difficult to interpret. For example, how is a 60-year-old man to make sense out of a diagnosis that indicates he has a 1 in 84 chance of developing prostate cancer in the next 5 years? Does this imply a high risk, a low risk, or an average risk? Is the risk sufficient to consider aggressive and sometimes dangerous treatments? He and his family may be alarmed by these odds until they learn that these are about the same odds of dying in an automobile accident. When you are confronted with a statistical assessment of risks, it is helpful and sometimes reassuring to ask for comparison benchmarks.

## Ask Questions About Information

Answers to four questions about the nature and type of study will help you sort through the contradictory findings and claims reported in the popular press.

### What Type of Study Was Used?

There are several types of studies and each has certain advantages and limitations. **Epidemiologic studies** are population studies (rather than scientifically controlled experimental studies) that observe the health habits and lifestyles of thousands of people for a period of time. The Framingham Study in Framingham, Massachusetts, is perhaps the longest-running and most famous epidemiologic study in the United States. It has yielded invaluable information in our understanding of the risk factors associated with many diseases, especially heart disease. Epidemiologic studies may be *prospective* or *retrospective*. In a prospective study, researchers follow a group of people at a specific point in time and identify relationships between lifestyle and diseases. In a retrospective study, researchers look back in time to identify possible disease relationships. Retrospective studies are generally considered less reliable than prospective studies. An advantage of epidemiologic studies is that they tend to be more generalizable to the population at large. A disadvantage is that they do not prove cause and effect.

**Scientifically controlled studies** are experiments conducted in controlled settings. The classic study is a **double-blind study** that includes at least two groups, one that is an experimental group and receives some form of experimental treatment and another that is a control group and receives no treatment. The double-blind feature of a study ensures that neither the researcher nor the subjects know who is receiving an experimental treatment and, therefore, will not influence the outcome with that knowledge. If a researcher wanted to prove, for example, that a particular brand of soap prevents athlete's foot, one group of subjects would use the experimental soap and the other would use a **placebo**, or soap substitute. Researchers administering the soap treatment would not know which soap each subject was using, nor would the subjects in the experimental and control groups know. If the experimental group had significantly fewer cases of athlete's foot, the results could then be attributed to the treatment.

The experimental control, double-blind requirement of scientific research is a difficult standard to meet. Such studies are costly and require considerable resources and manpower. Typically, they are referred to in the press as *clinical trials* or *population intervention studies*. The advantage of scientifically controlled studies is that they control the variables, so that it is often possible to establish cause-and-effect relationships. The disadvantage is that results usually apply to a narrowly defined population group and lack generalizability to the general population.

### What Were the Characteristics of the People Included in the Study?

Scientific studies require random sampling of subjects to represent the diverse racial, religious, gender, and cultural characteristics of the population at large. Medical breakthroughs should not be based on a small number of homogeneous, or similar, subjects. Broadly designed human clinical trials that are randomized (a systematic sorting of subjects according to the laws of chance), that are placebo controlled, and that include a double-blind trial are the "gold standard" of research studies.[15] If a study is limited to one gender or ethnic group, its findings will not apply to anyone of a different gender or ethnicity. If the study involves animals, avoid drawing conclusions until subsequent human studies are conducted.

If you are at low risk for a condition being studied, the results probably do not apply to you. The consumption of alcohol illustrates the point. A number of studies report that one drink per day for a woman and up to two drinks a day for a man may reduce the risks

associated with heart disease. These studies affect only people who have heart disease and consume alcoholic beverages. If you do not have heart disease and if you do not drink beverages that contain alcohol, the study findings are not relevant to you.

Remember, true breakthroughs in medical research are the exception rather than the rule.

### How Many People Were in the Study?

In general, the more people included in a study, the better. If a study reports findings that are based on a small number of subjects or patients, be cautious about drawing conclusions. Small-scale studies are seriously limited in their ability to generalize to the public, regardless of how tightly controlled they are. It is not unusual for the media, in their quest to be first to get the word out, to blow medical findings out of proportion. Sometimes small research projects give reason to be hopeful; sometimes they just lead to false hope. Large-scale studies involving many people and repeated over time lead to findings that are reliable and generalizable.

### Who Funded the Study?

Businesses stand to gain or lose substantial sums of money (and reputation) from headline stories featuring their products. Consider the huge upswing in profits experienced by businesses in the pharmaceutical industry when several studies reported the weight-loss benefits of new diet drugs. Profits were staggering; so were the losses when the drugs were later pulled off the market.

The potential conflict of interest between a funding sponsor and the results of a study is obvious but not always made public. For example, in a review of press releases issued by journals on scientific studies, only 23% identified the name of the funding sponsor.[16] Before jumping to conclusions, inquire about the funding source.

### Consider the Sources of Information

Valid and reliable health information comes from respected journals, magazines, and newsletters. Such publications have experienced health or medical editors who subject their articles to peer review and criticism by other scientists. To determine if a study or an article has been subjected to the rigors of scientific review, check whether it can be found in the National Library of Medicine's PubMed database **www.ncbi.nlm.nih.gov/sites/entrez?db-pubmed**.[17] Because little or no space is devoted to advertising, these sources are less inclined to be influenced by the need to protect the reputation or promote the product of a sponsor or an advertiser. Several of these sources are available free online (see Just the Facts: Health Help You Can Trust on the Internet).

# [ JUST THE FACTS ]

## Health Help You Can Trust on the Internet

The Internet has grown so rapidly that it would take volumes to list all of the available websites that offer health information. Even if that were feasible, there would be little assurance that the information could be trusted. Fortunately, several respected health organizations have reviewed selected websites and identified the ones that are useful and reliable. A few of these sites are listed here. Remember that many more excellent sites are available. (A $$ sign indicates that the website may charge a fee for use.)

### Newsletters

- Harvard Medical School publications at www.harvardhealth.org
- Health News at www.webmd.com
- Aetna with Harvard Medical School Inteli-Health Newsletter at www.intelihealth.com
- Mayo Health Oasis at www.mayoclinic.org
- Nutrition Action Health Letter at www.cspinet.org
- Tufts University Health and Nutrition Newsletter at http://healthletter.tufts.edu

### Medical Database, Links, and/or Search Engines

- Centers for Disease Control and Prevention at www.cdc.gov
- Hardin Meta Directory of Internet Health Sources at www.lib.uiowa.edu/hardin/md/pharm.html
- Health-Resource at www.thehealthresource.com ($$)
- HealthAtoZ at www.Healthatoz.com
- Medical Matrix at www.medmatrix.org
- MedicineNet at www.medicinenet.com
- National Institutes of Health at www.nih.gov
- National Library of Medicine's PubMed database at www.ncbi.nlm.nih.gov/sites/entrez?db-pubmed
- MEDLINE (also National Library of Medicine) at www.medlineplus.gov
- Medscape at www.medscape.com
- WebMD at www.webmd.com

### Other Health Sites

- American Cancer Society at www.cancer.org
- American Dental Association at www.ada.org
- American Heart Association at www.americanheart.org
- American Medical Association at www.ama-assn.org
- American Psychiatric Association at www.apa.org
- Clinical trials at www.clinicaltrials.gov
- Drugs at www.drugs.com
- Health at www.healthology.com
- Health at www.realage.com
- Institute for Safe Medication Practices at www.ismp.org
- Medicine at www.emedicine.com
- OncoLink cancer information at www.oncolink.upenn.edu
- Prescription medicines at www.rxlist.com
- U.S. Food and Drug Administration at www.fda.gov
- U.S. Pharmacopeia (pharmaceutical information) at www.usp.org

### Other Health Sites

- Alternative medicine at www.wholehealthmd.com
- Children's health at www.kidshealth.org
- Department of Health and Human Services at www.healthfinder.gov
- Mayo Clinic at www.mayoclinic.com
- Medical Library Association at www.mlanet.org
- Ratings of physicians at www.healthgrades.com
- The Merck Manual at www.merck.com
- The Merck Manual Home Edition at www.merckhomeedition.com

## Health Information and the Internet

People who have access to a computer and an Internet service provider can obtain health and medical information that once was available only to those in the medical profession who had user privileges at major medical libraries and research centers. Websites provide information regarding most diseases and health conditions. Some sites provide access to news groups, chat rooms, bulletin boards, support groups, and even med-ical specialists (see Nurturing Your Spirituality: Support Is Just a Click Away). The Internet is a powerful tool for people who want to become actively engaged in their health care. Much of the information available online is accurate, reliable, and trustworthy and as good as you'll find in a library. Often information is explained more thoroughly and understandably than might be expected when you talk to your physician. However, the Internet is a double-edged sword in that

## Nurturing Your Spirituality

### Support Is Just a Click Away

Online patient support groups can be useful, especially for people with chronic illness. With the click of a mouse it is possible to interact with others who share health problems. One of the most direct methods of communicating with others on the Internet is through newsgroups. Newsgroups are locations where electronic messages (e-mail) related to a medical topic are posted. These are usually plain text messages rather than sophisticated, color-graphic presentations. Newsgroups are not a collection of news items. Essentially, they are virtual bulletin boards open to anyone who wants to participate. Newsgroups make it possible to locate other people experiencing the same health concerns you are and to hear about their experiences, as well as tell about yours.

More than 100,000 newsgroups are available on the Internet. To locate the name of a specific newsgroup that might be helpful to you, visit one of the following websites:

- Deja News at www.dejanews.com
- Dictionary.com at www.dictionary.com
- Self-Help Sourcebook at www.mentalhelp.net/selfhelp/
- Healthfinder at www.healthfinder.gov

Following are some popular newsgroups devoted to specific health issues:

- AIDS at www.aids.org/atn/a-233-07.html
- Arthritis at arthritis.boomja.com/Arthritis-Newsgroups-23405.html

- Asthma at www.faqs.org/faqs/by-newsgroup/alt/alt.support.asthma.html
- Cancer at www.faqs.org/faqs/by-newsgroup/sci/sci.med.diseases.cancer.html
- Depression at www.faqs.org/faqs/by-newsgroup/alt/alt.support.depression.html
- Diabetes at www.alt-support-diabetes.org/charter.php
- Eating disorders at www.winternet.com/~terrym/eating.html
- Headaches at www.faqs.org/faqs/by-newsgroup/alt/alt.support.headaches.migraine.html
- Infertility at www.fertilityplus.org/faq/infertility.html
- Stop smoking at www.faqs.org/faqs/by-newsgroup/alt/alt.support.stop-smoking.html

A newsgroup may receive dozens and even hundreds of new postings each day. You can read all of them or select those that seem to be most relevant. Messages on a related topic often are grouped together in a *thread*, making it easier to follow a conversation. Often, participants share practical tips for daily living. Sometimes, experts offer medical advice. Some groups are managed by administrators who screen submissions. However, most groups are uncontrolled, which means that they may contain inaccurate information.

it is also a source of misleading, outdated, and incorrect information. Some people have referred to the Internet as a "wild frontier" mixed with all sorts of truths, half truths, and blatantly false information. Others have called the Internet "the world's bazaar, delivering virtually anything you might want, day or night. And, like any marketplace, the Web is populated by thieves and pickpockets who are happy to take your money if you give them half a chance."[18] Some information may not be managed by knowledgeable sources or has not been subjected to peer review or has not been updated. Some websites are ruses for hawking products or services. How can you tell if the information on the Internet can be trusted? The following guidelines[19] will help:

1. Check the date of Internet postings. Reputable websites provide dates of entry of their content. If dates are not included, it's probably because the website sponsor doesn't want you to know.

2. Identify the source or owner of the website. Established health and medical institutions usually provide valid and reliable information. They also disclose contact information including telephone numbers and address. Institutions that have earned a good reputation for the quality of programs and services they deliver to customers and patients can usually be counted on to go the extra mile to ensure quality websites. Websites ending in "gov" and "edu" are managed by governmental and educational institutions, respectively, and can usually be trusted.

3. Determine whether the website promotes products or procedures. Be skeptical if the website overwhelms you with ads. Also exercise caution if the website relies on testimonials and anecdotes to promote its products and services. Avoid websites that don't explain their privacy policy. There's a good chance they don't have one because they sell your information to other websites.

## Managing Health Care

A major theme throughout this text is that you can control many factors that influence your health. An outgrowth of this attitude is the **self-care** movement, the trend toward becoming an active partner in the management of one's health rather than a passive recipient of medical treatment. Armed with correct information, you can manage many aspects of your health care that were once thought to be solely within the realm of a physician. An added bonus of becoming actively involved in self-care is a shift from feelings of helplessness and despair to feelings of control, responsibility, and involvement.

Answers to the following questions guide the use of health care services, providers, and products and facilitate the self-care approach to wellness:

- When should you seek health care?
- What can you expect from a stay in the hospital?
- How can you select a health care professional?

### When to Seek Health Care

Many people tend to fall into two extreme groups regarding health care: those who seek health care for every ache and pain and those who avoid health care unless experiencing extreme pain. Both groups unwisely use the health care establishment. Those in the first group fail to understand that too much health care can be ineffective or even harmful. They also fail to recognize the powerful recuperative powers of the body. The reality is that most people who seek medical care are unaffected by the treatment. Most of the time the body is capable of healing itself. Of course, sometimes medical treatment is essential, but for every person who gets better from treatment, another person experiences an **iatrogenic condition.** An iatrogenic condition is a health problem or condition caused by medical treatment. Several examples include drug reactions, medical mistakes, and infection. Sometimes the iatrogenic condition is worse than the presenting symptom. This does not mean that symptoms should be disregarded on the assumption the body will heal itself or that if treatment is sought there is a 50:50 chance of an unnecessary complication. People who avoid health care at all costs fail to recognize the value of early diagnosis and detection of disease. The challenge, therefore, is to know when to seek health care and when to allow for the natural course of events that occurs in the healing process.

Perhaps the best way to find a balance between too much and too little health care is to establish a physician-patient relationship with a general practitioner. The general practitioner may be a family practice physician or an internist who specializes in internal medicine.

Visit your doctor while you are in good health. This permits your doctor to serve as a facilitator of wellness and provides him or her with a benchmark for interpreting symptoms when they occur.

A second important way to balance health care is to trust your instincts. Nobody knows when something is wrong with your body better than you do. Health and illness are subject to a wide variation in interpretation. If you are attuned to your body, you are your own best expert for recognizing signs and symptoms of illness. For example, you, more than anyone else, will know if you experience a symptom for the first time, or if it gets more severe or chronic over time, or if it doesn't respond to therapy or medication in the usual way, or if it requires you to make changes in your daily activities.

Some signs and symptoms almost always require immediate medical attention. For example, unexpected shortness of breath; severe chest pain; sudden weakness of part of the body; sudden paralysis; loss of speech; sudden intense "explosive" headaches, especially in people over 50; poisoning; head traumas; and uncontrolled bleeding and internal bleeding as shown by blood in the urine, bowel movement, sputum, or vomit; or blood from any of the body's openings suggest a medical emergency and should be treated as soon as possible.[20,21,22] Injuries from falls and accidents, and first aid emergencies, also often require a trip to a medical emergency facility (see Just the Facts: When a Cut or Scrape Requires a Doctor at **www.mhhe.com/anspaugh8e** Student Center, Chapter 14, Just the Facts). Many other signs and symptoms may require medical help, especially if they persist longer than usual, become more intense, or are unlike any previous symptoms you have experienced. Symptoms associated with headaches, dizziness, disorientation, nausea, abdominal pain, rashes and skin infections, unexplained weight loss, loss of appetite, unusual thirst, and unexplained changes in bowel habits are difficult to diagnose and often require the expertise of one or more medical specialists. They may indicate any number of conditions including heart attack, cancer, stroke, diabetes, herniated disc, serious infections, and inflammatory bowel disease, to mention a few.

There is debate about when medical care is needed in the case of fever. Normal body temperature is 98.6 °F. What may be normal for one person may be slightly different from that of another person. Body temperature may also fluctuate during the day. It is usually lowest when you get up in the morning and higher, by as much as 1 degree, in the evening. Exercise and ambient temperature may also cause body temperature to rise, and for women an increase in body temperature may signal ovulation (see Just the Facts: What is Your "Normal" Body Temperature?). The only way to know what is normal for you is to take your temperature when you're feeling well. (See Assessment Activity 14–1.) An elevated temperature may also indicate the presence of an infection. A *fever* is an elevated temperature,

The so-called normal body temperature of 98.6 °F is an overall average temperature based on 19th-century research. Current methods of assessing body temperature reveal a large variance from one person to another, depending on the time of day, age, whether or not you're participating in physical work or activity, gender, and fertility status. Determining what's normal for you requires an assessment of body temperature at least three times a day for 3 days. Take your temperature, using an oral thermometer, before getting out of bed in the morning, in the late afternoon, and before going to bed at night. Calculate the average temperature at each time of the day and save for future reference when you're sick. (See Assessment Activity 14–1.)

defined as an oral temperature of 100 °F or a rectal, ear, or forehead temperature of 101 °F.[23] A fever is a sign that the body's immune system is working to destroy pathogens or disease-producing organisms. In other words, a fever is the body's own adaptive response that helps fight disease. However, if left untreated for an extended time, a fever may cause harm to sensitive tissues in the body, such as connective tissue found in joints and tissues in the valves of the heart.

It is not usually necessary for an adult to seek medical care for a fever. Home treatment includes the use of fever-reducing medicines such as acetaminophen and ibuprofen. Aspirin is another medication for fever but should not be given to anyone younger than age 20 due to the risk of Reyes syndrome.[24] A bath or shower with lukewarm (not cool) water may also lower body temperature. Cold-water baths or showers should be avoided because they constrict superficial blood vessels, which will increase body temperature rather than lower it.[25] You should consult your physician if fever remains above 102 °F despite your actions or, in the case of a low-grade fever (99 °F to 101 °F), if there is no improvement in 72 hours.[26] Some ailments, such as sore throat, ear pain, diarrhea, urinary problems, and skin rash, may be the cause of a fever and should be treated. Fever in young children should be discussed with a physician. (See Real-World Wellness: When to Seek Treatment for a Fever.)

## Entering a Hospital

Hospitals are driven by the goal of saving lives. They range in size and service from small units that provide general care and low-risk treatments to large, specialized centers offering dramatic and experimental thera-

pies. You may be limited in your choice of a hospital by factors beyond your control, including insurance coverage, your physician's hospital affiliation, and the type of care accessible in your location.

Approximately 35 million Americans benefit annually from the care and services provided by hospitals.[29] The average length of stay in a hospital is 4.8 days[30] and includes procedures ranging from elective cosmetic

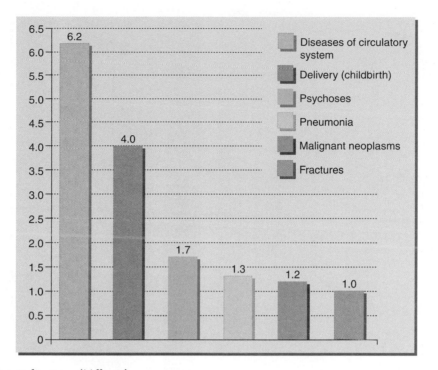

**FIGURE 14-1**   Inpatient Hospitalizations (Millions)

**Source:** DeFrances, C. J., K. Cullen , & L. Kozak. (2007. National Hospital Discharge Survey: 2005 annual summary with detailed diagnosis and procedure data. National Center for Health Statistics. *Vital Health Statistics, 13,* (165).

surgery to leading edge transplant surgery. The six most common health problems that require inpatient hospitalization are heart disease, childbirth delivery, psychoses, pneumonia, malignant neoplasms, and fractures (see Figure 14–1).[31] People usually check in, receive treatment, and leave better off than they were when they were admitted. The length of stay varies according to many factors, such as the health and age of patients, the seriousness of the health problem, the presence of multiple risk factors, and insurance coverage. Figure 14–2 on page 462 presents the average length of hospital stay for seven common conditions.

While Americans enjoy the benefit of some of the world's best hospitals, you should still be aware of possible dangers. Well-known hospital hazards are unnecessary operations, unexpected drug reactions, harmful or even fatal blunders, and hospital-borne infections. An estimated 100,000 people die each year in the United States as a result of hospital-infection-related deaths, many of which are preventable by the simple practice of hand washing.[32]

What can laypeople do to ensure proper and safe care while in the hospital? The following guidelines should be considered:

• If you have a choice of hospitals, inquire about their accreditation status, reputation, and ratings from consumer groups (see Just the Facts: Grading Hospitals). Hospitals are subject to inspection to make sure they are in compliance with federal standards.

• Before checking into a hospital, you need to decide on your accommodations. Do you want to pay extra for a single room? Do you need a special diet? Do you need a place to store refrigerated medicine? If someone will be staying with you, will he or she need a cot? You should try to avoid going in on a weekend when few procedures are done. When you get to your room, speak up immediately if it is unacceptable.

• You need to be familiar with your rights as a patient (see Just the Facts: Do You Know Your Medical Rights?). Hospitals should provide an information booklet that includes a Patient's Bill of Rights. The booklet will inform you that you have the right to considerate and respectful care; information about tests, drugs, and procedures; dignity; courtesy; respect; and the opportunity to make decisions, including about when to leave the hospital.

• You should make informed decisions. Before authorizing any procedure, you must be informed about your medical condition, treatment options, expected risks, prognosis, and the name of the person in charge of treatment. Your agreement to a procedure based on your having been informed of these matters is called **informed consent**. The only instances in which hospitals are not required to obtain informed consent are life-threatening emergencies, cases involving unconscious patients when no relatives are present, and compliance with the law or a court order, such

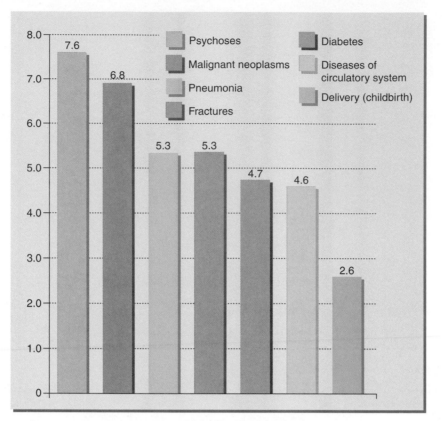

**FIGURE 14-2** Average Length of Hospital Stay for Selected Health Conditions (Days)[34]

**Source:** DeFrances, C. J., and M. J. Hall. 2004. *2002 national hospital discharge survey*. Hyattsville, MD: National Center for Health Statistics.

as those regulating sexually transmitted diseases. If you are asked to sign a consent form, you should read it first. If you want more information, you should ask before signing. If you are skeptical, you have the right to postpone a procedure and discuss it with your doctor.

- Authorization of a medical procedure may be given nonverbally, such as through your appearance at a doctor's office for treatment, your cooperation during the administration of tests, or your failure to object when you could easily refuse consent. Your agreement to a procedure in such situations is called **implied consent.**

- You need to weigh the risks of drug therapy (see Just the Facts: "Brown Bag" Solution to Polypharmacy Problems on page 464), X-ray examinations, and laboratory tests against their expected beneficial results. When tests or treatments are ordered, you should ask about their purpose, possible risks, and possible actions if a test finds that something is wrong. Finally, you should inquire about prescribed drugs. It is not unusual for a patient to be on more than a dozen drugs, often prescribed by different specialists who don't necessarily communicate with

each other. Some of these drugs may be similar and lead to an overdose. Others may counteract each other. Still others, when combined, may cause serious side effects. Up to one-half of patients encounter drug errors after being discharged from a hospital.[35] One of the most important things a patient can do before leaving the hospital is to take a careful inventory of medicines being prescribed, check the labels, know how much to take and when, and know what the medicines are treating. Make a list of these drugs and carry it with you. Include supplements and over-the-counter drugs, too. Discuss any questions you might have with your pharmacist. Remember the age-old advice: "The best dose of any medication is the lowest one that works."[36]

- When scheduled for surgery, prepare for anesthesia. In rare cases, general anesthesia can cause brain damage and death. One cause of such catastrophes is vomiting while unconscious. To reduce the risk, avoid eating or drinking anything after midnight the night before surgery.

- You need to know who is in charge of your care, record his or her office number, and note when you can expect a visit. If your doctor is transferring

# [ JUST THE ] FACTS
## Grading Hospitals

The following websites rate, rank, and compare U.S. hospitals.

1. *U.S. News and World Report*
   a. Lists the top 50 hospitals in 17 specialties
   b. Website: www.usnews.com

2. Leapfrog Group
   a. Develops a safety score based on survey results of 30 safety practices
   b. Website: www.leapfroggroup.org

3. Consumer Checkbook
   a. Lists hospital ratings based on surveys of physicians, mortality rates, and adverse outcome rates for surgery
   b. Website: www.checkbook.org

4. Health Grades, Inc.
   a. Grades hospitals on a five-star rating system that is based on mortality data from Medicare
   b. Website: www.healthgrades.com

5. Health Care Choices
   a. Identifies hospitals by state and provides general information, financial information, and indicators of performance
   b. Website: http://www.healthcarechoices.org

6. U.S. Department of Health and Human Services
   a. Provides a tool to compare patients' assessment on the quality of care they received during a recent hospital stay.
   b. Website: www.hospitalcompare.hhs.gov/

7. Consumer's Health Ratings
   a. Provides a comprehensive listing of organizations that rate or report performance on specific hospitals, health plans, physicians, nursing homes, home health agencies and other health care providers in the United States. The ratings information is free.
   b. Website: www.consumerhealthratings.com/

8. Consumer Reports
   a. Provides patients' ratings regarding how well doctors communicate, how attentive the hospital staff is, and how reliably a hospital performs recommended steps before and after surgery to prevent infections. Hospitals are presented by state.
   b. Website: www.consumerreports.org/health/doctors-hospitals/hospital-ratings.htm

# [ JUST THE ] FACTS
## Do You Know Your Medical Rights?

The following is a short list of some of your rights as a patient in the health care system:

- You have the right as a parent to stay with your children during tests and treatments, provided you don't interfere with medical treatment or are not suspected of child abuse.

- You have the right to request that a relative or friend accompany you during a test, treatment, or hospitalization unless you're in a semiprivate room.

- You have the right to see your medical records if your state law permits it. Some states allow you to copy parts of your record under certain conditions[37] (see Just the Facts: Are Your Medical Records Yours? at www.mhhe.com/anspaugh8e Student Center, Chapter 14, Just the Facts).

- You have the right to emergency care, whether you have insurance or not.

- You have the right to refuse to sign any form. The health care provider can also refuse to provide treatment in the absence of your signed authorization.

- You have the right to a second opinion, but your doctor can also stop treating you for challenging him or her.

- You have the right to leave the hospital at any time, even against medical advice or without paying the bill.

- You have the right to refuse or stop any treatment, whether or not it is experimental.

- You have the right to an itemized, detailed bill for all medical services.

- You have the right to know the results of all tests unless the doctor has reason to believe that the information will be harmful (for example, cause you to commit suicide).

your care to someone else, you need to know who it is. If your doctor is not available and you do not know what is happening, you can ask for the nurse in charge of your case. Your care may be turned over to a **hospitalist**, an emerging medical specialist who is board certified and trained specifically to practice in-hospital medicine.[39]

- You should keep a daily log of procedures, medicines, and doctor visits. When you get your bill, compare each item with your written record. Insist on an itemized bill.

- You should stay active within the limits of your medical problem. Many body functions begin to suffer

## [ JUST THE FACTS ]

### "Brown Bag" Solution to Polypharmacy Problems

**Polypharmacy** refers to the administration of many drugs at the same time. If prescribed indiscriminately, the combined interaction of multiple drugs has the potential to cause problems that are worse than the disease being treated. Doctors are often unaware of all the drugs their patients are taking. And it is not uncommon for hospitalization to lead to drug side effects. Many factors contribute to polypharmacy:

1. Patients' expectations that a doctor's visit ends with a prescription.
2. Direct marketing of prescription drugs.
3. Increased use of herbs and supplements that interact with medicines.
4. Many people go to several doctors and pharmacies at the same time. No one claims ownership for the overall administration of medicines.
5. Many people save unused medicines and take them on their own when symptoms return.
6. Side effects from one drug may lead to the prescription of another drug and promote a vicious cycle of multiple drug use.

What can patients do to prevent complications from polypharmacy? Some experts suggest a "brown bag" approach, in which patients put all their pills, including vitamins and herbal medications, in a bag and take them to the doctor for review.[38]

from just a few days' inactivity. Moving about, walking, bending, and contracting muscles help clear body fluids, reduce the risk for infections (especially in the lungs), and minimize the stress of hospital procedures, which can add to the depression and malaise of hospitalization.

- Eating habits change for many people following surgery, and it is not uncommon to experience a deficiency in nutrients. This is particularly true if you are on a sodium-restricted or calorie-restricted diet. Some medical experts recommend a complete multivitamin/mineral supplement when hospitalized, whether it is added to your IV fluids or taken as a pill.[40]
- Ask questions until you know all you need to know. Know the three Ps: Be polite, be pleasant, and most of all be persistent. According to some experts, the best way to avert hospital errors can be summarized in two words: "Speak up!"[41] The more you assert yourself and the more questions you ask, the fewer mistakes will result.

- Arrange for a family member or friend to stay with you during procedures such as surgery and some tests that require anesthesia, especially during the first 24 hours when you might experience sickness and are not fully capable of monitoring your care. Make sure your companion records medicines and procedures in the log mentioned previously.
- Plan ahead for your discharge from the hospital. It is not unusual for people to make meticulous plans to ensure a smooth admission to the hospital, which is important, but give little thought to their release from the hospital. This is unfortunate because according to a survey of hospital nurses, the discharge presents the highest risk of your hospital stay.[42] In the rush to return home, patients often leave without a full understanding of their drug regimen and follow-up medical care they are to receive. What can you do? First, check for medical reconciliation in your discharge papers. *Medical reconciliation* is a written comparison of medications administered during your hospital stay with the ones you were taking before being admitted to the hospital.[43] This is important because half of discharged patients experience drug errors, in part because of the failure to check for drug interactions.[44] Second, review discharge instructions with your physician. Twenty percent of patients discharged from the hospital are readmitted within a month because of inadequate or incomplete discharge instructions.[45] Ask about services or equipment you might need when you return home. Determine who should be contacted if you experience a complication. Third, schedule an appointment with your primary care doctor during the week following your discharge to make sure there are no complications. Fourth, if you have unanswered questions before leaving the hospital, ask for an exit conference with the hospital's patient advocate, social worker, or case manager. Fifth, discuss when you will be discharged. If you feel ready to go home, let your doctor know. Conversely, if you think you're being discharged prematurely, also speak up. You have the right to leave on your own, but doing so without your doctor's approval comes with risks. People who leave the hospital without their physician's approval stand a much greater chance of experiencing a serious medical consequence that requires readmission to the hospital.[46] Doing so also undermines the relationship between you and your physician.

## Selecting a Health Care Professional

Choosing a physician for your general health care is an important and necessary duty. Only physicians are discussed here, but this information applies to the selection of all health care practitioners. You must select one who will listen carefully to your problems and diagnose them accurately. At the same time, you

# [ JUST THE FACTS ]

## Selected Health Care Specialists

The following list shows the fields of specialty of selected health care specialists.

| Name of Specialist | Field of Specialty |
| --- | --- |
| **Medical Specialists** | |
| Allergist | Allergic conditions |
| Anesthesiologist | Administration of anesthesia (such as during surgery) |
| Cardiologist | Coronary artery disease, heart disease |
| Dermatologist | Skin conditions |
| Endocrinologist | Diseases of the endocrine system |
| Epidemiologist | Study of the causes and sources of disease |
| Family practice physician | General-care physician |
| Gastroenterologist | Stomach, intestines, digestive system |
| Geriatrician | Diseases and conditions of the aged |
| Gynecologist | Female reproductive system |
| Hematologist | Study of blood |
| Hospitalist | In-hospital medical care |
| Immunologist | Diseases of the immune system |
| Internist | Diseases in adults |
| Neonatologist | Newborns |
| Nephrologist | Kidney disease |
| Neurologist | Nervous system |
| Neurosurgeon | Surgery of the brain and nervous system |
| Obstetrician | Pregnancy, labor, childbirth |
| Oncologist | Cancer, tumors |
| Ophthalmologist | Eyes |
| Orthopedist | Skeletal system |
| Otolaryngologist | Head, neck, ears, nose, throat |
| Otologist | Ears |
| Pathologist | Study of tissues and the essential nature of disease |
| Pediatrician | Childhood diseases and conditions |
| Plastic surgeon | Use of material to alter or rebuild tissues |
| Primary-care physician | General health and medical care |
| Proctologist | Disorders of the rectum and anus |
| Psychiatrist | Mental illnesses |
| Radiologist | Use of X rays |
| Rheumatologist | Diseases of connective tissues, joints, muscles, tendons |
| Rhinologist | Nose |
| Surgeon | Surgery |
| Urologist | Urinary tracts of men and women and reproductive organs of men |
| **Dental Specialists** | |
| Dentist | General care of teeth and oral cavity |
| Endodontist | Diseases of teeth below the gum line (root canal therapy) |
| Orthodontist | Teeth alignment, malocclusion |
| Pedodontist | Dental care of children |
| Periodontist | Diseases of supporting structures |
| Prosthodontist | Construction of artificial appliances for the mouth |

need a physician who can move you through the modern medical maze of technology and specialists (see Just the Facts: Selected Health Care Specialists).

For most people, good health care means having a **primary care physician,** a professional who assists you as you assume responsibility for your overall health and directs you when specialized care is necessary.

Your primary care physician should be familiar with your complete medical history as well as your home, work, and other environments. You will be better understood in periods of sickness if your physician has also seen you during periods of wellness.

For adults, primary care physicians are usually family practitioners, once called "general practitioners," and internists, specialists in internal medicine. Pediatricians often serve as primary care physicians for children. Obstetricians and gynecologists, who specialize in pregnancy, childbirth, and diseases of the female reproductive system, often serve as primary care physicians to women. General surgeons may offer primary care in addition to the surgery they perform. In some states, osteopathic physicians also practice family medicine. (Doctors of osteopathic medicine are licensed medical physicians whose approach to health care emphasizes the treatment of the whole person, not just signs and symptoms of disease.)

There are several sources of information about physicians in your area:

- Local and state medical societies can identify doctors by specialty and tell you a doctor's basic credentials. You should check on the doctor's hospital affiliation and make sure the hospital is accredited. Another sign of standing is the type of societies in which the doctor has membership. The qualifications of a surgeon, for example, are enhanced by a fellowship in the American College of Surgeons (abbreviated as FACS after the surgeon's name). An internist fellowship in the American College of Physicians is abbreviated FACP. Membership in academies indicates physicians' special interests.
- All physicians board certified in the United States are listed in the *American Medical Directory* published by the American Medical Association and available in larger libraries.
- The American Board of Medical Specialists (ABMS) publishes the *Compendium of Certified Medical Specialties* (**www.ama-assn.org**), which lists physicians by name, specialty, and location.
- Pharmacists can be asked to recommend names.
- Hospitals can give you names of staff physicians who also practice in the community.
- Local medical schools can identify faculty members who also practice privately.
- The American College of Surgeons (**www.facs.org**) can identify doctors who are a fellow of the college. This suggests that the surgeon has passed a peer-reviewed evaluation and is staying current with the latest developments in his or her field.
- Many colleges and universities have health centers that keep lists of physicians for student referral.
- Friends may have recommendations, but you should allow for the possibility that your opinion of a doctor may differ from theirs.
- Detailed reports on doctors, including credentials, degrees, and possible disciplinary actions and malpractice judgments, are available online (**www.consumerinfocentral.com**) for a fee. You can also check your state department of health website for information on licensure for all health professionals.

Once you have identified a leading candidate, you can make an appointment. You need to check with the office staff about office hours, availability of emergency care at night or on weekends, backup doctors, procedures when you call for advice, hospital affiliation, and payment and insurance procedures. You should schedule your first visit while in good health. Once you have seen your doctor, reflect on the following: Did the doctor seem to be listening to you? Were your questions answered? Was a medical history taken? Were you informed of possible side effects of drugs or tests? Was respect shown for your need of privacy? Was the doctor open to the suggestion of a second opinion?

## Patient-Physician Communication

Most doctors are not disinterested in you, but they are busy. Most doctors have to see many more patients today than they did 5 years ago to maintain the same income, and on some days they report seeing too many patients to spend adequate time with them.[47] It's not surprising therefore that patients often complain that doctors cannot or will not listen to them. On average, patients get 10 to 20 minutes with the doctor to describe symptoms or the reasons for their appointment.[48] The time crunch facing doctors creates a challenge for the patient because correct diagnoses depend largely on what you tell your doctor. Good, open communication between doctors and patients leads to more accurate diagnoses, fewer tests, increased adherence to treatment, and greater satisfaction with care. It also helps to prevent medical mistakes that have become so commonplace that the medical profession itself says medical errors are now epidemic.[49] Good communication is more likely to occur when we view health care as a "team sport" where the patient and primary care physician are co-captains (see Assessment Activity 14–2). Stated another way, the physician and patient form a partnership where there is shared decision making (see Just the Facts: Characteristics of the Ideal Physician).

Patients can do much to facilitate the development of a physician-patient partnership. Understanding the meaning of commonly used medical words, abbreviations, suffixes, and prefixes can enhance this communication (see Just the Facts: Communicating with Health Care Professionals). The following are some tips to ensure good communication:

- Take along a family member or close friend. According to one highly respected health newsletter, this is the single most important piece of advice anyone can give.[51] It is not unusual for a patient who is unaccompanied at the doctor's office to return home unable to explain what was said, done, or recommended. The patient benefits from a second pair of eyes and ears, and the physician benefits because patients are usually calmer, and the family member or close friend can provide insight into the patient.

## [ JUST THE FACTS ]

### Characteristics of the Ideal Physician

What qualities do most people seek in their physician? According to a recent survey,[50] the terms used to describe the ideal physician are not unlike those that might be expected of people in other professions. The seven characteristics most often cited are:

- Confident
- Empathetic
- Humane
- Personal
- Forthright
- Respectful
- Thorough

"Thorough" was the quality identified most often by survey participants. The most disliked characteristic was disrespectful behavior.

- When you see your physician about a problem, you should state the most important problem first. Doctors tend to believe that the first thing a patient says is most important.
- You should be specific. If you have a headache, where does it hurt? How long does it last? How often does it occur?

- You should know your family history. Because many illnesses run in families, you may be at higher risk for certain diseases. Before your first visit, you should contact your parents and close relatives to learn of their health problems, especially heart disease, cancer, stroke, arthritis, diabetes, alcoholism, and tuberculosis.
- You need to list medications and treatments you are receiving, including over-the-counter drugs. The possibility of overdosing on either prescription or over-the-counter drugs is a growing problem, especially for older people—those over 65 years of age (see Wellness for a Lifetime: Older Adults Can Go Too Far with Self-Care).[52] You will also need to identify any allergies and drug reactions. Remember the "brown bag" approach to polypharmacy.
- Ask your doctor if his or her office is set up to retrieve personal health records electronically. A **Personal Health Record (PHR)** is an electronic file or record of your health information that can be stored on the Internet and, with your permission, can be accessed by your doctor.[55] Some health insurance plans provide PHRs to their members. Some doctors also offer password-protected Web pages that allow you direct access to your own electronic medical file.
- You should tell about dietary supplements, including herbs, vitamins, and minerals. Just because supplements are advertised as "natural" doesn't mean

## Wellness for a Lifetime

### Older Adults Can Go Too Far with Self-Care

In an effort to assume responsibility for their own health care, people sometimes go too far. This is especially true for older people—those over 65 years of age—who are taking medications, both over-the-counter and prescription drugs. Common mistakes include the following: (1) taking larger doses of over-the-counter medicines than called for on the label; (2) mixing different types of medicines, both over-the-counter and prescription, without understanding the potential impact of taking two different drugs at the same time (such as analgesics and alcohol); and (3) taking someone else's medicine.

The risks and potential dangers for self-medication mistakes increase for the elderly. Drug companies typically set dosages for new drugs high enough to be effective for 90% of the intended population. Many times this dosage is too high even for people under age 65, and for those over 65, the risk for harmful side effects increases significantly.[53] Three characteristics are used to determine dosages by drug companies: (1) how much of the drug is absorbed into the bloodstream from the intestine; (2) how much of the drug is broken down in the body; and (3) how quickly the drug is eliminated from the body. The tests used to determine these characteristics are usually

completed on healthy, young volunteers with healthy, young intestines, livers, and kidneys.

Unfortunately, as humans age, their organs tend to decline in function and the processes responsible for eliminating drugs decrease, thus allowing an "overloading" effect on the user. This problem is made worse when an elderly person is taking more than one type of drug, as many elderly people do. The more drugs ingested, the greater the possibility of drug interactions. Drug interactions can increase the potency of a drug, render it ineffective, or cause other side effects that might be life-threatening. Older people in particular seem to be highly sensitive to drugs that affect the central nervous system, such as tranquilizers, antidepressants, and sleeping pills. Generally, older people are at increased risk for side effects if they are taking antidepressants, arthritis medications, blood thinners, dementia drugs, diabetes drugs, muscle relaxants, pain relievers, or sedatives or tranquilizers.[54]

To avoid potential overdoses, elderly patients should make both the physician and the pharmacist aware of all medications being taken, so that more appropriate dosages can be prescribed and closer monitoring of effects can occur.

# [ JUST THE FACTS ]

## Communicating with Health Care Professionals

Following are some words, abbreviations, suffixes, and prefixes often used in health and medical care.

| Term | Meaning |
| --- | --- |
| A– (prefix) | Without |
| Aberration | Different from normal action |
| Acute | A condition that occurs suddenly |
| Adult | Developed fully |
| Affinity | Attraction |
| –algia (suffix) | Pain in |
| Angio– (prefix) | Vessels (veins or arteries) |
| Arrest | Stopping, restraining |
| Arthr– (prefix) | Joint-related |
| Asymptomatic | Without symptoms |
| Bowel | Intestine |
| BP | Blood pressure |
| Cardiac (cardio–) | Relating to the heart |
| Carpo– (prefix) | Wrist |
| CAT | Computer-assisted X-ray |
| CCU | Coronary care unit |
| Chronic | A condition that occurs for a long time |
| Coma | Complete loss of consciousness |
| Congenital | Existing at or before birth |
| Contraindication | A reason for not prescribing a drug, procedure, or treatment |
| Coronary | Relating to the heart |
| CVA | Cerebrovascular accident (stroke) |
| Degenerative | Deterioration of a part of the body |
| Diagnosis | Determining of a disease |
| Dilation | Stretching, increase in size |
| Distention | Widening or enlargement |
| DO | Doctor of osteopathy |
| Dose | Amount of medication to be given at one time |
| Dys– (prefix) | Bad, difficult |
| Dysfunction | Impairment of function |
| Edema | Swelling from accumulation of fluid |
| EEG | Electroencephalogram |
| EKG, ECG | Electrocardiogram |
| Embolus | Blood clot floating free in the bloodstream |
| Emia– (prefix) | In the blood |
| Endemic | Disease prevalent in a particular area |
| Entero– (prefix) | Intestine |
| Epidemic | Disease prevalence that is higher than normal |
| ER/ED | Emergency room/emergency department |
| Etiology | Reference to the cause of a disease |
| Extra– (prefix) | Outside of |
| Gastr– (prefix) | Stomach |
| GP | General practitioner |
| Hem– (prefix) | Blood |
| Hemorrhage | Bleeding |
| Hyper– (prefix) | Excessive |
| Hypo– (prefix) | Insufficient |
| Indication | Condition that leads to a prescribed drug, procedure, or treatment |
| ICU | Intensive care unit |
| Innate | Hereditary, congenital |
| Innocuous | Harmless |
| Insidious | Refers to a disease that does not show early symptoms of its advent |

*continued*

# [ JUST THE **FACTS** ]

JUST THE FACTS
*continued*

| Term | Meaning |
|---|---|
| –ism (suffix) | Condition, theory, method |
| –itis (suffix) | Inflammation |
| IV | Intravenous (within a vein) |
| Jaundiced | Yellow |
| Macro | Large |
| Mal– (prefix) | Bad, deficient |
| Malady | Illness |
| Malaise | Uneasiness |
| MD | Medical doctor |
| MI | Myocardial infarction |
| Micro– (prefix) | Small |
| MRI | Magnetic resonance imaging |
| Myo– (prefix) | Muscle |
| Nephro– (prefix) | Kidney |
| –opathy (suffix) | Cause unknown |
| Pandemic | Disease that is prevalent over a large region |
| Pernicious | Severe, fatal |
| Phag– (prefix) | To eat |
| –philia (suffix) | Attraction, affinity |
| Presby– (prefix) | Old |
| Primary | Principal, most important |
| Prognosis | Medical outlook of a disease |
| Pulmo– (prefix) | Lung |
| Renal | Kidney |
| Sepsis | Infection |
| Sign | Something tangible that can be observed |
| Stenosis | Constricted, decreasing in size |
| Symptom | Intangible evidence of a disease |
| Symptomatic | Relating to symptoms |
| Syndrome | Set of symptoms that occur together for unknown causes |
| Systemic | Affecting all systems of the body |
| Thrombus | Solid blood clot |
| TIA | Transient ischemic attack |
| TPR | Temperature, pulse, respiration |
| Trauma | Injury from external force |
| Tumor | Growth |
| –uria (suffix) | Urine, urination |

they're safe. Like drugs, supplements can have side effects and interact with each other and medicines.

- You should ask questions. You can take a written list of questions, but try to make them brief and specific. You should ask about anything that is unclear and repeat the answers in your own words.
- Before leaving the doctor's office, you need to make certain you know the diagnosis or how to follow the recommended treatment. If drugs are prescribed, you should inquire about the possible **contraindications** (reasons for not using a drug), side effects, and generic substitutions.
- When appropriate, ask your physician to write down instructions or recommend reading material

for more information on a particular subject. Inquire about the next steps in the treatment, if and when a return visit is required, and danger signs to look for and report to your physician.

- If you go to your doctor for a medical test, ask him or her when you can expect to get the results. It's important to remember that a large number of missed medical diagnoses occur simply because someone in the doctor's office fails to communicate test results to patients.[56] Rather than blaming the doctor's staff, it's more instructive and helpful for patients to assume responsibility for their own health care and take the initiative to follow up with a phone call to the office.

- Be honest with your doctor, and don't underestimate the importance of lifestyle habits such as smoking, consumption of alcohol, and diet supplements. Potentially sensitive subjects related to sex, incontinence, drug experimentation, eating disorders, depression, anxieties, and stress should also be discussed.

- Ask your doctor if he or she communicates with patients by e-mail. There is a trend toward e-mail communication between doctors and patients and in some states insurers pay doctors for online consultations. If your doctor encourages e-mail communication, inquire about confidentiality and security issues. Ask if anyone else reads messages directed to the doctor. Also ask about the turnaround time for responding to messages. If you are impatient by nature and can't wait the required time for a response, don't write. Your impatience will likely lead to subsequent e-mails, possible telephone calls, and then a visit for the same problem. This is overkill and, except in emergency situations, is wasteful of both your time and your doctor's. Some guidelines for facilitating e-mail communication include the following:[57,58,59]

  - Keep messages brief. If this isn't possible, you need to see the doctor face-to-face.

  - Write a subject line that is descriptive, such as "surgery question."

  - E-mail messages may not accurately describe who you are. In the body of your message, indicate your full name, birth date, and address.

  - Edit your message before sending it. A good suggestion is to print your message, let it sit for a couple of hours, check it again for errors, revise it as needed, and then send it. Ask about the turnaround time.

  - If a follow-up visit to the doctor's office is required, take a copy of your message(s) and the doctor's responses with you.

  - Don't expect a doctor to respond to your questions if he or she hasn't seen you or doesn't have a medical file on you.

  - Don't use e-mail for emergencies. By the time you get a response, it may be too late. If you have an emergency, call 9-1-1 or immediately go to the emergency room.

  - Ask if e-mail is stored on a secure site. Otherwise, your message may be as open as a postcard.

  - E-mail, like any other form of communication, can be misused and abused. It is ideal and efficient for many circumstances. Still, it is no substitute for periodic office visits.

## Second Opinions

Chronic pain, recurring illnesses, and conditions involving elective surgery often benefit from a second opinion. A second opinion is often appropriate, and peace of mind is a sufficient reason for seeking it.

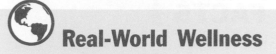

## Real-World Wellness

### How to Get a Second Opinion

*I am considering elective surgery and want a second opinion. What are some good sources for referral?*

Following are some options for finding second opinions:

- Ask your primary care physician for the names of two or three experts in the field.

- Call a medical center or hospital and ask to talk to the chief of surgery for a surgical opinion or to the chief of medicine for a nonsurgical question.

- Call the county medical society.

- Call the Second Surgical Opinion Hotline (800-638-6833) for medical organizations, which provides referrals on surgical questions.

- Call the Health Benefits Research Corporation, which offers a Second Opinion Hotline (800-522-0036, 800-631-1220 in New York) and referral service. Consultation with a board-certified specialist is available for a fee.

- Call the American Board of Medical Specialists to determine if the opinion you're getting is from a board-certified physician. The number is 800-776-CERT.

In some cases, such as elective surgery, your health insurer may require a second or third opinion before authorizing payment for certain treatments. (See Real-World Wellness: How to Get a Second Opinion for advice on getting a second opinion.)

If you decide to ask for a second opinion, common courtesy dictates that you discuss it with your physician. Your physician may suggest bringing in a consultant to assess your situation and discuss it with you and your physician. You can also ask your physician for the name of someone to see separately.

A physician may feel that a second opinion is a waste of time or money. Regardless, your wish for more information should be respected. Reputable physicians do not feel threatened by another opinion; to the contrary, they welcome another perspective on a difficult case. If your physician expresses displeasure for or resists your wish to have a second opinion, you may want to consider looking for another doctor. Exercise caution in changing doctors. The more you change doctors, the more likely your medical care will become fragmented and the better chance it will become unnecessarily confusing and complicated. If you decide to make a change, your new doctor will need a detailed explanation of previous treatments and medications. You are within your legal rights to request a copy of your medical records, and doing so is not only helpful to your new doctor but also will likely spare you the expense, inconvenience, and pain associated with previously administered medical tests and procedures.

Another good, and often overlooked, resource for a second opinion is your pharmacist. As experts on drugs, drug interactions, contraindications, and side effects, pharmacists can help you navigate through a myriad of drug options associated with treatments. If your pharmacist recommends a particular medication, it will still require your doctor's approval.

## Alternative Medicine, Complementary Medicine, Integrative Medicine

Laypeople often refer to alternative medicine, complementary medicine, and integrative medicine as one and the same. Actually, there is a distinction between the terms. The differences are based on how each compares with traditional medicine, which is referred to as allopathic medicine. **Allopathic medicine** refers to medical practice that is based on science and treats disease by using remedies that produce effects different from those caused by the disease under treatment.[60] Medical doctors, along with many of the medical specialists listed on page 465 (see Just the Facts: Selected Health Care Specialists) who have earned MDs, practice allopathic medicine, which is also called conventional medicine. **Complementary medicine** is unconventional treatments used *in addition to* treatments by your medical doctor. These treatments include a diverse group of medical services and products not currently considered a part of mainstream medicine. An example is using meditation in addition to a prescription medication to manage anxiety.[61] **Alternative medicine** includes treatments used *in place of* conventional medicine. An example is seeing an acupuncturist instead of your regular medical doctor.[62] **Integrative medicine** is a combination of allopathic, complementary, and alternative medicine and emphasizes the treatment of the whole person—mind, body, and spirit—not just the disease or a symptom. An example is a medical doctor prescribing a medication to treat a migraine and also recommending biofeedback training to reduce stress.[63]

Nearly 40% of adults use some form of complementary and alternative medicine (CAM, see Table 14–1).[64] CAM treatments vary considerably in their approach and include natural products, deep-breathing exercises, meditation, chiropractic manipulation, massage, yoga, and many more (see Figure 14–3). The use of natural products is the most common CAM treatment; echinacea, fish oil/omega-3, herbs, and flaxseed top the list.[65] The diseases and conditions for which adults are most likely to use CAM therapies are those related to pain in the back, neck, and joints (see Table 14–2).[66] The

practitioners most likely to be visited by patients seeking CAM therapies are those who provide manipulative and body-based therapies such as chiropractic or osteopathic specialists.[67] This is not surprising, because chronic pain, lower-back problems, neck pain, and osteoarthritis don't respond well to conventional medical approaches. If at first conventional treatments aren't effective, CAM therapies may offer some benefit.

Should you consider using CAM therapies? While scientific evidence supports the use of some CAM therapies in some instances, for most therapies there are questions about their safety and whether they work as intended. The National Center for Complementary and Alternative Medicine investigates CAM therapies using rigorous scientific methods. The Center provides a database on the safety and effectiveness of various therapies (see http:// http://nccam.nih.gov/). Two CAM therapies that are supported by research include acupuncture for osteoarthritis pain and a combination of acupuncture and meditation to relieve chronic pain.[68] Ongoing research on many other CAM therapies is promising but still under investigation. CAM therapies should not be used indiscriminately, because many of them come with risks and others may interfere with medical therapies prescribed by your physician. A good example is the use of "natural" products. The perception is that if a product is "natural," it is safe and risk-free. This may be a false perception. Take the drug cyclosporine, a powerful drug used to suppress the body's immune system in patients who receive organ transplants. The consumption of grapefruit, a "natural" food, interacts with cyclosporine in ways that increase its effects and may cause potentially harmful results.[69] Many other herbs may negate or interfere with important medicines. If you decide to use a CAM therapy, it is important to talk to your physician. If a CAM practitioner recommends discontinuing a prescription drug or modifying a prescribed therapy, check with your physician first. Doing so promotes communication with your physician, an important theme of this chapter, and also improves the chances of a good medical outcome.

## Assessing Your Health

Many tests, procedures, gadgets, and machines assess various aspects of health and wellness. They range from the hands-on physical examination to the use of sophisticated diagnostic tests.

### The Physical Examination

Until recently, the annual physical examination was viewed as a normal and necessary part of health care.

**TABLE 14-1** Selected Complementary and Alternative Approaches to Medicine

| Name/Type* | Proposed Therapeutic Applications | How It Works |
|---|---|---|
| 1. Acupuncture | Nausea, fibromyalgia, osteoarthritis, chronic pain management, smoking cessation | The body has energy pathways, known as meridians, that are accessible at approximately 400 different locations. Very fine sterilized stainless steel needles are inserted at specific points in these locations. Usually the procedure isn't painful. The needles are gently manipulated or stimulated with electricity or heat. Some people are energized by the needles; some people feel relaxed. Acupuncture may stimulate endorphins and relieve pain. |
| 2. Guided imagery (visualization) | Stress management, pain, side effects of cancer treatment | Imagery is the thought process that invokes and uses the senses. It relies on memories, dreams, fantasies, and visions to connect the mind with the body. Imagery activates the part of the brain that turns on the relaxation response or reduces fear and anxiety. |
| 3. Ayurvedic medicine | Heart disease, cognitive function, diabetes, hepatitis, osteoarthritis | *Ayurvedic,* which means "science of life," is a system of medicine that uses natural therapies personalized to each individual to achieve balance in body, mind, and spirit. |
| 4. Meditation | Anxiety, stress, fibromyalgia, high blood pressure, asthma | Different types of meditation (e.g., analytical, breathing, mindfulness, transcendental, visualization, walking) are used to focus attention on relaxation, mental calmness, alertness, and psychological balance. |
| 5. Spinal manipulation | Low back pain, neck pain, headache symptoms | Practitioners such as chiropractors use massage, stretching, exercise, ultrasound, electrical stimulation, and manual manipulation to relax muscles that are in spasms. Spinal adjustments are used to treat restricted spinal mobility. |
| 6. Homeopathy | Allergies, influenza, pain, vertigo, and acute childhood diarrhea | Illnesses are treated with trace amounts of a disease component or with mild doses of a substance that produces the symptoms of the illness. |
| 7. Hypnosis | Pain management, headache, anxiety, smoking cessation, sleep disorders, behavior change | Artificially induced state of relaxation is induced with the goal of opening the unconscious mind to the power of suggestion that can be acted on. |
| 8. Magnetic field therapy | Arthritis, bone fractures, depression, fibromyalgia, high blood pressure, stress | Magnetic fields produced by static magnets or electromagnets are used to penetrate the human body. |
| 9. Reflexology | Stress and tension, headache symptoms, premenstrual syndrome | Based on the belief that the hands and feet contain reflex areas that correspond to every part of the body, even the organs and glands. These parts can be affected by stimulation of the appropriate reflex areas. |
| 10. Yoga | High blood pressure, heart disease, depression, stress, anxiety | Form of exercise that teaches mind-body unity through breathing, meditation, posture, and precise movement exercises. |

*Selected from more than 30 complementary and alternative therapies listed in the source below.

**Source:** Mayo Foundation for Medical Education and Research. (2007). *Mayo Clinic: Book of Alternative Medicine.* New York: Time Inc. Home Entertainment Books.

Now, considerable debate exists among medical experts as to who needs a physical examination, how often it is needed, and what it should include. The emphasis today is on the use of selective health examinations and periodic examinations. **Selective health examinations** are specific tests used for specific problems. The assumption of this approach is that tests are more useful if they are matched to specific complaints. **Periodic**

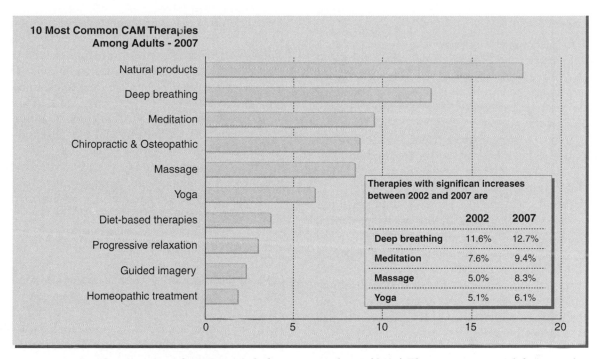

**FIGURE 14-3**  Most Common Complementary and Alternative Medicine (CAM) Therapies Among Adults—2007*

*The findings from the 2007 National Health Interview Survey (NHIS), an annual in-person survey of Americans regarding their health- and illness-related experiences. The CAM section gathered information on 23,393 adults aged 18 years or older.

Source: Barnes, P., B. Bloom, R. Nahin, (2008). *CDC National Health Statistics Report #12. Complementary and alternative medicine use among adults and children: United States, 2007.* http://nccam.nih.gov/news/camstats/2007/72_dpi_CHARTS/chart4.htm

**examinations** are assessments given according to age, health habits, predisposition for certain conditions, and/or risk factors.

The periodic exam includes only those tests warranted by the information coming from a thorough medical history and discussion of those lifestyle factors related to diseases. The assumption is that behavior and habits are the best criteria for predicting disease risk.

Criticisms of the comprehensive annual physical examination for a healthy adult are not meant to undermine the doctor-patient relationship. They simply cast doubt about the efficacy of the physical examination. However, this does not nullify the value of regular visits to the doctor. To the contrary, seeing a physician for a limited examination at regular intervals can be good preventive medicine.

**TABLE 14-2**  Diseases/Conditions for Which Complementary and Alternative Medicine (CAM) Is Most Frequently Used Among Adults—2007

| Rank | Disease/Condition | Percentage of Adults* |
|------|-------------------|-----------------------|
| 1 | Back pain | 17.1% |
| 2 | Neck pain | 5.9% |
| 3 | Joint pain | 5.2% |
| 4 | Arthritis | 3.5% |
| 5 | Anxiety | 2.8% |
| 6 | Cholesterol | 2.1% |
| 7 | Head or chest cold | 2.0% |
| 8 | Other musculoskeletal | 1.8% |
| 9 | Severe headache or migraine | 1.6% |
| 10 | Insomnia | 1.4% |

*The findings are from the 2007 National Health Interview Survey (NHIS), an annual in-person survey of Americans regarding their health- and illness-related experiences. The CAM section gathered information on 23,393 adults aged 18 years or older.

Source: Barnes, P. B. Bloom, & R. Nahin. 2008. *CDC National Health Statistics Report #12. Complementary and alternative medicine use among adults and children: United States, 2007.* http://nccam.nih.gov/news/camstats/2007/72_dpi_CHARTS/chart4.htm.

## How Often?

The need for a complete physical exam depends on a person's age, health, and lifestyle. People over the age of 65 benefit from a checkup every year. People in good health and between 40 and 65 should see their physicians for routine tests at least every 1 to 5 years.[70] Healthy people between the ages of 18 and 39 should have two complete physical exams in their twenties.[71] During the first exam, ask to have your blood profile checked (cholesterol, LDLs, HDLs). Height, weight, body mass index, and blood pressure should also be checked.

Regardless of their age, people with family histories of heart disease, stroke, high blood pressure, cancer, and diabetes can benefit from periodic checkups, even if they are in good health. The same is true for people whose health habits or occupations put them at higher than normal risk for chronic diseases and disabling conditions. Even in these cases, good judgment and discretion should rule the choice of tests to be included in the physical examination.

## Components

The three basic tools for completing a physical examination are medical history, hands-on examination, and diagnostic/laboratory tests. A medical history includes information about health habits, lifestyle, family history, and symptoms. Many physicians use health-risk appraisals, detailed questionnaires that provide information about health habits. This is one area of the physical examination for which a patient can prepare. A useful tool for recording your family's health history is provided online by the U.S. Department of Health and Human Services at **www.hhs.gov/familyhistory**. By following the guidelines for communicating with your physician presented earlier in this chapter, you can help your physician obtain an accurate health profile.

The hands-on examination is the second part of the physical examination. It consists of touching, looking, and listening. Physicians can feel, or palpate, for enlarged glands, growths, and tumors with procedures such as the breast examination, pelvic examination, rectal examination, and hernia examination. Thumping the back and chest lets the physician know whether any fluid has built up in or around the lungs. Tapping a knee for reflexes may reveal nervous system damage. A stethoscope is used to listen to the heart, lungs, abdomen, and glands located near the surface of the skin. Possible problems that can be detected with the stethoscope range from a heart murmur to poor circulation, a lung infection, intestinal blockage, blood-flow restrictions, and an overactive thyroid gland.

Physicians have a number of instruments with which to inspect visually for problems. An ophthalmoscope is used to view the brain through the eye. The first sign of

some brain diseases is an unhealthy-looking optic nerve. Leakage in the blood vessels of the eye may be a sign of diabetes or hypertension. An otoscope is used to inspect the ear, particularly the tympanic membrane. The proctoscope and sigmoidoscope are used to examine the rectum and colon. The laryngoscope and bronchoscope provide a look at the larynx and bronchial tubes.

The last part of the physical examination includes **diagnostic laboratory tests,** which vary from a simple urinalysis to invasive dye tests. The effectiveness of these tests is being debated. Tests conducted for specific symptoms may be invaluable in pinpointing disabling conditions. They may be just as valuable for what they do not reveal as they are for what they do reveal. This can be reassuring to the patient and physician. On the negative side, many physicians rely too heavily on laboratory tests. Patients often demand or acquiesce to more tests than are necessary and sometimes more than are good for them.

Many times tests are recommended more for the purpose of protecting the doctor against medical malpractice suits than for their diagnostic value. This practice, called **defensive medicine,** paints a sobering picture of the difficulty in making medical decisions for doctors and patients. A doctor may know with 99% certainty a particular diagnosis but order a test or procedure anyway, as protection against liability, should he or she be sued later. Malpractice suits are a reality; many hospital patients experience injuries, some leading to death, as a result of medical mistakes. To avoid the threat of a malpractice lawsuit, it is not unusual for physicians to order a battery of extra tests. Of course, patients always have the right to decline prescribed tests. The decision must be made by patient and doctor and should be based on the test's potential for contributing to an effective medical intervention.

Thus, when you go for a physical examination, you can determine which tests you are willing to be subjected to by asking the right questions:

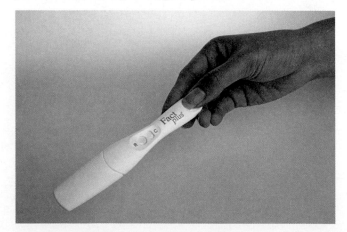

Self-care medical kits, such as home pregnancy tests, allow you to become more involved with your health care.

• *What do you expect to find?* You should start by asking why you need the test. How will it help facilitate a diagnosis? You need to ask about alternatives and the disadvantage of waiting and not testing. Sometimes the best test is the test of time. Agreeing to a test because it is routine procedure is not a satisfactory explanation.

• *What risks are associated with the test?* No test is risk-free; you should compare potential benefits and risks. One problem with tests is that they are not 100% accurate. An inaccurate result can lead to a wrong diagnosis. A **false positive,** in which a test incorrectly reveals an abnormality, may occur. False positives provoke needless anxiety, causing some people to feel and even act sick. Conversely, normal results do not necessarily indicate good health. A **false negative,** in which a test indicates normality even though a person is sick, may occur. These results may lead to a false sense of health and may delay much-needed treatment at critical stages of a disease. Statistically, test results are accurate for about 95% of the population. Thus, 5% of patients can be expected to have false positives or false negatives on any laboratory tests. Other factors that may cause test errors are the taking of certain medications, exercise, stress, diet, time of day, and mistakes in handling or processing specimens.

Another problem with tests is that they may involve physical risks. Some of the more common risks are infection; bleeding; damage to vital structures; and reactions to anesthetics, drugs, and dye-contrast materials. Again, it is important to ask questions.

• *What are the options after the test?* The bottom-line question to ask is, "So what?" If a test is positive, so what? That is, what are the treatment options, and what do these treatments entail? If none of the options is plausible to you, why have the test administered? If it is impossible to treat a disease that a test reveals, the test is not justified.

• *Where can I get more information?* The more patients know about a test and treatment options, the more likely they are to choose conservative treatments, as opposed to more aggressive treatments such as surgery.[72] Your doctor may have materials in his or her office that explain the pros and cons of various tests and treatments. The Internet can also be a good source of information (see page 457, Just the Facts: Health Help You Can Trust on the Internet). If you are seeking information on a new test, remember that just because it is new and takes advantage of cutting-edge technology doesn't mean it's more justified than established tests.

• *What are the risks of doing nothing?* This question need not be perceived as confrontational. If approached with sincerity and courtesy, answers to this question should prove helpful in determining if a test is really necessary. Sometimes a disease does not have many good treatment options, and in other cases the risks associated with a particular treatment comes with more risks than the condition being tested for. Of course, the diagnosis of a treatable disease usually justifies the test.

## Common Diagnostic Laboratory Tests

Americans are having many diagnostic tests performed. Home medical tests, available from most pharmacies, allow you to monitor a growing list of medical conditions including high blood pressure, high body temperature, asthma, allergies, urinary tract infections, pregnancy, diabetes mellitus, colon cancer, high cholesterol, and HIV infection. The tests should not be viewed as substitutes for your doctor. The accuracy rates and reliability of over-the-counter medical kits vary considerably, and their instructions do not always explain how to interpret the results. These test procedures are also subject to human error, but they provide a useful way to get involved in your health care.

Regardless of the number and types of self-care, home medical kits you may want to use, some other inexpensive items should be included in your medicine cabinet (see Just the Facts: Essentials for Your Medicine Cabinet). These items should help you cope with most common minor aches and pains.

Depending on your health status, gender, age, symptoms, and risk for a disease, some of the more common tests may be recommended when you go to your physician for a checkup. *Multiple blood screening tests* check for high blood sugar, which indicates diabetes; blood urea nitrogen, an indicator of kidney function; an overactive parathyroid gland; blood count, a screen for anemia; and much more (see Assessment Activity 14–3).

A *complete blood lipid profile* checks for high LDL cholesterol, low HDL cholesterol, and triglyceride levels. (See Chapter 2 for a thorough discussion of cholesterol and lipoproteins—HDLs and LDLs.) This assessment is recommended every 5 years, starting at age 34 for men and 44 for women.[73]

*Fecal occult-blood tests,* also called *hemoccult tests,* are used to detect hidden blood in bowel movements. If a test is positive, it may indicate signs of an early cancer of the colon. People over 50 should either test themselves (home screening kits are available in most pharmacies) or have their stools tested for blood every year.[74] (See Just the Facts: Fecal Occult-Blood Tests: Reducing False Positives at **www.mhhe.com/anspaugh8e** Student Center, Chapter 14, Just the Facts.) Another option, which is invasive and recommended in combination with or in place of the fecal occult-blood test, is a *colonoscopy.* This procedure involves the insertion of a long, thin, flexible tube with a viewing scope attached to it to examine the entire colon. In addition to checking the colon for growths and signs of cancer,

## [ JUST THE **FACTS** ]

### Essentials for Your Medicine Cabinet

Except for personal items and prescription medicines, what should you keep in your medicine cabinet? The following are the essentials, according to experts:

1. A *thermometer* to assess body temperature (oral, rectal, ear, and electronic models available)
2. *Ipecac* to induce vomiting in case of poisoning
3. *Acetaminophen* to reduce fever and pain (in liquid form for children; aspirin should not be given to anyone under 20 years of age because of its link to Reye syndrome)
4. An *antiseptic,* such as hydrogen peroxide, for cleaning open wounds
5. *Gauze* and *tape* to treat minor wounds
6. An *ice bag* to reduce swelling
7. *Ace bandages* to wrap pulled muscles or twisted ankles or to bind a splint
8. *Nonprescription antihistamine* to reduce allergic reactions. Examples are Benadryl, Claritin, and Alavert. The last two items are less sedating than Benadryl.
9. *Hydrocortisone cream or ointment* for minor skin irritations and rashes.
10. *Antibiotic cream* to prevent infections from cuts.
11. *Swim-Ear* or similar medicine for mild outer ear infection that occurs after exposure to water.
12. *Murine Earwax Removal* or similar medicine to dissolve wax in the outer ear.
13. *Antiacid* such as Tums for indigestion. Proton pump inhibitors such as omeprazole and lansoprazole, which block the production of stomach acids, are now available as nonprescription medicines for indigestion that is chronic and persistent.
14. *Antidiarrheal medication,* such as Imodium, to treat diarrhea.
15. *Variety package of bandages* for open wounds and cuts.
16. *Cold medicines* including lozenges with glycerin or honey for cough; pseudoephedrine pills, such as Sudafed, or nasal sprays, such as Afrin, for nasal congestion; nonprescription antihistamines for runny nose or watery eyes; and throat spray, such as Chloraseptic Spray, for sore throat.

this procedure permits the removal of polyps, some of which might be precancerous. The colon should be checked at age 50 and then every 10 years if a colonoscopy is used in combination with an annual fecal occult-blood test.[75] A noninvasive option is the use of a CT scanner that pro-

duces 3-D images of the colon. However, this option is not widely available and may not be covered by health insurance. If this option is used, it should be repeated every 5 years, starting at age 50.[76] If it yields suspicious results, it may be followed by a colonoscopy.

*Pulse rate* may be an indicator of a health problem. The normal resting heart rate is between 60 and 80 beats a minute. Resting heart rates above 80 beats per minute put a person in a higher risk category for heart attacks and sudden death. The high heart rate does not increase the risk but is an indicator of basic problems, such as cigarette smoking, too much caffeine, stress, anxiety, hyperthyroidism, and most commonly a poor level of physical fitness. Slow heart rates are normally found in physically fit people; in them, slow heart rates are a sign of good health. Very slow rates below 50 beats per minute can occur in people who are not fit and who have heart problems. These people should seek medical advice.

*Blood pressure* measurements should be monitored regularly, especially for people who have had previously high readings or have family histories of hypertension (high blood pressure). Inexpensive, accurate home blood pressure kits can be purchased at most drugstores. Because all kits are not equally reliable, you should ask your pharmacist for a recommendation. People who have measurements higher than 140 over 90 mmHg or lower than 100 over 60 mmHg should keep records of their blood pressure and present them to their physicians during periodic checkups.

*Mammography,* an X-ray examination of the breast, detects early signs of breast cancer. There is some controversy associated with mammography screening. The American Cancer Society (ACS) recommends breast screening every year for women beginning at age 40. A clinical breast exam should be performed before mammography. For women in their twenties and thirties, a clinical breast exam should be part of a periodic health examination, preferably at least every 3 years. Asymptomatic women aged 40 and over should continue to receive a clinical breast exam as part of a periodic health examination, preferably annually.[77] A U.S. government advisory panel makes a different recommendation. It advises women in their forties and those 75 and older to discuss the pros and cons of the test with their doctor, rather than automatically undergoing a mammography. This is because mammograms are associated with an increase in false positives for women in their forties, and false positives may lead unnecessarily to more mammograms, biopsies, or radiation, not to mention worry and anxiety.[78] A conversation with your doctor regarding your risk of contracting breast cancer along with your family history should help you to choose between the ACS recommendation or the more conservative recommendation of the U.S. government advisory panel. You can assess your risk online at the National Cancer Institute's test at **www.cancer.gov/bcrisktool.**

*Pelvic examinations and Pap smears* detect abnormalities of the ovaries, uterus, and cervix. ACS recommends cervical cancer screening approximately 3 years after a woman begins having vaginal intercourse, but no later than 21 years of age. Screening should be done every year with conventional Pap tests or every 2 years using liquid-based Pap tests. At or after age 30, women who have had three normal test results in a row may get screened every 2 to 3 years. Women 70 years and older who have had three or more consecutive normal Pap tests in the last 10 years may choose to stop Pap tests. Women who have had a total hysterectomy (removal of the cervix and uterus) may choose to stop cervical cancer screening.[79] The American College of Obstetricians and Gynecologists (ACOG) offers a slightly different recommendation. Because there is a very low chance that cervical cancer will occur before age 21, ACOG recommends Pap smears starting at age 21. Women younger than 30 years old should get them every 2 years. Women 30 and older can get one every 3 years, with the option of combining it with a test for the human papillomavirus (HPV), which can lead to cervical cancer.[80] Since ACS and ACOG have different recommendations, you should discuss your risks of contracting cervical cancer with your physician to determine which recommendation is most appropriate for you.

A complete *eye examination* includes a test for visual acuity; *tonometry,* a painless test for glaucoma; and a cataract (a clouding over the lens) check. If you have vision problems, an eye exam is recommended every 2 years, regardless of age. Everyone (with or without eye problems) should have an eye exam every 2 years after age 40. Beginning no later than age 45, glaucoma screening should begin.[81]

*Electrocardiograms (ECGs)* are used to detect irregularities of the heart. Although there is some debate about the use of ECGs as routine screening procedures for *asymptomatic* (without symptoms), low-risk people. Chest pain, hypertension, and symptoms of cardiovascular disease justify earlier ECGs. *Stress tests* use ECGs to assess how the heart functions under the stress of exercise. They are routine when symptoms are present.

*Chest X-ray examinations* are valuable diagnostic tools for people with chest symptoms, respiratory diseases, and heart problems. In the absence of symptoms, their routine use is questionable. Avoid chest X-ray if there is a chance you are pregnant.

*Prostate cancer tests* check for the possibility of prostate cancer usually by combining two procedures: a digital rectal exam and a PSA test, a blood test that looks for prostate-specific antigens. You should discuss with your physician the potential benefits and limitations of prostate cancer early detection testing, beginning at age 50 for men who are at average risk for prostate cancer and who have a life expectancy of at least 10 years.[82] Men who are at high risk for prostate cancer, including African American men and those with a family history of prostate cancer, should start testing at age 45.[83]

An *HIV test* is recommended for people who think they may have been infected with HIV. This includes people who have had unprotected sex or a blood transfusion, have used IV drugs, or have participated in high-risk behaviors. After the blood test, these people should avoid high-risk behavior for 6 months to a year and then retest.

A *visual skin test* for skin cancer is recommended as part of any periodic health examination for men and women beginning at age 20. Individuals with a history of melanoma should have a full body exam at least annually and perform regular self-exams for new and changing moles.[84]

A *blood glucose test* is recommended to detect diabetes mellitus. There are two different tests to determine whether you have prediabetes: the fasting plasma glucose test (FPG) or the oral glucose tolerance test (OGTT). The blood glucose levels measured after these tests determine whether you have a normal metabolism or whether you have prediabetes or diabetes. If your blood glucose level is abnormal following the FPG, you have impaired fasting glucose (IFG); if your blood glucose level is abnormal following the OGTT, you have impaired glucose tolerance (IGT).[85] A blood glucose test is recommended for people who have a strong family history of diabetes, or have symptoms of diabetes, including excessive thirst and frequent urination, and who are overweight. People, with or without symptoms, should have a fasting blood glucose test every 3 years, starting at age 45.[86] You can take a test online to determine if you are at risk of having prediabetes or diabetes by going to **www.diabetes.org/diabetes-basics/prevention/diabetes-risk-test/.**

A *bone mineral density test (BMD)* detects bone thinning that increases the risks of developing osteoporosis, a disease in which bones become fragile and more likely to break. It is recommended for postmenopausal women under age 65 with one or more risk factors for osteoporosis, and women age 65 or older and men age 70 or older, even without risk factors. A woman or man after age 50 who has broken a bone and postmenopausal women who have stopped taking estrogen therapy or hormone therapy may need a bone mineral density test. The test is noninvasive and involves the use of an X-ray-type machine at two sites: spine and hip. A person remains fully dressed, and the test usually takes less than 15 minutes. Test results are reported in terms of a T-Score, which describes how much the bone density varies from what's considered normal. "Normal" is based on the typical bone mass of people in their thirties, when bone mass is at its peak.[87] (See Just the Facts: Interpreting Your T-Score.)

## Direct-Access Testing (DAT)

**Direct-access testing**, or **DAT,** is a trend in medical testing that offers patients convenience, privacy, and a sense of control. Patients simply order a particular test, go to a commercial or hospital lab affiliated with the DAT vendor, and submit a blood test; within a couple of days, test results are mailed or made available online. This is done without a visit to the physician's office or a prescription. Convenience is the number one reason patients seek DAT; "no need to see a physician" is the number two reason.[89]

DAT providers offer medical tests for chronic conditions, such as diabetes and heart disease, and acute conditions, such as infections. Some tests are modestly priced (e.g., less than $25), while others cost several hundred dollars or more. DAT is not available in some states, and it is not usually covered by health insurance.

The American College of American Pathology, the professional group that oversees medical testing, warns against the indiscriminate use of DAT. However, it does not restrict its members from offering DAT. Here are some criticisms of DAT:

- A "positive" will require a follow-up appointment with a doctor and probably a repeat of the same test.
- DAT may raise patients' anxiety levels and ultimately result in more tests, more visits to health care providers, and ultimately higher costs. This is particularly true for false positives.
- If doctors are not in the loop during the testing phase, neither are they in the loop to interpret test results and plan follow-up treatment options.
- Some test results will be false negative and therefore lead to a false sense of well-being.
- Patients who think they have a little knowledge about a particular health issue may use the results of DAT to mistakenly self-diagnose and actually exacerbate their condition.

Regardless of these criticisms, DAT is an option for patients who demand privacy and convenience and have the financial resources to pay for it. Advice for DAT users includes the following:[90]

- Use DAT discriminately; it is not intended to be a substitute for your physical or your physician. To quote the editors of the highly respected *Tufts University Health and Nutrition Letter,* "Testing should never be an entirely do-it-yourself project."[91]
- Investigate and ask questions about the test just as you do for those administered in the doctor's office.
- If DAT yields abnormal results, consult with your doctor.

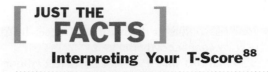

## [ JUST THE FACTS ]
### Interpreting Your T-Score[88]

A bone density test for possible signs of bone thinning and/or loss may signal the development of osteoporosis. Test results are presented as T-Scores and can be interpreted as follows:

- T-Scores ranging from $-1$ to $+1$ or higher mean that bone density is "normal" and suggest low risk for bone fractures due to osteoporosis.
- T-Scores ranging from $-1$ to $-2.5$ indicate low bone density (*osteopenia*) and a greater risk for bone fractures.
- T-Scores of $-2.5$ and lower indicate the presence of osteoporosis.

## Immunizations for Adults

Many people believe that **immunizations** (administrations of preparations or vaccines, usually in the form of injections, for providing immunity or preventing a disease) are only for children. Consequently, many thousands of adults die every year of diseases they would not have acquired if they had received standard vaccines. Adult immunization is recommended to prevent or ameliorate influenza, pneumonia, some forms of hepatitis, measles, rubella (German measles), tetanus, diphtheria, chicken pox, and shingles.

People born after 1956 may need to be reimmunized for measles, mumps, and rubella (MMR) because the earlier vaccine may not have provided complete coverage.[92] A booster is not suggested for those born before 1957 because of the likelihood that they have natural immunity.

Booster shots should be given for tetanus and diphtheria every 10 years (tetanus and diphtheria vaccines are usually combined). A booster shot is required annually for protection against common seasonal strains of influenza, whereas a pneumonia vaccine is usually good for life if administered after age 65. If administered before the age of 65, a booster shot is recommended at least 5 years after the first shot.[93] Anyone older than 18 who smokes should also get a pneumonia vaccine.[94,95]

A vaccine for preventing *shingles,* a painful disease of the skin and certain nerve pathways that is caused by the chicken pox virus, is recommended for people 60 years old or older. This vaccine is recommended even if shingles has occurred, because it can recur.

Girls and women ages 11 to 26 should be vaccinated against human papillomavirus (HPV) to prevent a virus that can cause genital warts and cervical cancer. Ideally, the vaccine should be administered before potential exposure to HPV through sexual activity; however, females who are sexually active should still be vaccinated.[96]

Varicella vaccination protects against chicken pox. Anyone who has not had chicken pox should get this vaccination.[97]

Hepatitis A and hepatitis B vaccinations protect against liver disease and are recommended for adults at risk because of their jobs, travel, or exposure to susceptible children or infected people.

## Summary

- Health information that can be trusted is based on scientifically controlled studies that yield consistent results over time.
- A study is considered reliable if its findings can be confirmed in repeated studies conducted over the course of many years.
- The *provocative effect* refers to the tendency to adopt certain behaviors as a result of being asked about it. It often occurs when people are asked to complete questionnaires or serve as participants in survey research. It may lead to the adoption of either positive or negative health practices.
- Scientifically controlled studies involve experimental and control groups, use randomly selected participants, and feature double-blind procedures.
- *Statistical significance* is a term health journalists and researchers use to indicate probability. If a finding is statistically significant, 95 of 100 times similar studies yield similar findings.
- *Statistical relationship* is a term used to indicate the degree of association between two or more variables (e.g., dietary fat and heart disease). Statistical relationships do not demonstrate cause and effect.
- In the health literature the term *absolute risk* refers to the actual number of people affected by a risk factor. *Relative risk* refers to the percentage of people affected by a risk factor in comparison with some benchmark. Relative risks are often used in the news media because they tend to produce more sensational headlines but they are more prone to deception than absolute risks.
- Epidemiologic studies are population studies that observe the health habits and lifestyles of many people over time. They may be prospective or retrospective.

- The discriminating use of the Internet can yield helpful information for most health conditions.
- Signs and symptoms that warrant immediate medical attention are unexpected shortness of breath; severe chest pain; sudden weakness of part of the body; sudden paralysis; loss of speech; sudden intense headaches, especially in people over 50; poisoning; head traumas; injuries from falls and accidents; first aid emergencies; and uncontrolled bleeding and internal bleeding as indicated by blood in the urine, bowel movement, sputum, or vomit; or blood from any of the body's openings.
- People can help ensure proper and safe care while in a hospital by checking on the hospital's accreditation status, deciding on accommodations before admission, knowing their patient rights, discussing treatments and procedures with their physicians, asking questions, and staying active. (See Assessment Activity 14–4.)
- Americans have the benefit of some of the world's best hospitals. However, hospitalization carries some risks, such as medical errors, unexpected drug reactions, and hospital-borne infections. Many hospital-related infections could be prevented by the simple practice of hand washing.
- *Polypharmacy* refers to the administration of many drugs at the same time. Prescribed indiscriminately, the combined interaction of multiple drugs has the potential to cause problems worse than the disease being treated.
- *Medical reconciliation* is a written comparison of medications administered during a hospital stay with the ones you were taking before being admitted to the hospital.
- Good health care means establishing a doctor-patient relationship while in good health.

- The doctor who manages the general care of patients and directs patients to specialized services is the primary-care physician.
- A *personal health record (PHR)* is an electronic file or record of your health information that can be stored on the Internet and, with your permission, can be accessed by your doctor.
- *Allopathic medicine* refers to conventional or traditional medical care provided by doctors trained in medical school. *Complementary medicine* is unconventional treatments used in addition to treatments by your medical doctor. *Alternative medicine* refers to treatments used in place of conventional medicine. *Integrative medicine* is a combination of allopathic, complementary, and alternative medicine.
- When telling a physician about a problem, you can enhance good communication by presenting the most important problem first, being as specific as possible, being familiar with your family medical history, knowing the names of medicines you are taking, and asking questions. If possible, take a friend or close relative when seeking medical care or treatment.
- The three major components of a physical examination are the medical history, the hands-on examination, and diagnostic laboratory tests.
- A medical history is an important part of the physical examination, especially during the initial visit to a doctor.
- A selective health examination involves the use of specific tests for specific problems. A periodic exam involves the use of tests and procedures after a complete medical history and a discussion of personal lifestyle factors and risk factors.
- *Defensive medicine* is the practice of prescribing tests and procedures for

the purpose of protecting doctors from medical-malpractice lawsuits.

- *Direct-access testing (DAT)* empowers patients with the ability to purchase medical testing without a prescription or a trip to the doctor's office. DAT may be more convenient than scheduling an appointment with a doctor, but it is also expensive (not usually covered by insurance) and if the test results are not favorable the doctor is left out when he or she is needed the most.
- The eight diseases for which adults need to maintain immunization are influenza, pneumonia, hepatitis, measles, rubella, tetanus, diphtheria, and chicken pox. In addition, people 60 years old or older should be immunized to prevent shingles. And, females 11 to 26 should be immunized to prevent cervical cancer, preferably before becoming sexually active.

## Review Questions

1. How does the availability of so much information in the printed, electronic, and video press contribute to misinformation and misunderstanding of matters related to health?
2. To what does the phrase "medical contradiction" refer? What are some examples, in addition to those mentioned in this chapter?
3. What do you think was the purpose of the discussion of coffee consumption and how the research community appears to have reversed its position on its benefits and dangers? Elaborate.
4. What criteria must a research study satisfy before its claims can be trusted?
5. What are some techniques and strategies that manufacturers and producers of health products use to mislead and deceive the public?
6. Explain the meaning of *provocative effect*. Discuss ethical issues related to the influence of the provocative effect on health behavior.
7. Explain the meaning and significance of scientifically controlled, double-blind studies. Cite an example.
8. What do the terms *statistical significance* and *statistical relationship* mean in reference to health studies?
9. Differentiate between the terms *absolute risk* and *relative risk*. Which of these two terms tends to be misleading? Why?
10. How do epidemiologic studies differ from scientifically controlled studies?
11. Explain why it is important to know the funding source of a study that makes some promising claims regarding a medical procedure or product.
12. How can you tell if health information on the Internet can be trusted? Identify three criteria or guidelines.
13. The Internet has been described as a "wild frontier" and "the world's bazaar." Explain what these terms mean in reference to health.
14. Identify signs or symptoms that require immediate medical attention.
15. A high body temperature, a fever, is described in the chapter as "an adaptive response." What does this mean?
16. Why is it important to see a physician while in good health?
17. What can laypeople do while in a hospital to ensure that they receive safe and proper care?
18. Define the term *polypharmacy*. What can people do to prevent health complications caused by polypharmacy?
19. To what does the "brown bag" solution to polypharmacy refer?
20. Identify the health conditions that are responsible for the greatest number of inpatient hospitalizations.
21. What is the major role and function of a primary care physician?
22. Differentiate between informed consent and implied consent. Give an example of each.
23. Differentiate between allopathic medicine, complementary medicine, alternative medicine, and integrative medicine. Give an example of each.
24. What does medical reconciliation mean? Why is it an important process for a successful experience in the hospital?
25. List four sources of information for researching physicians and specialists in your geographical area.
26. Identify four techniques that facilitate communication between patient and physician.
27. List four guidelines for facilitating e-mail communication between you and your health care provider.
28. Identify six rights patients have when in a hospital.
29. Differentiate among selective health exam, periodic exam, and comprehensive physical examination.
30. Identify five items that should be included in the home medicine cabinet. What is the purpose of each?
31. In reference to medical tests, differentiate among the terms *positive, negative, false positive, and false negative*.
32. Define *defensive medicine*. Discuss its impact on both the quantity and the quality of health care provided to patients.
33. Identify five commonly used alternative medical therapies. Differentiate between each therapy in terms of application and how it works.
34. What does the acronym DAT mean? What are the pros and cons of DAT?
35. Identify immunizations for adults.
36. List five questions you should ask before undergoing an invasive medical diagnostic test.

## References

1. Antinoro, L. (2009). What you worry about . . . but shouldn't vs, things that are worth your worry. *Environmental Nutrition, 32*(1), 1,4.
2. Schardt, D. (2009). You must remember this: How to keep your brain young. *Nutrition Action Healthletter, 36*(3), 1, 3–8.
3. Editor. 2010. Coffee, tea, or diabetes? *Nutrition Action Healthletter, 37*(2), 9.
4. Harvard Medical Information Publications Group. (2009). Putting the

joie de vivre back into health. *Harvard Health Letter, 34*(1), 1–3.

5. Sandroff, S. (2000). Frustrations of science. *Consumer Reports on Health, 12*(8), 2.

6. Levi, J., C. Juliano, & L. M. Segal. (2006). *F as in fat: How obesity policies are failing in America 2006.* Washington, DC: Trust for America's Health.

7. Ibid.

8. Tufts Media. (2006). Medical-meeting news lost in media translation. *Tufts University Health and Nutrition Letter, 24*(7), 6.

9. Latifi, S. (2006, July 23). Study: Survey alters behavior. *The Commercial Appeal* p. A3.

10. Williams, P., L. G. Block, & G. J. Fitzsimons. (2006). Simply asking questions about health behaviors increases both healthy and unhealthy behaviors. *Social Influence, 1*(2), 117–27.

11. Latifi (2006).

12. Ibid.

13. Ibid.

14. Knight Ridder Washington Bureau (KRT) via Thomson Dialog NewsEdge. (2006). Survey questioning can alter subjects' behavior, study says. Retrieved from www.tmcnet.com/usubmit/2006/07/20/1722651.htm.

15. Tufts Media. (2006). Studying research studies: 10 questions you need to ask. Tufts University Health and Nutrition Letter, 24(4), 4–5.

16. Levi, et al. 2006.

17. Tufts Media. (2009). The bad news about products "too good to be true." *Tufts University Health and Nutrition Letter, 27*(7), Special Report, 4–5.

18. Schardt, D. (2009). Web self-defense. *Nutrition Action Healthletter, 36*(3), 9, 11–12.

19. Consumers Union. (2005). Making sense of medical news. *Consumer Reports on Health, 17*(5), 8.

20. Mayo Foundation for Medical Education and Research. (2009). News and our views: Avoiding the emergency department. *Mayo Clinic Health Letter, 27* (5), 4.

21. Consumers Union. (2009). When you need care fast. *Consumer Reports on Health, 21*(4), 6.

22. Consumers Union. (2008). Emergency-room survival tips. *Consumer Reports on Health, 20*(7), 6.

23. Davis, B. (2010). Body temperature. Retrieved March 16, 2010, from http://firstaid.webmd.com/body-temperature.

24. Ibid.

25. Ibid.

26. Tufts Media. (2000). When nagging symptoms should trigger a doctor's visit. *Tufts University Health and Nutrition Letter, 18*(5), 4–5.

27. Consumers Union. (2004). Fever: Eight burning questions. *Consumer Reports on Health, 16*(11), 8–9.

28. Consumers Union. (2002). When to treat a fever. *Consumer Reports on Health, 14*(9), 10.

29. DeFrances, C. J., K. Cullen , & L. Kozak. (2007. National Hospital Discharge Survey: 2005 annual summary with detailed diagnosis and procedure data. National Center for Health Statistics. *Vital Health Statistics, 13*, (165).

30. Ibid.

31. Ibid.

32. Consumers Union. (2010). Deadly infections. *Consumer Reports, 75*(3), 16, 17–21.

33. DeFrances, et al. (2007).

34. Ibid.

35. Santa, J. (2009). How to get out of a hospital safely. *Consumer Reports on Health, 21*(6), 11.

36. Consumers Union. (2005). Are you taking too much prescription medication? *Consumer Reports on Health, 17*(8), 1, 4–6.

37. Sandroff, Ronni. (1997). AHAdvocate. *American Health, 16*(6), 41–43.

38. Consumers Union. (2001). Medication errors—yours and theirs. *Consumer Reports on Health, 13*(11), 1, 4–6.

39. Lipman, M. (2008). The hospitalist fills a crucial gap. *Consumer Reports on Health, 20*(9), 11.

40. Editor. (2004). Hospitalized? Insist on getting a multi. *Environmental Nutrition, 27*(8), 3.

41. Consumers Union. (2001). Doctor, can we talk? *Consumer Reports on Health, 13*(7), 7–8.

42. Consumers Union. (2009). Patients beware. *Consumer Reports, 74*(9), 18, 19–23.

43. Ibid.

44. Santa (2009).

45. Consumers Union (2009).

46. Lipman (2008).

47. Consumers Union. (2007). Get better care from your doctor. *Consumer Reports, 72*(2), 32–36.

48. Ibid.

49. Santa, J. (2009). Doctors, admit your mistakes. *Consumer Reports, 74*(11), 12.

50. Editor. (2006). Seven characteristics of the ideal physician. *HealthNews, 12*(5), 12.

51. Harvard Medical Information Publications Group. (2004). Nine tips for patients. *Harvard Health Letter, 29*(9), 1–2.

52. Consumers Union. (1998). Special report on health guide to medication. *Consumer Reports, 63*(4), 1–8.

53. Ibid.

54. Ibid.

55. Mayo Foundation for Medical Education and Research. (2009). Personal health records. *Mayo Clinic Health Letter, 27*(2), 7.

56. Consumers Union. (2009). Don't be a diagnostic error. *Consumer Reports on Health, 21*(9), 1, 4–5.

57. Lipman, M. (2004). E-mailing your doctor *Consumer Reports on Health, 16*(4), 11.

58. Consumers Union. (2002). Take two aspirins and e-mail me in the morning. *Consumer Reports, 67*(1), 59, 61.

59. Sands, D. (2008). E-mailing your doctor. *Consumer Reports on Health, 20*(6), 12.

60. Medicine.net. (2010). Definition of allopathic medicine. Retrieved March 19, 2010, from www.medterms.com/script/main/art.asp?articlekey=33612.

61. Mayo Foundation for Medical Education and Research. (2007). *Mayo Clinic: Book of alternative medicine.* New York: Time Inc. Home Entertainment Books.

62. Ibid.

63. Ibid.

64. Nahin, R., P. Barnes, B. Stussman, & B. Bloom. (2009). Costs of complementary and alternative medicine (CAM) and frequency of visits to CAM practitioners: United States, 2007. *National Health Statistics Reports*, No. 18: Hyattsville, MD: National Center for Health Statistics.

65. Barnes, P. B. Bloom, & R. Nahin. (2008). *CDC National Health Statistics Report #12. Complementary and alternative medicine use among adults and children: United States, 2007.* Retrieved March 20, 2010, from http://nccam.nih.gov/news/cam-stats/2007/72_dpi_CHARTS/chart4.htm.

66. Ibid.
67. Nahin, et al. (2009).
68. Tufts Media. (2008). Exploring the alternatives. *Tufts University Health and Nutrition Letter,* 26(7), Special Report), 4–5.
69. Ibid.
70. MedlinePlus. (2010). Physical exam frequency. Retrieved March 20, 2010, from www.nlm.nih.gov/medlineplus/ency/article/002125.htm.
71. Ibid.
72. Consumers Union. (2010). When doctor doesn't know best. *Consumer Reports on Health,* 22(4), 8–9.
73. MedlinePlus (2010).
74. American Cancer Society. (2009). Cancer facts and figures 2009. Atlanta, GA: American Cancer Society.
75. Ibid.
76. Ibid.
77. Ibid.
78. Consumers Union. (2010). Rethinking women's health issues. *Consumer Reports on Health,* 22(2), 7.

79. ACS (2009).
80. Consumers Union (2010).
81. MedlinePlus (2010).
82. ACS (2009).
83. MedlinePlus (2010).
84. American Academy of Dermatology. (2010). Skin cancer fact sheet. Retrieved March 22, 2010, from www.aad.org/media/background/factsheets/fact_skincancer.html.
85. American Diabetes Association. (2010). How to tell if you have diabetes. Retrieved March 22, 2010, from www.diabetes.org/diabetes-basics/prevention/pre-diabetes/how-to-tell-if-you-have.html.
86. Consumers Union. (2009). Screening tests you can live without. *Consumer Reports on Health,* 21(1), 8–9.
87. National Osteoporosis Foundation. (2010). BMD testing. Retrieved March 22, 2010, from www.nof.org/osteoporosis/bmdtest.htm.
88. Ibid.
89. Editor. (2003). What's DAT? *Health-News,* 9(7), 5.

90. Ibid.
91. Tufts University. (2003). Putting home tests to the test. Tufts University *Health & Nutrition Letter,* 21(8), 1–4.
92. Centers for Disease Control and Prevention. (2010). Recommended adult immunization schedule—United States, 2010. *Morbidity and Mortality Weekly Report,* 59(1).
93. Consumers Union (2009).
94. Harvard Medical Information Publications Group. (2009). The shoulds—and the shouldn'ts—of getting your shots. *Harvard Health Letter,* 34(5), 3.
95. CDC. (2010).
96. Ibid.
97. Ibid.

# Suggested Readings

Brownlee, S. (2007). *Overtreated: Why too much medicine is making us sicker and poorer.* New York: Bloomsbury USA.

This is a must-read book for anyone interested in the economics of health care. Award-winning medical author Brownlee illustrates why and how Americans get too much medical care, surgery, diagnostic tests, and medicines. The author challenges every assumption regarding health care and shows why overtreatment, like undertreatment, is bad medicine.

Mayo Foundation for Medical Education and Research. (2007). *Mayo Clinic: Book of alternative medicine.* New York: Time Inc. Home Entertainment Books.

Doctors from the world famous Mayo Clinic provide answers to questions about the effectiveness of complementary and alternative medicine and when it is appropriate to use natural remedies. More than 30 therapies are presented and include dietary supplements, mind-body medicine, energy therapies, hands-on therapies, and many other approaches. Each therapy is defined and explained, and research findings regarding its effectiveness to treat certain conditions are presented in laypersons' terms.

Mitchell. D. (2009). *25 medical tests your doctor should tell you about . . . and 15 you can do yourself.* New York: St Martin's Press.

An easy-to-use, up-to-date, A-to-Z guide, this book contains comprehensive, accessible information on medical tests that doctors don't usually have time to discuss with their patients. Features 15 tests that readers can administer themselves at home. The author includes simple screenings that could save your life, specialized tests for every member of your family, how to tell if the risks of a test outweigh the benefits, tips on choosing the best home testing kits, the latest in prevention and diagnosis of common medical conditions, and the best way to prepare for tests and how to interpret the results.

Schneider, Edward. (2006). *What your doctor hasn't told you and the health-store clerk doesn't know.* New York: Penguin.

This book provides an overview of the latest medical research on alternative medicine. It describes an integrative therapy approach to treat common health issues including sleep problems, joint pain, depression, anxiety, premenstrual syndrome, prostate health, back pain, heart disease, cancer, and memory loss.

Thompson PDR. (2009). *The PDR pocket guide to prescription drugs,* 9th ed. New York: Simon and Schuster.

This pocket-sized book provides FDA-approved information on drugs according to brand name and generic cross-reference along with benefits, risks, and side effects. Possible food-drug interactions and overdose information are included. Drug profiles are based on information from the *Physicians' Desk Reference.*

# Assessment Activity 14-1

## Assessing Your "Normal" Body Temperature

Use this assessment to determine the body temperature that is normal for you. Do this assessment when you are feeling well. Take your temperature three times on three successive days: (1) before getting out of bed in the morning, (2) in the late afternoon, and (3) before going to bed at night. If you exercise, wait several hours before taking your temperature. Wait at least 10 minutes after eating or drinking hot or cold food or beverage. Use a digital, electronic, or mercury *oral* thermometer, depending on your personal preference. Calculate the average temperature for each column. These averages represent your normal range of temperatures.

| Date: | | | |
|---|---|---|---|
| **Day** | **Morning** | **Afternoon** | **Bedtime** |
| 1 | | | |
| 2 | | | |
| 3 | | | |
| 3-day average | | | |

# Assessment Activity 14-2

## Are You Communicating with Your Physician?

**Directions:**  Using the following scale, circle the appropriate number for each question. Total your responses and find your score at the end of the activity.

| When I go to my physician for a health problem, | Almost Always | Very Frequently | Frequently | Occasionally | Never |
|---|---|---|---|---|---|
| I plan ahead of time how I am going to describe my problem. | 5 | 4 | 3 | 2 | 1 |
| I describe my most important problem first. | 5 | 4 | 3 | 2 | 1 |
| I check with my immediate family to determine if my problem runs in the family. | 5 | 4 | 3 | 2 | 1 |
| I take a list of medications, over-the-counter drugs, and treatments I am receiving. | 5 | 4 | 3 | 2 | 1 |
| Before the visit, I prepare a written list of questions to ask. | 5 | 4 | 3 | 2 | 1 |
| I ask about anything that is unclear to me. | 5 | 4 | 3 | 2 | 1 |
| I repeat in my own words the physician's answers to my questions. | 5 | 4 | 3 | 2 | 1 |
| I understand the doctor's diagnosis of my problem. | 5 | 4 | 3 | 2 | 1 |
| I make sure I know the benefits and risks of prescribed treatments. | 5 | 4 | 3 | 2 | 1 |
| I know if and when to return for a follow-up visit. | 5 | 4 | 3 | 2 | 1 |

## Scoring

46–50 = Excellent communication
41–45 = Good
36–40 = Average
31–35 = Fair
Less than 31 = Poor

# Assessment Activity 14-3

## Assessing the Results of Diagnostic Tests

**Directions:** Use this assessment to record the dates and results of commonly administered diagnostic medical tests. Refer to information in this chapter to review the purposes of these tests.

| Test Name | Typical Reference Range | What's Being Tested | Your Results | Date |
|---|---|---|---|---|
| 1. Alanine aminotransferase (ALT) | 10–40 U/L | Heart, liver, muscle damage | | |
| 2. Albumin | 3.5–5.2 g/dL | Kidneys | | |
| 3. Alkaline phosphate | 35–128 mg/dL | Liver, parathyroid glands, bone disease | | |
| 4. Aspartate aminotransferase (AST) | 10–59 U/L | Liver, heart, muscle damage | | |
| 5. Bilirubin | 0.3–1.5 mg/dL | Liver, kidneys | | |
| 6. Blood urea nitrogen (BUN) | 8–22 mg/dL | Kidneys | | |
| 7. Calcium | 8.6–10.0 mg/dL | Parathyroid glands, cancer, bone disease | | |
| 8. Carbon dioxide | 22–28 mEq/L | Lungs and heart | | |
| 9. Chloride | 98–107 mEq/L | Dehydration | | |
| 10. Cholesterol (total) | < 200 mg/dL | Heart and artery disease | | |
| 11. Creatinine | 0.7–1.3 mg/dL | Kidneys | | |
| 12. Free T4 hormone | 1.0–4.3 mg/dL | Thyroid gland | | |
| 13. Globulin | 1.5–3.8 g/dl | Infections | | |
| 14. Glucose | < 120 mg/dL | Diabetes mellitus | | |
| 15. Hematocrit | 42–52% | Anemia | | |
| 16. High-density lipoprotein (HDL) | > 40 mg/dL | Heart and artery disease | | |
| 17. Iron (total) | 50–175 mg/dL | Anemia | | |
| 18. Lactic dehydrogenase | 100–190 U/L | Liver | | |
| 19. Low-density lipoprotein (LDL) | < 130 mg/dL | Heart and artery disease | | |
| 20. Lymphocyte | 20–40% | Immune deficiency disorder | | |
| 21. Phosphorous | 2.3–4.6 mg/dL | Kidneys | | |
| 22. Potassium | 3.4–4.4 mEq/L | Kidneys | | |
| 23. Protein | 6.4–8.3 g/dL | Kidneys, nutrition | | |
| 24. Red blood cells (RBC) | 4.2–6.1 m/mL | Anemia | | |
| 25. Sedimentation rate | (< 50) 15–20 mm/h | Infections | | |

**Name** _____ **Date** _____ **Section** _____

# Assessment Activity 14-4

## Self-Care Inventory

**Directions:** Using the following scale, circle the appropriate number for each statement. Total your responses and find your score at the end of the activity.

| Statement | Never | Occasionally | Most of the Time | Almost All of the Time |
|---|---|---|---|---|
| 1. I read health-related advertisements in a critical and careful manner. | 1 | 2 | 3 | 4 |
| 2. I maintain a suspicious attitude about health claims. | 1 | 2 | 3 | 4 |
| 3. I have a primary care physician. | 1 | 2 | 3 | 4 |
| 4. I know which hospitals my physician recommends. | 1 | 2 | 3 | 4 |
| 5. I ask about fees before using health care services. | 1 | 2 | 3 | 4 |
| 6. I ask about the risks and benefits of a medical test before its use. | 1 | 2 | 3 | 4 |
| 7. I seek second opinions when I feel uncertain or uncomfortable with a recommended treatment. | 1 | 2 | 3 | 4 |
| 8. I maintain adequate health insurance coverage. | 1 | 2 | 3 | 4 |
| 9. I ask about the contraindications and side effects of prescription drugs before taking them. | 1 | 2 | 3 | 4 |
| 10. I thoroughly read labels before taking nonprescription drugs. | 1 | 2 | 3 | 4 |
| 11. I look for evidence of scientifically controlled studies when reading sensational health claims. | 1 | 2 | 3 | 4 |
| 12. I am familiar with the medical history of close relatives. | 1 | 2 | 3 | 4 |
| 13. I follow directions when taking medicines, including continuing their use for the prescribed duration. | 1 | 2 | 3 | 4 |
| 14. I keep a supply of essential items in my medicine cabinet. | 1 | 2 | 3 | 4 |
| 15. I keep records of the times, dates, and results of medical tests. | 1 | 2 | 3 | 4 |
| 16. I keep a record of my immunizations. | 1 | 2 | 3 | 4 |
| 17. I engage in appropriate medical self-care screening procedures. | 1 | 2 | 3 | 4 |
| 18. I understand which health conditions are covered in my health insurance policy and which are not. | 1 | 2 | 3 | 4 |
| 19. I know the deductible amount of my health insurance policy. | 1 | 2 | 3 | 4 |
| 20. I go for selective health examinations according to the recommended schedule. | 1 | 2 | 3 | 4 |

## Scoring

70–80 = A highly skilled, discriminating, and assertive health consumer
60–69 = An adequately skilled health consumer
50–59 = A health consumer who tends to be passive
 0–49 = A passive consumer

# Glossary

absolute risk the actual number or percentage of people affected by a risk factor.

abstinence to refrain completely from engaging in a particular behavior.

acesulfame a nonnutritive sweetener that is 200 times sweeter than sucrose and marketed as "sunette" in many food products.

acquaintance rape forced sexual intercourse between people who know one another well.

acquired immunodeficiency syndrome (AIDS) viral destruction of the immune system, causing loss of ability to fight infections.

acute illness an illness that occurs suddenly, often has no identifiable cause, is usually treatable, and often disappears in a short time.

addiction a pathological need for a substance that has life-damaging potential.

addictive behavior behavior that is excessive, compulsive, and psychologically and physically destructive.

adipose cells fat cells.

adrenocorticotropic hormone (ACTH) a hormone released by the hypothalamus during periods of stress that initiates various physiological responses.

aerobic literally "with oxygen"; when applied to exercise, activities in which oxygen demand can be supplied continuously by individuals during performance.

aerobic capacity maximum oxygen consumption.

alcohol a socially acceptable drug.

alcoholism the disease in which an individual loses control over drinking; an inability to refrain from drinking.

allergens substances that cause allergic reactions.

alternative medicine the body of therapies that are not taught in U.S. medical schools and are generally unavailable from doctors or hospitals.

amenorrheic the cessation of menstruation.

amino acids chemical structures that form protein.

anabolic steroids drugs closely related to testosterone that increase muscle mass in humans.

anaerobic literally "without oxygen"; when applied to exercise, high-intensity physical activities in which oxygen demand is greater than the amount that can be supplied during performance.

android the deposition of fat that is characteristic of men; fat tends to accumulate in the abdomen and upper body.

aneurysm a weak spot in an artery that forms a balloonlike pouch that can rupture.

angina chest pain that is the result of ischemia (see ischemia).

angioplasty a procedure in which narrowed arteries are dilated through the use of a catheter.

anorexia nervosa a serious illness of deliberate self-starvation with profound psychiatric and physical components.

antioxidants compounds that block the oxidation of substances in food or the body (vitamins C and E and beta-carotene are examples).

arthritis inflammatory disease of the joints.

asthma a chronic respiratory condition characterized by difficulty breathing.

asymptomatic without symptoms.

atherosclerosis a slow, progressive disease of the arteries characterized by the deposition of plaque on the inner lining of arterial walls.

ATP adenosine triphosphate, the unit of energy used for muscular contraction.

atrophy a decrease in the size of organ, muscle, and body tissues from disease or disuse.

autogenics the form of suggestion that precipitates relaxation.

autoimmune disease a disease in which the immune system fails to recognize the body's own parts and produces antibodies against them to the point of causing injury.

autonomic nervous system the part of the nervous system that is concerned with control of involuntary body functions.

avoidance a behavioral strategy that emphasizes eliminating circumstances associated with undesirable behavior.

ballistic stretching  repetitive contractions of agonist muscles to produce rapid stretches of antagonist muscles.

balloon angioplasty  a surgical procedure that involves the insertion of a catheter with a balloon at the tip used to compress fatty deposits and plaque against the walls of the artery.

bariatric surgery  surgery to reduce weight.

basal cell carcinoma  the most common type of skin cancer; it grows slowly and usually does not metastasize (spread).

basal metabolic rate (BMR)  the number of calories needed to sustain life.

behavior assessment  the process of counting, recording, observing, measuring, and describing behavior.

behavior substitution  a lifestyle change technique in which an incompatible behavior is substituted for a behavior being altered.

behavioral contract  a written agreement in a lifestyle-change program.

benign  noncancerous; refers to a growth that is unable to spread.

binge drinking  consuming five or more drinks in a single session at least once during the previous two weeks, with the intent to become intoxicated.

binge-eating disorder  the practice of eating large amounts of food in a short period of time.

biofeedback  an educational tool used to provide information about an individual's physiological actions.

blood alcohol concentration (BAC)  the percentage of alcohol content in the blood.

body composition  the amount of lean versus fat tissue in the body.

body dysmorphic disorder (BDD)  a psychiatric disorder characterized by a preoccupation with perceived imperfections in physical appearance that cause

the person to withdraw from social activities.

body image  the perception of and about the body.

body mass index (BMI)  the ratio of body weight in kilograms to height in meters squared.

botanicals  plants that are thought to have medicinal properties (also called herbs and phytomedicinals).

bulimia nervosa  an eating disorder characterized by episodes of secretive binge eating and purging.

caesarean section delivery  the surgical removal of the fetus through the abdominal wall.

caffeine  a stimulant that increases the heart rate.

caloric deficit  a deficit that occurs when the number of calories burned exceeds the number of calories consumed.

caloric expenditure  calories expended by physical activity and metabolism.

caloric intake  calories supplied by food.

calorie  short for kilocalorie, which is the unit of measurement for food energy; a calorie is the amount of heat required to raise the temperature of 1 gram of water 1 degree Centigrade.

cancer  a group of diseases characterized by uncontrolled, disorderly cell growth.

capillaries  the smallest vessels transporting blood from the heart to the tissues.

carbohydrate loading  the practice of increasing carbohydrate intake for six days before an event, while decreasing exercise duration.

carbon monoxide  a colorless, tasteless, odorless gas that is the product of incomplete combustion of carbon-containing fuels.

carcinogens  substances that cause cancer or enable the growth of cancer cells; cancer-causing agents.

carcinoma  cancer of a body surface or body cavity, such as

cancer of the breast, lung, skin, stomach, testis, or uterus.

cardia dysrhythmia  an irregular heart rate that is sometimes intractable.

cardiac output  the amount of blood ejected by the heart in 1 minute.

cardiorespiratory endurance  the ability to take in, deliver, and extract oxygen for physical work.

cariogenic  promoting of dental caries, or cavities.

catheterization  the process of examining the heart by introducing a catheter into a vein or an artery and passing it into the heart.

cause and effect  in medical research, the type of a relationship in which one variable is scientifically proved to cause a certain effect.

cerebral hemorrhage  the bursting of a blood vessel in the brain.

chemoprevention  nutritional intervention to prevent diseases, such as cancer, by bolstering the immune system.

chemotherapy  the use of drugs and hormones to treat various cancers.

child abuse  the physical, emotional, or sexual mistreatment of a child.

chlamydia  one of the most common sexually transmitted diseases.

cholesterol  a steroid that is an essential structural component of neural tissue and cell walls and is required for the manufacture of hormones and bile.

chronic disease  a disease that usually begins gradually and persists for an indefinite period of time, usually months or years.

chronic effects of exercise  the physiological changes that result from cardiorespiratory training.

circuit resistance training  a total of 8 to 15 exercises are usually used in a circuit; the exerciser goes through the circuit three times, with minimum rest between exercise stations.

cocaine a stimulant used in powdered form.

cognitive dissonance an internal conflict that occurs when a person's behaviors are inconsistent with his or her beliefs, values, or knowledge.

colonoscopy a procedure involving the insertion of a flexible viewing scope that examines the entire colon.

communicable diseases diseases that can be transmitted from one person to another.

complete protein a protein that contains all the essential amino acids.

complex carbohydrates polysaccharides, including starch and fiber.

concentric contraction the shortening of a muscle as it develops the tension to overcome an external resistance.

condyloma warts on the genitalia.

contracting a behavior change strategy that involves a written statement of health goals, target dates for completion of each goal, intervention strategies, rewards, and incentives.

contraindication a reason for not prescribing a drug or treatment.

control group in health research, the group receiving no treatment.

coping effort(s) made to manage or deal with stress.

coronary artery bypass surgery a procedure involving the removal of a leg vein, which is used as a shunt around the blocked area in the coronary artery.

countering substituting a new behavior for an undesirable one.

crack a smokable form of cocaine that is extremely dangerous and very addictive.

Crohn's disease a type of inflammatory bowel disease whose cause is unknown; Crohn's disease is characterized by frequent and intense diarrhea, abdominal pain, gas, fever, and rectal bleeding.

cross-training the attainment of physical fitness by participating in a variety of activities regularly.

crude fiber residue of plant food following chemical treatment in the laboratory.

cunnilingus oral sex performed on the female genitalia.

daily values (DVs) nutritional guidelines for the ingestion of carbohydrate, fat, saturated fat, cholesterol, sodium, potassium, and dietary fiber.

date rape forced sexual intercourse between people who are in a dating situation.

deceptive advertising advertising that misleads consumers by overstating or exaggerating the performance of a product.

deductible the amount paid by a patient before being eligible for benefits from an insurance company.

defensive medicine the practice of prescribing medical tests to protect doctors against malpractice lawsuits.

dehydration the excessive loss of body water.

delta-9-tetrahydrocannabinol (THC) a major psychoactive drug found in marijuana.

depressants sedatives and tranquilizers; these agents slow the central nervous system.

designer drugs illegally manufactured drugs that mimic controlled substances.

diabetes mellitus a metabolic disorder involving the pancreas and the failure to produce insulin; a risk factor for cardiovascular disease.

diagnostic laboratory tests tests conducted for specific symptoms during a physical examination.

dietary fiber the residue of plant food after digestion in the human body; 1 gram of crude fiber equals 2 to 3 grams of dietary fiber.

Dietary Reference Intakes (DRIs) the replacement for the Recommended Dietary Allowance as the standards for presenting nutrient recommendations.

diet resistance the inability to lose weight by dieting.

direct-access testing (DAT) testing in which a patient purchases a particular test online or at a participating lab, submits blood, and receives results without visiting a physician.

disability insurance insurance that pays for income lost because of the inability to work due to an illness or injury.

disordered eating sporadic eating, poor nutrition, unnecessary dieting, or occasional bingeing and purging, but not classified as full-blown problem areas by the American Psychiatric Association.

distress the form of stress that results in negative responses.

diuretics substances that increase water output and the body's need for water.

diverticulitis an infection of the diverticula of the intestines.

diverticulosis the condition of having saclike swellings (diverticula) in the walls of the intestines.

domestic violence violence that occurs when an individual is in some way hurt by a person whom he or she knows.

double-blind study the type of health research in which neither the researcher nor the subjects know who is receiving an experimental treatment.

drug a chemical substance that has the potential to alter the structure and functioning of a living organism.

eating disorders eating disorders that meet specific criteria established by the American Psychiatric Association.

eccentric contraction the lengthening of a muscle as the weight or resistance is returned to the starting position.

echocardiography a noninvasive technique that uses sound waves to determine the shape, texture, and movement of the valves of the heart.

ectomorph the body shape characterized by a thin body frame.

elderly abuse  physical, emotional, sexual, or medical abuse of an elderly person; most often the abuser is an adult child of the victim.

electrocardiograph (ECG)  a device for recording electrical variations in action of the heart muscle.

embolus  a mass of undissolved matter in the blood or lymphatic vessels that detaches from the vessel walls.

endomorph  the body shape characterized by rounded physical features and large body frame.

endorphins  mood-elevating, pain-killing substances produced by the brain.

energy nutrients  nutrients, such as carbohydrates, fat, and protein, that provide a source of energy for the body.

enhanced food  food that has been modified and/or supplemented for the purpose of achieving or facilitating a health benefit.

environmental dimension of wellness  aspects of wellness that improve quality of life in the community, including laws and agencies that safeguard the physical environment.

epidemiologic studies  population studies that observe the health habits and diseases of large numbers of people.

epinephrine  a hormone produced by the adrenal medulla that speeds up body processes.

essential fat  fat that is indispensable for individuals to function biologically and necessary to support life.

essential hypertension  high blood pressure caused by unknown reasons.

essential nutrients  nutrients that cannot be made by the body and must be supplied in the diet.

ethyl alcohol  the intoxicating agent in alcoholic drinks; a colorless liquid with a sharp, burning taste.

eustress  stress judged as "good," positive stress or stress that contributes to positive outcomes.

exclusion  a medical service that is not covered by an insurance policy.

experimental group  in health research, the group receiving some form of experimental treatment.

false negative  a test result that incorrectly shows a person is healthy when an abnormality actually exists.

false positive  a test result that incorrectly shows an abnormality when a person is actually healthy.

family practitioner  a medical doctor who serves as a general practitioner for an individual or a family.

fasting  complete starvation; avoidance of food consumption.

fat  a mixture of triglycerides.

fellatio  oral sex performed on the male genitalia.

female athletic triad  a condition characterized by disordered eating, lack of menstrual periods, and low age-adjusted bone density.

fiber  substances in food that resist digestion; formerly called roughage.

fight or flight syndrome  the initial phase of the general adaptation syndrome (GAS); when a stressor is encountered, the body responds by preparing to stand and fight or run away, depending on the situation; also called the alarm phase of the GAS.

fixed indemnity benefits  specified amounts that are paid by an insurance company for particular medical procedures.

flexibility  range of motion at a joint.

folate  a vitamin B nutrient found primarily in leafy vegetables.

foodborne illness  illness caused by ingestion of foods containing toxic substances produced by microorganisms.

fraternal twins  twins who emanate from separate eggs and do not have identical genes.

freebasing  smoking liquefied cocaine.

free radicals  naturally produced chemicals that arise from cell activity.

fructose  fruit sugar.

functional foods  foods that provide a specific health benefit above and beyond their inherent nutritional value.

gastroplasty  bariatric surgery performed to limit the size of the stomach.

general adaptation syndrome (GAS)  a series of physiological changes that occur when a stressor is encountered; the GAS is conceived of as having three phases: alarm, resistance, and exhaustion.

genital warts  warts on the genitalia.

glucose  the primary source of energy used by the body; blood sugar.

Glycemic Index (GI)  an assessment of food in terms of its ability to increase blood sugar in the two to three hours after eating.

glyceride  fat compound, including triglyceride, monoglyceride, and diglyceride.

Golgi tendon organ  a proprioceptor that responds to muscle stretch and tension.

goniometer  a protractor-like instrument used to measure the flexibility of various joints.

gonorrhea  a bacterial disease that is sexually transmitted and can lead to serious complications if left untreated, including sterility and scarring of the heart valves.

gynoid  a fat deposition characteristic of females, in whom fat tends to accumulate on the hips and thighs.

hardiness  the label used in describing the type of personality that tends to remain healthy even under extreme stress; the three components of hardiness are challenge, commitment, and control.

hate crimes  crimes directed at individuals or groups solely because of their racial, ethnic, or religious background, sexual orientation, or other differences from the perpetrator.

headache a common discomfort that is often caused by distress, tension, and anxiety; may be the result of injury or brain disease.

health the balancing of the physical, emotional, social, and spiritual components of personality in a manner that is conducive to optimal well-being and a higher quality of existence.

health behavior gap a discrepancy between what people know and what they actually do regarding their health.

health care providers people and facilities, such as physicians and hospitals, that provide health care services.

health disparities the disproportionate prevalence of diseases and health problems among certain population groups.

health fatalism in health information, the view that new information cannot be believed or trusted because it will inevitably be refuted.

health insurance a contract between an insurance company and an individual or a group for the payment of medical care costs.

health maintenance organization (HMO) a prepaid group insurance program that provides a full range of medical services.

health-promoting behaviors things done to maintain and improve one's level of wellness.

health promotion the art and science of helping people change their lifestyle to move toward a higher state of wellness.

health-related fitness the components of fitness that include cardiorespiratory endurance, muscular strength, muscular endurance, flexibility, and body composition.

health risk appraisals questionnaires used to provide information about health habits, lifestyle, and medical history.

heat exhaustion a serious heat-related condition characterized by dizziness, fainting, rapid pulse, and cool skin.

heat stroke a heat-related medical emergency characterized by high temperature (106° F or higher) and dry skin and accompanied by some or all of the following: delirium, convulsions, and loss of consciousness.

hemoglobin the substance in blood that carries oxygen.

hepatitis B one of five types of viral hepatitis; hepatitis B is the most serious type and can be transmitted sexually.

herbs see botanicals.

herpes simplex virus (HSV) the virus responsible for herpes genitalis, a sexually transmitted disease.

highly polyunsaturated fat a fatty acid composed of triglycerides in which the carbon chain has room for many hydrogen atoms.

homeostasis a state of balance or constancy; the body is continually attempting to maintain homeostasis.

homicide the intentional taking of another person's life; murder.

homocysteine an amino acid that is thought to increase the risk for heart disease.

homogeneous group a group of subjects with similar characteristics.

human immunodeficiency virus (HIV) the virus that is the source of AIDS.

human papilloma virus (HPV) the causative agent of condyloma (genital warts).

hydrogenation the process of adding hydrogen to unsaturated fatty acid to make it more saturated.

hyperglycemia high blood sugar.

hyperplasia an increase in the number of cells.

hypertension high blood pressure.

hyperthermia an excessive buildup of heat in the body.

hyperthyroidism a disease caused by an overactive thyroid gland.

hypertrophy an increase in the size of organs and muscle tissue.

hypokinesis physical inactivity.

hypothalamus the part of the limbic system that contains the center for many body functions; in stressful situations, the hypothalamus releases specific hormones to elicit appropriate body responses.

hypothermia a cold weather–related condition that results in abnormally low body temperature.

hypothyroidism a disease caused by an underactive thyroid gland.

iatrogenic condition a condition caused by receiving medical care.

identical twins twins who emanate from the same egg.

immunization a vaccine or another preparation administered to prevent disease.

immunotherapy in relation to cancer, a technique for stimulating the body's immune system to destroy cancer cells.

implied consent the nonverbal authorization of a medical procedure, such as cooperation during the administration of tests.

incomplete protein protein that does not contain all the essential amino acids in the proportions needed by the body.

infarction the death of heart muscle tissue.

inflammatory bowel disease (IBD) a variety of diseases that cause inflammation of the intestines; the two most common types are Crohn's disease and ulcerative colitis.

influenza an illness commonly called flu; caused by a virus.

informed consent a legal provision requiring a patient's authorization of any medical procedure, therapy, or treatment.

inhalants substances that cause druglike effects when inhaled.

insoluble fiber fiber that does not dissolve in water; comes from wheat bran and vegetables.

insulin  a hormone, secreted by the pancreas, that increases the use of glucose by the tissues of the body.

intensity  the degree of vigorousness of a single bout of exercise.

internist  a medical doctor specializing in internal medicine and sometimes serving as a primary care physician.

ischemia  a diminished supply of blood to the heart muscle.

isoflavones  the phytoestrogens in soybeans that are thought to help prevent breast cancer by blocking natural estrogens.

isokinetic  a method for developing muscular strength that involves a constant rate of speed and changes in the amount of weight resistance.

isometric  the use of static contractions to develop strength.

isotonic  a method for developing muscular strength that involves a variable rate of speed and a constant weight resistance.

lactic acid  a metabolite formed in muscles as a result of incomplete breakdown of sugar.

lactose  a simple sugar; milk sugar.

lactovegetarian  a person who eats plant foods and dairy products but excludes eggs, fish, poultry, and meat from the diet.

Leading Health Indicators (LHIs)  healthy lifestyle issues identified in the document Healthy People 2010 as health priorities for Americans.

legumes  foods that come from plants with seed pods that split on two sides when ripe.

leptin  a protein made in fat cells that controls weight gain and loss.

leukemia  cancer of the blood-forming tissues, including the bone marrow and spleen.

life insurance  insurance that pays a death benefit.

lifestyle diseases  diseases and/or health conditions largely caused by health habits and practices under the control of the individual.

limbic system  a large, C-shaped area in the brain that contains the centers for emotions, memory storage, learning relay, and hormone production (the pituitary gland, thalamus, and hypothalamus).

lipid  the class of nutrients more commonly referred to as fat.

lipoprotein  fat-carrying protein.

liposuction  the surgical removal of fat tissue.

locus of control  the perspective from which an individual views life; individuals with an internal locus of control believe that their decisions make a difference and that they have control over their lives; people with an external locus of control see themselves as "victims" and consider other people, situations, and conditions as being the controlling factors in their lives.

low-calorie diet  a diet that limits intake to 800 to 1,000 calories a day; results in atrophy of heart muscle.

low-carb diet  a diet that limits carbohydrate intake to below the recommended 45 to 65 percent of calories in daily intake.

lymphoma  cancer that develops in the lymphatic system, including the neck, armpits, groin, and chest.

macronutrients  nutrients required by the body in large amounts; usually refers to the energy nutrients: protein, fat, and carbohydrates.

mainstream smoke  smoke that is inhaled and exhaled by the smoker.

major minerals  minerals required in large amounts (more than 5 grams a day).

malignant  cancerous; refers to a growth that has the ability to spread to other areas of the body.

mammography  X-ray examination of the breast to detect cancer.

marijuana  cannabis; a plant that produces mild effects similar to both a stimulant and a depressant; also labeled as a mild hallucinogen.

megadose  a large dose, usually in the form of supplements.

melanoma  a dangerous form of skin cancer that has a strong tendency to spread to other areas of the body.

mesomorph  a body shape characterized by a muscular, athletic body build.

metabolism  all chemical reactions that occur within the cells of the body.

metastasis  the process by which cancerous cells spread from their original location to another location in the body.

micronutrients  nutrients required by the body in small amounts; usually refers to vitamins and minerals.

migraine headaches  headaches characterized by throbbing pain that can last for hours or days, sometimes accompanied by nausea and vomiting; migraines are thought to be the result of dilation of blood vessels in the head.

minerals  inorganic compounds in food necessary for good health.

mitochondria  the cell's "powerhouse."

moderate-calorie diet  a diet that limits caloric intake to 1,300 to 1,600 calories a day.

monocytes  white blood cells that grow into macrophages, which protect the body by ingesting foreign material.

monounsaturated fat  fatty acid composed of triglycerides in which the carbon chain has room for two hydrogen atoms.

morbidity  the incidence of disease and/or sickness.

mortality  the incidence of death.

muscular endurance  the application of repeated muscular force developed by many repetitions against resistances considerably less than maximum.

muscular strength the maximal force that a muscle or muscle group can exert in a single contraction.

myocardial infarction a heart attack; the death of heart muscle tissue.

narcotics powerful painkillers.

negative reinforcers avoidance of something unpleasant.

neoplasm an abnormal mass of cells; also called a tumor; can be benign or malignant.

net carbs the total grams of carbohydrate per serving after subtracting grams of fiber and sugar alcohols.

neutraceuticals natural ingredients intended to promote and maintain health.

newsgroup a location on the Internet where electronic messages related to a medical topic are posted.

nicotine the addictive substance and alkaloid poison found in tobacco.

novelty diets fad diets often based on gimmicks that typically promote certain nutrients or foods as having unique weight-loss qualities.

nucleoside analogs a combination of drugs (AZT & ddl) that seems to prevent the development of opportunistic infections associated with AIDS.

nutrient a substance found in food that is required by the body.

nutrient density the ratio of nutrients to calories; also called the index of nutritional quality.

nutrition the science that deals with the study of nutrients and the way the body ingests, digests, absorbs, transports, metabolizes, and excretes these nutrients.

obesity an excessive amount of storage fat.

ob gene a gene found in fat cells that produces leptin; also called the fat gene.

occupational dimension of wellness aspects of wellness that help achieve a balance between work and leisure in a way that promotes health and a sense of personal satisfaction.

Olestra a synthetic fat that has the flavor and taste of real fat but yields no calories.

omega-3 fatty acids the type of fatty acid found in cold-water seafood and thought to lower the risks for heart disease.

oncogene a cancer-causing gene.

osteoarthritis the most common form of arthritis, characterized by the deterioration of the articular cartilage that covers the gliding surfaces of the bones in certain joints.

osteophyte a bone spur.

osteoporosis a progressive decrease in the mineral content of bone, making bones brittle.

overcompensatory eating an eating pattern characterized by overconsumption of low-fat foods, which causes an increase in total caloric intake.

overfat may or may not be within normal guidelines for weight but with an excessive ratio of fat, compared with lean tissue.

overweight excessive weight for one's height without regard for body composition.

ovolactovegetarian a person who eats plant foods, eggs, and dairy products but excludes fish, poultry, and meat from the diet.

partner abuse physical or emotional abuse committed by an adult against his or her partner.

passive smoking the inhalation of environmental cigarette smoke by a nonsmoker.

pathogen a disease-producing organism.

pelvic inflammatory disease (PID) a chronic infection in the uterus, fallopian tubes, and upper reproductive areas; the leading cause of infertility in women.

performance-related fitness sports fitness; composed of speed, power, balance, coordination, agility, and reaction time.

periodic examination a physical exam in which tests and assessments are prescribed according to risk factors.

pescovegetarian a person who eats plant foods, eggs, dairy products, and fish but excludes red meat from the diet.

phytochemicals plant chemicals that exist naturally in foods.

phytoestrogen the plant hormone (estrogen) that exists naturally in foods.

phytomedicinals see botanicals.

placebo an inactive substance, such as a fake drug.

point of service (POS) a type of health insurance plan in which subscribers use approved providers who have agreed to accept fixed co-payments.

pollovegetarian a person who eats plant foods, eggs, dairy products, fish, and poultry but excludes red meat.

polypharmacy the administration of many drugs at the same time.

polyunsaturated fat fatty acid composed of triglycerides in which the carbon chain has room for four or more hydrogen atoms.

positive reinforcers rewards earned for achieving goals in a lifestyle-change program.

preferred provider organization (PPO) a group of private practitioners who sell their services at reduced rates to insurance companies.

preventive health behaviors health practices associated with the promotion of wellness and the prevention of sickness and death.

primary-care physician a medical doctor who is responsible for an individual's overall health.

primary site in reference to cancer, the original site of cancer cell formation.

proprioceptive neuromuscular facilitation (PNF) several stretching techniques that involve a combination of contraction and static stretching and holding agonist and antagonist muscle groups.

prospective study an epidemiologic study in which researchers predict possible disease relationships and patterns among groups of people.

protease inhibitor inhibits the enzyme protease, which allows HIV to develop.

protein complementing combining plant protein with cereal/grain protein to provide complete protein.

psychoactives drugs that can alter feelings, moods, and/or perceptions.

psychoneuroimmunology (PNI) the medical discipline whose philosophy rests on the connections among brain function, the nervous system, and the body's response to infection and abnormal cell division.

psychosomatic disease a disease (physical symptom) caused by psychological and emotional stressors.

radiotherapy the use of radiation to either destroy cancer cells or destroy their reproductive mechanism so they cannot replicate.

rape trauma syndrome psychological reactions following a rape; characterized by fear, nightmares, fatigue, crying spells, digestive upset, and perhaps impaired sexual desire/functioning.

reactance motivation a behavioral response to force or coercion in which the behavior is the opposite of that intended (e.g., a child refuses to eat a particular food because of parental force).

recidivism the tendency to revert to original behaviors/conditions after completing a behavior change program.

Recommended Dietary Allowances (RDAs) daily recommended intakes of nutrients for normal, healthy people in the United States.

Reference Daily Intakes (RDIs) minimum standards for essential nutrients; replaces the U.S. recommended daily allowance established in 1968.

relative risk the number or percentage of people affected by a risk factor in relation to or comparison with something else.

relaxation techniques techniques used in coping with and managing stress.

reliability the extent to which health studies yield consistent results.

reminders a behavioral strategy used to formulate action goals.

residual volume the amount of air remaining in the lungs after expiration.

retrospective study an epidemiologic study in which researchers review previously gathered data to identify possible disease relationships and patterns among groups of people.

reward deficiency syndrome a variety of disorders that have in common the traits of impulsiveness, addiction, and compulsiveness.

rheumatoid arthritis the most crippling form of arthritis, characterized by inflammation of the joints, pain, swelling, and deformity.

risk factors conditions that threaten wellness and increase the chances of contracting a disease.

road rage overly aggressive driving, which includes physical or verbal assault against another driver after a traffic dispute.

saccharides sugars.

safer sex a pattern of behavior in which steps are taken to protect oneself and one's partner from pregnancy and infection with HIV and sexually transmitted diseases; these steps can include using condoms or dental dams and having periodic medical tests and examinations.

sarcoma cancer of a connective tissue, such as bone and muscle.

saturated fat a fatty acid composed of triglycerides in which all the fatty acids contain the maximum number of hydrogen atoms.

scientifically controlled study a study conducted in a controlled setting that involves a treatment (experimental) group and a placebo (control) group.

secondary site in reference to cancer, the location of cancer cells after they have spread from the primary site.

sedentary physically inactive.

selective health examination a specific test used in response to specific symptoms or for diagnosing a specific problem.

self-care the movement toward individuals taking increased responsibility to prevent or manage certain health conditions.

self-efficacy people's belief in their ability to accomplish a specific task or behavior; that belief then affects the outcome of the task or behavior; the theory that individuals who expect to succeed tend to succeed and those who expect to fail tend to fail.

self-help the approach to lifestyle change that assumes individuals can plan and execute their own plans.

set point theory the theory that the body has a preference for maintaining a certain amount of weight and defends that weight quite vigorously.

sexually transmitted diseases (STDs) diseases spread through sexual contact, such as AIDS, chlamydia, gonorrhea, and herpes.

shaping up a behavioral strategy in which a person acclimates to desired behaviors in small increments.

sidestream smoke smoke given off by burning tobacco products.

sigmoidoscopy the insertion of a flexible viewing scope into the lower third of the colon.

skinfold measures the method for determining the amount of body fat by using skin calipers.

sleep apnea a condition characterized by loud snoring and brief periods during which breathing ceases.

soluble fiber  fiber that dissolves in water; comes from fruit pectins and oat bran.

squamous cell carcinoma  the second most common type of skin cancer; it rarely spreads to other areas, but it grows more quickly than basal cell carcinoma.

starch  plant polysaccharides composed of glucose and digestible by humans.

static stretching  the passive stretching of antagonist muscles by slowly stretching and holding a position for 15 to 30 seconds.

statistical relationship  an association between two or more variables or events.

statistical significance  the probability that a study's findings are reliable and are not due to chance.

stimulants  drugs that speed up the central nervous system.

stimulus control  the technique in lifestyle management involving the elimination and/or manipulation of stimuli related to a specific behavior.

stress  the body's nonspecific response to any demands made on it.

stressor  any physical, psychological, or environmental event or condition that initiates the stress response.

stretch reflex  the myotatic reflex.

stroke volume  the amount of blood that the heart can eject in one beat.

subliminal advertising  a technique in which messages, words, and symbols are embedded or hidden in advertisements.

sucrose  table sugar.

syndrome X  a combination of high blood pressure, high blood sugar, high blood lipids, and abdominal obesity.

syphilis  a sexually transmitted disease.

tar  a black, sticky, dark fluid composed of thousands of chemicals and found in tobacco.

tension headache  the most common kind of headache; caused by involuntary contractions of the scalp, head, and neck muscles; may be precipitated by anxiety, stress, and allergic reactions.

thermic effect of food (TEF)  the amount of energy required by the body to digest, absorb, metabolize, and store nutrients.

thrombus  a stationary blood clot; can occlude an artery supplying the brain.

trace minerals  minerals required by the body in small amounts.

trans fatty acids  saturated fat found in processed food that has been hydrogenated.

transmit time  the time it takes food to move through the body.

transtheoretical model of behavior change  a self-help approach to lifestyle change consisting of six well-defined stages; it is based on the principles of the behavior change model developed by James Prochaska.

triglyceride  a compound composed of carbon, hydrogen, and oxygen with three fatty acids.

tropical oils  oils that come from the fruit of coconut and palm trees.

ulcerative colitis  chronic inflammation of the colon lining; the symptoms are the same as those of Crohn's disease, but the only area affected is the colon lining.

unintentional injury  any injury that occurs as a result of an accident or reckless behavior.

unsaturated fat  fatty acid composed of triglycerides in which the carbon chain has room for more hydrogen atoms.

validity  the extent to which the research design of a health study permits the assertion of certain health claims.

variable resistance  provides increasing resistance as a weight is lifted through the full range of motion.

vegan  a person whose diet is limited to plant foods; also called a strict vegetarian.

very low-calorie diet (VLCD)  a diet containing fewer than 800 calories a day.

viral hepatitis  an inflammation of the liver caused by one or more viruses.

visualization  a form of meditation that makes use of the imagination.

vital capacity  the amount of air that can be expired after a maximum inspiration.

vitamins  organic compounds in food necessary for good health.

vitamin supplements  natural and synthetic compounds taken orally to supplement the vitamins consumed in food.

water intoxication  the consumption of more water than the kidneys can excrete.

weight cycling  a potentially harmful pattern of repeated weight loss and weight gain.

weight maintenance  the consistent maintenance of weight within certain limits between any two points in time.

wellness  engaging in activities and behaviors that enhance quality of life and maximize personal potential.

# Index

COUNTY COLLEGE OF MORRIS